Nursing Ethics

For Churchill Livingstone:

Senior Commissioning Editor: Sarena Wolfaard
Project Development Manager: Mairi McCubbin
Project Manager: Derek Robertson
Design Direction: George Ajayi

Nursing Ethics

Ian E. Thompson BA(Hons) PhD
Professor of Ethics and Philosophy, University of Notre Dame Australia,
Fremantle, Western Australia

Kath M. Melia BNurs(Manc) PhD
Professor of Nursing Studies, Department of Nursing Studies,
University of Edinburgh

Kenneth M. Boyd MA BD PhD
Director of Research, Institute of Medical Ethics;
Honorary Fellow, Faculty of Medicine, University of Edinburgh

FOURTH EDITION

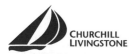
CHURCHILL
LIVINGSTONE

EDINBURGH LONDON NEW YORK OXFORD PHILADELPHIA ST LOUIS SYDNEY TORONTO 2000

CHURCHILL LIVINGSTONE
An imprint of Elsevier Science Limited

First published 2000
Reprinted 2001, 2003

ISBN 0443 06147 5

British Library Cataloguing in Publication Data
A catalogue record for this book is available from the
British Library.

Library of Congress Cataloging in Publication Data
A catalog record for this book is available from the Library
of Congress.

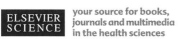

ELSEVIER
SCIENCE

your source for books,
journals and multimedia
in the health sciences
www.elsevierhealth.com

The
publisher's
policy is to use
**paper manufactured
from sustainable forests**

Printed in China

Contents

Acknowledgements

In preparing this fourth edition of *Nursing Ethics*, we are very conscious of the debt we owe to the many people, who, over the years, have taught us what we know of ethics in theory and in practice, who have enriched our understanding of applied ethics in general – specifically in health care – and those who by their skills and example have helped us learn to be more effective ethics educators. These people include our original teachers, our professional colleagues, academic scholars and critics, with whom we have shared the enjoyment and trials of working in this area, and in particular our students, from whom we have probably learned the most. We would also like to express our gratitude to those who have reviewed the book for the nursing press, and those many colleagues who have taken the trouble to give constructive and critical feedback on the value or limitations of the book, based on their experience of using it in the classroom.

If, as we hope, each edition has been an improvement on the last, then those improvements are as much due to this friendly advice and criticism as to any special insight or expertise of our own. Here we should mention two people in particular, whose friendly, penetrating, but constructive criticism of the third edition has helped us produce what we hope is a better book. These are Dr Heather McAlpine, Associate Professor of Nursing, University of New Brunswick, and Dr Alex Robertson, Reader in Social Policy, University of Edinburgh. Many improvements to the book can be attributed to their insights, and any weaknesses of argument or oversight that remain are our responsibility.

We appreciate the confidence shown in us by the staff at Churchill Livingstone, and the publishers Harcourt, in supporting the three previous editions of this book, and thank them for the patience, professional support and encouragement they have shown in the long process of appraising and refining, editing and preparing this fourth edition for publication.

Finally, we dedicate this edition to our nearest and dearest, without whose support we could not have begun, continued and finished this project, and especially to all those nurses and others who read and use this book. We hope that they will share with us the excitement and challenge of engaging with the ethical issues that confront us as we move into the third millennium. As ethical beings we do not exist in isolation, but draw strength and wisdom from sharing with other people in the moral communities in which we live and work. This book has grown organically out of such sharing of experience, first between us as collaborators in the authorship of the book, and then with many other people. We seek to share this common wealth of experience with you for our mutual enrichment and service of the common good and the common weal.

Preface to the fourth edition

NOTES TO READERS – TEACHERS AND STUDENTS

The primary aims of this preface are:

- To explain how changes in biomedical ethics and nursing practice, and findings from research on nursing and nursing ethics have made an updated fourth edition of Nursing Ethics necessary
- To re-state and justify the particular philosophical standpoint we have adopted towards practical ethics and the study of nursing ethics
- To explain the general educational approach and methods we would recommend for the teaching of nursing ethics, based on our experience over 25 years.

Facing the challenges of nursing ethics in Y2K

To be requested by the publishers to prepare a fourth edition of *Nursing Ethics* is something to celebrate. However, as we stand on the threshold of the third millennium, the task is both daunting and challenging. It is rewarding that the book is still in demand and exciting that there have been requests for it to be translated into Hungarian and into Spanish for the Mexican market. This means that our experience in Scotland is perceived to be relevant to nurses in other parts of the world. In this era of globalisation, in international trade and political cooperation, nursing itself has become part of a global health care workforce. While we may continue to 'act locally' we are obliged to 'think globally' both as teachers and as practitioners. However, on the brink of a new era, the task of anticipating the needs of the next generation of nurses is daunting, because of our uncertainty about future trends and the unpredictability of world health needs in the next century.

Since the first publication of *Nursing Ethics* in 1983, reflecting as it did our research and practical experiments in teaching ethics to nurses in Edinburgh in the late 1970s, so much has changed that we recognise the need to revise and update it to take account of changes at four levels:

- To do justice to developments in nursing and 'nursing ethics' as a distinct area of study
- To reflect on both the perennial and new ethical issues confronting nurses today
- To apply what we have learned about methods for teaching ethics in nursing in the book
- To meet the expectations of a more ethically sophisticated nursing audience by our treatment of ethical theory and practical research on ethics in nursing.

Nursing ethics as a valid area of study in its own right

While we hope the fourth edition will break new ground and be relevant to nurses of the 21st century, we also hope to preserve and consolidate what was good in previous editions and has proved useful to nurses in the past. As we attempt to be relevant to the contemporary scene and to look to the future, we must also seek to preserve what has served us well in the past. Tradition and innovation always stand in tension with one another in any living, developing moral community. This is reflected in the changing ways in which we view individuals and their rights and duties relative to other people and the community at large in different cultures at different times. Kant points out, in his great work on the foundations of ethics (Paton 1969), that the *concept of a person* (or responsible moral agent) and the *concept of a moral community* (a body of people who share common principles) are logically connected with one another, and both concepts are necessary for and presupposed in any discussion of ethics. Given this function of ethics to explore the nature of the boundaries between people relating to one another in community, the process by which a community develops its sense of identity and articulates its common values and goals is as important to its continuing identity as a moral community, as innovation and adaptation to change are necessary to its survival in a changing world. This applies as much to nursing as to any other community.

In this edition we not only look back at the process by which individual nurses are formed by their education and training, within a profession and health systems that have a history of their own, but we also attempt to anticipate some of the challenges the nursing profession and nurse education must face as we enter the 21st century. Developments and changes in nursing, as the profession defines and redefines itself, have an impact on the scope and nature of nursing ethics. It is a sign of vitality in nursing that it is not stuck in a particular image of the nurse, e.g. as a Nightingale 'doctor's handmaiden' or the 'angels' of media fiction. On the one hand, nurses are vigorously debating the nature and role of nursing, within the profession, in dialogue and competition with medicine and the paramedical professions, and on the other hand, nursing must engage with society and the media, as nurses strive to change public expectations and break out of the confines of an oppressively patriarchal past. Nursing ethics, now and in the future, will have to grapple with gender-related politics in a profession where women predominate numerically, but where, in proportion to their numbers, men enjoy disproportionate power and influence.

This reflection on past experience and attempt to discern the most appropriate way to move forward into the future is in some ways a model of ethical decision-making itself, for we make decisions based on *evaluative* judgements – we evaluate the past, assess the needs of the present and project ourselves forward into the uncertainty of the future. We apply our values to appraisal of these different kinds of facts: (1) as we examine how the present context is shaped by the past; (2)

as we examine what particular challenges or crises confront us in the present, and what means are available to us for dealing with them; and, finally, (3) by identifying and striving to achieve those goals that are defined by our *values* in the first place. Sound ethics must involve proper valuation of tradition and past experience, but ethical decision-making is not retrospective, it must be prospective. It requires courage to move forward into the future, to engage with uncertainty, the unpredictable and the unknown. It cannot just be reactive to the demands of the past, to established conventions, rules and practice. Competence in ethics means having the knowledge, skills and confidence to be proactive, take risks and accept responsibility for difficult decisions (Thomson 1976).[1]

Although nursing, as the activity of caring for those who are sick, injured, weak and vulnerable, is as old as human society itself, as a formally recognised profession it is barely 100 years old. As we move into the third millennium, it is almost impossible to predict where nursing will be by the end of the next century. If the pace of change in the past century is anything to go by, we can be pretty sure that the pace of change in the future is likely to accelerate. Nursing, throughout its history, has had to adapt to changing social conditions, changes in the patterns of morbidity and mortality, advances in medicine and applied medical technology, changes in the modes of health care delivery, and associated changes in the roles and responsibilities of nurses in health care administration. As an occupational group, nurses have proved remarkably resilient in their ability to adapt to change. This has perhaps been a distinctive mark of their professionalism and fidelity to their vocational ideals.

Social, demographic, economic and epidemiological changes have brought challenges to nurses, to improve their knowledge and repertoire of skills; but they have also brought new challenges of an ethical nature – both in terms of new problems to be addressed and in terms of increased personal and professional moral responsibility. Nursing ethics itself has undergone a revolution from an early focus on nursing etiquette to a serious exploration of the knowledge and skills required by nurses to enable them to bring the same professionalism to their ethical decision-making that they seek to apply to their clinical, educational and managerial roles. Nursing ethics is now a rapidly developing area of professional ethics, and nurses in their own right are increasingly making a significant contribution to academic debate, research and teaching in ethics (Benjamin & Curtis 1986, Johnstone 1994, Bandman & Bandman 1995).

The perennial and current issues in nursing

In the attempt to be contemporary and relevant, to address the extraordinary challenges presented by new developments (e.g. in genetic engineering), there is a risk that we will fail to address the ordinary routine issues and ethical problems that all nurses must face. We realise that some issues that were highly topical in 1975 are less the focus of debate today. This may be because people's attention has shifted, or been focused by the media on different issues, or the issue has in some sense become 'settled', or because changes in the law have shifted the locus of debate. Thus, decriminalisation of abortion and attempted suicide, the passing of legislation enabling research on and the use of human tissue for transplants, and changes in mental health legislation more effectively protecting the rights of the mentally ill have all helped to change the ethical agenda, or at least how we address the issues. We attempt in the book to identify and discuss some of the new problems confronting nurses at the frontiers of medical advance and research, but are convinced that we must not neglect the ordinary everyday moral problems which are perennially part of the care and treatment of people made vulnerable by disease, injury, mental disorder, infertility or frailty.

Life is characterised by both continuity and change, and while we must address the challenges of present and future change, we believe there are certain features of human life and the human condition that do not change. For example the processes and problems, pleasure and suffering related to birth, maturation, adulthood, reproduc-

tion, parenting, maintenance of physical and mental health, ageing and death apply to all human beings, past, present and future. While individuals may change, for good or ill, it is questionable whether human nature changes. In fact, the problems of making sense of living, of pain and suffering, facing death and bereavement, and the meaning of happiness will remain, whatever advances are made in medicine and the human sciences. The role of the nurse in providing professional care and emotional and spiritual support to people in times of personal crisis around some of the most critical of 'life events' is probably something that will never change, although the resources and skills available at different times and in different places will undoubtedly change (Bevis 1988, Campbell & Bunting 1991, Johnstone 1994).

The relevance of research in nursing and applied ethics

Finally, because of the rapid changes in nursing over the past half century in particular, with the development of tertiary level education and training for nurses, and the establishment of nursing as a recognised subject of academic study and research, it is imperative that discussion of ethics in nursing takes proper account of the advances in nursing research. The application of the behavioural and social sciences, as well as the clinical sciences, to the study of the theory and practice of nursing has changed the profession's perception and understanding of itself and the image of the nurse in society. Nursing research has become multidimensional, ranging from research into the efficacy of nursing procedures routinely used in patient care, through studies of nurse–patient communication, the social dynamics of hospitals and life on a hospital ward, to research to establish appropriate indicators for appraisal of nursing performance, quality assurance and the economics of nursing within the context of hospital- and community-based health care. Like any other research involving human subjects, directly or indirectly, nursing research must be subject to objective monitoring in order to maintain rigorous scientific and ethical standards, and the experience of nurses is increasingly sought on ethics of research committees dealing with both clinical and administrative practice in health care.

Nursing research has thus come of age as an area of applied research in its own right. Research on ethics in nursing and the effectiveness and/or ineffectiveness of various approaches to teaching ethics in nursing is relatively new and underdeveloped, but recent work in this area is taking the discussion beyond the anecdotal, or the opinionated grandstanding of untried theories, into an era of more systematic application of tried and tested methods of appraisal from other human sciences. From educational research, and health education research in particular, nurses and others have begun to apply objective measures to appraise education and skills training in ethics, both formative and summative evaluation of the training of nurses. This book attempts to apply what has been learned from these sources to the way our material is presented, and teachers are offered some practical guidance on appropriate methods, and students are directed to the sources from which they can gain access to further information on this research for their own purposes (Fry 1989a, McAlpine 1996).

Much has changed in the past quarter of a century, since we co-authors were first appointed to conduct practical research in ethics and experimental teaching in Edinburgh University Medical School, the Department of Nursing Studies, and the associated Colleges of Nursing in Lothian Region. We have witnessed a major change from the previous exclusive focus on 'medical ethics' to a recognition that nursing ethics represents a proper domain of study in its own right. There have been changes in the range of 'fashionable' issues which have been the centre of ethical debate in nursing, and a related shift from a narrow focus on clinical nursing ethics to study of the many levels at which nurses exercise moral responsibility – including critical study of the whole culture and organisation of nursing management and service delivery. Our own attempts to apply adult education and group learning methods to ethics teaching in health care has been part of ongoing research on educational methodology as applied to nursing which has led to some revolutionary new approaches to teaching and learning. We have progressed from segregated and didactic courses to multidisciplinary, interactive and participative learning; and from an overly theoretical approach to ethics to a focus on case-based, self-directed and experiential learning in appropriate learning environments. Further, as there has been much progress in the sophistication of nurses in ethics – with their increased general familiarity with the literature in ethics, nursing and health care – so there has been more emphasis on wider familiarity with logic and philosophy of science as well as philosophical ethics. Many colleges of nursing now teach ethics and the philosophy of medicine as part of the required curriculum, and consequently nurses are more expert in the area than when we began. Finally, there is a burgeoning literature in the field of nursing ethics – written by nurses as well as other experts in the social sciences, psychology, law and philosophy.

How do we teach ethics in nursing?

In the circumstances, the challenge in teaching ethics is not to teach a body of rules that may change or doctrines that will inevitably go out of fashion, even if they are not superseded by new rules and new teaching. The pedagogical challenge is to find ways to help people develop practical understanding of the ideals and standards of the profession, and to equip them with the tools or skills that will enable them to apply general principles intelligently to changing situations, in such a way that they choose competently and confidently the right means to achieve good outcomes. By this we arrive back at Aristotle's definition of prudence or practical wisdom as the foundation for responsible moral living and sound ethical decision-making.[2] The task of teaching practical ethics cannot be achieved by a textbook, however good. It requires the maieutic skills of the intellectual midwife (Rouse 1984);[3] the educator's skill to nurture and draw out the potential of the trainee; the counsellor's skill to assist students to develop insight and a capacity for self-criticism; and good role models to stand by them in the experience of life and actual practice to provide support and a context in which learners can practise and master the skills they require to be competent moral agents. In particular, we argue that we all need to develop the core skills required of competent members of a moral community, namely skills in *values clarification*, in *sound ethical decision-making*, and in *collaborating with others to determine sound ethical standards or policy*.

This book is not a training manual for those responsible for the education and training of nurses. That is a task for a different kind of publication. However, in response to many requests from nurse teachers, we are adding to each chapter a statement of the aims and objectives of the chapter, and the learning outcomes that may be achieved through its proper application in an appropriately structured teaching programme. Based on our experience of teaching ethics, we give some hints and guidance on methods that may be of assistance to teachers. We give with each chapter an agenda of suggested questions that nurse educators might use as a basis for tutorial discussions, essays or projects. Further reading on these selected topics is provided to assist lecturers and students with planning assignments.

The place of moral theory in practical nursing ethics

Ethics, as Aristotle observed over 2000 years ago,[4] is a *practical science*. It is practical in two senses: first, it must be rooted in actual practice, and second, it must help us to make more soundly based decisions so as to deal effectively with real problems in life. If a book on nursing ethics is to be practical in the first sense, then it must address the specific context of nursing practice and deal with the specific problems faced by nurses. For this reason we have not attempted to write a book for nurses on general moral philosophy, but we have sought deliberately to address the specific contexts of nursing practice and nursing experience directly. If ethics is to be practical in the second sense, then it must help nurses develop the practical wisdom and skills that will enable them not only to become more competent in decision-making, but also to develop as responsible moral

agents. For this reason, general discussion of moral theory is kept to a minimum, and more emphasis is placed on dealing with cases and the management of problems taken from actual nursing.

However, given queries from a number of reviewers as to why ethical theory is not dealt with 'up front' and is left to the final chapters of the book, perhaps a few words need to be said about this matter before we outline the contents of the book. There are two kinds of approach to teaching ethics with which we would take issue here. The one we might call 'the philosopher's gambit', and the other 'the postmodernist feminist manoeuvre'.

'The philosopher's gambit' reflects the preoccupation of academic philosophers with moral theory, and the relative neglect of practical decision-making. It seeks to explain concrete moral experience not in its own terms but analysed in terms of some general moral theory, and the justification of specific ethical decisions as based on one or another of the classical moral theories. This seems to us to be misguided – partly for practical pedagogical reasons and partly for philosophical reasons. On the former, our experience is that attempting to teach moral theory to medical and nursing students is a complete turn-off, for above all they want help with practical decision-making, and discussion of ethical theory in their words 'just leads to head talk'. The philosophical objections are similar to Aristotle's insofar as he maintains that ethics is a practical discipline requiring the development of practical skills. Alternatively, we might apply to ethics Marx's general claim that 'praxis drives theoria', and argue that moral theory arises out of reflection on everyday experience of action and decision-making, rather than the other way around, and that justifying general moral judgements and justifying specific moral actions are different kinds of activity.

A number of influential textbooks on nursing ethics adopt the approach that in order to justify moral judgements we need prior knowledge of ethical theory (e.g. Davis & Aroskar 1983, Tschudin 1986 and Kerridge et al 1998). This seems contrary to both common sense and the traditions of ethical realism. Even Beauchamp &

Childress (1994), in their widely used textbook on biomedical ethics, seem to presuppose that we need understanding of philosophical categories and moral theory in order to be able to justify our ethical decisions. The authors set out to avoid the problems of either a simple *deductivist* approach based on ethical theory, or an *inductive* approach based on individual case studies or casuistry, by advocating a *coherence theory of justification*. However, the whole way they categorise different approaches to justification, and the heavy emphasis given to moral theory in the succeeding chapter reinforce an overly theoretical approach to justification of ethical beliefs and policies, rather than the practical task of making sound ethical decisions and being able to give a reasonable account of how we reached our conclusions in a particular case. We argue that two different levels or types of 'justification' are being confused and conflated here, namely the first-order level at which we may have to justify specific decisions or actions to someone else (e.g. sedating a particular disturbed patient in a crisis) and the second-order level of 'moral judgement' where we are concerned to justify our general approach to *types* of situations of this kind (i.e. in defining our general policy on sedating patients).

'The postmodernist feminist manoeuvre' involves the identification of traditional philosophical ethics as 'patriarchal' and, with its emphasis on universal principles and rational justice, as driven by a 'will to control' the world and other people (particularly women). In opposition to this, the 'caring perspective' of feminist ethics is recommended, because it avoids the 'totalising' and 'dominative critical' approach of a 'masculinist' ethic (Gilligan 1982). Instead of attempting to base ethical decision-making on universal rational principles and logical methods of problem-solving (which are supposedly the natural tendencies of the 'master discourses' of men), we are urged to listen to the 'different voice' of feminine sensibility – with its emphasis on 'narrative and contextual accounts, that encourages respect for the differences between persons and sensitivity to the complexity of our interconnections' (Bowden 1997, p. 10). While the empty formalism and impersonal nature of rationalist ethics invites

this kind of criticism, and an emphasis on the concrete and particular needs of the situation is important, it must also be argued that the great moral philosophers have all sought to give due weight to the emotions and people's desires and loves, and this type of critique caricatures the moral tradition and sets up 'straw men' that are all too easy to knock down.

Both these approaches will be dealt with in more detail when we come to discuss models for practical decision-making that are flexible enough to accommodate these criticisms in Chapter 10.

Because we believe that ethics is essentially a practical discipline, we have deliberately proceeded *a posteriori* rather than *a priori*; that is, we have started with nurses' ordinary moral experience rather than with theory, in order to show how moral theories seek to explain, after the event, why difficulties arise in moral practice. The more common approach is to start by setting out the various moral theories, as if they were dogmas that we have to choose between before we can address our moral experience. This, we believe, is like 'putting the cart before the horse'. We are then faced with the twin difficulties of how to justify our choice of moral theory and how to relate the theory or theories back to actual practice. This is contrary to our common sense experience, where the majority of people manage to make reasonably competent moral decisions in blissful ignorance of moral philosophy, unaware of the classical moral theories, or even their names.

If we start the teaching of ethics with instruction in moral philosophy and critical study of the various ethical theories debated by philosophers through the ages, the illusion is created that moral theory is directly relevant to ethical decision-making, whereas it only becomes relevant when we are faced with disputes about the general rationale for moral rules, or conflicts of ethical policy, or ideological differences between people. When in dispute about ethical policy, we may appeal to higher-level moral theories in order to justify our overall moral position. It would not, however, be considered either necessary or appropriate in justifying a specific action or decision to a court, e.g. by saying: 'I gave the dying patient an overdose of diamorphine because I am a utilitarian!' or 'I told the patient that he was dying because I am a deontologist!' (Rachels 1993).

However, in a theoretical debate, far removed from the situation in which we have to make real decisions, we may engage in discussion of the relative merits of these different ethical theories as a means of justifying or explaining why we opt for certain general policies or rules of action.

If, however, we are challenged to explain or justify a specific moral decision to a friend, to a nurse manager, or before a formal enquiry, then we would ordinarily be expected simply to outline:

● *what* the main facts of the case were
● *which* principles or rules we applied to the problem
● *why* we acted as we did, i.e. what goal or purpose we set out to achieve
● *how* we chose the means or methods used to achieve the goal
● *what consequences* we anticipated on the basis of past experience
● *whether or not* our action was successful in reaching its intended goal.

Such an explanation or justification for an action would normally suffice to satisfy a court and our standard tests of a responsible person's ability to give a coherent account of what they have done, why they acted as they did, and whether or not their desired outcome was achieved.

We believe then that the proper place for ethical theory, and debate about the strengths and weaknesses of different ethical theories, is not in determining or justifying specific decisions or actions, but that moral theory becomes relevant when we come to justify rules or policies. The relevance of ethical theory to practical action is limited, as most students find when they emerge from the classroom into real life. However, once the basis for our assent to rules, trust in authority, or our general ethical approach to problems is challenged, then the relevance of ethical theory becomes apparent. Another way of expressing this is to say that debate about ethical theory belongs to the *second-order* level of debate about ethics in general, rather

than to debate about the rights and wrongs of a particular action, or even whether a specific action is good or bad.

The consequence of placing the primary emphasis in teaching on ethical theory is that it creates, or reinforces, the belief that everything in ethics is contestable, and simply a matter of opinion (or rhetorical debate about our opinions). To the degree that this happens, it encourages the view that ethical decision-making is either so difficult that it must be left to experts, or an area where 'anything goes' (and where one person's opinion is as good as another's). The object of teaching ethics, as distinct from moral theory or moral philosophy, is to help people reach ethically sound and justifiable decisions and to develop relevant life skills in related areas to operate with confidence as responsible moral agents. Instead of 'putting the cart before the horse', we work up to and end with moral theory, rather than begin with it, for we start where Aristotle suggests we should, with everyday practice, rather than in the speculative world of theory.[5]

Virtue ethics and competency based training in ethics

One crucial lesson we have learned from the debate about the nature of nursing ethics, and from personal experience in teaching ethics, is that the question of *how* ethics is taught may be of greater importance than *what* is taught. In line with concern in other areas with defining competence and the competencies required of nurses to practise, more attention needs to be given not only to how we create the sort of learning opportunities and environments where nurses can acquire the knowledge and skills in ethics to make competent decisions, but also to how we can ensure that student nurses develop the personal attributes or competencies that will make them confident and responsible moral agents. Here the revival of interest in *virtue ethics* in academic circles, and even in the business world, reflects a growing awareness that in appraising our own or other people's performance, it is not enough to assess people's knowledge of ethics. We must be able to assess how well people have acquired and internalised the core skills in applied ethics and how well they can apply them in their work and responsible practice in the workplace; these core skills are:

- skills in personal and professional values clarification
- skills in prudent individual and team ethical decision-making
- skills in negotiating sound ethical policy or performance standards.

The acquisition of both scientific knowledge and practical expertise is not sufficient to ensure that we can act responsibly as moral agents. Neither is it sufficient that we are good decent people with a capacity for self-insight and self-mastery, courage and integrity, or that we show respect and deal fairly with others, for if we do not have the necessary professional competence, we can be of little help to people in need. Professional integrity or competence requires a balance between the former, which Aristotle called the *intellectual virtues*, and the latter, which he called the *moral virtues*.[6] What he believed holds them together is *prudence* or *practical wisdom* which not only enables us to integrate theory and practice and to apply our expertise in a responsible ethical way for the benefit of ourselves and others, but also represents the only way in which we can achieve the kind of consistent and coherent moral character that we refer to when we speak of the virtuous, integrated person.

 end notes

1 These requirements for sound ethical judgement were spelled out by Aristotle in 330 BC in defining the nature of the intellectual and moral virtues and explaining the part played by practical wisdom in making sound prudential decisions. See Aristotle: *Nicomachean Ethics*, Book III.
2 This is a paraphrase of Aristotle's definition of prudence. See note 1 above.
3 Plato has Socrates describe himself as an intellectual midwife, whose task is to draw out or help people give birth to their own ideas. See Plato's dialogues the *Apology* and the *Meno*.
4 Aristotle: *Nicomachean Ethics*, Book I.
5 Aristotle: *Nicomachean Ethics*, Book I.
6 Aristotle: *Nicomachean Ethics*, Book III.

The social context of nursing values

SECTION CONTENTS

1

Ethics in our everyday life and decision-making

AIMS

This chapter has the following aims:
1. To clarify what we mean by ethics and some of the basic concepts such as 'right', 'wrong', 'good' and 'bad' that we use in our everyday ethical life and discussion
2. To distinguish between ethical problems and ethical dilemmas, and personal and shared social values
3. To examine the foundations of common ethical principles and how we deal with cultural and personal differences
4. To explore some of the connections between religion and morality and how ethics can be distinguished from religion.

LEARNING OUTCOMES

When you have read and worked through this chapter, you should be able to:
■ Give a critical account of the nature of ethics, and how it is distinguished from social convention, customs and etiquette

■ Distinguish between the different types of discourse in which we: (a) judge things to be 'right or wrong', and (b) judge things or actions to be 'good or bad'

■ Give examples of and explain the difference between an ethical 'dilemma' and an ethical 'problem', and explain how we attempt to deal with them

■ Explain in what sense justice, respect for persons, and protective beneficence are fundamental and universal principles

■ Discuss the nature of 'ethical relativism' and give examples to explain the value and limitations of relativism in ethics

■ Give a critical account of the relationship between ethics and religion.

WHAT DO WE MEAN BY ETHICS?

Nursing is only one area of life in which we face moral choices, and while it has many special features which we will consider later, it also has much in common with the rest of our moral experience. By way of introduction, therefore, we will begin by defining some terms and discussing what we mean by them in the context of this book: 'ethics' and 'morals', 'moral problems' and 'moral dilemmas', 'moral choice', and 'moral values' (see also Box 1.1). We will discuss these first in the context of ordinary life, noting how perceptions of moral issues and choices are related to the ways in which moral values may change over time.

What, in the first place, do we mean by *ethics* and *morals*? These terms originally meant much the same thing, 'ethics' coming from Greek and 'morals' from its Latin equivalent. Both words referred to social custom regarding the rights and wrongs, in theory and practice, of human behaviour. In everyday usage, the terms 'moral' and 'ethical' can still be used more or less interchangeably, but a distinction has grown up between the two terms in more formal usage. Morals (and also morality) now tends to refer to the standards of

---

> **Box 1.1**   Defining etiquette, morals, ethics and meta-ethics. (Adapted from Hawkins 1996)
>
> **Etiquette** (French: ticket)
> Etiquette refers to the written or unwritten rules of a society or group relating to:
>
> ● Conventional manners or rules of behaviour in public
> ● Social customs relating to gender roles, dress and people of different status
> ● Court ceremonial, rules of 'professional' conduct
>
> **Morals and morality** (Latin: *mores* = custom or convention)
> 'Morals' or 'morality' are generally taken to refer to the following:
> ● The domain of personal values and rules of behaviour
> ● Conventional rules of conduct regulating our social interactions
> ● Culture-specific mores, grounded in our religious and ideological beliefs
>
> **Ethics** (Greek: *ethos* = custom or convention, or the spirit of a community)
> ● 'An ethic' refers to the collective belief-and-value-system of any moral community, social or professional group.
> ● Ethics (the science of morals) studies how we determine what is good for the flourishing of individuals and society, and what rules we need to put into place to prevent people from being harmed. It is also concerned with the education and training process by which people are assisted to develop the competencies required for responsible moral action
>
> **Meta-ethics or moral philosophy**
> Moral philosophy is the systematic and critical study of the different kinds of theory that we invoke or fall back on when challenged to justify the ethical policies on which we base our moral lives and decisions. This kind of study of the theoretical underpinnings of our systems of moral beliefs is sometimes called 'meta-ethics' because it represents a 'second order' or higher level study of our basic or 'first order' moral rules and principles.

---

behaviour actually held or followed by individuals and groups, while ethics refers to the science or study of morals – an activity, in the academic context, also often called moral philosophy.

This distinction, however, is complicated by three popular ways of using the words. 'An ethic' can also be used to refer to the morals or morality of certain groups, such as 'a nursing ethic', or sometimes to the morals or morality of individuals, e.g. 'her personal ethic'. The implication behind this usage is that the morals or morality involved either

Table 1.1   What ethics is, and what it is not

What ethics is not	What ethics is
Ethics is not about negative codes of conduct, moral prohibitions, disciplinary rules or 'managing fraud'	*Ethics is* about commitment to positive values to ensure the well-being and flourishing of individuals and society
Ethics is not a private matter, nor just about subjective feelings, personal attitudes and choices	*Ethics is* a communal activity, of applying rational principles and universal standards to social life
Ethics is not introspective self-examination, judging one's moral state or that of other people	*Ethics is* about real power relations between people and responsible power-sharing, not abuse of power, in society
Ethics is not about personal reliance on experts, lawyers, philosophers, religious authorities or gurus	*Ethics is* about our active participation in a moral community and ownership of the policies it develops
Ethics is not theoretical 'head-talk', 'grandstanding' opinions, interminable disputes or insoluble 'dilemmas'	*Ethics is* a problem-solving activity, based on knowledge of ethical principles and their skilled application to life
Ethics is not about occult processes, 'feelings in the gut', 'voices in one's head' or privileged access to moral truth	*Ethics is* an educational process in which by experience we learn what it means to be responsible moral agents

have been codified or carefully worked out, or are, in some sense, high-minded. Associated with this kind of high-mindedness is the second popular use – that of both 'moral' and 'ethical' as terms of approval, the opposite of 'immoral' or 'unethical'. The third popular use derives from the idea of ethics as the impartial study or science of morals. This use is seen when 'ethics' and 'ethical' seem to be preferred to 'morals' and 'morality' because the latter are thought of as having some connection with either sexual conduct, on the one hand, or religious dogmatism on the other; 'ethics' and 'ethical', by contrast, are thought of as involving something more cerebral and objective. However, there is no substantial reason for these associations of ideas, which are largely a matter of preference, only slightly (if at all) more justifiable than the habit of preferring 'ethical' to 'moral' apparently for no better reason than that it sounds more impressive (Audi 1995).

In Table 1.1, we attempt to distinguish between what ethics is and what it is not.

We now suggest the following summary definition of ethics as a starting point for our discussion:

Ethics is concerned with the study and practice of what is good and right for human beings.

First, in ethics we seek to determine what conditions will promote what is *good* or *bad* for the flourishing of individuals, communities, businesses and organisations. Ethics is thus concerned with clarifying the general values and practical means

required to ensure the well-being, health, prosperity and happiness of people; and with identifying the kind of things that are likely to prevent this happening. This was recognised, for example, in the early ICN *Code for Nurses: Ethical Concepts Applied to Nursing* (ICN 1973):

The fundamental responsibility of the nurse is fourfold: to promote health, to prevent illness, to restore health and to alleviate suffering. The need for nursing is universal. Inherent in nursing is respect for the life, dignity and rights of man. It is unrestricted by considerations of nationality, race, creed, colour, age, sex, politics or social status. Nurses render health services to the individual, the family, and the community and co-ordinate their services with those of related groups.

Secondly, ethics is concerned with the formulation of rules defining what is *right* or *wrong*, e.g. to state what regulations are necessary to foster individual and community well-being, and what is required to protect the safety or integrity of individuals, communities and organisations.

Nurses have a general responsibility to 'hold in confidence personal information and use judgement in sharing this information' and to 'maintain the highest standards of nursing care possible within the reality of a specific situation' and 'should at all times maintain standards of personal conduct which reflect credit upon the profession' (ICN 1973).

The *Statement of Nurse's Role in Safeguarding Human Rights* (ICN 1983) further asserts that:

Health care is a right of all individuals. Everyone should have access to health care regardless of financial, political, geographic, racial or religious considerations. The nurse should seek to ensure such impartial treatment. Nurses must ensure that adequate treatment is provided – within available resources – and in accord with the ICN *Code of Nursing Ethics*, to all those in need of care.

However, local codes of ethics will often emphasise more particular legal and/or ethical obligations and rules applicable to nurses in that specific country.

RIGHT AND WRONG, GOOD AND BAD[1]

We are all born into a morally structured world, and encounter rules and regulations wherever we turn. Parents lay down rules for us to obey, and religious communities seek to impose all kinds of rules on us. Schools seem to be rule factories. Society is governed by rules, laws and regulations. Not surprisingly we are inclined to believe that: 'In the beginning was the rule!'

Adopting this perspective in nursing makes us focus on regulations and the law, rather than on moral principles and values or on the virtues of prudent judgement.

However, we may always question whether or not a rule is a *good* rule. As adolescents, we challenge family rules in this way, and will not 'own' a rule unless we feel that the rule benefits us as well as others. In this sense, judgements of value have to be made about rules, as to whether they are fair, respect the rights of all parties, and protect those who cannot defend their rights. Value judgements are therefore more fundamental than rules. Like the law – sound statutory law must be based on and consistent with common law and natural justice. Legislation alone does not make a law just or fair; it must serve to promote human well-being.

To be a mature and responsible moral agent means that we do not simply do our duty because we are ordered to do so by some authority or because the law says we must. We have to make our own commitment to the law (or conscientiously object to unjust laws) and we have to take full responsibility for our actions. To make conscientious moral choices means that we have internalised the moral law and made it our own. This is

the true meaning of moral autonomy; it is not a licence to do what we please or to be 'a law unto ourselves'.

Deciding what things are good or bad for us is not something other people can do for us. Parents and other people may well try to tell us that smoking or lazing about too long in the sun on the beach is 'bad' for us, but we are unlikely to be convinced until we have examined the facts or tried these things for ourselves. We may learn from bitter experience to avoid certain things that hurt us and to strive for others that bring us pleasure or fulfilment.[2]

We can only be said to be independent moral agents when we can challenge our inherited attitudes and test these by the light of reason and experience. In this way we come to adopt beliefs as our own. In the light of tested beliefs about ourselves and the world around us, we may come to change our attitudes to many things, to challenge the prejudices of our parents or teachers, and to begin to react differently to people.

We cannot inherit values from other people, nor have them imposed on us, as is the case with attitudes and unquestioned beliefs. Values must be of our own choosing, or they are not values. Values determine our choice of means to achieve our life goals. While we make testable truth claims for our beliefs, we need not act on them. Value judgements embody commitments we make, lifestyle choices, things on which we stake our decisions and perhaps even our lives. The differences between 'right/wrong', rule-governed thinking in ethics and thinking in terms of personal values and social goals defining what is 'good' or 'bad' are summed up in Table 1.2 (see Curtin & Flaherty 1982).[3]

MORAL PROBLEMS AND MORAL DILEMMAS

Given this background of different usage of ethical terms, what do we mean by 'moral problems' and 'moral dilemmas'? Both terms confront us with choices which involve our beliefs and feelings about what we fundamentally regard as good or right – our moral values or moral principles. We must distinguish between moral problems and moral dilemmas because there is a

Table 1.2   Right and wrong versus good and bad

Right and wrong	Good and bad
'Right' and 'wrong' are terms that relate to and presuppose a system of *formal rules*, laws and regulations	'Good' and 'bad' are terms that relate to *value judgements* about what does/does not promote our well-being or that of others
'Right' and 'wrong' belong to a *binary system* where things must be *either* 'right' *or* 'wrong'. They are mutually exclusive and collectively exhaustive terms	'Good' and 'bad' are *polar terms in a continuum* and (like 'health' and 'disease') are not mutually exclusive opposites, but admit degrees of comparison
'Right' and 'wrong' only *appear 'absolute' and 'objective'* so long as one does not question the system of rules that apply	'Good' and 'bad' may *appear 'relative' and 'subjective'* because we have to make personal appraisals of things/experience
Justification of judgements that things are 'Right' or 'Wrong' is based on *appeal to authority*, that of the rule or rule-giver	Judgements that things are 'good' or 'bad' have to be based on *appeal to evidence, facts and experience* (not authority or rules)
A system of rules defining what is to be 'right' or 'wrong' also serves to define our *rights and obligations* within that system	'Good'/'bad' are *normative terms*, by which we judge the degree things approximate to or deviate from a norm or ideal standard
'Right/wrong' thinking *seems to offer moral certainty* and security but is often associated with authoritarian dogmatism	Judgements that things are 'good' or 'bad' involve making *our own riskful decisions* based on personal experience

tendency in popular discussion in the media and the nursing press to refer indiscriminately to all difficult situations requiring moral decisions as 'dilemmas'. There is also a risk that, when confronted with a situation which presents such a dilemma, people will avoid taking responsibility for making hard decisions – regarding the 'dilemma' either as insoluble or simply as a matter of personal opinion or preference. We argue that if the issue can be reframed as a 'problem', there may be things that can be done, provided someone is prepared to take responsibility to find a practical solution that meets the needs of the situation (Box 1.2 gives definitions of 'problem', 'dilemma' and 'quandary').

In everyday life we often deal with *problems* which require us to make moral decisions. These may involve completely new and unfamiliar situations, but more often we are dealing with day-to-day problems which tend to recur. Past experience of similar situations equips us to face specific problems with some confidence because we have knowledge of how to deal with them, however painful or difficult they may be. Because problems, clearly defined and understood, usually have solutions, or possible solutions, they are not of the same kind as moral dilemmas, although we may also need courage to tackle them.

Box 1.2   Problems, dilemmas and quandaries

Problem (Greek: *problema* from *pro-ballo* = throw at or towards)
A doubtful or difficult matter requiring solution, 'thrown up' by life or experience, something hard to understand or to deal with, an exercise, test or challenge set for us, but something soluble in principle, with appropriate effort.

Dilemma (Greek: *di-lemma* = double argument with conflicting assumptions)
A specific situation in which a choice has to be made between alternatives that are both undesirable, or, in ethics, a situation involving a real or apparently irresolvable clash of principles or duties, where there are no rules or precedents to follow.

Quandary (origin unknown)
A perplexed state, a state of practical uncertainty or puzzlement over alternative choices, sometimes loosely called a dilemma.

A *dilemma*, on the other hand, is a choice, of whatever kind, between two equally unsatisfactory alternatives. Not all dilemmas are moral dilemmas; some dilemmas are the result of not knowing the best means, in theory or practice, to an agreed end. Nor are all moral choices moral dilemmas, since in many cases we may well know what we ought to do and the real question is whether we are willing do it. What makes the choice a moral dilemma, rather, is the fact that it involves conflict between competing moral principles or values applicable to the situation – what we believe we ought to do, or what we believe to be fundamentally good or important. We feel, in other words, that certain moral values or principles would make us adopt the one alternative, while others would make us adopt the other alternative, but we cannot adopt both. Choosing the one alternative means not only not choosing the other, but actually going against what the value or principle it represents would require us to do in the circumstances.

Moral dilemmas arise from time to time in the lives of most people. Consider, for example, Case History 1.1 – the experiences described present as moral dilemmas because a choice between conflicting moral values or principles seems to be involved in each case. The first experience involves, on the one hand, the moral principle that we should keep our promises; on this side of the dilemma there is also the moral value of being a good or dutiful student. On the other side, there is the moral value of being a good friend; there is also the moral principle that we should help others in need. The conflict here is not between different things the student wants to do (her best friend

case history 1.1

Some everday dilemmas

A student has promised her classmates that she will write up their group project, which must be handed in to their tutor the next morning. Just after she has started to write, her closest friend telephones in great distress, demanding to see her right away because her fiancé has just broken off their engagement. A few days later the student is approached on a bitterly cold morning by a beggar who asks her for the price of a cup of tea. The student can easily afford to give him this, but the beggar clearly has alcohol on his breath and it is only 10 o'clock in the morning. Later in the day the student meets her married sister who is worried about her 14-year-old daughter. The daughter has asked if she can go to the next town tomorrow with a girlfriend to see a new film and come back on the late train. She says that the other girl's parents have agreed, but her mother is unable to contact them and is not sure that her daughter has told her the whole story.

or the group project may each in their own way be tiresome and the alternative a welcome excuse) but between different things which she feels she ought to do.

Meeting the beggar, the student may want to give him the money – perhaps to get him out of the way, perhaps to make herself feel virtuous – but she may also feel that she ought not to, because it would not be in his interest to continue drinking himself to death. On the other hand, she may not want to give him the money in the first place – perhaps because she is afraid the beggar may recognise her and pester her again. She may also feel that she ought to give it, because as another adult, the beggar has a right to decide what is best for himself – and because one ought to help others in need.

The sister's dilemma, too, involves the right of other people to decide what is best for themselves, but in this case is complicated because the other person is a child. If teenagers are to become responsible adults, parents have to learn to trust them to be responsible, even if this means letting them make their own mistakes. On the other hand, some mistakes can have serious consequences, and parents also have a responsibility to protect their children. If the mother values responsibility, that value will exert considerable moral force on both sides of her dilemma.

The examples in Case History 1.1 all seem to be genuine irresolvable moral dilemmas. But certain facts may emerge which could question this. The student might have failed to read a notice from the tutor postponing the project deadline for a week. The beggar might have been at a crucial stage in voluntary psychiatric treatment for alcoholism. The other girl's parents might have agreed to her going to the cinema on the condition that one set of parents collected the two girls by car. In each case, this vital information, if it had come to light, might well have resolved (or dissolved) the respective dilemmas. In the case of the project, this would be for obvious reasons. In the case of the beggar, the student might be able to argue that because his psychiatric treatment was voluntary, her refusal of money was supporting his own prior decision about what was best for himself. As far as the girls were concerned, the information might allow the mother to negotiate an agreed compromise with her daughter about the degree of responsibility appropriate to the circumstances.

Possibilities of this kind illustrate the importance of good communication and adequate information about the circumstances, when facing moral quandaries in everyday life. Quite often, what appears to be a moral dilemma is the result of a breakdown in, or absence of, relevant communication between different people. This is certainly true of some areas of interprofessional and professional–patient communication, where the absence of clear procedures may give rise to 'dilemmas' that have more to do with poor professional practice than ethics in the narrower sense. If a nurse does not know what a doctor has told a dying patient, she may be left in a quandary about what to say if the patient asks her directly what is happening to him. When the bed of a patient awaiting discharge is urgently needed for another patient, and the nursing staff fail to discover, for example, that a relative has just arrived at home to look after the first patient, the misconception that this patient has nowhere to go could create an avoidable moral dilemma about priorities. So when the same kind of difficult moral choices recur, rather than agonising over each 'dilemma', it may be worth asking whether institutional or personal networks of communication cannot be improved in some appropriate way, either by some organisational means or by those involved cultivating a greater degree of tact or ingenuity.

MAKING SOUND MORAL DECISIONS

Improvements in communication clearly have a part to play in avoiding certain unnecessary moral dilemmas. On the other hand, there may be a temptation, particularly among practically minded people, to overestimate what can be achieved in this way. The student's difficulty, we might say, could have been avoided either if the college had had a better system of informing students or if the student herself had cultivated the habit of checking noticeboards more carefully. Her sister's problem, too, might have been avoided had she worked harder, over a longer

period of time, at communicating with her daughter. Even the moral quandary involving the beggar might have been avoided if the student, on meeting him, had talked to him and elicited the vital information. A way round the apparent moral dilemma can be found in each of these situations, just as, often enough, it can be found in everyday life. On the other hand, there are many situations in everyday life for which no such way exists; and even when it does, difficult moral choices and moral conflicts may remain.

To illustrate this fact, consider the examples in Case History 1.1 again. Meeting the beggar, the student might have started to talk with him and he might just possibly have given her the vital information. But in thus delaying any decision about whether to give him the money until she had more information, the student was already acting in a way which, at that time, with the information she had, went against what on one side of her 'dilemma' she felt she ought to do; it went against, that is, another adult's right to decide what was best for him. Her decision to seek more information in this case was not a neutral matter: she had come down on one side of the dilemma and made a moral choice.

Prior moral choice might equally have been involved in any means by which the other two apparent dilemmas could have been avoided. A better system of informing students might have been possible for the college only at the cost of choosing not to spend its limited resources on, say, library facilities or student amenities. Again, in cultivating the habit of checking noticeboards more regularly the student might have been opting for a general style of living which gave greater priority to the demands of work than to the demands of friendship. Here, too, moral choices would have been involved, as they would have been in the sister's decision to spend more time with her daughter – which might well have been at the expense of time spent on her own work or with her husband.

Thus, even when ways exist of avoiding painful conflicts between moral principles, this does not mean that moral choices are not being made. Such choices may have been made over a long period of time, as the characters of individuals, relationships or institutions were being formed. But the succession of small choices made every day by everyone, or collectively, is no less significant than the large choice presented by an acute moral dilemma. In this sense, every purposeful moral choice we make, in principle at least, is the result of some earlier moral choice we have made as individuals or as part of present or past society.

What all this suggests is that moral problems and even dilemmas, which we may reasonably wish to avoid in everyday life, can nevertheless play a useful part in our understanding of the moral dimension of our experience. The point about moral dilemmas, in particular, because they appear to confront us with irresolvable conflicts of duties, is that they demonstrate, more dramatically than anything else, the complexity of moral experience and the inescapability of moral choice in life.

A moral dilemma brings into sharper focus the moral values and principles which matter to us even when they conflict with one another – because of our previous moral choices. Many of these will have been everyday choices that were relatively unconsidered but which, cumulatively, have gone to make up what we may call our moral character. Confronted by a genuine moral dilemma, the fact that we recognise it as such challenges us also to recognise the strength of our conflicting values, and in making (or not making) a moral choice, to adopt, change or re-inforce the nature of our moral character. In studying moral issues, then, while it is reasonable enough to look – as we would in everyday life – for ways round or out of the dilemma, it is also useful to consider the dilemma on the assumption that there are no such ways, and to ask, if that is the case, which option we would choose and how we would defend our choice in the light of the values involved. When we have begun to do that, it might be added, we have begun to explore the nature of ethics.

Most people in the course of their lives learn to make ethical decisions, mainly by imitating others or by a process of trial and error rather than by learning systematic ways of doing so. As a result, people tend to believe it is 'all a matter of common sense' or 'intuition'. Alternatively, people say that when making moral decisions they go by 'gut feelings' or are guided by 'the voice of conscience'. Is this satisfactory? Without wanting to belittle these claims by people about how they take decisions, one can hardly say that they are convincing explanations, nor do they comprise adequate justifications for their actions. They are not the kinds of explanation that would stand up in court, for instance, as justifications for why someone did something that caused harm to someone else. For example, 'I shot the man because *I had a gut feeling* that he would attack me', or '*My conscience told me* to tell my boss of his secretary's dishonesty, despite having no hard evidence'.[4]

To treat every moral quandary as a 'dilemma' that necessarily leads to endless disputes and disagreement, or to treat all moral judgements as subjective, arbitrary or capricious, is a 'cop-out'. It is a refusal to take responsibility for making sound ethical decisions. Such talk leads all too easily to cynicism about ethics and scepticism about finding a rational basis for making moral choices. If every moral quandary is a dilemma, in the sense that it involves an irresolvable conflict of duties, then the study of ethics would be pointless. If it is possible, as we said earlier, to reframe an apparent dilemma as a problem, then we can begin to think of applying problem-solving methods to it and may possibly find a 'solution' to the difficulty confronting us.

Ethical decision-making is not some kind of occult process, but is just one kind of problem-solving process among many others. There is no mystery about applying common-sense methods of problem-solving to *ethical* problems. However, we usually do not give the same time and effort to ethical decision-making as we do to learning to apply problem-solving methods in the technical aspects of our professional work. Thus we do not take the trouble to learn about different methods of ethical decision-making, or make the time to learn and master the skills involved.

In many different types of situation in life, people have learned to apply systematic ways of dealing with problems. Part of our fascination with detective thrillers lies in being drawn into the problem-solving process and methods of the detective hero. Conan Doyle has his famous detective hero, Sherlock Holmes, reflect with Dr Watson on the logic of 'deducing' the right conclusions from the evidence. Whether we are detectives, lawyers, scientists, doctors, counsellors, nurses, accountants or public servants, we follow broadly the same steps in problem-solving:

● Collect and assess the evidence and define the problem
● Consider what principles and values apply to the case
● Review the options and choices available in the situation
● Devise an action plan, with clear objectives
● Act effectively to implement the plan and observe the process
● Analyse and learn from the results.

What this process does is to get away from simplistic 'right/wrong' answers to every situation. Even in those areas where rules and regulations or laws apply, most of the time and effort involved has to do with the appraisal of evidence for and against a case, and not with automatic application of a rule. In fact, the first issue to be decided in a court trial is whether a case falls under the rule or not.

Problem-solving demands careful appraisal of all relevant evidence. It involves reflection on alternative courses of action and their possible outcomes, and what kinds of reasons can be given in justification for a course of action chosen. A problem-solving methodology also builds the 'feedback loop' into the learning process. The value of using systematic and standard methods of decision-making is that they help us to deal with immediate problems. However, they also equip us to deal more effectively with future problems because we can repeat the process, learning from the results of past decisions and actions. This knowledge enables us, to some extent, to predict what will happen in future situations of the same kind and helps to guide our future actions. Carol Gilligan (1977), in her classic book *In a Different Voice*, suggests, however, that women are less inclined than men to adopt purely formal and rational models of problem-solving. Her research suggests that women tend to take greater account

than do men of questions of the bearing of decisions on personal relationships and interpersonal trust, and the likely emotional impact of actions on people. Whether or not we agree with Gilligan that men and women tackle ethical decision-making in different ways, we cannot afford to overlook those things she maintains are important to women.

SHARED AND CHANGING VALUES

In what has been written so far, moral values have been discussed mainly in terms of the values of individuals. But values, of course, are something we share with others. This can be seen in the fact that morals and politics are not distinct activities but part of a continuum. People, it is true, sometimes talk about politics as if it were only a matter of power for power's sake. However, while power is clearly of importance in politics generally, and to some politicians in particular, politics is also concerned with ideals and social goals, and values play an important part in political as well as moral decision-making. Some of the earliest moral philosophers, e.g. Aristotle in c.330 BC, considered that the study of ethics was part of the study of politics; and clearly enough, the purposes, values and principles we have as individuals cannot be properly studied in isolation from those of the society and culture that have made us what we are (Thomson 1976).

The fact of shared as well as individual values is of obvious importance in considering practical moral issues in nursing and the ethics of nursing care in general. Some of the ways in which becoming a nurse may create shared values among members of the profession, and also conflicts with the individual's values, will be discussed in Chapter 2, and the relationship between moral rules and roles will be mentioned in Chapters 3 and 10. In Chapters 4 and 5, the relationship between power and values, values and fundamental principles, and values in health care will be discussed further. In this discussion, in the broader context of everyday moral choice, however, it may be worth asking how our shared values have been changing, and what effect

---

> **Box 1.3** Attitudes, beliefs and values. (Adapted from Hawkins 1996)
>
> **Attitude** (Latin: *aptus* = fitting)
> An uncritical or unexamined position one adopts about something, a conditioned way of regarding or behaving towards someone, towards ideas or things. Positive or negative feelings, dispositions or reactions towards someone or something.
>
> **Belief** (Old French: *beleafe* = trusted, dear)
> Beliefs form a subset of acquired opinions and attitudes to which we give personal assent and for which we are prepared to make truth-claims, i.e. we make judgements based on our beliefs that are open to testing by others.
>
> **Value** (Latin: *valere* = to be strong, worthy)
> The basis from which we assess the importance or worth of something, estimate the relative salience of various things or actions, for the achievement of our life goals, or the well-being of others/society. Values are beliefs which we often share with others, to which we are personally committed and on which we are prepared to act, to stake our decisions and our futures.

this may be having on our contemporary moral decision-making (see Box 1.3).

One of the major changes which seems to have taken place in our society during the past century is a shift from general public agreement about moral values to a much greater variety of expressed moral opinion and tolerance of diversity. Of course, not everyone 100 years ago agreed about what was morally right and wrong, nor today is society without consensus on some moral issues. But the variety of moral viewpoints that it is acceptable to express and possible to justify in public does seem to have become greater. This situation of moral pluralism may well be one reason why we are particularly aware today of moral conflicts and dilemmas. How we view this situation will depend on our moral presuppositions: some of us will see it as symptomatic of moral liberation, others of moral decay. The truth is probably, as usual, more complex and, because we are living through it, largely hidden from us. On the basis of what has happened to societies in the past, one way of interpreting what is happening now may be by comparing it with the transition from childhood to adolescence.

An obvious aspect of this comparison is the way in which many people today look back nostalgic-ally to the lost moral certainties of the past. This nostalgia is reminiscent of what, in retrospect, seems so attractive about childhood – its security and particularly the certainty of childhood ideas. Grandmother is a saint, father can do anything, our family's ways are the best ways, the others' are rather odd. The pain, but also the excitement, of adolescence lies in discovering that things are really much more complicated and often not what they had seemed. Grandmother can be an emotional tyrant, father has not conquered the world, other families' ways and moral standards may be as good as, if not better than, ours. The change experienced in adolescence, in other words, is from a world in which things are morally black or white to one in which we discover an infinite variety of moral shades of grey. In this situation, we are faced with two major temptations. One is to deny that the shades of grey exist, possibly by adopting a new black and white morality supplied by some dogmatic moral, religious or political ideology. The dangers of this are those of moral short-sightedness about the complexity of real-life decision-making and moral insensitivity towards those with different convictions. The other temptation is to accept the infinite variety of moral shades of grey and to say that they are all the same. The dangers here are those of moral indifference and moral indecisiveness.

One way of understanding what has been happening to morality in our society, then, is to compare it with this transition from the moral certainties of childhood to the uncertainties, temptations and dangers of adolescence. Similar changes have taken place in the past, when individuals or societies have experienced the transition from tribal or village life to the life of large cosmopolitan cities. In the tribe or village, morality was a matter of shared fixed conventions which gave people considerable security – but at the price, often, of hypocrisy, guilt and even open cruelty towards those who deviated from the moral norm. The shift to city life, where people from different origins with different moral views lived together, made it difficult to maintain the old black-and-white certainties, revealed the moral shades of grey and exposed individuals and society to the adolescent's temptation to question all values or take refuge in dogmatism. In our time, something of the same kind seems to have been happening to society generally through experiences of war, the growth of travel, international communications, the mass media and public education. These changes have made more people than ever before aware of the variety of moral viewpoints that it is possible to hold, and consequently of the difficulty, in the face of this, of maintaining that any one traditional moral viewpoint is right or the best. Here we face the same risks, of moral dogmatism – the uncritical acceptance of a particular moral position as infallible – or moral relativism, the view that any moral position is as good as another.

Against this background, one particular value that has fallen in public esteem is that of paternalism and the principle that 'father knows best'. This shift is associated with greater respect for the value of self-determination (or autonomy) and the related ideal of human rights – especially the rights of women and minorities. Also involved in this change is an emphasis on the individual which favours such values as self-expression rather than self-sacrifice, tolerance rather than conformity, and flexibility rather than strict obedience to moral rules. Changes of this kind seem to be reflected today in changing attitudes within nursing, traditionally a female, obedient, self-sacrificing and sometimes rigid profession. These changing attitudes focus on questions about the authority of the traditionally male profession of medicine, the separate identity of nursing as a profession in its own right and the need for more flexible ways of providing care. Changing values also seem to be reflected in contemporary concern for such things as the patient's right to know and the right to choice and self-determination in health care.

CULTURAL DIVERSITY AND COMMON ETHICAL PRINCIPLES

In the study of ethics we set out to study the underlying principles common to all types of personal and social morality. But are we justified in assuming that there are common underlying principles? And what do we mean by 'principles'?

Many people think of *principles* as dogmatic beliefs, statements of absolute or infallible truths. This is unhelpful to ethics, for it removes the making of moral judgements from the domain of what can be debated on rational terms. Ethics from this standpoint becomes either an appeal to subjective intuition or a slanging match between competing fundamentalisms. We wish to use the term in its classical meaning, where the original meaning of the word 'principle' is a 'beginning' or 'starting point' for reasoning. Thus 'principles' refer to where you start, not where you end up, and refer to the basic questions you must ask, rather than providing you with ready-made answers. Unfortunately for those who believe in absolute moral truths, being able to recite a list of moral principles does not help you to decide which principle is applicable in a given situation, nor how to apply it, nor how to resolve conflicts between principles when these arise. Principles help give us direction; they point the way, but do not tell us where we will end up, or what will happen along the way (see Box 1.4).

We often hear it said, 'When it comes to morality, everyone seems to have different views of what is right and wrong', and 'Who are we to say that one person is right and another wrong?'. In an increasingly multicultural Britain and in other European countries with a colonial past, colonialism brought European 'Christian' culture into contact, and sometimes conflict, with other cultural and religious traditions. The massive social upheavals resulting from wars and revolutions in the 20th century, causing the dislocation of millions of people, and creating refugee populations on a scale previously unseen, has also brought people into contact with migrants from all over

---

Box 1.4 Principles and rules

Principle (Latin: *principium* = source or beginning)
A fundamental truth or doctrine that is the source of inspiration or direction for moral action, or used as the starting point for moral reasoning.

Rule (Latin: *regulare* = to rule or govern; cf. regulation)
A public statement of what can or should be done, a prescription which governs what we do, or defines our duties.

the world. These changes, coupled with global trade, travel, emigration and immigration, have left few cultures unchallenged by interaction with others. We are thus confronted with a rich variety of different religions and philosophies competing for our allegiance – i.e., besides Christianity, Judaism, Islam, Hinduism, Buddhism and Taoism as well as secular ideologies such as Marxism and Humanism – offering different systems of values to live by and different means of salvation.

The reality is that few of us live any longer in isolated or culturally homogeneous societies. Britain itself has become a multicultural society (and perhaps always has been) and is increasingly a multi-ethnic society too, so that not only does the UK National Health Service have to deal with patients from an incredible variety of religious, political and cultural backgrounds, but its health care staff represent the same variety and diversity as well.

On the one hand, this diversity and confusing variety of traditions of religious and social morality seem to make the talk of common principles appear naive and moral consensus an unrealistic dream. On the other hand, if we are not overwhelmed by the relativities and driven to moral scepticism, we can only wonder at the richness and variety of forms in which human beings have sought to express what they believe it means to be human and what values they see as necessary to make possible a full life (Downie 1971, Veatch 1981, Downie & Calman 1987). Moral relativism and scepticism are also useful challenges to thinking about ethics. As the German philosopher Kant pointed out in the 18th century, when we say that something is right or wrong, we are making an implicit or explicit claim that this is, or should be, true for everybody (Paton 1969).

This claim to universal validity implicit in our ordinary moral judgements is challenged by the evidence of moral disagreements between individuals and the diversity of moral rules in different systems of social morality. This may lead us to make dogmatic claims for the universal applicability of our own moral values and traditions; or lead us to sceptical relativism. In the face of scepticism based on moral relativism, namely that all moral beliefs are relative either to each individual or to their culture, we either take refuge in cynicism or are driven to find more fundamental principles which underlie these apparent individual and cultural differences.

The challenge represented by moral scepticism is to provide some kind of rational justification for these fundamental principles, once we have found them. The rational debate about the foundations of ethics as such takes us into the sphere of moral theory – a subject we will return to in the final chapter. We can pursue the demand for rational justification for moral principles only as far as is reasonable. If nothing will satisfy us but absolute certainty, then perhaps nothing will satisfy us, and we are left with paralysing scepticism or apathy. In practice, we do manage to get along more or less well with people of other religious and cultural traditions and we share enough common ground to do business with one another, intermarry and even vote for the same political parties. Moral scepticism has to make sense of this creative interaction between widely different human cultures, or it simply leads to a kind of cul-de-sac of thought and action.

For some people, the quest for the foundations of morality leads back to belief in a transcendent God who is the source of universal norms, or to metaphysical beliefs about the ultimate meaning of human being-in-the-world. Historically, most systems of social morality have evolved from metaphysical and religious beliefs, so it is always interesting, and often instructive, to trace their pedigree. However, it can be argued that ethics can, or should be able to, stand without the supports of religion and metaphysics, that it should be grounded in rational criteria based on reflection on the given structures and dynamics of human being-in-the-world, and the conditions that are necessary for us to fulfil our potential species nature. For many people, on the other hand, those who are less bothered by sceptical doubts, the matter is more pragmatic – how to reconcile their moral beliefs with those of other people in such a way that conflict can be avoided or reduced and cooperation made possible (Mitchell 1970).

If we are to avoid giving unnecessary offence to or injuring other people's moral sensibilities, we need to develop tolerance and an understanding, even respect, for moral standpoints which differ from our own. This is not easy. We are born into particular families and societies with their own unique traditions and values. Commitment to these values and a willingness to live by them, to fight for them and, in some cases, to die for them are vital sources of cohesion and solidarity in families and communities. Moreover, such values serve to define our identity as members of such social groups. For children born of parents of widely different cultural and religious views or ethnic origin, the conflict of values can be both painful and a source of enrichment. For people working in the caring professions, awareness of cultural and religious differences is not only important for dealing with their own confusion or disagreements with colleagues of a moral nature, but may also be vital in understanding what factors (dress, diet, genetic differences, customs relating to birth, reproduction and death) are directly relevant to the sense of dignity and identity, physical and mental health, of their patients or clients.

At a broader level, Christianity, Marxism and Islam, as three great 'religions', have sent out missionaries to spread their respective 'gospels' and to make converts. In the course of their endeavours, they have often treated with contempt the traditional religion and customs of the societies they have penetrated. At best, they have been guilty of a kind of cultural imperialism – the arrogant and often self-righteous claim to proprietorship of the truth or privileged access to moral wisdom. At worst, they have been guilty of forced conversions, witch-hunts, massacres, persecution and suppression of religious practices other than their own. Against this, the painstaking studies of anthropologists and sociologists, and the cross-cultural comparisons made on the basis of more objective and scientific analyses have brought to light not only the diversity and relativity of social customs and mores, but also the many common features shared by different cultures. They have helped us to become more tolerant and to gain insight into the rich wisdom and dignity of many cultures we might be tempted to call primitive.

Moral relativism has therefore helped to challenge cultural imperialism, religious and moral dogmatism, intolerance and arrogance. However, it must also be pointed out that there have been thinkers and leaders among Christians, Marxists and Muslims, who have also criticised religious intolerance among their co-religionists or party supporters. For Christians, it has been in the name of a God who transcends and judges all human institutions. For some Marxists it has been in the name of a science that is experimental and tentative, not dogmatic, and recognition of the need for ongoing reform even after the Russian revolution. For the great philosophers of Islam, it has been in the name of an uncompromising ethical monotheism and a belief in universal human values. The recognition of some kind of transcendent ideal itself may be grounds for a kind of moral relativism – the humility to recognise the limited and fallible nature of our own moral systems or personal insights.

The argument based on moral relativism can, however, be so exaggerated as to make nonsense of moral argument and the reality of human intercultural cooperation. If there were no common ground between the moral beliefs of different individuals or different peoples, then no rational debate and intelligent disagreement about ethical and political concerns would be possible. The reality is that even people with the most widely divergent views continue to debate moral principles and values in a way that they are not prepared to do when it comes to mere matters of taste (*de gustibus non est disputandum*). This suggests that there is sufficient common ground for each disputant to at least understand (or partially understand) what the other is saying, and thus attempt to marshal arguments, feelings and evidence in the effort to persuade the other. The reality is that, throughout history, diverse nations and cultures have been able to form pacts and alliances, cooperate in peace and war, and even develop the basis of public and international law. *The United Nations Declaration of Human Rights* (UNO 1948) (though not signed by the USSR and South Africa in 1947) was signed by the official representatives of all member states. The further elaboration of this Bill of Rights and the growing body of international law, together with the enhanced authority of the International Court of

Human Rights, suggest that there is in fact more agreement about fundamental principles and human rights than might first be apparent from the seemingly interminable wrangles in public debate and in forums such as the European Parliament or the United Nations General Assembly (Eide 1992).

This should not altogether surprise us, for, despite the seemingly infinite variety of individual human beings and their forms of social, cultural and political organisation, some things are universally common to all members of our species. For example, in all human societies, babies are born through the fertilisation of sperm and ovum from parents of different sex; children are initially very small and vulnerable – needing to be fed, nurtured and protected. With luck, good management and effective health care, they may survive the infections and traumas of childhood, reach maturity, reproduce themselves and decline into old age; and sooner or later all will die. These universal features of human life suggest that there are bound to be features of all systems of social morality that are similar. If certain general conditions must be satisfied before human life can develop and flourish, then the principles of morality will seek to protect vulnerable human life and promote the conditions necessary for human flourishing (Maritain 1944, Finnis 1999).

This question can be approached in two different ways: either by attempting to clarify the fundamental values by which we seek to direct human action and social organisation to protect human beings and to promote human flourishing, which leads to the formulation of *fundamental principles*; or by attempting to define the essential conditions that must be satisfied if human life is to be human, which leads to the formulation of *fundamental human rights*. We will discuss the first of these options in this chapter; the question of fundamental human rights will be examined in more detail in the next.

FORMATIVE AND REGULATIVE PRINCIPLES IN ETHICS

In his *Groundwork of the Metaphysic of Morals*, the German philosopher Immanuel Kant (1785) set out to clarify what he called the principles presupposed in and necessary to ethics as such.

He argued, for example, that the concept of 'person' or 'person-hood' is fundamental to ethics and is a formative or *constitutive principle* of ethics (Paton 1969). Without the concept of a person – defined as an individual who is a bearer of rights and responsibilities – ethics cannot get started. Such individual persons must always be treated as ends in themselves and never simply as instrumental means to an end. The concept of a 'person' defined as 'a bearer of rights and duties' also serves to define the membership and boundaries of the 'moral community'. 'Respect for persons' thus functions as a *regulative principle* for our ethical conduct by requiring us to respect the rights of others and to avoid the exploitation or abuse of persons in our everyday practice.

The concept of a person, as a bearer of rights and responsibilities, implies an individual who is able to exercise some degree of self-determination, who can understand the requirements of membership of the moral community to which he belongs, and who is free and able to act, to exercise his rights and to recognise his duties to others. Kant points out that this freedom and moral independence are necessary for any moral agent to qualify as a moral agent, or to be held responsible for his actions. He calls this moral independence 'autonomy', in contrast to 'heteronomy' which is subjection or forced submission to externally imposed authority. Thus, he argues that the *principle of autonomy* is a necessary theoretical and a practical presupposition for any functioning system of ethics or law. Responsibility and accountability, rights and duties do not make sense unless we can assume that people are capable of self-determination and of making a personal commitment to a set of values. Respect for persons also requires that we respect this autonomy in others.

However, the concept of a person, or even a derived list of personal rights, would not alone be sufficient to establish a coherent system of ethics. Personal rights alone would not provide an adequate basis for a system of social ethics unless these rights could be justified, promoted and protected as rights for all. This demand for universal human rights or the universal applicability of moral principles requires a second kind of constitutive principle, namely the *principle or criterion of universalisability*, as Kant called it. The principle of universalisability in ethics seeks to ensure that, as individuals, we act consistently and that the rights we claim for ourselves are applied to all without discrimination. This demand for equity or universal fairness is a demand of the regulative ethical principle of justice.

Justice and respect for persons together would make for a reasonably satisfactory combination of pillars for any system of ethics but for the fact of given inequalities – the fact that there are wide discrepancies in size and age, wealth and power, intelligence and skill, health and strength among human beings. To ensure a workable system of ethics we require another constitutive principle, which we might call the *principle of reciprocity* (do unto others as you would have them do unto you). This principle, or criterion, is necessary because at certain times in our lives we all experience extreme vulnerability – when we are infants, sick, injured, mentally disordered, senile or dying. Unless we build in a principle of reciprocity – the recognition of a reciprocal duty to care for one another – we cannot ground the social obligation to care for or protect the interests of the weak. The regulative moral principle of beneficence (the duty to care or to do good) and the principle of non-maleficence (the duty to do no harm to those in your care) thus complement respect for personal rights and justice, and complete the minimum requirements for a coherent system of ethics.

FUNDAMENTAL ETHICAL PRINCIPLES

If ethics is to have any credibility, it must be based not only on our shared and changing values, but on principles that are universally acknowledged and respected. Here, as we have already indicated, we seem to be up against an immediate difficulty. The popular view of ethics is that everyone has different ethical principles. Everything is relative and no agreement is possible in ethics. Is this really true, or is this just a 'cop-out'?

In a liberal society, tolerance of religious, moral and cultural diversity is encouraged. Living in 'multicultural societies' we are taught that:

- everyone is entitled to their own opinions about matters of ethics and politics
- people should not be prevented from expressing these views
- people should not be discriminated against because of the views they hold.

Now, this seems to imply that all points of view have equal validity, or that all moral points of view are relative. If all moral beliefs are just that (points of view), then it would not seem to be possible to talk of moral truth or of universal moral principles.

However, arguing that we *ought* to allow everyone the right to express their views on ethical and political matters is based on an unstated ethical principle, namely that of *respect for persons and their rights*.[5] This principle informs the whole of the ICN *Code for Nurses* (and many others) and is specifically expressed in the preamble (as quoted above), namely 'Inherent in nursing is respect for life, dignity and the rights of man'.

To argue that we *ought not* to discriminate against people with moral, political or religious views different from our own is based on appeal to the *principle of justice*.[6] Again, this principle of justice, universal fairness and non-discrimination is manifested in the statement: '[Nursing] is unrestricted by considerations of nationality, race, creed, colour, age, sex, politics or social status'.

Other elements in the code which arise out of the demands of justice are such obligations as the requirement that nurses accept responsibility to maintain their level of competence and that they share with other citizens the responsibility to 'initiate and support action to meet the health and social needs of the public', play 'a major role in determining and implementing desirable standards of nursing practice and nursing education', and participate 'in establishing and maintaining equitable social and economic working conditions in nursing'.

Historically, the liberal tradition has used relativist arguments both to attack religious and political bigotry on the one hand, and to defend civil liberties like freedom of speech and association on the other. However, underlying the liberal defence of personal rights and freedoms is an appeal to the more fundamental and universal principles of justice and respect for persons.

Linked to these arguments are similar arguments about our duty to defend the rights of those who are too young or too weak to defend their own interests, including ethnic and religious minorities. Here, appeal is being made to the underlying *principle of beneficence*[7] or the protective duty of care the strong owe to the weak. The basis for this moral demand for reciprocity in mutual care and protection is the need to recognise that we are all weak and vulnerable at different times of our lives and need others to care and advocate for us, classically expressed in the *golden rule*: 'Treat other people as you would like them to treat you'.

Nurses usually encounter people when they are sick, at their most vulnerable, injured or mentally ill, and when they, as nurses, are in an inherently more powerful position – based on their supposed knowledge, expertise and professional skills. Thus, nurses are said, in both law and ethics, to have a *fiduciary responsibility* not only to care for and to advise patients, but also to act on behalf of and advocate for those who are less well informed or actually incompetent. The nurse has a fundamental duty of care to protect the interests of the patient and not to take advantage of his naivety, ignorance or vulnerability.

The *principle of beneficence* – to do good – and the corresponding principle of *non-maleficence* – not to do harm – are fundamental to all moral communities. Parents have a basic duty of care, of protective beneficence towards their children (as well as to elderly and dependant relatives). Teachers exercise a legal duty of care *in loco parentis* (in place of the parent) towards the children in their care. Doctors and nurses, social workers and counsellors and all members of the caring or consulting professions (including lawyers and accountants) have to exercise a similar duty of care or protective beneficence towards their clients. This is by virtue of the relationship of trust or fiduciary responsibility in which they stand relative to their patients or clients.

The fact that the principle of reciprocity, or 'golden rule', crops up in virtually every known system of community morality is because it is universally true that while we are strong today we may be vulnerable tomorrow; we may be nurses today and patients tomorrow. As such, the requirement that we should do good and not harm to one another, the principle of protective beneficence and/or non-maleficence, is the necessary foundation for membership of any moral community. Without this principle, no society could survive or function very well.

Fundamental ethical principles in the context of health care (see Box 1.5)

The principle of respect for persons

In the context of health care, respect for persons basically means treating patients as people with rights. It means further respecting the autonomy of individuals and protecting those who suffer loss of autonomy through illness, injury or mental disorder, and working to restore autonomy to those who have lost it. It means recognising that patients have such basic human rights as the right to know, the right to privacy and the right to receive care and treatment. Clearly, there may be a tension between the patient's rights and the helper's duty to care, just as there may be practical difficulties in determining adequately informed and voluntary consent to treatment; or in setting sensible limits to confidentiality, or physical privacy, in institutions where care may be shared by a team of nurses, paramedics, social workers and doctors; and distinguishing between 'care' and 'treatment' (or the choice of therapies). Paul Ramsey (1970), in his classic book *The Patient as Person*, pointed out that for the carers, respect for persons in their care means working to maintain the optimum degree of independence for the patient and sharing knowledge, care and skills in such a way as to empower the patient and avoid creating and perpetuating dependency. Following in this tradition, the British Royal College of Nursing stressed that the primary duty of the nurse is to work to restore the optimum degree of autonomy to the patient that is compatible with what has been lost as a result of disease, injury or mental disorder (RCN 1979).

Box 1.5   Fundamental ethical principles

The principle of respect for persons
- The duty to respect the rights, autonomy and dignity of other people
- The duty to promote their well-being and autonomy
- The duty of truthfulness, honesty and sincerity (honour = respect), for deceit is dishonourable

The concept of a 'person' (i.e. as a bearer of rights and duties) and the principle of autonomy (i.e. a person should be free to determine his own choices) are here both constitutive principles essential to legal, ethical and political discourse.

The principle of justice
- The duty of universal fairness (equal opportunity for individuals) and equity (equality of outcomes for groups)
- The duty to treat people as ends in themselves, never simply as means to an end
- The duty to avoid discrimination, abuse or exploitation of people on grounds of race, age, sex, class, gender or religion

The principle of justice requires of us that any personal rule of action we use should, in principle, be capable of being universalised for all people. For this reason it is sometimes described as the constitutive principle of universalisability.

The principle of beneficence (or non-maleficence)
- The duty to do good and to avoid doing harm to others
- The duty of care, to protect the weak and vulnerable
- The duty of advocacy, defending the rights of those incompetent or temporarily unable to defend their own

Like the golden rule (do unto others as you would have them do unto you), this principle is sometimes referred to as the constitutive principle of reciprocity, and is a necessary condition for any moral community to survive or function.

The principle of justice

Justice, or the demand for universal fairness, stands in a relationship of tension with respect for the rights of individual persons. The exercise of our individual rights (such as freedom of movement or association) may have to be curtailed in times of crisis, in the interests of the common good – as in cases where public health measures have to be introduced to control epidemics. Action is taken here in the interests of distributive (not retributive) justice, but the restriction of individual liberties may appear punitive to infected individuals; for example, the way people with AIDS

have been segregated or incarcerated in some societies is reminiscent of past treatment of lepers or the mentally ill. When we consider the social controls imposed on mentally disordered people and the loss of rights of people in institutional care generally, or the policing role which nurses and other health care workers may have to perform, the analogy with retributive justice seems close (as the sociological analysis of sickness behaviour as a kind of deviance illustrates) (Freidson 1970a, 1994). However justified public health measures may be, we must not lose sight of the rights of individuals. Justice to individuals also means non-discrimination on the basis of sex, race or religion (or because of youth, old age, having a contagious disease, mental handicap or mental illness). It means equal opportunity to benefit from, or have access to, preventive medicine and treatment health services and the fruits of research.

Justice also means equality of outcomes for different groups. This raises questions of the broader 'political' duty of health professionals to contribute through research to informed debate on justice in health care and to contribute to fairer distribution of and access to health resources, by sound research and policy development. The well-documented evidence by health researchers of inequalities in health status of people in Britain during the so-called Thatcher 'boom years' (Townsend & Davidson 1982) and the growing health divide between rich and poor (Whitehead 1987) showed that to ensure justice in health care, political action was required to get the state to shift greater resources to deprived areas, even at the expense of more privileged sectors. Campaigning for resources to improve services or to defend standards of care is demanded of health professionals committed to the principles of justice and equity. This is also the theme of the World Health Organization Report *The Health Burden of Social Inequalities* (Illsley & Svensson 1984) and the World Bank World Development Report *Investing in Health* (1993).

The principle of beneficence

Beneficence has had a bad press recently. Attacks on paternalism in medicine and nursing, lay resentment of the medicalisation of life, the emphasis on patients' rights by militant pressure groups, as well as action by politicians concerned with social justice and the political economy of health care, have resulted in health professionals becoming defensive about beneficence. Certainly, beneficence, the duty to care, may be exercised in a way that 'infantilises' people and creates dependence, but it need not do so. In fact, it has been argued that patient advocacy, defending the rights of the vulnerable patient, or acting on behalf of those unable to assert their rights, is a requirement of beneficence. Beneficence is indispensable wherever there are dependent, severely disabled or helpless people in need of support or urgent care and attention. The reciprocity in our duty to care for one another should make us realise that we all need others to speak for us, to do things for us, or to defend our rights, when we are too weak to do so for ourselves. But if knowledge is power, the power of the true carer is aimed at sharing knowledge and skills with vulnerable individuals so as to empower them to reassert control over their own lives, if this is humanly possible (May 1983, Campbell 1984a, 1985).

CONFRONTING THREE TYPES OF MORAL RELATIVISM

The claim we make here is that all moral communities share at least these three fundamental ethical principles, as the basis for coexistence and cooperation. This runs counter to the popular relativist argument that 'everyone has different values' and 'ethics is a personal matter and just a matter of taste'. The view that all ethical values and judgements are relative to the individual, or to the societies within which they operate, is so widely held that it deserves further comment. (Thompson 1987b, Beauchamp & Childress 1994).

First of all, it must be said that the opposite to moral relativism is not moral absolutism or fanatical fundamentalism, of either the religious or moral variety. The movements associated with the self-styled 'moral majority' often (but only thinly) mask new types of moral bigotry of the right, while arguments about what is or is not 'morally

or politically correct' are often driven by ideologues of the left.

Against these forms of authoritarian thinking, ethical relativism and sceptical realism are refreshing antidotes. In the past, and in opposition to European cultural imperialism of the past, social scientists, historians and psychologists have rejoiced in pointing out the variations between the beliefs and values that form the foundations of different societies and the lifestyles of individuals. There are indeed interesting and often profound differences in the way various cultures (e.g. Anglo-Saxon, Asian, American or African) articulate themselves as moral communities, and how they come up with different social customs and conventions for behaviour in various circumstances. 'Ethical relativism' in one sense can be a safeguard against ethnic chauvinism, religious intolerance and cultural arrogance. However, maintaining that certain ethical principles are universal and applicable to all moral communities on this planet is not incompatible with a sincere recognition of this cultural diversity or of the individual differences in moral beliefs and values which exist.

It is of the nature of principles that they are just that, namely starting points from which we have to derive duties and rights and specific moral rules. It is part of the interest of comparative ethics that we can study the incredible variety of forms and practices in which different human societies have expressed their intuitions of beneficence, justice and respect for persons.

However, ethical relativism can lead to ethical scepticism and cynicism about the possibility of moral agreement and the applicability of universal rights or moral duties. For this reason, we need to address three types of ethical relativism:

● *Interpersonal relativism* emphasises that different people (even within the same family) may base their lives on different values and belief-systems. Does this disprove the universal nature of moral principles? Of course not. A brother and sister may be brought up in the same family traditions and one become a priest and another an atheist Marxist, but this does not mean that they abandon faith in universal ethical principles. Instead, what happens is that each of the positions they adopt results in a different emphasis or priority being given to justice or beneficence, or respect for persons as human values, or to their primary life goals in different belief systems. Like navigation instruments, principles help us orientate ourselves. They do not provide us with a map, or dictate a particular course to us. We have to choose our own destinations and routes for getting there. The articulation and adoption of our own moral beliefs, values and ethical rules are necessary to enable us to chart a personal course through life and to achieve our life goals.

● *Cultural relativism* is a healthy alternative to dogmatic fundamentalism, smug parochialism, gender-based sexism or chauvinistic nationalism. As we have seen earlier, the basis for the moral demand that we show tolerance and respect for cultural differences is appeal to underlying universal moral principles. These principles each express different modalities of power and power relations that are common to our relations with people in any and every kind of society. For these fundamental ethical principles deal with the different ways that power can be expressed or shared in relations between people. For example, the basis of the principle of justice is equitable power-sharing between people. Beneficence has to do with the responsibility of the powerful to protect the weak and vulnerable. Respect for persons expresses our duty, as members of a moral community, to assist or empower others to achieve their full potential and to claim and exercise their rights.

● *Philosophical relativism* is the argument that there cannot be agreement between people who hold different moral theories, such as a utilitarian or duty-based theory versus one that emphasises personal virtue or integrity. We pointed out earlier that there are some significant differences between thinking about ethics in terms of right and wrong – of principles and rules, rights and duties – and

thinking about ethics in terms of good and bad, where we are more concerned with values and goals, costs and benefits. While some philosophers ('deontologists') have attempted to develop a complete account of ethics in terms of the former, others ('teleologists') have been exclusively concerned with the latter. Recently, some philosophers have reaffirmed 'virtue ethics' as a third type of ethical theory which focuses on the moral agent as having to mediate in reality between principles and outcomes.

As we shall see in Chapter 11, these different moral theories do not necessarily contradict one another, unless they are interpreted absolutely, i.e. as the only possible way of determining whether or not our actions are ethical.[8] We will argue that they each emphasise complementary aspects of human acts and relate to different aspects of our moral experience. If we wish to give a complete or comprehensive account of moral action, then we must pay attention to each of these different

---

Box 1.6   Three types of ethical theory

The ***deontologist*** (Greek: *deon* – duty) argues that what makes actions right or wrong is their consistency with unconditional moral principles, or rules, and that these alone are the necessary foundation for a responsible ethics. The deontologist develops a system in which our moral duties and rights are clearly defined by rules. Sometimes referred to as 'principalism', deontology emphasises the priority of principles and rules, rights and duties

The ***teleologist*** (Greek: *telos* – goal or purpose) stresses that what makes an action good or bad (rather than right or wrong) is not the principle someone professes but the actual consequences, benefits or costs, of their action. Teleologists are hence often called 'consequentialists' or 'utilitarians', as they consider to be what is morally important the usefulness of the consequences in achieving good results

However, ***virtue ethics*** is another tradition which has an ancient history and has recently gained more attention, namely the tradition which attaches crucial importance to the integrity of the moral agent who has to decide how to act in a specific situation in the light of principles to achieve good ends. 'Virtue ethics', or 'prudential ethics', which is related to it, focuses on the crucial role of moral competence and the moral integrity of the agent

dimensions. These ethical theories each seek to justify our moral beliefs and ethical policies by reference either to principles or to means or consequences. In this book we argue that each type of moral theory has its own value within a broader theory of the nature of moral action and that they are not mutually exclusive. These three types of moral theory are briefly defined in Box 1.6.

SOURCES OF INSPIRATION FOR ETHICS

In almost every human culture, the connection between religion and ethics has been very close, and many people still assume that the roots of ethics are in religion. Some people would go so far as to claim that there is a necessary connection between them – that there must be a divine source and guarantee for the authority of the moral law, and that without religion there can be no ethics. Alternatively, some anti-religious thinkers have maintained that if God is dead or there is no God, then there is no pre-established moral law or ethical principles and we have to make up our own morality.[9]

Now, while there is plenty of evidence for the historical association between the emergence of ethical thought from within religious traditions and culture, there has also been a history of tension between philosophers or prophets, on the one hand, and the guardians of the religious traditions of the people, on the other. We see this in the case of Socrates' critique of traditional Greek polytheistic religion, of Confucius in relation to Chinese Taoism, of Buddha in relation to Indian Hinduism, and the critical stance of the Old Testament prophets and Jesus in relation to the religious law and practices of the Jews.

Because ethics springs out of the social customs and religious traditions of a country, this does not imply that ethics is confined to the boundaries of that culture. On the contrary, because ethics is a reflective discipline (as the rational science of morals), it involves critical exploration of the fundamental questions of human life – the questions of the meaning of being and what values should ultimately determine our individual lives and social goals. As a philosophical discipline, ethics involves both a quest and a continual questioning.

It is a spiritual quest, in the sense that it is a quest for the ultimate meaning and purpose of human life. It also necessarily involves questioning the traditions imposed on us by family, religion and society. For, as we have seen, we cannot develop as mature human beings or independent moral agents unless we make a personal commitment to a set of values and corresponding way of life. This may involve a personal re-appropriation of the religious vision and values of our upbringing, or it may involve rejection or adaptation of our inherited cultural traditions to our own needs and times. Either way, this requires critical questioning and serious commitment to the quest for truth.

Many ethical traditions around the world appeal to 'the gods', 'God' or 'the ancestors' as the source and inspirational foundation of morality. These 'divine command theories', as they are called, either appeal directly to divine revelation to justify ethical rules or commandments, or claim that the earthly representative(s) of the Deity has the ability to communicate moral truth to us. Alternatively, within the traditions of religious ethics, it is argued that the order we perceive in the world and try to imitate in human society is a divinely created moral order, and that this order is discernible by human reason. By applying our reason to understand the basis of order in the world, we are led to understand that we can only be happy or lead fulfilled lives if we live in accordance with the built-in moral imperatives of this created order and our own given nature.

We will have more to say about the issues raised by such ethical theories in Chapter 11, but it is important to note in this introductory chapter that ethics is not simply concerned with the regulation of conduct, but also with the deepest human longings and our quest for physical, mental and spiritual fulfilment as human beings. For nurses, as for other human beings, concern with ethics is part of a larger quest for spiritual and moral truth. The importance of the study of ethics for nurses is not merely for the knowledge it gives of moral rules and codes of conduct, or the skills we learn in clarifying our values in ethical decision-making and setting standards. To study ethics is to engage with some of the most profound philosophical questions asked by human beings.

Nurses often ask for training in how to give 'spiritual support' to patients faced with various kinds of personal distress, unrelieved pain or terminal illness. Here training in listening skills may be more important that attempting to tell people what they should think. Counselling patients in these contexts is less about giving answers than about learning how to listen attentively to people's questions and personal stories, and helping them to discover their own solutions to their problems. If 'answers' are demanded, this requires, more than anything else, that we are honest with ourselves and our patients about the difficult and painful nature of our quest for the meaning and purpose of human existence, the quest for moral and spiritual truth. Our own sincerity and honesty about these matters, our own integrity and willingness to explore difficult questions with them, rather than to give them 'flip' answers, may be more helpful and comforting than trying to give the appearance of having solved life's problems. As G. K. Chesterton said of the suffering of Job: 'Job found more comfort in the puzzles of God than the answers of men.'

The inescapability of the questions concerning the meaning of being for us all, and for nurses in particular, relates to the fact that it is not only patients who have to confront the question of the meaning of suffering or how to cope with it. Given the nature of their intimate involvement with pain and suffering, death and bereavement, nurses, perhaps more than any other group of professionals, have to wrestle with these questions themselves. Because we are all potentially vulnerable, nurses included – we may be well one day and critically ill the next – we do well to note the counsel of the poet John Donne (*Devotions XVII*):

No man is an Island, entire of itself; every man is a piece of the Continent, a part of the Main. Any man's death diminishes me, because I am involved in Mankind; and therefore never send to know for whom the bell tolls; it tolls for thee.

CONFLICT, CHANGE AND STABILITY IN HUMAN LIFE AND VALUES

In this introductory chapter we have pointed to the fact that there are features of our lives that are changing and others that remain constant. Human

life is being impacted on dramatically by rapid cultural change, especially in the area of scientific and technical advance, in medical science and understanding of our genetic and psychological make-up. On the other hand, there are universal features of the human condition that remain constant and invariable in time across human cultures:

Birth, copulation and death.
That's all the facts, when you come to brass tacks
(T. S. Eliot, *Samson Agonistes*)

We are all subject to the processes of growth, maturation, expression of sexual and reproductive potentialities, and will all eventually have to face suffering, death and bereavement. As St Augustine remarked: 'When a man is born, you might as well say his condition is fatal. He will not survive!'

We have argued in this chapter that certain values are common to all moral communities and are necessary for their functioning and survival, namely the values of beneficence, justice and respect for the dignity and rights of others. These values underlie and shape the way we prioritise other more personal values and our life goals, and just as the relative importance of these values may change in family life, from a preponderant emphasis on protective beneficence towards us as children, to a struggle for justice and equal treatment in adolescence, to a mature mutual respect for one another in adult life, so the priority we give to different values will change with changes in our economic and social circumstances and with wider changes in society.

The account we have given of changing attitudes and moral values in our society is merely one impression of what has been happening, and it can be immediately conceded that the changes suggested are far from universal. That this is so is, in fact, part of the point, since a major difficulty in moral decision-making today is the unpredictability of the values held by other people. Frequently, it is not possible when making difficult moral choices to rely on an appeal to values which, in the past, might have been expected to command general support. In nursing, for example, there is still considerable reluctance to go on strike. But this reluctance cannot be relied upon as much as in the past, and it is likely to be defended only in some cases by an appeal to the traditional values of duty and obedience. In other cases, the defence is more likely to be in terms of the value of care or concern for patients, or even of the profession's self-interest where strikes are thought to be counterproductive.

As this example suggests, the variety of moral values which people hold today is a matter of practical concern as well as of theoretical interest. Conflict between moral values exists not only on either side of the moral dilemmas confronting individuals, but also within society and between different societies. The great divisions in today's world are not only about material issues of power, wealth and poverty, but also about which moral values should have priority in the ordering of society. Should liberty be put first as we attempt to do in Western societies, or equality as in socialism, or the law of God as in resurgent Islam? Moral conflicts of this kind, clearly, can spill over into social, economic and even physical conflict within societies as well as between them. While political bargaining can play some part in the attempt to reconcile different interests, the purposes, ideas and values which move individuals and societies to action must also be taken into account in our decision-making, if the harmful consequences of conflict are to be avoided.

In seeking to avoid these harmful consequences, it is important to remember that moral conflict in itself is not bad. Indeed, it is only through moral conflict that society can resist tyranny or individual moral dogmatism and moral relativism, and thus remain responsive to the variety of moral values in personal and communal life which makes life fully human. To resist these temptations and at the same time avoid the harmful consequences of conflict is not easy, and not even possible, unless individuals and societies have some way of communicating with one another which helps each to understand the importance of the other's moral values without thereby diminishing the importance of their own. In human life, there are many ways of establishing such communication, ranging from marriage, negotiation and industrial bargaining, to international diplomacy. But one useful way, we would suggest, is through the kind of informed and rea-

soned public debate about moral issues which we undertake in the study of ethics. Such debate provides a framework within which people can communicate with one another about the values and principles which move them to action. Ethics provides a framework within which we can give one another reasons why we believe these values and principles to be important, can offer and listen to reasonable criticism and can, on occasion, find ways of establishing public consensus about the rights and wrongs of particular conflicts. In an area such as health care, at a time of increasing recourse to the courts and to political bargaining, ethics would seem to have a particularly useful contribution to make.

Of course, this is not to suggest that we all need to become philosophers any more than we are all able to be saints. Nor is it to suggest that someone who has mastered the technical language of ethics is necessarily thereby a better person or even someone better able to resolve moral difficulties in practice – indeed, the opposite is sometimes the case. But it does suggest that to make ourselves vulnerable to, and critical of, the ethical arguments and moral sentiments of others is a more creative and constructive way of responding to the moral complexity and conflicts of our time than by retreating into either moral dogmatism or moral relativism. Vulnerability is probably the key word here. Moral dogmatism and moral relativism are each in their own way attempts to be invulnerable to moral conflict, by pretending either to have no doubts or that none of it matters. The point we have been trying to make in this introductory chapter and which, we hope, will be apparent in the following chapters is that moral conflict does matter and that, in practice, we can rarely be entirely sure that our actions have always been right or for the best. This is particularly true in the field of health care, where professionals are frequently required to act quickly and decisively in matters affecting the vital interests of patients. To ask such professionals also to be vulnerable to such knowledge, and thus to the pain and guilt it may involve, is no doubt hard. But it is only in accepting such vulnerability, perhaps, that any of us has the courage to be ourselves and to escape from moral adolescence into precarious adulthood (Tillich 1952).

further reading

The meaning and scope of ethics
Frankena W K 1973 Ethics, 2nd edn. Prentice-Hall, Englewood Cliffs, NJ – *a brief and helpful but more advanced introduction to ethics and moral philosophy*

Macintyre A 1993 A short history of ethics. Routledge, London – *an illuminating and popular analysis of the history of ethical ideas in Western philosophy*

Preston N 1996 Understanding ethics. The Federation Press, Sydney – *a helpful non-technical introduction to ethics, with useful practical applications*

The nature of ethical decision-making
Hare R M 1981 Moral thinking; its levels, methods and point. Oxford University Press, Oxford – *an overview of theoretical approaches to analysing moral discourse and reasoning*

Stevens E 1980 Making moral decisions. Paulist Press, New York – *a helpful practical guide to making well considered and justifiable decisions*

Toulmin S 1986 The place of reason in ethics (re-issue). University of Chicago Press, Chicago – *a much used discussion of the role of practical reasoning in reaching moral decisions*

Fundamental principles and ethical relativism
Beauchamp T L, Childress J F 1994 Principles of biomedical ethics, 4th edn. OUP, New York – *involves a*

reflected discussion of 'principalism' after two decades of applying this approach

Thompson I E 1987 Fundamental ethical principles in health care. British Medical Journal 295: 1461–1465 [Reproduced as in Phillips C (ed) Logic in medicine. BMJ Publications, London] – *an explanation of the Hippocratic roots the Principles of Beneficence, Justice and Respect for Persons*

Veatch R 1981 A theory of medical ethics. Basic Books, New York – *an historical and philosophical analysis of the origins of the fundamental principles*

Practical connections between ethics, religion and nursing
Melia K M 1989 Everyday nursing ethics. Macmillan Education, Basingstoke – *a practical examination of how matters of ethics and personal belief impact on day-to-day nursing*

Mitchell B 1970 Morality religious and secular. Oxford University Press, Oxford – *sympathetic exploration of interrelationships and differences between religious and secular ethics*

Rumbold G 1993 Ethics in nursing practice, 2nd edn. Baillière Tindall, London – *a readable introduction to ethics for nurses, by an experienced nurse and hospital chaplain*

Steele S M, Harmon V M 1983 Values clarification in nursing, 2nd edn. Appleton-Century-Crofts, Norwalk, CT

end notes

1 This section on right and wrong, good and bad is adapted, with permission, from Thompson & Harries (1997), *Putting Ethics to Work*.
2 Although attempts to make the pursuit of pleasure and avoidance of pain the basis for ethics are as ancient as Plato and Aristotle in the 4th century BC and Epicurus in the 3rd century BC, it was Jeremy Bentham and John Stuart Mill in the 19th century AD who gave particular prominence to the pleasure/pain principle as a basis for ethics.
3 Leah Curtin, in examining the concept of conscience, discusses the relationship of right and wrong in an interestingly different way (Curtin & Flaherty 1982).
4 The remainder of this section is adapted, with permission, from Thompson & Harries (1997), *Putting Ethics to Work*.
5 Emphasis on freedom of conscience and expression for individuals and respect for others' personal rights gained prominence in the struggles for religious and political freedom in Europe, following the Protestant Reformation and in the 18th century Enlightenment. Great philosophers of this period who championed

individual rights were John Locke, Jean Jacques Rousseau, Immanuel Kant and John Stuart Mill. Kant, in particular, built his whole system of ethics on the principle of respect for persons as fundamental to any moral community.
6 See in particular the classic work *A Theory of Justice* by J Rawls (1971).
7 See Chapter 4 where it is observed that traditional codes of ethics have been based on the primacy of the duty of care of professionals responsible for clients who seek their help with personal problems and difficulties. Discussions relating to the value and limitations of the principle of beneficence have been most intense in medicine and nursing, because patients are particularly vulnerable and liable to infantilisation by overprotective health professionals (cf. Beauchamp & Childress 1994, section 1)
8 In Chapter 11 we argue that an adequate account of any moral judgement must take account of prior conditions and basic moral principles, choose the best means and methods to achieve our goal, and assess the likely consequences, costs and benefits of our action.

'Deontological' moral theories tend to emphasise prior conditions and principles as being of paramount importance. 'Pragmatism' emphasises the efficacy of the method used and 'virtue' ethics emphasises virtue as an essential means to achieve a moral outcome. 'Teleological', 'consequentialist' and/or 'utilitarian' theories focus attention on ends or goals and outcomes. In reality, we need to take account of all three aspects to give an adequate account of moral acts.

9 Cf. Dostoevsky F (1821–1881) *Brothers Karamazov*, part 1, book 1, ch. 6: 'If God does not exist, then everything is licit'; Nietzsche F (1844–1900) *The Anti-Christ*, where Nietzsche asserts that 'God is dead'; Sartre J P (1905–1980) makes a similar point in his *Existentialism and Humanism*.

some suggestions on method

Exploring the nature of ethics
In teaching ethics we should try to model what we are talking about. A good way to start is to get the class to work in small groups to develop ethical ground rules for the course itself – for their public and confidential relationships with you as teacher, their dealings with one another, commitment to the course and to personal development. You may then proceed to develop a course contract with the class to which you may refer later, e.g. to illustrate how it embodies the different fundamental principles.

What's right and what's good?
In small groups, a class can be set the task of first brainstorming examples of situations where we use the right/wrong distinction and the good/bad, and then to attempt to explain the difference themselves between rule- and rights-based judgements and evidence- or value-based judgements.

Following feedback from the groups, Table 1.2 (p. 7) can be used as an overhead to draw the discussion together and to introduce the distinction between deontological and teleological approaches to ethics. This also provides material to which you can refer in explaining how virtue ethics tries to bridge the gap between the other two theories.

Ethical 'dilemmas' and 'problems'
One could start by asking the class to identify examples of everyday problems that we solve by applying common-sense methods, and then go on to identify examples of situations where they have to make difficult choices involving conflicting loyalties or duties – e.g. putting your relationship with a close friend at risk by refusing to be a passenger if he or she is driving after having a few drinks.

Then it can be helpful to draw analogies between the examples produced by students and the difficult decisions nurses have to make in the course of their practical work – e.g. to contrast the students' examples with examples where a nurse is caught between the patient and the relatives, or the patient and the doctor. (It may also be useful to have some prepared case-studies for the class to analyse and discuss.)

Exploring ethical principles
A simple but effective way in which students can be assisted to understand how beneficence, justice and respect for persons stand in a relation of tension to one another and connect with the changing power relations between people is to get them to role-play (or discuss in small groups) the changing relations of parents and children as they grow from infancy to adulthood, from dependence on total care and protection to struggle for equal treatment and respect for their individual rights. The analogy can be drawn between this and the changing dynamics of nurse–patient relations as the patient moves from acute dependency through recovery and rehabilitation to restored autonomy.

Ethics and religion
Given adequate trust and confidence in assurances of confidentiality, students might be asked to write an autobiographical essay describing the way they perceive the development of their personal ethics.

Mature students might be willing to role-play a patient and nurse discussing the ethical and religious aspects of the meaning of suffering.

2

Becoming and being a nurse

AIMS

This chapter has the following aims:
1. To explore the processes by which nurses are socialised into their professional roles and how this differs from lay nursing
2. To help nurses understand the extent to which nursing and health care are social constructs reflecting social beliefs and prejudices about health and disease
3. To explore how medical and nursing practice defines the way in which people are regarded and the role of patients, and how the status of the patient can be both helpful and stigmatising for the person involved
4. To illustrate the need for objective research by examining two cases relating to the needs of minority groups and dying patients.

LEARNING OUTCOMES

When you have read and worked through this chapter, you should be able to:
■ Give a personal account of the various ways in which training as a nurse has changed you and the way you look at the world

- ■ Give a critical account of the practical social organisation of nursing and the impact on staff and patients of institutionalisation of health care services
- ■ Demonstrate ability to put yourself in the place of the patient, at the receiving end of nursing care, and to explain how relationships and patterns of interaction change
- ■ Give evidence of having explored, by research or objective means, the needs of specific groups of vulnerable patients, and of having checked out your assumptions about them against the facts.

ON ENTERING THE NURSING PROFESSION

The decision to become a nurse may well be made in much the same way as a decision to become anything else – an architect, a secretary or a market gardener.

In the case of becoming a nurse, however, the word 'become' is more apt than it is for many other occupations. 'Becoming a nurse' is not simply a matter of acquiring knowledge or learning particular skills, or what forms of behaviour to adopt in particular contexts. It is also a matter of assimilating the attitudes and values of the nursing profession. This process can have a profound influence on the thinking, personality and lifestyle of the individual concerned. In other words, being a good nurse demands not only theoretical knowledge and practical expertise, but also growth in moral experience in the application of this knowledge and skill in an ethically responsible way. This combination of acquired knowledge, skill and moral responsibility is what Aristotle called 'virtue' (Thomson 1976). Virtue and vice are defined by him as dispositions and actions that have 'become second nature' by habit and practice. In competent and virtuous behaviour, knowledge, skills and moral experience are integrated and so become the basis of reliable responsible action.[1]

It is now well understood in nursing that professional education continues beyond the initial preparation and qualification of the nurse, and that the development of competence and those personal qualities or virtues that make the good nurse demand continuing education. The acquisition of both clinical and moral experience is an important part of nursing education, in both basic training and continuing professional development. Being a nurse means having the confidence to act wisely and responsibly on the basis of acquired clinical and moral experience.[2]

In this chapter we shall discuss some aspects of what it means to be and become a nurse, considering both the practical and ethical aspects of this process. To do this, some ideas from sociology will be drawn upon in order to set the individual nurse making moral decisions in the social organisational context which shapes and influences those decisions. Because ethics is not merely an individual matter, but concerns our participation in a variety of social contexts or moral communities, sociology can help to throw light on nursing practice. The sociological outlook which sees the world in terms of roles, processes of socialisation, social organisation and social structure may not appear to be directly relevant to the nurse at a personal level, but it does provide us with some understanding of where individuals come from and what social factors are likely to influence or constrain their actions.

Within sociology there are traditions which are helpful to us in our attempts to understand interpersonal behaviour. Interactionism (Mead 1934, Goffman 1969) focuses upon the face-to-face interactions of everyday social activity. Other theoretical concerns of sociology have to do with the relationship of human action to social structure. As Giddens (1993) puts it: 'Are we creators of society, or created by it?' Questions of power, consensus and conflict are addressed by sociology. All those issues serve as a useful backdrop to the debates in nursing ethics. As we have already indicated, traditional ethics may be said to be too individualistic, and if we are attempting to examine the activities of a professional group providing a public service, we need to understand the social context of nursing ethics better.

By examining both the personal and social dimensions of nursing, we aim to strike a balance between the two and to look at the moral aspects of nursing from both the standpoint of the individual nurse and in the actual context of the nurse's work with other colleagues in an institutional setting. At an individual level, we might think that nurses are motivated mostly by an ethic of caring. When students are asked at interview why they want to become nurses, a common response is that they want to 'care for people'. However, when we look at the way in which nursing care is organised and delivered in public health services, it becomes clear that professional nursing has to be operated on principles which are rather less individualistic than the notion of simply caring for individual patients. The idea that nursing care should be based on sound knowledge of behavioural and social sciences is now well accepted, as is the idea that they are also important for nursing ethics.

In this chapter on becoming and being a nurse, we will consider first the difference between lay nursing, on the one hand, and professional nursing on the other, together with some of the moral conflicts that arise in the sphere of the nurse's relationship with other health professionals.

NURSING – LAY AND PROFESSIONAL

Those entering the nursing profession may not realise that their chosen sphere of work (e.g. midwifery or intensive care) will involve difficult decisions which may call into question their own personal convictions and values. The lay conception of nursing does of course involve some appreciation of the difficulties and conflicts faced by health professionals. Discussion in newspapers and on television has made the general public aware of ethical issues in health care. Nevertheless, it is probably true to say it is difficult for someone to appreciate from the outside what moral responsibilities and conflicts are encountered by nurses in dealing not only with patients, but also with doctors and the nursing hierarchy. The popular public image of medicine and nursing is changing as societies become more knowledgeable, the media more critical and litiga-

tion more commonplace. The continuing popularity of television hospital soap operas and 'fly on the wall' documentaries means that some version of medicine and nursing is constantly in the public eye. Based on such media coverage, doctors are generally regarded as skilled professionals who routinely deal in matters of life and death. The lay view of nursing, by contrast, is simultaneously less glamorous and more idealised (cf. the 'angels' of a popular BBC series). Nursing, moreover, is thought to be more easily understood for it is something which lay people themselves do. It is, after all, carried out by members of the family at home and by untrained as well as trained personnel in hospitals. The lay view of nursing, in other words, may make it difficult for the public or newcomers to the profession to appreciate the level of knowledge and skill and complex responsibilities involved, and hence the true nature of the moral conflicts they will encounter.

In order to appreciate these responsibilities, complexities and conflicts, it is necessary to look a little further at the similarities and differences between lay and professional nursing. Looking after sick relatives at home involves doing things for people which they cannot do for themselves because of their illness or incapacity (e.g. lifting, turning, bathing, toileting, feeding); preventing patients from undertaking anything which will impede recovery (e.g. confining them to bed, regulating their diet or access to alcohol); and administering any treatment or medication which has been prescribed. Leaving aside some of the technicalities of modern hospital care and allowing that professionals have a greater degree of relevant information and resources, these are essentially the same activities a qualified nurse would undertake either in the home or in hospital (Henderson 1966). In terms of what nursing involves at a practical level, therefore, it is difficult to establish how the care given by a lay person differs from that provided by nurses.

Nevertheless, the two types of care do differ, in at least three fundamental ways. First, nurses undertake their work not on the basis solely of duty, altruism or necessity, but on a contractual basis. Professional nurses look after patients in return for payment and, in the case of trainee nurses, to gain their professional qualifications

(Campbell 1985). Secondly, nurses and patients are not normally involved in one another's lives in any sphere other than the nurse–patient relationship. Lay nursing, by contrast, usually takes place within the context of a family or friendship, thus involving a different kind of carer–patient relationship. Thirdly, the nurse and patient in the professional setting may well come from different backgrounds and thus not share the same outlook, culture, values and expectations.

THE TRANSITION FROM LAY TO PROFESSIONAL

During the transition, or the socialisation process, the individual learns and adopts the professional approach to nursing by acquiring knowledge and practical skills and also learning a set of attitudes and values. In family life, differences in attitude and values may cause particular difficulties, either across generations or between individuals. But such difficulties arise against the background of a lifetime of experienced family differences and agreed ways of negotiating them. The needs of the individual within the family, rather than the demands of a large organisation, are the pivot of decision-making. In professional nursing, by contrast, there exist not only institutional pressures but also the need for some degree of congruence between the values of an individual and those of the profession or the institution. The risk of conflict between these personal, professional and institutional values is at its height during the early years of training, when the new recruit has not yet been socialised to the extent of having adopted the values of the profession.

The risk of such conflict is particularly acute in nursing because, while socialisation may be incomplete, the transition at a functional level has to happen quickly. Whatever preparation a student may have, both inside and outside the ward, there is always that first time when a patient calls 'nurse' and it dawns upon the student that in the patients' eyes the students are nurses. At this functional level, the student abandons lay status almost overnight. What, though, of the deeper adjustments to be made? When does the student feel like a nurse? It is in such experiences of being and yet still becoming a nurse that the learners

case history 2.1

The reactions of instinct and experience

A learner is being shown round her new ward by the staff nurse. It is care of the elderly ward, and clearly a busy one. She has been told that after a quick tour she is to work with a third-year student and that by such an arrangement they should 'get straight by lunchtime'. Halfway down the ward there is a woman in her 80s, sitting by her bed. As they approach, she asks the learner to tell her the time and what is for lunch, and while speaking she secures a firm grip on the learner's uniform skirt. The staff nurse announces loudly that Mrs B is always asking the same questions because she is demented and has a grossly impaired memory. She gives no indication as to how the newcomer is to extricate herself from the situation, while conveying clearly the message that she is to be followed down to the dayroom to complete the tour of the ward.

meet their first conflicts. They have to confront, on the one hand, their own personal feelings and reactions to the situations in which they find themselves and, on the other, the values and attitudes of the professional group they have joined (see Case History 2.1).

In the situation described in Case History 2.1, the personal moral code of the learner might dictate that she should stay and talk to the patient. At this level it matters little to the learner whether the patient is demented: she is another human being who has started a conversation with her. All the learner's past experience of life suggests that she should provide an answer and conduct the conversation as one might any other. However, within the context of nursing, this elderly woman's request for information has been reinterpreted as the product of her dementia and, as such, can and should be legitimately ignored so that the 'real' work of nursing may progress.

SOCIALISATION AND SENSITIVITY

A situation such as the one described in Case History 2.1 demonstrates the initial sensitivity which newcomers to the nursing profession possess, while at the same time indicating how, once the professional approach to the work is adopted, this initial sensitivity becomes threatened. This desensitising process is to a large extent synony-mous with the socialisation process. Much of the difficulty involved in 'becoming' a nurse is bound up with feelings of inadequacy and inability to cope with the reactions (e.g. to death or psychotic illness) which the introduction to nursing pro-vokes in an individual. The newcomer has no stock of responses or repertoire of skills to deal with these new encounters – such as with patients in extreme pain, highly dependent sick adults, young cancer sufferers and the victims of road traffic accidents. Past experience, values and per-sonal moral convictions might yield a set of emo-tional responses to these new encounters, but they do not provide any prescription for action or reac-tion. The new recruits tend therefore to adopt the ways of nursing they see around them. This can be said to be due, in part, to their lack of alternatives and, in part, to the efficiency of the socialisation process.

One of the consequences of an efficient social-isation process is the appearance of well ordered professional behaviour, with everyone assuming an air of confidence and security in the knowledge that their behaviour is in line with the 'profes-sional way'. This makes life even more difficult for the newcomers, as they tend to feel that everyone is coping except themselves. Learners might well think that they are the only ones to feel shocked by some of the sights they meet, e.g. the soon to be taken-for-granted sight of so much nakedness, the lack of privacy and a seemingly matter-of-fact approach to human suffering. These feelings of shock, revulsion or simply of inadequacy are fur-ther evidence of the naivety and sensitivity of the new recruits to nursing. Yet the concurrent sug-gestion, often made by learners themselves, that they should not register any such feelings, reveals the fact that already they have some notion of the professional attitude towards such feelings. It is more probably these early observations which make student nurses aware that they are weigh-ing up nursing against their own standards. The first sightings of a surgical wound, a colostomy, an amputation or a demented patient, and above all the experience of caring for dying patients can profoundly shock the newly arrived learner. It is in terms of such encounters that the students con-front personal feelings and values with the profes-sional values of nursing.

The speed with which the new recruits adopt the prevailing mode of nursing has both advant-ages and disadvantages. On the positive side it affords the learners some fairly immediate ways of coming to terms with what they see, and of finding a way of functioning. By looking around them they see what others do – others who are seemingly coping and who are not distressed by what they see – and follow suit. Indeed, the new-comer learns how to carry out nursing work with more confidence and competence and so the socialisation process serves the common good, as well as enabling nurses to cope with crises and emotionally stressful situations. The disadvant-age in the newcomer's so readily adopting the 'professional' approach to nursing is, as has already been suggested, that it puts at risk the ini-tial sensitivity, where personal moral values dom-inated. An example might be the way in which the toilet needs of patients in a care of the elderly set-ting are met. Students might well be initially offended by the idea of several elderly people being supplied with commodes en masse and with little privacy. As the weeks go by, however, they will become accustomed to such practices, even if they do not come fully to accept them. As one student nurse put it when asked how her practice had altered during her first year as a stu-dent nurse: 'I pull fewer screens'.[3] In other words, this student nurse had become used to the lack of privacy which may be encountered on hospital wards.

Because newcomers are at a loss to know how to behave when faced with patients, they will often feel silly and incompetent. Their major concern might well be to find some way to avoid this and meet the expectations of the trained staff. In so doing, learners can be well aware that they are compromising their own value systems in the way that they feel they must behave towards patients. For example, hospital mealtimes are often rushed affairs, where the main nursing objective might well appear to a newcomer to be to serve meals and collect in plates, empty or otherwise, in the shortest space of time. Learners, given the task of feeding a reluctant patient, are often placed in a situation where they feel obliged to hurry the patient in order to satisfy the expectations of the staff. At the same time, learners feel a natural response of sympathy for the patient and, following their own instincts, might be disinclined to hurry the patient or, if the patient is very reluctant, even to try to offer food at all. Again, there is a conflict between the preferred individual behaviour of the learner and that of the experienced nurse.

THE ORGANISATION OF NURSING

The distinction between lay and professional approaches to nursing can be elaborated in terms of the organisation of nursing in order to provide some further understanding of the conflicts which the professional style of nursing presents. Lay nursing is essentially organised on an individual basis – one patient with one or more carers who know one another. The way in which nursing is carried out is thus constrained, for the most part, only by the needs of this small group of people. The lay activity of nursing is able to follow a pattern based on a set of values normally worked out over a long period of time. Professional nursing, on the other hand, is usually carried out on a larger scale and involves people who do not know each other. Even taking account of the moves towards individualised care introduced into nursing under various banners – team nursing, patient allocation, nursing process, primary nursing – the fact remains that professional nursing is organisationally oriented and operates along the lines of routine approaches to care. Routines are less accommodating for individuals with regard to their personal needs or particular values. This lack of emphasis upon the individual is true for both patients and nurses. It should perhaps be noted that nursing curricula still lay stress upon the individual. The patient is the focus and the learners are taught to plan care according to individual needs. This denies the reality of the routinised approach to nursing found on many wards (Melia 1984). The student is then left to reconcile the individualised care ideology that the educators put across and the reality of ward life, which is often at odds with that ideology. There are

instances, of course, where the two coincide and patient care is truly individualised. Nonetheless, due to a variety of circumstances – lack of resources or thought – it is often the case that care as experienced in the ward does not match the rhetoric of individualised care.

ROLES AND INDIVIDUALS

Professional nursing within an organisation relies upon the notion of fulfilling a role rather than exercising individual initiative. That is to say, there are several stereotypical roles, e.g. 'nurse', 'patient', 'relative', 'doctor' and so forth, into which individuals are placed. Their expected behaviour within the organisation is determined by the rules applying to the role and not by the individuals themselves. This is how institutions and organisations are made to work. These role-based arrangements mean that a certain uniformity is introduced into the system, for along with each role goes a set of expectations, responsibilities and privileges. In practical terms, this means that certain standard forms of behaviour can be expected of the incumbents of different roles: the nurse is expected to care for patients in a way that the whole body of professional nurses would recognise and deem fit.

Similarly, patients, whoever they are, are expected to follow the dictates of their carers, to be grateful for their care and to do their best to comply with the treatment (Parsons 1970). In this way an organisation such as a hospital can function without every individual having to start from first principles at every encounter. The rules of behaviour are laid down, and adherence to role expectation is the key to the success of such an organisation.

There remains one problem. That people adopt roles is only one side of the coin: they also retain their individuality. The person who adopts the role of a nurse takes on the legal and moral obligations of nursing as defined by statute and the profession. But at the same time nurses do not relinquish their individual character or their personal beliefs and values. It is the coexistence of and potential conflict between personal values and professional values that presents many practical and ethical problems for nurses. The nurse may ask himself: 'What ought I to do, feel or think?' Emmet (1966) in *Rules, Roles and Relations*, explored the question of what 'is' and what 'ought to be' and suggested how one determines what the 'ought' might look like. Much of what people think they ought to do is governed by how they see their roles. Nurses as individuals may want to act in one particular way, yet in their role as nurse may feel they ought to act differently.

ROUTINE AND COMPROMISE

Despite the ideology of individualised care, it remains the case that the mainstay of the professional approach to nursing is routine. Nursing care can be reduced to a set of routines designed to meet the needs of a group of patients. Whatever system of care is the one of the moment – patient allocation, primary nursing and so on – from the patient's viewpoint there is always an element of routine involved, such is the nature of institutions, however well professionals aspire to work within them. Patients have individual needs, but in their role of 'patient' they can be added to other patients and have their overall needs provided along organised professional nursing lines rather than lay individual lines. In this way the nursing care of a group of patients can be conceived of as a workload to be got through. One of the most efficient ways to do this is to divide the care into a series of tasks and to share them, and incidentally the patients, among the nurses. This practice confronts students with a further kind of conflict – to decide whether they should hold on to the principles of 'good' nursing they have been taught and proceed along the individualised lines of care put forward by the college, or simply join in the routine care being practised. In the event, they have little choice since, being student nurses, they will invariably do as they are told as they have agendas to follow, such as surviving their clinical placements, beyond the immediate situation in which they find themselves. However, this does not remove the conflict, since learners have the added problem of living with their consciences if they feel that they have compromised judgement and acted against the interests of patients.

Unfortunately, at this early stage, while students are still able to see with new eyes what goes on in nursing, they are also preoccupied with becoming nurses, i.e. with behaving as other nurses do. By the time the students have become accustomed to the work and are less frightened and perplexed by the realities of nursing, they have probably also lost some of that initial innocence. To return again to an earlier example, new nurses are often struck by the dehumanising aspects of hospital care (Melia 1987). Patients appear to have little control over their lives in hospital; there is greatly reduced privacy and intimate procedures and issues are often treated lightly. The new nurse's perspective in all of this is in some ways closer to the lay perspective of the patient than it is to that of the professional nurse. Still in the process of transition from the lay to the professional perspective, they can empathise with the patient. At this early stage, however, the learner is in no real position to influence the style of care given. By the time learners reach a stage when they feel that they might exert their own views and carry out their nursing according to their own judgements, there is a danger that the sights that initially offended and provoked a desire to respond in a way that was not congruent with professional values will be commonplace. This may not necessarily mean that the learner has lost touch with the lay approach to nursing and its attendant personal values. It may mean that the actual consideration of the ethical implications of seemingly straightforward nursing work must now be a deliberate and critical activity, rather than a spontaneous reaction.

The process of becoming a nurse is in some ways similar to that of becoming a patient. The loss of a certain amount of identity, taking on a generalised role and behaving accordingly are experiences common to nurses and patients. The student has a uniform, the patient nightwear; decisions about day-to-day living have been taken from the person and placed in the hands of the organisation, e.g. mealtimes, off-duty for the nurse, waking and sleeping times for the patient. New nurses often feel that they are in a rigid hierarchy which relies upon rank rather than rationality and reason. Their freedom to act and question what they see is sometimes restricted. This leaves many of the conflicts of personal and professional values unresolved.

The process of becoming a nurse, then, requires the student to adopt an approach to nursing consistent with that adopted by the profession as a whole. The socialisation process is by and large an efficient one, since few lay people have the resources to cope with the demands of nursing at an individual level, and newcomers tend to opt for the security which goes with adopting the profession's values. It takes a very special kind of persistence to maintain a position that is not in line with the profession's viewpoint. Although 'whistleblowing' is becoming more common, nevertheless it takes a good deal of personal conviction and moral strength to speak out about things you believe to be wrong, or to stand firm on a matter of principle in the face of disapproval from the profession and the health care system.

The socialisation process is not perfect; if it were, nurses would behave in entirely predictable and uniform ways. The adoption of professional nursing values can only go so far. There may always be some residual tension for the individual between personal values and the expectations that go with the role of the nurse who operates according to professional ethical mores. There are clearly positive advantages to be gained from adopting the standard modes of behaviour of the nursing profession, rather than relying upon individual moral judgements; but each individual nurse must then cope with any discontinuities which may exist between personal values and those of the profession. Such discontinuities do not cease with qualification.

Up to this point we have studied two kinds of moral question facing the student. How can personal and professional values be reconciled? And how can the individual nurse practise 'good' nursing in the face of accepted compromise? Having become a nurse, the individual finds that these questions, although sometimes now easier to avoid, do not go away.

RELATIONSHIPS AND FEELINGS

One area in which questions continue to arise is that of building up relationships with patients.

From their earliest days as students, nurses are made aware of the importance of building good relations between themselves and patients. If patients are to gain the maximum benefit from nursing care, they must trust the nurse who gives it. Ramsey's (1970) exhortation that patients must be considered as persons is as relevant as ever it was, but how does the total patient care approach work out in practice? This approach suggests that the nurse should become intimately acquainted with a number of patients. But these patients will be people towards whom the nurse is likely to have the normal range of human feelings. And alongside the advice to build relationships with patients as people, the nurse is also likely to receive advice not to become too involved with patients.

In formal terms, the advice to treat patients as persons involves respect for the individual patient's rights as well as for what the nurse or the health care system may consider to be the patient's interests. The socialisation process lays much emphasis upon acting in a professional manner and not getting too involved with patients. Such considerations tend to detract from the central issue, which has to be respect for the patients' rights (discussed more fully in Ch. 6).

There may be difficulties and conflicts when it comes to the individual with whom the nurses come into contact. The nurse may well feel much more sympathy for, say, a young leukaemia patient of the same age than for an elderly demented patient at the end of life – or, for whatever reasons, it may be the other way around. In the everyday life of nurses outside their sphere of work, the fact that there are some people they take to, some they dislike, and many about whom they have no strong feelings is something they may take for granted on the assumption that it takes all sorts to make a world. But when much the same mixture of people arrive as patients, the demands of building good relationships and treating them as persons are much more difficult. Clearly, nurses cannot be forced to like people to whom they may feel an aversion, any more than the patients with similar feelings towards nurses can be forced to like them. Under these circumstances the nurse may adopt the Hippocratic maxim 'first, do no harm',[4] to ensure that an instinctive dislike is not reflected in overt attitudes. Nurses may also be grateful for the positive feelings which make it easier to treat certain patients as persons. In the end, the nurse will still remain prey to a range of different feelings towards other people, and these feelings will have a potential for harm as well as good. Furthermore, these feelings are never entirely suppressed or removed by the process of socialisation, so it is important that they are recognised.

The fact that nurses have perfectly natural feelings of like and dislike for particular patients, and that these feelings can do both good and harm, clearly lies behind the advice not to become involved. How far nurses heed this advice, and how far they find it incompatible with building good relationships with patients as persons must ultimately be a matter for individual judgement. However, judgement is not formed in isolation, and there are factors in the interaction of nurses with seniors, peers and patients which may exert an unrecognised influence. One such factor is the effect on nurse–patient relationships of the practice of labelling patients.

LABELLING PATIENTS

The theory of labelling comes from the sociology of deviance and has to do with our attitudes to people with attributes that we do not consider normal (Lemert 1951, Becker 1963). These attributes may relate to their health problems, physical or mental pathology, their physical appearance, personality type or other particulars. Sociological analysis of diagnostic labelling in medicine and its significance in the clinical management and social control of patients emphasises both the privileges and obligations of the 'patient' within the 'sick role' (Freidson 1970a, Parsons 1970). A diagnosis of renal failure, schizophrenia or alcohol-dependent syndrome has benefits for patients, in legitimating their access to resources for care or treatment and allowing them to adopt the 'sick role' and then get time off work, claim sickness benefits/insurance and so on. However, even these medical labels are potentially stigmatising and impose obligations on patients to cooperate in

 case history 2.2

The 'awkward' patient

A patient who is used to working shifts does not settle early to sleep and prefers either to watch late night television or to read. The nurse whose job is to follow hospital policy and turn the ward lights out by 22.30 h finds this patient difficult to cope with. Because the patient feels strongly about staying up, he makes a great fuss each night and wins his fight to watch the late television film. The nurse, when handing over shifts, reports that he is 'being awkward' again. In the patient's terms, this simply means going to bed at his usual time.

the prescribed forms of treatment even if these are inconvenient or distressing. In this context, however, we wish to examine the way nurses label patients, and the significance this has for nurse–patient relationships (Bond & Bond 1994). For example, nurses may refer to patients as 'difficult' or 'uncooperative' or to their behaviour in terms such as 'she won't help herself', 'just trying it on', 'doesn't want to get well', and so forth. In this way, behaviour which makes the nurses' work more difficult is deemed to be deviant. By implication, this makes the nurse the innocent party in any encounter – a position strengthened by drawing upon the support of colleagues in the use of the label (see Case History 2.2).

When nurses use this technique of labelling, then, it serves to legitimise the feelings that individual nurses may have towards a patient. Nurses can then think in terms which make, say, their own impatience with a patient seem not their own fault. In the case, for example, of a patient who is making slow progress from a stroke, the nurses may have applied the label of 'doesn't try', which in turn shields the nurse who tries to get the patient dressed in the morning from his own feelings of frustration or even anger. When labelling is used in large institutions such as hospitals, moreover, the labelled behaviour can take on the character of a stereotype. The term 'awkward patient', for example, is then more than simply a description of one individual; it conjures up for the nurse a whole set of forms of behaviour expected from any patient thus labelled. To some extent, of course, such labelling and stereotyping are an inevitable part of social interaction. But the patient's vulnerability and dependence on the nursing staff mean that it has more far-reaching effects in this case than in everyday life. It is therefore particularly important that nurses should be aware of what they are doing in applying or agreeing to a label. Is the label really accurate? Or is it simply a way of defending or excusing nurses at the patient's expense?

Not all labels are of the kind described so far. A patient might be labelled as 'dependent', 'a child', 'dying' or 'mentally retarded', and labels of this kind can have some significance. They are not necessarily labels with which the patient would agree; and again, even category labels of this kind can be used in ways which are less in the interests of the patient than in that of the professional's own self-justification. There are, however, a number of category labels whose use has achieved a degree of consensus among health carers, and in discussing the moral questions we are concerned with further, it may be useful to look at one or two of these in greater detail.

DIFFICULT SITUATIONS AND UNPOPULAR PATIENTS

Patients can be labelled as 'difficult' for a variety of reasons. A demanding elderly patient, a private patient who treats nursing staff as paid servants or a non-compliant patient all tend to attract this description. The elderly woman who rings her bell every time the nurse leaves the room is clearly as entitled to the services of the nurse as the person in the next room who hardly ever asks for anything. Nevertheless, nurses are likely to feel annoyed with such a person who wastes their time and they may often be tempted to use minor sanctions against her or to resort to delaying tactics. Any attempt to justify this understandable kind of response, however, must overcome the objection that the nurse, being the stronger party in the relationship, has a greater responsibility to act in a just or fair way towards the weaker. Treating patients as people, in other words, involves respecting their rights – even when they seem to abuse them.

The nurse's problem in handling personal feelings is more complicated when conflicting demands arise. The nurse may feel antagonistic towards an alcoholic or 'overdose' patient, who seems to have brought her troubles upon herself. When a young woman who has taken an overdose is brought in to a casualty department – followed within minutes by the victims of a serious road accident – the nurses who are left to look after her may well feel that they could be better employed working with the more 'deserving' accident victims. Similar problems may arise among nurses working in gynaecological wards, where those having terminations may be nursed alongside infertile women who desperately want children. In situations of this kind, judgemental labelling may be a strong temptation for those whose personal moral values create antagonism. Health care professionals must avoid falling into the trap, encouraged by media representations, of referring to some HIV patients as 'victims', while others are seen to have brought the condition upon themselves through adopting a particular lifestyle. Unpopular patients may consequently be at some risk of having their psychological if not physical needs undervalued. The principle of justice is important here, for not only is the patient in danger of having her rights to proper physical and psychological treatment compromised, but there is a danger that she will not be respected as a person.

The nurse–patient relationship is a complex power relationship, the patient being in the weaker position. The nurse's stronger position is derived to a great extent from special knowledge. This has many consequences for the patient in relation to labelling and may involve more than simply giving the patient a bad name in such terms as 'difficult', 'rude' or 'demanding', which might be used by anyone. Nurses, because of their special knowledge, are in a position to misuse as well as use legitimate clinical labels. Typical examples of this come from the field of psychiatry. Patients who are unsettled in hospital surroundings may well display strange behaviour: they may be rather aggressive towards people or emotionally very labile, or they may refuse to talk to anyone. The words nurses use to describe

case history 2.3

When 'low spirits' become 'depression'

If a patient is rather low in spirits one evening because her husband is away on business and cannot visit her for a few days, the nurse might write in the Kardex, 'feeling low tonight'. At the morning report she may say that the patient is 'a bit depressed'. The label 'depressed' then finds its way into the Kardex. The changeover of staff the next day means that the original user of the 'feeling low' term is no longer on duty, so that the reason – the husband's absence – gets lost and the 'depression' label gains momentum to the extent that the house officer is asked to prescribe something for the patient.

this behaviour to one another may easily take on the apparently objective overtones of a clinical diagnosis. An example of this is given in Case History 2.3.

The dangers of using clinical labels which have quite specific meanings in psychiatry in this way are clear. Labelling of this kind is not in the best interests of either patients or nurses. If nurses are prepared to describe individual patients in derogatory or misleading terms, this is likely to affect the kind of care they give. It also seems clear, from the literature on deviance, that persons are often labelled as deviant simply because they do not conform to the norm. How do nurses decide what should be classed as normal? Even if a consensus about normality can be arrived at by nurses, what right does one group have to decide that the behaviour of another is not acceptable and thus refuse to tolerate it? The issue is not merely a clinical or social one, but one that has ethical implications relating to justice, in the sense of non-discrimination, and respect for persons, e.g. the right to adequate care and treatment.

THE NURSE AND DYING PATIENTS

One of the most difficult aspects of nursing, and one which many nurses will admit they have never fully come to terms with, is the care of dying patients.

The first dying patient encountered by first-year students may be the first dying person they have ever encountered, and even the experience of having to touch a dead human body may be something for which they are completely unprepared. Whether there are any adequate ways in which students can be prepared for such experiences is doubtful. There is, in the end, no substitute for the real thing. Nor is there any way of avoiding the feelings of pain, grief, guilt and helplessness which can be evoked in encounters with the dying, with death and with those who are left behind. Under these circumstances, the moral pressure to put a brave face on things must usually, for practical reasons, be heeded. There are occasions, however, when nurses cannot do this; and perhaps they should not, for the very good reason that some direct experience of their own human fallibility and frailty may be required to help individual nurses recognise and accept the feelings of pain, grief, guilt and helplessness in the face of death. Without recognition and acceptance of feelings of this kind, they may lie unspoken and denied, so that either they resurface in the future in irrational and inappropriate ways which are difficult to control, or, if they are controlled, it is at the cost of suppressing in the nurse those sensitivities which are essential for good nursing care.

Lay nursing and professional nursing of dying patients are obviously different experiences, not least by virtue of the ties of family or friendship which normally bind the dying to their lay carers. Even when death is a relief, the experiences of a lifetime's closeness, together with the memories of happiness and hurt, have to be worked through. When the inevitability of death is recognised, the working through may begin before death itself takes place. Professional nursing, by contrast, normally has no such fund of experiences to work upon. This does not mean that the professional nurse is not vulnerable to the hopes, fears and present experience of the dying individual. The experience of being in hospital is one which can allow people to speak more freely about themselves than they might normally; and the relationship between nurse and patient, however temporary, can be important to the patient, not least because of her dependence on the nursing staff. How important the relationship is to the nurse will depend, of course, on how far the nurse heeds the advice not to become involved. Clearly, nurses cannot build up close relationships with all of their patients, even when nursing is undertaken on a patient-centred rather than a task-oriented basis. Inevitably, for many reasons – perhaps because the patient reminds the nurse of a parent, or perhaps because the patient chose to confide in this nurse about domestic troubles – some patients will be of particular importance to some nurses. Their encounter with one another, however brief, will leave unfinished business which nurses must work through in their own emotions.

Nurses' own emotional demands should not get in the way of skilled caring. This may be particularly difficult if the death of such a patient occurs when the nurse is feeling low for reasons rooted in domestic or personal life. Under the circumstances, the pressure of other work may either give the nurse the strength to postpone working through emotions until some time alone can be found or it may be the final straw. Thus, the need to act in a professional way, given advantageous circumstances, may be what enables the nurse to get through this experience. On the other hand, the nurse's professional identity may itself complicate the pain of a patient's death – even where no particularly close nurse–patient relationship existed – by adding feelings of guilt and failure. The nurse's role, after all, is to sustain life and alleviate suffering. When it has not been possible to do either or both of them, it is natural enough to ask why; and it is not unnatural, sometimes, to be less than rational about one's own possible errors or omissions.

The death of a patient may be difficult, then, because unfinished emotional business concerning a particular patient has to be worked through, or because anything less than a 'good' or timely death may create a sense of guilt and failure among professionals. The death of a patient may also be disturbing when, for whatever reason, it brings home to those around a profound awareness of finality – that this is something no one can do anything whatever to alter. This knowledge brings with it the awareness of our own mortality and finite powers. It is difficult for many of us to come to terms with this finality, for one measure of our achievement as human beings is our capacity to live in the past and the future as well as the present. In the face of death, however, the past – much of which was preserved in the brain now dead – becomes much more tenuous, dependent now on the memories of others; while the present is empty, and the future, for the dead person at least, no longer exists. Some way of working through this experience may be found by many people in religion, while for others the experience of death and bereavement may result in disillusionment with religion, or may provide the impetus to different kinds of action. The realisation of finality and finitude, when a particular death evokes it, does need to be worked through in some way that provides a tolerable and sustaining equilibrium between accepting this realisation and straining against it.

There is a variety of reasons, then, why the death of a particular patient may evoke strong feelings in a particular nurse, which may need to be addressed. Field (1984, 1989) and Field & James (1993) give some moving accounts of nurses' experiences with dying patients. If the deaths of all patients evoked such feelings, or if all nurses responded to one death in this way, professional nursing care of the patients, their relatives and other patients would not be possible. Yet, if nurses never gave expression to their feelings, it would indicate that they were less than human, rather than just human. The extent to which individual nurses do or do not allow themselves to express their feelings openly in such circumstances may be beyond their control, or a matter of professional judgement or personal moral choice.

Some degree of detachment from the situation has its positive aspects. Nurses have to continue to care for other patients when one patient has died. Distancing themselves from the death helps nurses to continue to function. It affords some emotional protection and leaves them free to work according to the dictates of their professional knowledge rather than being entirely at the mercy of their own emotions. But sometimes tears are inevitable, and sometimes, when a whole ward has been aware of what has been happening behind the screens, it may be comforting to patients to know that nurses care enough to cry, provided that this does not cast doubts on their competence.

From the patients' points of view, evidence that the medical and nursing staff have 'failed' in another patient's case may be disturbing. For this reason it is understandable, when a patient has died in the night, that other patients, on asking where the patient is, may be told by a nurse that he has been moved to another part of the hospital. There are moral pressures on both sides of the argument here. If evasion is chosen, the case for not telling the whole truth cannot simply be taken for granted as being in the best interests of the patients (as the patronising attitudes of the past would have assumed), as it may be helpful to talk through with patients their fears about what has happened. Similarly, there may be good reasons for not giving information about a patient's death over the telephone to enquirers outside the immediate family, where there is doubt about whether all the family have been informed or whether they have had time to assimilate the knowledge. Related considerations also apply to summoning the family of a patient who may have died sooner than was expected. In subsequently breaking the news of a patient's death to her family, the way in which the truth is told is clearly as important as what is told. The question of what to say to dying patients and their relatives is a difficult one and there are no straightforward answers. Glaser & Strauss (1965) indicated the complexity of the issues involved for nurses. They showed some of the key issues surrounding the nursing of dying patients. One such issue was the question of truth telling and being open with dying patients and their relatives. Another issue was dealing with the condition known as 'persistent vegetative state'. In such situations, where the person is in many ways 'dead' but continues to be in need of care and is recognised as a patient, the condition presents difficulties for both carers and relatives alike. Aside from all the emotions that nurses feel in caring for the dying in these circumstances, they have to contend with the fact that these patients raise questions about the use of resources for what appears to be no good purpose.

EVIDENCE-BASED NURSING – HOW SCIENTIFIC CAN NURSING BE?

In distinguishing between informal lay nursing and professional nursing, we said that what they have in common is caring for patients as people with feelings, dignity and rights. Professional nursing, however, requires more than just caring and scientifically based knowledge. It also requires the nurse to use methods that have been tested in sound research. The medical profession has long determined the worth of a treatment on the basis of the results of randomised controlled trials (RTCs). The concept of evidence-based practice was first articulated at McMaster University in Canada. Evidence-based medicine has been described as 'a process of turning clinical problems into questions and then systematically locating, appraising, and using contemporaneous research findings as the basis for clinical decisions' (Rosenberg & Donald 1995). The aim of evidence-based medicine is to substitute 'objectively evaluated scientific evidence' for 'fallible subjective judgement'.

The benefits of this kind of objective scientific approach are clear in so far as it makes for more reliable predictions of the likely effectiveness or ineffectiveness of various drugs, interventions or therapies in dealing with a standard range of examples. It seeks to regulate practice by making it subject to universal standards and routines, more subject to comparative performance appraisal, quantitative analysis of results and cost–benefit or cost-efficiency analysis. It also offers a means of standardised processing and storage of the massive amounts of data, research findings and other types of information that are being produced in all areas of health care practice and research. Applied to nursing systems and procedures, evidence-based practice could be helpful in improving the efficiency and cost-effectiveness of some kinds of routine services or treatments; but it is a debatable question whether those uniquely personal aspects of caring for people in distress are susceptible to these kinds of quantitative study and analysis.

However, just as some clinicians have argued that the blanket application of such 'scientific' methods risks overlooking the specific or unique features of a particular patient's condition or circumstances, and detracts from the importance of clinical judgement in discriminating carefully between the needs of different patients, so the same arguments could be said to apply even more strongly to nursing practice. Of necessity, nursing practice has had to be standardised and routinised. However, there is a grave risk that further self-styled 'scientific' and 'cost-efficiency' requirements will result in nursing becoming over-routinised and impersonal to the detriment of both patient care and any personal satisfaction nurses get from patient contact. Here, as elsewhere in health care, it is important to reflect on the ethical significance of such innovations and what values are driving change.

Patricia Benner, who adopts a more qualitative and phenomenological approach to researching nursing practice, has emphasised certain distinctive features of nursing that tend to be overlooked if it is subjected to direct comparison with clinical medicine. Benner (1984) claims that if we pay attention to the specific features of the 'knowledge' and 'expertise' of the nurse, these arise in 'situated caring interactions'. She argues that it is the distinctive personal style of embodied and affective engagement of the nurse with the particular patient that provides 'the key to understanding the nature and significance of nursing care'. It is this specific and relational aspect of the engagement, rather than the objective scientific approach, which abstracts from the particular and attempts to isolate and control the variables in the situation in order to arrive at valid generalisations and reliable predictions. As Bowden (1997) remarks:

Her main point is that the decision-making and action required in the practice of nursing rely on kinds of 'perceptual awareness' and 'discretionary judgement' that cannot be pre-articulated or formulated according to abstract rules. While skilled nursing clearly depends on formal education with respect to knowing what to consider and how to organise information about patients, how to operate equipment and how to monitor vital signs, excellence in caring emerges through more intuitive understanding that 'responds to the demands of given situations' rather than rigid principles and rules.

Benner & Wrubel (1989) defend these ideas further in their later study *The Primacy of Caring: Stress and Coping in Health and Illness*, in which they analyse in depth a wide variety of concrete situations of interaction between nurses and patients in order to show that the progress from student nurse to experienced and confident professional is as much as anything the process whereby the nurse learns to integrate his real emotions and sense of embodied contact with patients with the academic knowledge and technical skills learned in training. They argue that the unique contribution of the nurse is to make observations and judgements about a patient's needs and condition, informed by an understanding attuned to the subjectivity and complexity of the patient's world and his unique self-understanding.

'Evidence-based practice' is not ethically neutral, as is often suggested. The values of 'objectivity', 'cost-effectiveness' and 'standardised patient care' are all legitimate values in their own right, and can serve to achieve more equity and accountability in the use of public resources. However, they can also serve the interests of managerial control and institutional bureaucracy (or even the commercial interests of private institutions), at the cost of appropriate forms of care, sensitive to the needs and rights of individuals, while also robbing nurses of their right (and duty) to make informed professional judgements in particular cases, based on their particular experience of working with the patient.

We have to bear in mind too that all methods of meta-analysis, such as 'evidence-based practice' and applied epidemiology, which allow us to make sense of great volumes of data, yielding statistically based guidance, are nevertheless reductionist and in some ways partial at the same time. The particular is lost in the universal, and the individual becomes a cipher in a statistical table. What is to count as 'evidence' is not unproblematic either, but rather based on certain prior assumptions and value judgements as to what is 'relevant' and what is not, whereas for the individual patient what is seemingly irrelevant may be of the greatest moment (e.g. to have access to a particular nurse). Systematic reviews, meta-analyses and RCTs may be applied as the 'gold standard' without realising that the selection of 'relevant evidence' may be biased or problematic. 'Scientific practice' should perhaps be more open to critical examination and revision than the current use of 'evidence-based practice' would seem to suggest. An unthinking commitment to evidence-based practice can lead to a rush from processed information to dogmatic 'truth', and as evidence-based practice requires such effort, once a conclusion about a particular treatment has been drawn, the practice in question tends to be 'set in concrete'. All these issues beg for further ethical and philosophical examination.

The fundamental ethical questions raised by evidence-based practice are those about the nature and scope of 'evidence' to be considered, and what value criteria are applied in determining what is to count as evidence. Focusing on what can be easily observed and subjected to quantitative analysis risks neglect of those areas where reliable evidence is difficult to obtain, because it is more qualitative in nature and requires alternative forms of data collection (such as personal interviews) and the application of non-quantitative analysis. Much 'evidence' gained by nurses through sensitive day-to-day interaction with patients is qualitative and intuitive, and yet it is critical to the assessment of the general state of their health or well-being. How do we incorporate evidence that does not come from RCTs? Well, of course, that is very difficult. And therefore there is still a need for professional judgement, even within evidence-based practice, for nurses as much as for doctors, and it is here that the moral dimension comes into play.

Related to these attempts to make hospital administration more effective, efficient and financially accountable are concerns that nurses as well as all health care staff should become cost-conscious and more responsible in the use of public resources. Hospital-based and community nursing require competent and efficient service administration, organised so as to provide equal access to services and fairness in the distribution of health care resources for all in need. Nurses, as individuals in their own right, as managers and as members of the profession, cannot ignore these moral questions of how to balance the needs of care for individual patients with justice for all. At a wider societal level, debates about the basis upon which care should be available to the whole population raise ethical issues of another kind about human rights and justice in health care. The escalating costs of the UK National Health Service, for example, led to concerns about the viability of state-administered health services in late 20th century society. The financing of health care is no less problematic in countries which rely more upon an insurance-based than a state-funded system. The issue is the same and it has to do with how nurses actually provide care for people, whether the context is private or state health care. This wider debate is addressed more fully in Chapter 9.

In this chapter we have explored some of the moral conflicts involved in becoming and being a nurse. We have considered the conflicts between personal values and routine practice in the transition from lay to professional status. We have also looked at the conflict between treating patients as people and not becoming involved, and discussed the dangers of labelling patients. These are, of course, only some of the moral issues which arise in patient care and the process of becoming and being a nurse. However, they give some indication of the variety of moral choices which nurses have to make on a day-to-day basis, not only during their training but throughout their professional careers. In the next and subsequent chapters, we shall examine a wide variety of other moral issues in nursing for the experienced and qualified nurse.

 further reading

On becoming and being a nurse
Benner P 1984 From novice to expert: excellence and power in clinical nursing practice. Addison-Wesley, Menlo Park, CA – *an analysis of the unique experience and perspective of the nurse*

Bishop A, Scutter J (eds) 1985 Caring, curing, coping: nurse, physician, patient relationships. University of Alabama Press, Alabama – *a work which focuses on how carers cope with caring*

Melia K M 1987 Learning and working: the occupational socialisation of nurses. Tavistock, London *– report of an interview-based research study on student nurses' experience of nursing*

Stevenson J, Tripp-Reimer T (eds) 1990 Knowledge about care and caring: state of the art and future developments. American Academy of Nursing, Kansas City, MO *– a critical appraisal of the future role of care in the developing 'science' of nursing*

On nursing people who are dying
Cousins N 1979 Anatomy of an illness. WW Norton, New York *– a classic account of being a patient from a patient's point of view*

de Beauvoir S (tr. O'Brian P) 1989 A very easy death. Penguin, Harmondsworth *– an account by a great feminist philosopher of the death of her mother*

Doyle D (ed) 1994 Domiciliary palliative care: a handbook for family doctors and community nurses. Oxford University Press, Oxford *– a practical book addressed to those working with the dying in the community and at home*

Lugton J 1987 Communication with dying people and their relatives (with illustrations by S Gaffney). The Lisa Sainsbury Foundation, London *– written by a nurse primarily for nurses*

Stedeford A 1984 Facing death: patients, family and professionals, Heinemann Medical Books, London *– a more general book on the stresses of facing death in professional work with patients*

Evidence-based health care in nursing
Friedland D J 1998 Evidence-based medicine: a framework for clinical practice. Appleton & Lange, Stamford, CT *– one of the first practical textbooks on the subject for health professionals*

NHS 1999 Evidence-based health care: an open learning resource for health care practitioners. CASP and HCLU, London *– a basic introduction to evidence-based methods in health care*

Rosenberg W, Donald A 1995 Evidence based medicine: an approach to clinical problem solving. British Medical Journal 310: 1122–1126 *– directed to doctors, but has a wider relevance*

end notes

1 See Aristotle's *Nicomachean Ethics*, Books 1–3 (Thomson 1976).
2 See *Post Registration Education and Practice Project*
(UKCC 1993).
3 Personal communication.
4 See Appendix 1 – the Hippocratic oath.

some suggestions on method

The social role of the professional nurse
Students might be encouraged to keep a journal in which they note specific ways in which their common assumptions about health and disease are challenged and changed in training. This could involve a few simple questions which encourage reflection on the socialisation process and way the role of the nurse is defined.

Small groups of students could be encouraged to reflect upon and share their experiences in the classroom and on the wards – again using a simple list of questions to prompt discussion – and then to share the general findings with the class.

Social construction of health and disease
Students could be asked to write a brief autobiographical essay to describe their own childhood concepts of health and experience and fears of disease and death.

To explore lay concepts of health and compare these with their developing professional and scientific understanding, students could be set the task of constructing a brief questionnaire and conducting vox pop interviews with the general public or other non-nursing students.

Alternatively, they could be encouraged to conduct focus group discussion with small groups of people representing minorities or practitioners of alternative medicine.

Nurse's definition of the role of the patient
First, students could be encouraged to share, in small confidential groups, their own experiences of being patients at home and in hospital (or attending a clinic) and what the role of being a patient involved in each case.

Alternatively, a more ambitious project might be to track a couple of patients from admission through treatment to discharge home, and to conduct brief interviews with them on their perceptions of what happens to them as they are given an identity and status in terms of their medical complaint and mode of treatment.

Observing the needs of vulnerable patients
A class visit to a hospice or terminal care ward followed by a case presentation by a staff nurse and opportunity for group discussion might serve to bring out a number of important issues. However, the task would be for the class to identify kinds of investigation that might help to address some of the needs of dying patients.

An alternative might be for students to visit a home for children with learning difficulties and to be encouraged to interact with the children as best they can (under supervision) and then report formally on what they learned from the experience.

3

Responsibility and accountability in nursing

AIMS

This chapter has the following aims:
1. To explore the structure of power and authority in institutionalised nursing care, and the reasons why hierarchical or other forms of organisation are necessary
2. To examine the nature of management in nursing, the roles and responsibilities of nurse managers, and their own relationship with management and the medical hierarchy
3. To explore the responsibilities of the nurse within a system of organised authority and official duties, and the scope for conscientious objection or 'whistleblowing' when faced with unethical or unacceptable practice
4. To become familiar with the codes of ethics applicable to nursing and to explore the value and limitations of codes as a means of ensuring discipline and good practice.

LEARNING OUTCOMES

When you have read and worked through this chapter, you should be able to:

■ Map the structure of power in your health care setting, identifying the various roles and responsibilities of people in authority over you

■ Give a clear account of what qualities you would expect in a good nurse manager, and what competencies such a person would need to do the job well

■ Explain on what grounds you would be justified in taking a stand on a matter of ethical principle or objecting to practice

■ Give an account of the broad requirements of a sound code of ethics for nursing and demonstrate familiarity with your own.

THE SOCIAL CONTEXT OF NURSING VALUES

Nurses form an occupational group which provides a wide variety of services within society. As such, nursing has organised itself into a bureaucratic style of working which places individual nurses within a formal structure. This structure determines, to a large extent, the behaviour of individual nurses; it puts limits on their range of activities; and it holds nurses accountable for their actions both as individuals and as members of the occupational group.

The organisational structure of nursing raises several issues which are pertinent to ethical debate about nursing. These can be divided into at least three areas where ethical issues arise:

● issues concerned with the nurse as a part of the nursing hierarchy
● issues concerned with the nurse and other members of the health care team
● issues related to nurses' responsibility to their own profession.

In order to understand many of the difficulties which nurses confront in their day-to-day work, it may be helpful to begin by examining the hierarchical structure of nursing, and then to discuss the other two areas mentioned.

THE NURSING STRUCTURE

The nursing service, unlike medicine, has a history of being organised according to the principles of line management. Essentially this means that qualified nurses, from the grade of staff nurse upwards, are organised into hierarchical grades within which each nurse is responsible for certain work and accountable to a senior nurse. Clearly, this is potentially a formalised system for 'buck passing'. On the other hand, the system does not relieve individual nurses of responsibility for their own actions. We will return to this point later.

The nursing organisation currently found in the UK is, in general terms, a development of the Nightingale tradition which was established upon principles borrowed from military organisation. This description of nursing organisation is specific to the UK and its National Health Service (NHS); however, many of the issues arising from these structures and the professional organisation of nursing can be found in other health care systems. The organisation for the delivery of nursing care instituted by Florence Nightingale was designed to allow for a wide range of ability within the service, and it worked as long as obedience of the military kind prevailed. As Carpenter (1977) put it in his seminal paper on nurse management:

The beauty of this idea lay in its simplicity, serving in turn to unify the occupation into a single community stretching from the lowest ranking nurse to the highest ranking nurse. The crucial element in the situation was the power of the matron.

This early band of nurse managers and matrons, by insisting upon obedience from their nurses, achieved a nursing service which would follow doctors' orders unquestioningly, yet which would not allow itself to be disciplined by doctors. The nursing service came under the direct control of the matrons. In the 1960s, two administrative reorganisations replaced the matrons with a line management structure (Salmon 1966, Mayston 1969). This new structure resulted from the Salmon report's implicit call for an industrial model of professionalised management. Nursing was to be managed as might be any other workforce whose business it was to accomplish a task by means of group effort. The line management approach took the power held by the old style matrons and shared it, to some extent, 'down the line' by giving different 'ranks' appropriate areas of responsibility and making them accountable for their work to an immediate superior.

There have been some revisions of the original Salmon structure, but the line management principle still holds. Strong & Robinson (1990) note that 'nursing's hierarchy stemmed not so much from within nursing itself, as from the many powerful forces – medicine, gender, and the demands of an extremely labour intensive industry – which created, shaped and controlled the nursing trade'.

The Griffiths Inquiry (1983) focused on management practices rather than the structure of the NHS. The result was the introduction of general management with control of resources and extensive decision-making powers at every level. Here the introduction of the 'internal market' and the 'provider' and 'purchaser' roles into the health service was not without its problems.

Mays (1991) notes that 'a competitive contract system in health care cannot be guaranteed to produce high standards automatically'; also, that 'there remains the risk that the elderly and the chronically sick, who are less vocal in demanding services and difficult and expensive to treat, will be ignored or excluded'. The internal market lasted for 10 years until a more cooperative approach was introduced, removing the competitive element while retaining some of the cost efficiency that the market ideology had brought with it (see the discussion in Ch. 9).

The NHS then set out to provide continuity of care between hospital and community – a team approach to care with managers and practitioners equally responsible for the quality of the service. The restructured and managerially oriented NHS, then, presents problems for nursing. A new bureaucratic model of operation poses problems for an occupational group which claims to be a profession. Autonomy and control over one's work are important hallmarks of a profession. Nursing has severe problems in this direction, not only because of the presence of the dominant profession of medicine, but also because the bureaucratic line management approach threatens to stifle professional judgement on the part of the individual nurse (Freidson 1970a,b).

The medical profession gets around this difficulty by operating a collegial approach, which accepts each doctor as a professional who gives and seeks advice among colleagues and is open to judgement by her peers, but who is not held accountable for her day-to-day work to a management hierarchy. This difference in the organisational structures of medicine and nursing clearly presents problems when consultation and cooperation are required between individuals from the two professions. Strong & Robinson (1990) note, in their study of the NHS under new management, that:

there was, then, a quite extraordinary contrast in managers' eyes between the individual power of doctors and the collective feebleness of nurses; between medicine's influence at the highest level and nursing's national representation; between doctors' fierce syndicalism and nursing's massive internal hierarchy.

As well as the military influence on nursing there was, of course, an even earlier religious influence. The older meaning of 'profession' has to do with the vows taken, or 'professed', by members of religious orders, some of whom were responsible for the care of the sick and poor in medieval hospitals or hospices. These vows included obedience (also stressed in the military model), together with a strong sense of hierarchy. The religious model, too, emphasised the idea of the professed individual as a servant of others. This service emphasis was continued in Florence Nightingale's time. Nursing was not to be undertaken primarily for profit or financial gain. In practice, of course, 19th century nursing seems to have been a means of providing work for the unmarriageable daughters of the middle and upper middle classes. The religious origins of its ideals also held out the promise of work which provided some measure of social worth. In this connection, the introduction of a capitalist rationality, which the Salmon Report brought to the organisation of nursing, marks a further move away from its religious origins.

In the context of this discussion it is interesting to note how Florence Nightingale has been evoked in differing ways depending upon what image of nursing the author is trying to create. Whittaker &

Olesen (1964) discussed the roles of Florence Nightingale – 'the lady with the lamp', 'the politician', 'the occupational status enhancer for nursing' – and the different uses to which they are put.

The underlying rationale of the line management structure on which the Salmon and Mayston reorganisations were based provides a key to understanding the power and authority structures of nursing. The advent of primary nursing and the formalisation of leading roles for service staff that the clinical regrading exercise introduced are intended to replace, or at least displace, the hierarchical approach to nursing and nursing education. However, at a day-to-day level the implicit hierarchical organisation from the most junior learner to the charge nurse is obvious enough. Learners are made aware of the fact that they are the newest recruits; and as soon as another group arrives they immediately feel that they have moved up a rung on the ladder. From these early days, therefore, a sense of the authority structure is acquired.

Crucial to the functioning of this hierarchical organisation is an understanding by all nurses of the standard routines and expected ways of carrying out nursing procedures and how to handle situations which arise in the course of nursing work, in hospital or in the community. That is, nurses are made aware not only of their responsibilities in direct patient care, but also of the manner in which they should conduct themselves within the nursing hierarchy and in relation to it (Melia 1983). Within this routinised structure, individual nurses have to learn how to reconcile their personal values with the values of the profession and specific institution within which they have to make decisions and exercise responsibility as nurses.

ADVANTAGES AND DISADVANTAGES OF LINE MANAGEMENT

The hierarchical system of line management has certain obvious advantages. One advantage is that it brings some power of decision-making closer to the area of patient care. A charge nurse, for example, instead of having to ask the highest ranking nurse for extra help on a busy shift, might simply ask the immediate superior with whom

she is in closer contact. On the other hand, requests involving greater changes may have to go to a higher authority, while policy decisions may come down the line to the ward level and be put into practice whether or not they are thought to be acceptable. General management may have brought decision-making closer to the action and demanded more accountability from clinicians, but the hierarchical features of the organisation of nursing are deep-rooted and will no doubt be around for some time to come.

This form of management, then, puts nurses in a position where they are not always able to act in the way in which they, as individuals, might see fit. Depending upon the circumstances, this can be a positive or a negative feature of the hierarchical organisation of nursing. If, for example, the nurse involved is inexperienced or a learner, actions based on her own judgement might not be for the best. In such a case the hierarchical system and the restrictions it places upon the individual's behaviour may have advantages (see Case History 3.1).

In the example in Case History 3.1, the advantage of the hierarchical organisation of nursing is that it affords protection to a less experienced member of

 case history 3.1

When a patient decides to leave

A young patient decides that he is tired of waiting around the medical ward for the results of his tests and, despite his quite severe symptoms of a yet unknown cause, makes up his mind to take his own discharge. He waits until a quiet period in the afternoon when the charge nurse has gone for a break and only junior nurses are in evidence on the ward. A junior nurse sees him dressing and he tells her he is leaving. He is very articulate, telling her that he fully understands his condition and has every right to leave. The nurse knows that she should tell a qualified member of staff, in the hope that someone might be able to persuade the patient that it is in his own interest to stay. On the other hand, as an individual she can see his point; she feels, moreover, that he is a sensible young man who would get in touch with his general practitioner if he deteriorated in any way. Nevertheless, she follows the hospital's dictated procedure and, recognising that dealing with the situation falls outside her competence, informs the staff nurse.

staff. The junior nurse might well have thought that there would be no harm in simply letting the patient go – as indeed he had a legal as well as a moral right so to do. However, as a nurse she was expected to follow hospital policy, which dictated that she should inform a senior nurse and that the patient must be required to sign himself out in the presence of nurses, who in turn must sign as witnesses of his discharge. In the event of the patient thus leaving the hospital of his own will, the student would not necessarily feel that she had compromised her own values, or indeed the patient's, since he had achieved his end. What, though, if he had been persuaded by senior staff to stay? The student nurse might then have felt embarrassed at having let him down by not following her own instincts. As an individual she might have liked to see him go; at the very least she might have wanted his interests as well as his rights respected, and in the conflict between rights and interests she might well have felt that it would be in his best interests to stay. In this case, the solution was determined by the student's position in the nursing hierarchy – she passed responsibility 'up the line'. Having done so, however, she still has to come to terms with the fact that had it not been for her action the patient might well have got his own way.

CONSCIENTIOUS OBJECTION

Case History 3.1 illustrates some of the difficulties involved when the nurse's personal view of the patient's best interests conflicts with the official view the nurse is expected to follow. These difficulties are particularly acute if nurses feel that they really must oppose the official line taken by the nursing hierarchy, since if they lose the support of colleagues, they are placed in a vulnerable position. In this connection, the saying about there being safety in numbers is particularly true when it comes to making important decisions that affect other people's lives.

There is, however, a further difficulty which may arise when nurses decide to stand by their personal beliefs and perhaps refuse to participate in certain kinds of treatment (e.g. termination of pregnancy) or in a particular treatment for an individual patient (e.g. ECT). This difficulty lies in

the pressure the nurse's action places on those who do not exercise the right of conscientious objection. This applies particularly in the case of nurses who claim the right not to participate in abortions. In the theatre this is a reasonably straightforward administrative problem, since only those nurses willing (or not objecting) to work with abortion lists will be employed there, although with a general theatre list this can still create difficulties for the staff who are left to cope after the conscientious objectors have absented themselves. The issue is becoming increasingly problematic for nurses when abortions are being carried out on the wards. The clauses of the UK Abortion Act 1967 do not provide for the case where the nurse refuses to participate in the pre- or postoperative care of a patient having an abortion. What, then, is the nurse's position to be in the care of a patient undergoing an induced abortion on the ward? Perhaps the nurse might reasonably refuse to have anything to do with the administration of the drug. But what should she do when the patient requires help when vomiting as a result of the abortion-inducing drugs? It seems unlikely that a nurse would refuse to help a patient in distress, but this does illustrate the practical limits on the nurse's right to follow the dictates of conscience in this situation. One practical way out of such a problem might be to carry out ward-situated abortions only in areas where learners are not required to work; trained staff can choose where they will work. This solution, however, might open the way for a rather different kind of abortion service, not necessarily in the interests of either patients or staff.

The moral difficulty which arises in the above situation where a nurse exercises her 'right' to opt out of abortion work is that if one nurse will not undertake certain work to which patients are entitled, then another nurse must. A different aspect of this problem is illustrated in Case History 3.2.

This example illustrates the protection that may be afforded by the hierarchy to the junior members of staff. However, it also demonstrates that even when the junior nursing staff are prepared to stand together, they cannot always expect support from their seniors. In this case, had the charge nurse taken the view of the majority of the nurses,

case history 3.2

Treatment of a young man with renal failure

A 27-year-old man with a wife and small daughter had hepatitis and renal failure. He had been on machine dialysis for 3 days a week. He was an in-patient, and although his progress was steady, it was not as good as expected. The consultant decided that the dialysis machine could be used to better effect for other patients. A decision was therefore made to take the patient off the machine and put him on diamorphine. This was done without much discussion and when the staff nurse was told to give the diamorphine injection, she asked for time to discuss this with other staff. The nursing staff, except for the charge nurse, decided to refuse to be involved with this injection because of the patient's age and his prognosis since coming off the dialysis machine and being given diamorphine. The night staff also refused. The night senior nurse, a third-year student, was spoken to about her refusal, which upset her. Only the sister and the doctor gave the injection of diamorphine. The patient died before the next dialysis procedure was due.

then the doctors would have had to take both prescriptive and practical responsibility for their treatment. As it was, the senior nurses further up the line of management made the third-year student feel uncomfortable about the stance she took. This example raises considerations on both sides of the argument. If nurses are to decide on conscientious grounds how far they are prepared to go along with certain forms of treatment, the carrying out of patient care might well become a much more difficult matter than at present. Nursing still works according to the Nightingale premise that nurses will do as they are told. But as nurses become better informed, more vocal, more aware of their rights and more sensitive to the ethical implications of patient care, the nursing service may well need to look again at its terms and conditions of employment. A hard line which states that all care undertaken in a particular hospital will be undertaken by all nurses leaves the individual little scope for manoeuvre in moral matters. On the other hand, it would be administratively or operationally difficult to have a system of health care in which nurses could pick and choose which prescribed treatments or procedures they will administer.

Such issues were at stake in the case where a psychiatric nurse was dismissed for refusing to give a patient medication (Walsh 1982). This same nurse appealed against his dismissal and sought to take his case to the House of Lords, such was the seriousness of his disagreement with the medical treatment of a patient and his conviction that he and the junior nurses should have no part in it. Graham Pink was finally vindicated after a long and extremely costly battle. In the wake of the Pink case and in conjunction with the increase in NHS Trust hospitals (hospitals, which although within the NHS, can manage their own budgets, contracts and affairs generally), there has been a move towards the inclusion of so-called 'gagging clauses' within the contracts of NHS staff. These clauses make it clear that staff should not approach the media if they have concerns about standards of care or service. The Department of Health was forced to issue Draft Guidance Freedom of Speech for NHS Staff.[1] The guidelines have been thought to be very restrictive and present ethical quandaries for nurses, especially as they explicitly state that a health care worker 'may as a last resort contemplate the possibility of disclosing his or her concerns to the media'. The guidelines go on to say that 'such action may lay him/her open to the possibility of disciplinary action by the employer'.

KNOWLEDGE AND CONTROL IN NURSE MANAGEMENT

Problems of a different kind again may be raised by the hierarchical structure of nursing when more junior members of staff have in fact more knowledge about a particular situation and are thus better suited to take relevant decisions. One example of this might be in an intensive care unit, where the charge nurse and her senior staff nurses may be in a better position than is the unit manager to determine what staffing levels are required in the unit at any given time. The nursing manager may perhaps be out of touch with intensive care nursing, or may indeed never have had any clinical experience in the area. Managers are, nevertheless, in a position of authority which allows them to deploy staff in their units as they see fit. Even if this leaves the ward short-staffed, nurses are obliged to defer to the decisions of senior staff.

At ward level, the hierarchical order may also require a junior nurse to obey the instructions of a less well informed senior. Learner nurses encounter this problem when they come across a ward where the nursing care being carried out does not conform to the 'correct practice' they were taught in the college of nursing. A typical example of the problem is in the treatment of pressure areas. One might be excused for thinking that so long after Norton (1975) first published her research on the topic that such difficulties are a thing of the past. It remains the case, though, that practice varies enormously in this aspect of care. Some of the 'old school' approaches to preventive measures in skin care generally, and pressure areas in particular, have been shown to be not only ineffectual but possibly harmful. The learner nurses face difficult situations when a senior nurse asks them to carry out a procedure for a patient which the students know is not in the patient's best interest. The learners may well be able to cite the relevant research, to describe the preferred treatment and to justify the case. However, the fact remains that for unqualified juniors to question a senior, the position is awkward. The easiest practical solution to such a problem would probably be to follow the senior nurse's wishes rather than pursue the matter with their tutor, even though the tutor might be more sympathetic to the view that nursing practice should be based on research findings.

What about the nurse's legal responsibility to the patient in such cases? Nurses worldwide are becoming increasingly aware of the risk of facing litigation, as patients become more aware of their legal and moral rights as consumers. Legal proceedings can be instigated if patients or relatives feel that they have a case against the medical or nursing staff with respect to their treatment and care. If student nurses have reason to believe that the care they are being asked to give by seniors could be harmful to the patients, then a confrontation with the senior nurse might seem the only course open to them. Such behaviour might not be consistent with the demands of line management, but it might be morally and legally prudent in

such a case. The introduction of evidence-based practice is relevant here. It should, in principle, alleviate many of the problems of the kind described above. There remains, however, the question of who decides what counts as evidence, and what can be done about those areas where there is no 'evidence'?

RESPONSIBILITY, WARD ORGANISATION AND RECORD-KEEPING

As has already been mentioned, the style of organisation on a ward can have implications for the amount of responsibility an individual nurse carries, in particular where nurses are responsible for planning the care of one or more patients. The use of detailed care plans, in which individualised instructions for the patient's care can be found, is a characteristic of this style of ward management. These care plans may also be used if a more task-oriented routinised approach to care is in operation, where the care plans are translated into routine tasks in terms of the whole ward. Where the individual nurse is responsible for all the care of one or more patients, there is more pressure on the nurse than there would be if she were a part of the ward workforce with a share in the care of all patients.

If nurses are given specific tasks, e.g. responsibility for fluids and fluid balance charts for the whole ward, then they can go about their tasks in a fairly routine way without taking responsibility for any single patient: while one nurse takes care of fluids, others in turn will attend to baths, dressings, recording, etc. for the same patients. Thus the patients, or at least their needs, are fragmented and distributed among the nurses, who have collective responsibility for their care, but the weight of responsibility falls upon the nurses in charge who allocate the tasks.

Task-oriented nursing is regarded as an outmoded means of organising nursing care. However, its more recent replacements – patient allocation and primary nursing – have their critics. One of the common arguments against patient allocation is that more staff are required to put it into practice. But in a study of student nurses' views on nursing (Melia 1981), a number of students recorded a positive preference for routine and a task-centred approach because it represented a foolproof system for getting through the work without items of care being missed out. On these grounds it can be argued that the certainty which a routine provides can benefit the patients, who may rest assured that their basic needs will be met. Junior nurses may also gain security by avoiding the stress of being wholly responsible for any one patient. Against this view, however, must be set the possible therapeutic benefits of a patient-centred approach and its advantages in terms of work satisfaction for many nurses.

Whichever style of organisation is adopted, however, legal responsibility ultimately falls on one member or other of the nursing staff, whether it be the nurse wholly responsible for a particular patient or the nurse in charge of a task-oriented ward. In practice, of course, the nurse's employer, the health authority, is also vicariously responsible for a nurse's actions or omissions, and while individual nurses may be sued by patients or relatives along with the health authority, it is recognised that the health authority is most likely to be able to pay any damages awarded by the court.

On the other hand, it is worth noting that the employing authority is then entitled to try to recover its costs from the individual nurse. In such circumstances, record-keeping is clearly a crucial factor. How the patient has been treated can be seen from accurate notes kept and signed by the nurses involved in the case; then, should there be any dispute, a statement of the facts is available. The kind of issues involved are illustrated in Case History 3.3.

In this case the records concerned – the hospital accident forms – were additional to the nursing care records. The senior nurse manager looked at the situation in terms of wasted time and effort, but the nurse who was most immediately involved was anxious to follow the hospital procedure, not least for her own protection.

The question of whether a health visitor could be sued for omitting to tell parents about all the side-effects and possible dangers associated with vaccination has also arisen where parents have complained about a lack of information. Obviously, health visitors do not record every word of their conversation with clients, so that in court it could well be the client's word against the health visitor's. A history of clear and full record-keeping would be in the health visitor's interest if a case were to be brought; however, individual health visitors are far less likely to be sued than their health authorities. Aside from the legal issue, there is a more basic moral point to be made. Because health visitors have a prime professional responsibility for preventive health care, they may encounter difficulties when individual parents want to know what they personally think about vaccination. When asked, for instance, 'What if it were your child?', the health visitor has to balance her own personal concern for that particular family with her wider duty to achieve comprehensive immunity in the population (Whincup 1982).

The transfer of nurse education to the universities has led to much discussion about the different perspectives this has given to nursing. These are often described in terms of a change of ideology or philosophy of nursing. Nursing can be generally described as a planned activity which is based on assessment of patient (or client) needs and the evaluation of the care given. Although there is a good deal written on the philosophy of nursing, e.g. whether it is an art or a science, we would

case history 3.3

When accidents occur frequently

An elderly patient, who was unable to walk, persisted in getting out of bed unaided during the night and repeatedly fell to the floor. Because of the layout of the ward and the lack of staff, constant observation was not possible. Cot sides were not used in the unit and extra sedation was not recommended. The accident forms often amounted to three a night, although not every night. The senior nursing officer questioned the number of forms and recommended that it was not necessary to fill these in at each incident, because of the frequency with which these falls occurred. The nurse who had been filling in the forms then had to ask herself whether she should continue to do so, to cover herself from the legal aspect, or whether she should carry out her senior's instructions.

argue that the empirically based discussions of nursing are more likely to lead to a useful basis for practice and the production of knowledge than is reliance on customary practice and tradition.

THE NURSE AND THE HEALTH CARE TEAM

The greatest scope for conflict in nursing practice is possibly in the relationship between nursing and medical practice in the context of the health care team. Just as there is a power dimension to the relationship between patient and nurse, so there is in the relationship between nurse and doctor. The source of the medical profession's authority and power lies in the fact that doctors carry legal responsibility for most decisions about patient care and treatment. As we have seen in the earlier discussion of conscientious objection, conflict or disagreements between nurses and doctors arise over who has ultimate authority and control over patient care. Nurses may be left with responsibility for patients, yet have no authority to change doctors' orders, nor a legal right to refuse to carry out medical instructions even if they object.

There are two factors related to the structure of medicine and nursing which are potential sources of conflict. The first, which has already been mentioned, is the difference between the collegial organisation of medicine and the hierarchical organisation of nursing. The collegial mode is based upon professional trust, individual discretion and an informal system of regulation by one's peers; in practice, a junior doctor will seek advice from and be guided by his more experienced senior colleagues, but with much less need for a formal line of command than in nursing. At the ward level, this can create problems. If, for example, a registrar acts in some way which contravenes hospital policy, she enjoys greater freedom to do so than does the charge nurse who is associated with this action. Doctors may leave the ward and ask to be telephoned if a seriously ill patient's condition deteriorates. They may then find it perfectly acceptable to prescribe medication over the telephone, await the outcome and decide to return only if certain changes occur. This action may meet the approval of medical staff, and the charge nurse, as an individual, may consider it perfectly reasonable, not least because the patients will benefit from receiving the drug sooner than if they had to wait for the doctor's return. The charge nurses may also be aware that to order drugs over the telephone is against the hospital policy, which they have a duty to follow. If they comply with the registrar's wishes they will not enjoy the support of their seniors.

This is only one example of the kinds of conflict which arise when these two frontline professionals try to work together. At a day-to-day level, both must be able to cooperate in planning the care of the patients; the smooth and efficient running of the ward depends on a good working relationship between doctor and nurse at this level. The nursing staff, however, are to some extent bound by the rules involved in being what we might usefully think of as the hospital's 'clinical civil service'. This can bring them into conflict with doctors who have more of the status of free agents who practise their craft in hospitals. In much the same way as nurses can be seen as the 'clinical civil service' of the hospital, they might be said to be the 'moral housekeepers'. The ethical issues which arise in nursing care are very closely related to the way in which nursing is constructed. Nurses are responsible for the provision of safe and effective care and this includes the maintenance of a safe environment. In so far as there are ethical dimensions to many decisions about care and its day-to-day practice, so is there a routine ethical aspect to care. It is the need to build ethical thinking into the routines of nursing that makes the notion of 'moral housekeeping' so apt.

The second factor which is a potential source of conflict in the nurse–doctor relationship lies in the nature of nursing as an occupation. Nursing can be said to be partly dependent upon and partly independent of medical practice. There are, clearly, some areas of nursing work which mostly have to do with carrying out the care prescribed by doctors. In this sense the nurse is simply following orders. There are, however, other areas of care, mostly to do with the patient's comfort and social well-being, in which the nurse should take action independent of medicine. The introduction of nurse practitioners and nurse prescribing makes the issue of interprofessional power relationships even more complex. Doctors have a tendency to see nursing as an entirely dependent profession, which exists to help them. Some nurses are happy to go along with this working definition. Others prefer to develop their nursing skills, arrive at decisions on how best they think the patient might be cared for, and form what could be called a nursing opinion. Having formed an opinion, the nurse might then wish to question the word of the doctor; at a level more pragmatic than ethical, the nurse might, for example, question the wisdom of his prescription.

Often an experienced charge nurse will be in a position to advise a more junior doctor upon the best treatment in cases of which she has had past experience. If the doctor is not prepared to listen to her opinion or, having listened, ignores it, the nurse is then faced with a choice. Either she can let the matter drop, possibly to the detriment of the patient on the grounds that 'the doctor knows best', or she can press her opinion to the extent of calling in a senior doctor or refusing to cooperate in the treatment. On the military analogy, the charge nurse may then marshal troops and dictate to nursing staff what the nursing strategy will be. In the case of such confrontation, teamwork breaks down and the issue moves from the pragmatic area to the ethical and 'political'. The determining factor in the outcome of such conflicts often lies in the answer to the question about who is ultimately responsible. Nurses, to their own satisfaction, might have a right to a nursing opinion and also a right to challenge medical staff. But what of the legal responsibility? The 'contract' which the patient enters into when he is ill is between patient and doctor. The patient is ultimately the doctor's responsibility.

Difficulties of this kind are often most acute in areas such as geriatric medicine, terminal care, psychiatry and obstetrics where team decisions are often taken but where the responsibility is ultimately that of the doctor. Because of this, the teamwork ideal may be difficult to translate into practice. Further difficulties can be caused by the fact that health care professions and occupations other than medicine and nursing may each have their own hierarchies, lines of accountability, rules, regulations and working practices. Many decisions that directly affect the care of patients and the running of wards – from cleaning to hospital meals, portering to the ambulance service – are outside the control of the charge nurse and her ward staff, however much patients and their relatives may imagine that they are responsible.

Nurses are exhorted to 'care' for patients – in both a generalised and an emotional sense – while at the same time they have to make decisions about how and where to distribute their time and care. Nurses are thus largely responsible for seeing that patients get the care and personal attention that they require. However, judgements have to be made about how to spread nursing time among a group of patients. These are in part clinical and in part moral judgements, usually described as 'professional judgements'. A professional nursing service must make well-informed, fair and equitable decisions on the basis of nursing expertise and knowledge of available resources, not on some generalised emotive ethic of 'caring'.

Evidence-based practice is again relevant here, for nursing knowledge must be the product of empirical investigation. Assertions about what nursing is and is not are of little value to the profession unless there is some means of testing, or at least questioning, the propositions. Professional nursing, if it is to distinguish itself from lay nursing, must operate not only on a tried-and-tested knowledge base, but also on objective criteria of justice based on nursing experience, when it comes to determining how much time and care can be devoted to individual patients. The only real justification for having trained nurses (an expensive commodity) is the fact that they have specialist knowledge and skills upon which to base their judgements and practical work – as opposed to the altruism that guides lay carers.

This expertise allows professional nurses to meet the clinical needs of patients while also addressing the demands of justice and equity in the allocation of time and resources to groups of patients. To treat a ward full of patients justly requires both knowledge and skill, and an ability to make appropriate practical judgements in the light of experience. Justice does not have to do with an *equal* distribution of time and care among all patients; rather, it demands that sensible decisions are made about the *equitable* allocation of nursing time and effort relative to objectively assessed need. If, for example, there is a violent patient causing disruption on a ward, it is in the best interests of all patients that nurses concentrate their efforts on that patient until such time as he has been calmed down. This might mean that a meal is served late or a routine drug round is delayed. Even though the majority of patients do not receive attention for a period of time, when a disturbed patient takes the full attention of the available nurses, and this may mean that other patients have their meals and medication delayed, nevertheless, the nurses can be said to have acted in the best interests of all the patients. Professional nursing decisions, then, have in general to be made on appeal to evidence-based knowledge and to practical justice rather than to a more simplistic ethic of caring.

RESPONSIBILITY TO THE PROFESSION

Occupational groups which enjoy a professional monopoly in determining the service they provide must also accept responsibility for maintaining their standards of practice. Nurses, as a professional group, must therefore also be concerned about the quality, effectiveness and standards of care in the services they provide to clients.

One has only to look at the nursing press or reports from nursing conferences to see that a preoccupation with standards and the quality of patient care is one which many nurses share. Typically, the professions claim to have knowledge and skills which allow their members to give some form of service. The fact that the service is of a specialised nature with a theoretical base makes it difficult for a lay person to judge the performance of professionals. For this reason, the professions themselves seek to develop ways of assuring society that it will be protected from any undesirable consequences of the professional monopoly. To this end, the profession sets its own standards of practice, trains its own recruits, disciplines its members and strives to maintain its standards. The arguments for this practice centre on the fact that a specialist knowledge is required in order to understand professional behaviour, and so self-regulation is the most effective way to maintain standards. The difficulty, however, is that the 'closed shop' nature of such professional organisations prevents any independent critical viewpoint being brought to bear on the profession's practice.

The fact that no professional is above the law goes some way to alleviating any fears which society might have about abuse of privileged positions. The courts provide a means of holding professionals publicly accountable, and thus of regulating the conduct of professionals whose conduct moves outside the law. While the law may not be the most appropriate medium for resolving ethical issues, it does have the virtue of impartiality and can set limits to the harmful potential of monopoly power. On the other hand, while it would be undesirable to have a medical profession whose members were never required to justify their actions, the complexities of medical decision-making are such that a legalistic approach to a debate about its rights and wrongs may be unhelpful (see Case History 3.4).

If, in such a case, circumstances lead to a court hearing because a decision has been taken to terminate life support, then the complex series of events which led up to switching off the machine might appear very different in a courtroom from how they appeared in the ward. The way in which testimony is handled in court, and is

 case history 3.4

Taking the decision to switch off a life support machine

A nurse, as part of an intensive care team, has been involved in the care of a brain-damaged patient. After the patient has been on a respirator for a few days, the physicians establish that brain death has occurred. After discussion with the relatives and the nursing staff, the doctor in charge of the patient's case decides that the respirator should be turned off and the patient's heart left to stop. The whole team is in complete agreement with the decision and the nurse who has been looking after the patient turns off the machine.

subject to cross-examination by counsel for the plaintiff, often leaves little scope for an explanation by the nurse of all the surrounding circumstances. Thus the description of events might be interpreted by a lay jury in a way that is very different from that of informed medical and nursing opinion. On the other hand again, is it not right that an outside view should be sought? Is there not a risk that a professional group will 'close ranks' in defence of colleagues and simply approve its own conduct because of familiarity, failing to see the flaws in its practice which a lay person might see?

Doubts about the impartiality of 'professional self-regulation' cannot be dismissed out of hand, not least because when cases come to the courts, the profession's own 'evidence' and definition of events are influential. McCall-Smith (1977) remarked in his discussion of the legal aspects of the Royal College of Nursing (RCN) code:

The law may ultimately be called upon to define what is acceptable practice on the part of the professions but it tends to do so on the basis of what the professions themselves suggest. The law, then, looks for guidance to professional consensus, while the professions naturally look to the law for a statement of what they can or cannot do.

In the light of this circular relationship between consensus and the law, McCall-Smith concludes: 'The promulgation of a code of professional conduct is of major legal significance, in that it can be influential in the moulding of legal attitudes.'

The judge's summing up in the case of the late Dr Leonard Arthur, accused of murdering a Down's syndrome baby, underscored the point (Brahams & Brahams 1983). After hearing expert medical opinion on the treatment of severely handicapped neonates, the judge said:

Whatever ethics a profession might evolve they could not stand on their own or survive if they were in conflict with the law .... I imagine you will think long and hard before concluding that doctors of the eminence we have here have evolved standards that amount to committing a crime.

In the case of Tony Bland, a victim of the 1989 Hillsborough football stadium disaster, whose cerebral cortex was destroyed as a result of prolonged oxygen deprivation, the physician and the NHS Trust went to law in order to discontinue treatment.[2] This case was of particular concern to nurses as the 'treatment' in question was feeding by nasogastric tube. Again, the law courts were required to pronounce on essentially medical and moral matters.

From the profession's point of view, codes of ethics or codes of conduct are also important – both as ways of proclaiming publicly their trustworthiness and as a means of giving their members some guidance as to their practice. In this connection it is perhaps useful to think of a profession's standards as follows: at the *micro level*, regulating the conduct of individual members towards their patients, clients and colleagues; and at the *macro level*, setting out the values upheld by the whole profession. This is where the 'professional ethic' may be invoked by individual members to justify their behaviour. In discussing codes of ethics in nursing, we will be concerned with both levels at which codes operate.

CODES OF ETHICS

There are several professional codes of ethics to which we might turn in order to gain some idea of their form and purpose (UKCC 1992).

Until the 20th century, the medical profession in Britain never had an agreed code of ethics, although the Hippocratic oath (see Appendix 1) was commonly claimed to be the basis of its ethics. Following the World War II Nuremberg war crimes trials, the World Medical Association (WMA) adopted the oath, in a modified form, as its basis – known as the *International Code of Medical Ethics*. The British Medical Association (BMA), as a founding member of the WMA, is a signatory to this and the various other declarations of the World Medical Association (see Duncan et al 1981). The American Medical Association (AMA 1977), however, followed what it saw as a British lead when it adopted a code of ethics based on an earlier code drawn up by the Manchester physician, Thomas Percival, in 1849 (see Parker 1977).

The established professions tend to make explicit the moral standards which guide their professional conduct and then rely on the integrity of their members to carry out their work in the clients' best interests (BMA 1984). Wilding (1982) has described codes of ethics and conduct as simply 'campaign documents prepared in a search for privilege and power, or in their justification'. Few would go so far, but it has to be said that the practice of producing ethical codes is probably linked to the desire of certain occupations to claim professional status.

Today British doctors accept the *International Code of Medical Ethics* as providing general guidelines for medical practice (Veatch 1977). In recent times, written codes and declarations in medicine have been developed in order to deal with particular crises of public confidence in medical standards, or in response to challenges facing the medical profession, e.g. *The Nuremberg Code* (1947) was drawn up after revelations about Nazi war crimes involving medical experiments on human subjects. It, together with the later Declaration of Helsinki (1964 and 1975), sought to define the criteria for permissible ethical research involving human subjects. Others sought to set standards for the determination of the time of death (the Declaration of Sydney 1968); for therapeutic abortion (the Declaration of Oslo 1970); and for torture, degrading treatment and punishment (the Declaration of Tokyo 1975). Ethical guidelines for psychiatry were drawn up by the World Psychiatric Association in the Declaration of Hawaii (1977) (Duncan et al 1981).

Nursing and social work are two major caring professions which have followed the example of medicine and produced their own codes of ethics. Again, we have to look to America to find one of the earliest codes. In 1893, at the Farrand Training School for Nurses at the Harper Hospital of Detroit, Lystra Grecter, principal of the school, devised the Nightingale Pledge (Robinson 1946). By this pledge, graduates of the school promised '[to] pass my life in purity and to practise my profession faithfully. I will abstain from whatever is deleterious and mischievous and will not take or administer any harmful drug'. There was no connection between this pledge and Florence Nightingale; it would appear, however, that Lystra Grecter felt that the name of Nightingale would add weight to the pledge.

It was some time before the ethical codes in nursing with which we are familiar today were developed. In 1950 the American Nurses Association produced its *Code for Nurses*. The early versions of the code were mainly prescriptive, as Tait said, 'identifying codes of both personal and professional behaviour, describing appropriate relationships with physicians and other health care professionals', but the latest code, 'while remaining prescriptive, depends more upon the nurse's accountability to the client' (Tait 1977). Along with the code there are 'interpretive statements', which render the code more than a list of 'do's and don'ts'. The RCN adopted this approach in 1976 when it drew up its *Code of Professional Conduct* (RCN 1977a). The International Council of Nurses (ICN) first produced its *Code of Ethics* in 1953; this was revised in 1965 and replaced in 1973, when the Council adopted the *Code for Nurses: Ethical Concepts Applied to Nursing* (ICN 1973).

The most recent professional code for nurses in Britain is the UK Central Council's *Code of Professional Conduct* (UKCC 1992). This code, now in its third edition, was drawn up following the Nurses, Midwives and Health Visitors Act 1979, which gave the UKCC powers including 'that of giving advice in such a manner as it thinks fit on standards of professional conduct'. The authors of this code could be said to have taken a rather narrow view of a professional code in so far as it can be seen in large part to be a checklist against which alleged cases of professional misconduct might be judged. In many ways, the opening remarks in this code could have stood in its stead. The more detailed clauses which follow tend to undermine the professional idealism proclaimed at the outset. The council has, however, over the last few years put considerable effort into expanding upon the code and has produced a number of useful supplementary 'advisory papers'.[3]

If nurses are to work as members of multidisciplinary teams, it is perhaps relevant here to take a brief look at the social worker's approach to the question of professional ethics. The American National Association of Social Workers formulated its ethical code in 1960 (Morris et al 1971), but it was not until 1976 that the British Association of

Social Workers (BASW) adopted its code (BASW 1977). Clark & Asquith (1985) remarked:

…if the generations of American and British social workers who practised before these dates managed well enough without a formalised code of ethics, it is at least questionable that a formal statement adds anything to their inheritor's understanding. Whatever the improvements in knowledge that may have been attained by later generations, it is not suggested that the first social workers were less ethical than modern ones.

They went on to say, as has already been argued in the case of nursing, that the move towards a production of codes goes hand in hand with aspirations for recognised professional status. They discussed the BASW code and its similarities with the ICN *Code for Nurses*. They concluded that since much that is contained in these codes is descriptive rather than prescriptive:

It is unclear in what sense these can be ethical statements…the principles purportedly underlying the codes are not translated into any clear or complete statement of rights and duties, indeed the social work codes seem to have more to say about professionals' rights than clients'.

What, then, are the limitations of ethical codes? Let us, by way of illustration, examine just one part of the Declaration of Oslo, on therapeutic abortion, which states (Clause 6): 'If a doctor considers that his convictions do not allow him to advise or perform an abortion, he may withdraw while ensuring the continuity of (medical) care by a qualified colleague.'

At first sight this clause appears to provide a fairly straightforward guideline which the doctor might follow. This kind of conscience clause allows the doctor the right of conscientious objection, i.e. to refuse to perform any procedure which is against his principles. It does, however, leave the potential for practical difficulties. If no colleague is available to provide the care (either, say, in a routine case or if his colleagues are equally opposed to abortion), can the individual doctor demand the right to work according to his beliefs if these are at variance with those of many of his patients?

In practice, then, codes of ethics clearly have their limitations and cannot be seen as always providing the answer to day-to-day moral dilemmas. What such codes can do, however, is to set out aspirational ideals, and the general rights, duties, values and policies which should govern professional practice. As such, they provide a means of laying down standards of conduct which a profession might expect its members to meet. Indeed, this is recognised in the RCN (1977a) discussion document. The introduction states: 'No code can do justice to every individual case and therefore any set of principles must remain constantly open to discussion both within the nursing profession and outside it.' The same document supplies a further reason for having an ethical code: 'To provide a clear and comprehensive document for further discussion, particularly during training.'

The code thus states the ideal professional standards in a clear way which can be recognised as a description of the desired behaviour of professionals. If, as an individual, a nurse is unsure of the position that she should adopt in some situation, the code can supply some guidance. For example, if nurses are unhappy about a particular treatment which a dying patient is receiving, they might feel that as individuals they have no option other than to follow the doctor's instructions. However, not only do nurses have the right, but it is also their duty to express an opinion about the effect of treatment on patients. While nurses might feel diffident about making an opinion known, especially if they are expressing views which run counter to those of the doctor who is prescribing the care, they can find support for their action in the code of ethics. The RCN *Code*, for example, states: 'Measures which jeopardise the safety of patients, such as unnecessary treatment, hazardous experimental procedures and the withdrawal of professional services during employment disputes should be actively opposed by the profession as a whole.' Individual nurses must live up to this code and express opinions when they have them. Nurses can be said to have a duty to the profession to behave in such a way, even though the organisation within which they work historically gives more weight to doctors' opinions.

RESPONSIBILITY FOR PROFESSIONAL STANDARDS

If nurses are to be accountable for their care in a professional sense, they also have a duty to keep up to date in the knowledge base of their profession. It is not sufficient that a nurse pass her final examinations, qualify and then never consider it necessary to continue her education. Nurses must be responsible for the care they give, and it cannot be claimed that because nurses work according to doctors' orders they are exempt from any responsibility to keep up to date. For example, if a nurse thinks that a doctor's prescription contains the wrong dose of the drug, there is a duty to question it, and if there is still doubt, to refuse to give the drug. Nurses, along with the doctor, might be charged with negligence if they failed to recognise the incorrectly prescribed dosage of a commonly known drug such as digoxin.

One might, of course, argue that it is the doctor's business to get the prescription right and that the nurse cannot be held responsible. However, nurses take responsibility for their actions and must carry out patient care in an intelligent way, which includes recognising potential harm to their patients. Again, from a code of ethics, this time from the ICN (1973): 'The nurse takes appropriate action to safeguard the individual when his care is endangered by a co-worker or any other person.' The general point about responsibility for professional standards is also made by the RCN *Code* (1977a):

The professional authority of nurses is based upon their training and experience in day to day care of ill persons at home or in hospital; and the enhancement of positive health in the community at large. All members of the nursing profession have a responsibility to continue to develop their knowledge and skill in these matters.

In order to maintain professional standards, then, nurses must inform themselves of advances in knowledge of nursing care. Not only must the profession ensure that its new recruits achieve a certain standard before they are allowed to practise, but it must make certain that its established members maintain those standards. Indeed, because nurse training involves a substantial amount of learning on the job, it is imperative that qualified practitioners keep themselves up to date so that the learners are exposed to practice of the right standard. The UKCC proposals for PREP are evidence that the Council is taking seriously the requirement for a profession to ensure that its members keep their knowledge of practice updated.

Practice based on sound principles and established empirical evidence might distinguish a professional from a lay approach to activity in a given field. At a macro level the profession must ensure that its standards of practice are supported by a sound theoretical base. At a more individual or micro level, the practitioners must be sure their own practice is up to date.

In the case of nursing, much of the work that nurses undertake has tended to be based upon tradition rather than research. However, for some years now nursing research has been undertaken and its findings made available to the profession. This means that the individual nurse can no longer plead ignorance if she chooses to follow tradition rather than a proven form of treatment. A good example of this, which we have already mentioned, is the care of pressure areas and the treatment of pressure sores. Even after publication of condemnatory findings (Norton 1975) nurses continued to rub soap and water, spirit and a variety of other dubious applications on patients' skin. For learner nurses this particular example might pose ethical difficulties. In their lectures, students will have been supplied with the latest research-based information in relation to the care of pressure areas; yet on the ward they could be told that the charge nurse's policy involves a treatment which the students know has been shown to be harmful. Given that nurses are supposed to be not only responsible for their actions but also morally accountable for them, these students' choice between following the teachings of the college and obeying the charge nurse is a difficult one. In this particular example, because of the workings of the nursing hierarchy, it might also be hard for the students to invoke the professional code of practice to justify disregarding the charge nurse's instructions (RCN 1977a).

Clearly, professional and individual standards of practice converge at some point, as both share responsibility for advancing the knowledge of the discipline. Accurate and meaningful record-keeping on the part of the nurse can provide the data required to evaluate present practice. Thus, while each individual nurse will not be a researcher as such, she should take a responsible attitude towards her nursing record-keeping, in order that the effects of X upon Y in nursing care can be documented. The nursing process is an attempt to apply such an approach to nursing. For example, toilet practices with elderly incontinent patients could be recorded carefully and, after a period, the success of individual programmes could be assessed in terms of the degree of continence attained. Nurses might take a lead from their medical colleagues in this respect. Doctors do not all follow identical treatment patterns in patients with similar conditions. For instance, coronary care might vary from one doctor to the next with equally successful results. It matters little that the treatments are different; what does matter is that doctors take note of the effects of their treatment and thus build up a working medical practice, based, of course, upon the theory available to all those practising medicine, but refined according to their observations. Furthermore, if a doctor arrives at a particularly successful way of treating a condition, she will communicate this to her colleagues through the professional journals.

REPORTING ON COLLEAGUES

In addition to exercising personal responsibility for their own practice and maintenance of professional standards, nurses also have a wider responsibility to the nursing profession. This means that they should be prepared to report poor standards of care and nursing that is not practised in accordance with the professional standard, when they encounter them. This presents perhaps the most trying moral difficulties of all.

If poor practice is to be curbed it must be reported, and it is a fact of life that often the person best placed to observe and report bad practice on the part of a nurse will be another nurse. What price professional loyalty then? If a nurse sees a col-league maltreating a patient, e.g. an elderly patient or a vulnerable person, what should be her response? The nurse's own personal morality and professional standards will dictate that the action was wrong and that the correct line of action is to report the incident. Privately, the nurse might feel something of a 'sneak', telling tales about another individual's actions. However, nurses should be able to ignore these feelings because they have a duty to defend the rights of the maltreated patient – but they may still have to face their colleagues' charges of disloyalty.

Nurses are trusted by patients, indeed by society as a whole, to be caring and kind. They are put in a position of trust by virtue of having been put in charge of the care and, in some sense, the lives of other individuals. The nurse who witnesses a colleague's malpractice is then faced with a choice between exposing the colleague and risking publicity (and the damage to the image of the nursing profession which goes with it) or keeping quiet and betraying the patient's trust.

If a nurse faced with this choice is a learner, then the dilemma is more acute. Aside from the conflict for learners between maintaining the trust of patients and keeping solidarity with the profession, they have to consider the impact of any action on their future career as nurses (see Beardshaw 1981 for a discussion). They may thus feel forced to stand by when individual patients are ill-treated or when poor conditions deprive patients of adequate care. Their silence is reinforced by feelings of impotence and fears of reprisal. The victimisation of some nurses who have spoken up about abuse is a vivid illustration that these fears can be well founded.

If nurses complain about the conduct of other nurses, they have to consider whether they will be listened to or believed, whether their good faith will be questioned (they might, for example, be accused of acting on a grudge), and what it will do to other relationships within the hospital and ultimately to their career prospects. Even though it might be a patient's suffering which is at stake, it is a difficult thing to 'blow the whistle' on one's colleagues, as Beardshaw puts it. One DNE's comment sums it up: 'Students still comment as follows: "We would be told off for interfering";

"No one would take any notice of me"; "I need a job in the future". All worry about victimisation' (Beardshaw 1981).

Beardshaw (1981) pointed out the difficulties for student nurses which exist in the ICN *Code for Nurses*. How can the nurse follow the ICN *Code* and take appropriate action to safeguard the individual when his care is endangered by a co-worker or any other person, when the nurse is subject to the authority of both the medical profession and the nursing hierarchy? The position of the student nurse, she concluded, 'encapsulates an essential contradiction of nursing professionalism – a professional waiting for orders – where emphasis on obedience to authority dilutes the professional responsibility of individual nurses'.

Whistleblowing has in recent years become a vexed topic, appearing regularly in the nursing press. It has perhaps become an overused word and so is losing some of its power. Cole (1993) points out that even after winning his case, Graham Pink did not recover his job, nor has the massive publicity that his case attracted improved the staffing on the care of the elderly ward on which the case first arose.

SUMMARY

In this chapter we have looked at some of the ethical issues that arise out of working in a hierarchy, working as a member of a health care team and having a responsibility to a professional group. Some time has been spent considering codes of ethics and their utility. It is clear that the issues are so wide-ranging and complex that no code can be more than a guide to professional conduct. It can, to borrow the words of Florence Nightingale, do the profession no harm to have an ethical code, for in the code lie the means of safeguarding the public and a reminder to the profession of the need to maintain standards. Codes of ethics will, however, never provide a panacea. It is the prevailing moral climate within the profession that will exert the most influence at the end of the day. Nurses, along with their colleagues in the caring professions, must develop skills in applying ethical principles to their practice and a sound sense of moral judgement in their day-to-day work, demonstrating that they recognise that health care is both a scientific and a moral enterprise.

 further reading

On ethics in nursing in general
Curtin L, Flaherty M J 1982 Nursing ethics, theories and pragmatics. Robert J Brady, MD, section III – *a useful introduction to the issue of nurses' responsibilities towards patients and society*

Davis A J, Aroskar M A 1983 Ethical dilemmas and nursing practice, 2nd edn. Appleton Century Crofts, New York – *Chapter 5 is useful on professional ethics and institutional constraints in nursing*

The structure and operation of management in nursing
Carpenter M 1977 The new managerialism and professionalism in nursing. In: Stacey M, Reid M, Heath C, Dingwall R (eds) Health and the division of labour. Croom Helm, London – *a critical appraisal of nurse management*

Mayston 1969 Report of the working party on management structure of the local authority nursing services (Mayston report). HMSO, London – *official report and recommendations for introduction of the new pattern of management*

White R 1985 Political issues in nursing. Wiley, Chichester, vols 1 and 2 – *a useful overview of political issues in nursing, including those internal to nurse administration*

Conscientious objection and informed consent
Faulder C 1985 Whose body is it? The troubled issue of informed consent. Virago, London – *issues relating to privacy and access to one's body, of particular concern to women*

Johnstone M-J 1994 Bioethics: a nursing perspective. WB Saunders/Baillière Tindall, London – *in particular, Chapter 13, 'On taking a stand', is a most useful discussion of the issues for nurses*

Kerridge I, Lowe M, McPhee J 1998 Ethics and law for the health professions. Social Science Press, Katoomba, NSW – *adopts a more technical legal perspective, but is helpful in clarifying issues*

Kohnke M F 1982 Advocacy: risk and reality. Mosby, St Louis, MO – *the role of the nurse as patient advocate is not without its risks and complications for nurses*

Codes of ethics and issues of discipline
Boyd K M, Higgs R, Pinchin A J 1997 The new dictionary of medical ethics, BMJ Publishing, London – *a most useful dictionary of terms widely used in biomedical ethics and nursing*

McHale J, Tingle J, Cribb A 1995 Law and nursing. Butterworth-Heinemann, Oxford – *a valuable exposition for nurses of the essentials of law as it applies to nursing practice*

Pyne R 1998 Professional discipline in nursing, midwifery and health visiting – including a treatise on professional regulation. Blackwell, Oxford – *a useful*

overview of issues related to discipline and regulation in nursing by a consultant to the UKCC

Tingle J, Cribb A 1995 Nursing law and ethics. Blackwell Scientific, Oxford – *a practical study of the inter-relationship of ethics and law in nursing practice*

end notes

1 For the text of the guidance, which went out for limited consultation in 1992, see *Bulletin of Medical Ethics* 83: 9–11, 1992; and, for a discussion, see *Bulletin of Medical Ethics* 89: 3–4, 1993.
2 See *Bulletin of Medical Ethics* 85: 31, 1993.

3 UKCC advisory papers:
- *Confidentiality – an elaboration of clause 9 of the second edition of the code*, UKCC, London, 1987 (at the time of writing this is being updated to match the third edition of the code).
- *Exercising Accountability*, UKCC, London, 1989.

some suggestions on method

Understanding the structure of nursing
Students could be assigned to different types of hospital or hospital ward, to observe the different ways in which power and authority are shared in acute medicine and surgery, on the one hand, and chronic care and psychiatric nursing on the other. They should then be asked to reflect on why they are different.

Students could be asked to work in small groups to develop a detailed organisational chart of the hospital or college, in which they identify the roles of the various internal stakeholders and the framework of responsibility and accountability within which they operate. They could also be asked to reflect on whether or not the people who wield the most influence are those in positions of official power.

Understanding the nature of nurse management
Students could be asked to brainstorm the qualities of a good manager and to identify what kinds of training and experience managers might need to fill these roles. Having done this, they could be presented with evidence, based on organisational research, showing that good management involves qualities such as vision, integrity and ability to listen, exercise leadership and take risks, rather than merely asserting authority.

At a more senior level they might be required to work a placement in an administrative office, to give assistance and observe nurse managers at work and the way decisions are made.

Authority, obedience and conscientious objection
Students could be presented with examples, for guided group discussion, of cases where nurses have been faced with serious moral dilemmas in relation to their obedience to authority and their right of conscientious objection or duty to blow the whistle on unethical practice. The object would be to develop some ground rules for sensible action in such circumstances.

Exploring codes of conduct and their function
First, students could be set the task of collecting examples of other professional codes and comparing these with nursing codes of ethics. They should be required to identify similarities and differences between them in relation to the responsibilities of different professions. They should then be asked how they might improve their own code so that it might lead to better practice.

4

Ethics and power-sharing in nursing

AIMS

This chapter has the following aims:
1. To demystify ethics by demonstrating that it is about the relations of power and responsibility rather than subjective attitudes and feelings
2. To explore the different levels of power and responsibility in which we have to act as moral agents: the personal, team, corporate and political levels
3. To introduce two sets of models to clarify the different ethical responsibilities of nurses in the various kinds of situations in which nurses relate to patients, and in different kinds of nurse management.

LEARNING OUTCOMES

When you have read and worked through this chapter, you should be able to:
- Illustrate the inadequacy of a privatised view of morality by examples of power relations and power-sharing in nursing
- Discuss what 'virtues' are required if one is to be a competent moral agent, and give examples from nursing practice

■ Demonstrate insight into the different kinds of ethical demands involved in relating to patients in crisis intervention, and consultative, supportive and service roles

■ Demonstrate understanding of the various forms in which power and authority are expressed in teams, line management, community nursing and corporate planning

■ Demonstrate sensitivity to the ways in which gender–role stereotyping can affect both personal attitudes and behaviour and institutional practices in hospitals and community nursing.

POWER AND MORAL RESPONSIBILITY

Against the prevailing tendency to psychologise ethics, we would like to reaffirm the classical view that ethics is fundamentally about power and responsibility, about the conditions for power-sharing and the criteria for the responsible exercise of power in our relations with one another and, for nurses, in dealings with their patients. However, there are various ways we can analyse the forms in which power and responsibility exercised in health care have a bearing on our understanding of nursing ethics.

Sociological analysis focuses attention on the structure of power relationships in different social settings, e.g. in consulting relationships, in the home, in institutional settings, and in more public and political contexts. It will analyse the different ways moral values and personal or professional responsibility are interpreted in each situation, because each social setting will be governed by its own set of formal and informal rules. It is also concerned, for example, with critical examination of how gender–role stereotyping affects the public perception of the identity and role of nurses in health care, and reinforces what many analysts would regard as the institutional exploitation and oppression of women in an essentially patriarchal health service.

Philosophical analysis focuses in ethics more on the logical relationships between the fundamental ethical concepts and the principles which embody our basic moral values, and on clarifying the practical criteria we use in making moral judgements – applying our principles to the concrete situations which demand decisions from us. From a philosophical point of view we appeal to fundamental moral principles to legitimate our exercise of power and to define its scope and responsible use.

Historical analysis will look at the evolution of a given society (or societies) through time, and will seek to describe the way values have developed in the creation of its institutions and specialised roles in the division of labour. Thus, for example, historians may study how the development of medical science shapes the traditions of medical practice, or the increasing specialisation of nursing functions from lay, religious and military settings to those exercised in modern hospital and community settings. Historical analysis throws light on the evolution of a largely gender-based division of labour in health care, and on how ethical codes have evolved in each profession to reflect this. As the emergence of different professions has been marked by the formal differentiation of roles and demarcation of different areas of functional responsibility within health care, so each has developed its own peculiar set of values.

While we recognise that a great deal could be written, and has been written, about the history of health care and the nursing profession (e.g. Allan & Jolley 1982, Bullough & Bullough 1984, Maggs 1987), here we will discuss mainly sociological and philosophical models for interpreting moral issues in health care, and in nursing ethics in particular. As the sociological and philosophical analyses draw much of their material from the history of ideas and the general history of culture anyway, the historical dimensions of the subject are not being ignored and are implicit in much of what follows. Thus understanding of historical developments in Western society (as distinct from other societies) influences how we perceive health care institutions and the relationships among medical, nursing and other staff, and their dealings with patients or clients. It is also directly relevant to our understanding in different societies of the respective rights and duties of professionals and the rules and values which govern their relationships with one another.

DEMYSTIFYING ETHICS[1]

It is commonly implied in the popular media that ethics is concerned with our feelings, attitudes and personal preferences. While these are clearly important in life, and in our dealings with people, confusion and difficulty are likely to arise in ethics if we treat these psychological states as the primary subject matter of ethics. In fact, the mystification of ethics begins with the relegation of ethics to this realm of subjective and non-rational experience. When this happens, ethics ceases to be open to public scrutiny or debate, and it is difficult to see how ethical decisions can be judged by any kind of criteria that are inter-subjectively valid. This mystification of ethics in English-speaking culture arises because of certain pervasive popular misconceptions of ethics current today (cf. Table 1.1, p. **5**).

The common view that ethics is an intensely private matter, concerned only with one's subjective feelings, attitudes and personal preferences, is a dangerous aberration in the context of our Western tradition, which has insisted that ethics is a public and community enterprise and that the quest for justice and fairness is fundamental to that endeavour. Even the Judaeo-Christian love ethic is not based on how we feel about people, but about how we *demonstrate care* for their well-being and fulfilment, by what we do for them and with them.

Alternatively, ethics is privatised by making it into an occult process in which only an elect few have privileged access to moral truth by direct intuition, the 'voice of conscience', or divine guidance. This has the consequence of driving a wedge between ethics and law, ethics and politics, ethics and business – in each, the former belonging to the private sphere and the latter to the public domain. Restating the principle, as old as Aristotle, that ethics is about power and power-sharing – whether in the sexual politics of family life, in edu-

cation, business, professional life, health care, politics or international relations – puts ethics back squarely in the public domain.

Our experience of being subjected to the arbitrary moral authority of parents, teachers and religious figures lends credence to the view that ethics, and moral codes, like the Ten Commandments, are handed down from above by God or his self-appointed agents, and that they are infallible and set in stone. Such an approach tends to be absolutist and authoritarian, and infantilises people by denying them scope for the expression of their own moral autonomy and responsibility. Alternatively, it becomes the domain of experts – philosophers, theologians or gurus – and requires mastery of esoteric knowledge. However, if ethics is about how we articulate, negotiate and agree a set of common principles, and the skills we need to apply to them, then ethics must be about how we educate people for independence and personal responsibility.

An analogous difficulty arises, as indicated in Chapter 1, if all moral difficulties are treated as 'dilemmas'. In the strict sense, a dilemma has no solution, where there is an irresolvable conflict of duties. In the face of dilemmas we can either throw up our hands in despair and abrogate our responsibility for making difficult choices or treat the matter as one of arbitrary judgement. Dilemmas obviously do arise, but the overwhelming majority of our ethical difficulties turn out to be resolvable problems if we analyse them carefully enough. Those that prove intractable demand a particular kind of courage – to act responsibly in the face of painful conflicts of duty, doing the best we can, or the least harm, in the circumstances. This means accepting moral uncertainty and being prepared to accept responsibility for the results. If our 'dilemmas' can be reframed as 'problems', then we should be able to apply rational problem-solving methods to the resolution of most of our ethical quandaries.

Another variant of the privatisation of ethics is the treatment of ethics as a 'skills package' which can be marketed as a 'training product' – skills for improving our public relations, or techniques for 'winning friends and influencing people'. Ethics from this point of view becomes just a matter of technique, or manners, or knowing the right rules, possessing the right management competencies – which usually means being masterful in applying techniques to 'control' people. In contrast, our ethical tradition is that moral competence requires effort and growth in the development of personal integrity and virtue. Even the word 'conscience' in this tradition is not capricious or arbitrary judgement, but stands for a disciplined intellectual faculty in which theoretical knowledge of universal principles and practical experience are skilfully combined and expressed in application to real-life problems.

We have already pointed out the connection between the fundamental principles of beneficence, justice and respect for persons and different, changing modalities of power in human relationships. Thus the protective duty of responsible care for others (beneficence) has to do with *the duty the strong owe to the weak and vulnerable*, because we are all weak and vulnerable at different times in our lives and need the help of other people, particularly when we are very young or very old, seriously ill, injured or mentally disordered.

The principle of justice or universal fairness is fundamentally about different kinds of *power-sharing*. Distributive justice is concerned with how we share power, knowledge, skills and resources with those who lack them – for the common good of society. Protective justice is about how we prevent the abuse of power, by policing observance of the law, protecting people from violation of their rights, from insult or assault, exploitation or torture, discrimination or oppression. Retributive justice is about how we ensure that victims of crime or abuse have equal access to the courts to make complaints, to seek compensation or redress, or the punishment of offenders; and, if accused, have the right to due process, fair and public trial, and legal representation.

The principle of respect for the dignity and rights of other people has to do with *mutual empowerment* of one another within both our local and wider moral communities. Respect for the dignity of all persons, as fellow members of the human moral community, and as bearers of

rights and responsibilities, is ultimately in our own interests too, for it helps to protect our own dignity and moral autonomy, thus empowering us as moral agents. Ultimately we are diminished ourselves when we humiliate another person, or disregard the privacy or dignity of other people – particularly when they are vulnerable and dependent on us for care and protection.

Against the trend to privatise ethics, we wish to assert, therefore, that in a fundamental sense ethics is concerned with power, power relationships and power-sharing – with the responsible use (or the abuse) of power in one's personal life, professional work and in our social institutions. However, we also wish to assert that ethics is concerned with values – with those things which we value because they enable us to achieve our personal goals and fulfilment as human beings. In fact, the powerful attraction our values hold over us is what gives us the motivation and power to act.[2]

The connection between power and values should be evident in what we have said above about the nature of the fundamental ethical principles as power principles. It relates to both our striving for personal fulfilment and our service of other people.

Our personal quest for health, prosperity, fame and the respect or admiration of others is ultimately about our quest for power, for fulfilment of our potential powers of being – whether our quest is 'worldly' or 'spiritual'. The literal meaning of the term 'health' in most European languages connects it with two kinds of reality: the quest for fulfilment of our *potential* (power of being) as human beings, and the ideal or value of *the strength of wholeness*. Both are combined in the WHO (1947) definition of health: 'Health is complete physical, mental and social well-being, and not simply the absence of disease, or infirmity'. For nurses, as well as other health care workers, the responsible use of power, to promote their own health and well-being and that of their patients, combines both the need for the responsible exercise of power and its direction by appropriate values, which serve the interests of those dependent on them, and not just themselves.

DIFFERENT LEVELS OF POWER RELATIONSHIPS IN HUMAN AFFAIRS

How are the concepts of power and power-sharing, on the one hand, and values or ideals, on the other, related to one another, and what do they mean in more practical terms in nursing ethics? Let us attempt to unpack what is implied in these concepts, starting with the relevance of defining ethics in terms of its relation to individual human potential, power-sharing in interpersonal relationships, power structures within social institutions and power relations between different institutions:

- Ethics in our personal and professional life as nurses is about our *responsibility for developing our own individual potential* (traditionally called 'virtues') – both for our own sake and to be able to contribute more effectively to the service of others. It also means avoiding those things that prevent us from realising our full potential as nurses and human beings. Ethics in nursing relates to the power of the nurse, the degree of authority, or lack of authority, exercised by the individual nurse within the nursing hierarchy.
- Ethics as *power-sharing in the relations of nurses and their patients* or clients can be expressed in a number of different modes, which we refer to as code, contract, covenant and charter. In analysing these we explore the ethics of the caring role, the service role, the supportive role, and the role as accountable public officer (see also May 1975).
- Ethics as *power-sharing in interprofessional relationships* concerns the way power is shared (or not shared) in relationships between nurses, doctors and other health workers in hospital and community teams. While nurses have certain *power over* patients, they may have limited *power to* control their work, and even more limited *power to* decide what treatment or care patients should or should not be given. This has to do with their generally subordinate role, even in relation to junior doctors, but is also related to the identity and role of nurses as a mainly female profession within a male-dominated and largely patriarchal health service.

- Ethics as it relates to *corporate power structures* in social institutions, including hospitals and colleges of nursing, is concerned with the development of systems and procedures for the management of relations with and between the internal and external 'stakeholders' of the institution. Structures of power and authority are set up to ensure the flourishing of the corporate body and the well-being of its members and clients. They also have to direct policy and public relations with external stakeholders and institutions, including local and national government. To study the range and variety of these relations we examine four types of model: command management, critical expert, community development, corporate planning.

ETHICS IN THE PERSONAL LIFE OF THE NURSE

Intellectual and moral virtues, competence and competencies

First of all, nursing ethics relates to the responsibility individual nurses and the profession have for their personal and professional development as nurses. Thus nursing ethics (as emphasised in Ch. 3) must address issues relating to the academic and clinical training of nurses, their moral formation, personal growth and professional competence and their continuing education. We all need to develop critical insight into the 'moral prejudices' and personal moral values that we bring with us to our work. We also need to develop sound critical knowledge of moral principles, skills in ethical decision-making, skills in setting policy and standards with other people, and to cultivate what Aristotle would call the moral and intellectual virtues – specifically as they apply to us as nurses at all levels in the care and management of other people.

Aristotle's discussion of the virtues is of particular relevance to the contemporary discussion of 'competencies' and 'competency-based training' in the professional development of nurses.

Aristotle sums up the *intellectual virtues* as combining scientific knowledge with competence in the application of scientific method and technical expertise; also included are reflective and intuitive understanding, wisdom, insight and skill in judgement. Regarding the *moral virtues*, he considers the two virtues of courage and temperance as necessary for self-control and the exercise of moral responsibility, but the key social virtue is justice or fairness. Other moral virtues or personal competencies that he mentions are generosity, magnanimity, honour and a sense of style, good-temperedness and good humour, honesty, amiability, communication skills, and modesty or a realistic assessment of one's own worth. The intellectual and moral virtues represent, as it were, the two legs of an arch in which prudence or practical wisdom is the keystone. Prudence, for Aristotle, is the most essential virtue required by the competent and mature moral agent. Prudence is defined as competence based on skilled application of relevant moral and practical knowledge to specific situations, choosing the right means to a good end (Thomson 1976 [Bks III, VI], Macintyre 1981).

Nurse education has always involved both direct and indirect instruction in ethics; however, modern developments require much more thorough integration of practical training in ethics and scope for the moral formation of nurses in nurse education, as well as explicit integration of ethical review in all nursing processes. In the chapters 'Becoming and being a nurse' and 'Responsibility and accountability in nursing', it was argued that nurses are being subjected to various forms of moral formation through their induction into nursing and working in hospitals, whether consciously or unconsciously, deliberately or inadvertently. The challenge facing those teaching ethics to nurses is to ensure not only that the form and content of direct training in ethics facilitate the development of relevant skills and competencies in ethical decision-making, but also that appropriate learning environments are created where the moral formation of nurses can be nurtured. Besides a capacity for cognitive learning, other competencies relevant to nurses as moral agents include skills in individual counselling and sharing in groups, ability to supervise learning on the job, and skilled facilitation of performance appraisal at personal, team and institutional levels.

Talk about 'virtue' and 'vice' in professional ethics has been suspect for some time, unless it is in valedictory speeches praising a departing colleague's virtues, or in disciplinary hearings where someone's misconduct or negligence is at issue. However, recent stress on 'competencies', and attempts to define these, involve a return to something like the classical meaning of 'virtue' as 'proficiency or excellence in performance' and 'vice' as 'culpable incompetence'. The value of this form of language is that it gets away from moralising and focuses on what kinds of education and training could remedy the deficits of the individual(s) concerned. It follows, therefore, that in assessing the 'virtues' (or 'vices') of nurses, we are not attempting to measure their moral temperature, state of sanctity or moral laxity, but rather their competencies or standards of professional performance under normal working conditions. Some of the ethical competencies that we should be able to demonstrate if we are to act confidently and proficiently as moral agents are:

- an ability to clarify our own personal and professional values, and exhibit insight into the distinction between them, and to show sensitivity to the different values of other people
- an understanding of fundamental ethical principles shown in ability to apply these with discriminating judgement to specific practical cases in one's working environment
- proficiency in the application of relevant problem-solving and decision-making skills in dealing with general or nursing-specific situations
- interpersonal, groupwork and group leadership skills, relevant to teamwork, negotiation with management and other professional colleagues, and skills in supervision of junior staff
- an ability to give a reasoned account of one's decisions and actions (to set out clearly the key facts of the case and relevant principles applied in reaching a decision) and to show how one might justify one's principles.

Furthermore it is important to stress that ethics is concerned not only with how we exercise power and authority over other people, or exercise responsibility in caring for the health and well-being of other people, but also with striving to fulfil our personal potential as human beings. Ethics is not simply other-related. It is also about responsibility to develop our skills and talents, and our own personal fulfilment. If ethics is about how we share power in human communities, then it is also about how we protect one another's rights and promote one another's good. An egocentric ethics will place the emphasis on my right to fulfil my own powers of being as a person. An altruistic ethics will tend to sacrifice self-interest in the service of others, so that they may fulfil their potential, raising questions about the relations of love, power and justice in nursing. (Tillich 1954, Campbell 1984a).

In practice, nursing ethics needs to maintain a balance between the two. Job satisfaction and personal fulfilment in a nursing career are important ethically, for without adequate emphasis on the needs of the nurse, the quality of patient care is likely to suffer. Frustration and poor staff morale are likely to undermine competence and efficiency in the service. On the other hand, selfless service in the care and treatment of others, respecting their dignity and value as human beings, gives satisfaction to work, however menial. Mere careerism, or the attitude of 'it's just another job', deprives nursing of professional dignity if other-regarding values of care are neglected. However, some forms of care can be dependency creating, turning people into perennial 'patients', if nursing care is not directed to empower patients to 'stand on their own feet again', and to restore autonomy, where possible, to people who have lost it as a consequence of illness, injury or mental disorder (as required by the RCN *Code of Ethics for Nurses* 1979). Thus, the ethics of nursing, like that of other caring professions, is fundamentally about the sensitive sharing of power with vulnerable people, helping to facilitate their recovery of independence (Campbell 1985).

RESPONSIBILITY AND ACCOUNTABILITY, POWER AND AUTHORITY

Ethically, to be designated a 'responsible person' implies a number of things, namely that one is, or can be presumed to be:

- a self-conscious rational being *capable of making a response to other people*
- someone who *acknowledges a legal or moral obligation of some kind*
- someone who has *proved that he is reliable and trustworthy*
- someone who is *capable of acting as an independent moral agent*
- someone who is *competent to perform the task in hand*
- someone who can *give an account of what he has done and why*.

In the last-mentioned sense, responsibility is inclusive of accountability, the ability to *give an account* of one's actions, in particular to give a coherent, rational and ethical justification for what one has done. The main difference between responsibility and accountability is perhaps that the former is self-reflexive, namely relating to oneself as a moral agent, whereas accountability relates to one's relationship to other moral agents, in particular to those who have authority over us.

It may be useful in this connection to distinguish between two different kinds of *responsibility to* and two kinds of *responsibility for*, and to give their more technical names (see Box 4.1).

Personal responsibility

Ordinarily one is held responsible for one's own actions and praised or blamed for them, provided one knows what one is doing, has acted freely and voluntarily and provided one can distinguish between right and wrong. This includes awareness of the obligations one is under and one's liability to be praised or blamed depending on how one discharges one's obligations. It is this sense of responsibility which is involved when one's own

---

Box 4.1   Responsibility and accountability

- Responsibility *for* one's own actions (personal responsibility)
- Responsibility *for* the care of someone (fiduciary responsibility)
- Responsibility *to* higher authority (professional accountability)
- Responsibility *to* wider society (public accountability/civic duty)

moral actions are under scrutiny, or one has to appear before an investigating inquiry or one is being tried for negligence in a court. On the other hand, some of the *excusing conditions* which may be taken into account in determining the degree of guilt and/or possible diminished responsibility involved are:

- ignorance of the circumstances, the specific nature of the obligations involved, or the likely consequences of one's action
- acting under threat or duress, or compulsion of some kind
- the stress of the circumstances, shock or grief, or factors beyond one's control
- inexperience in the exercise of the relevant kind of responsibility (see also Ch. 10, pp. 281–286).

Fiduciary responsibility

When someone is entrusted into your care (e.g. a child, an unconscious or a mentally disordered patient), or when a patient voluntarily entrusts herself into your hands, whether as a nurse or in the context of lay care, you acquire 'fiduciary responsibility' (from Latin *fiducia* = trust). Thus, having responsibility for the care and treatment of patients, or for decisions about their individual and collective well-being, is a matter of fiduciary responsibility, and the moral authority or power of the nurse to do these things derives from the trust which the patient and society places in him.

Professional accountability

The professional responsibility vested in nurses by society is underwritten in Britain by the National Board for Nursing, Midwifery and Health Visiting (NBS) and the United Kingdom Central Council for Nursing Midwifery and Health Visiting (UKCC), and as a result nurses have an obligation to their colleagues of *professional accountability*, i.e. a duty, if required, to justify their actions to their peers, their superiors, to the NBS and UKCC, and to society – through the courts if necessary. This duty of professional accountability follows from the responsibilities entrusted to the nurse, as a nurse, by the profession, the health care system and society.

Many nurses will feel both *responsible for* and *responsible to* their patients, and to relatives as well. Because nurses are responsible for the well-being of their patients, they may feel guilty if things go wrong and consider that some kind of explanation or apology is due to the patient or relatives. The sentiment might be right, and in some circumstances explanations or apologies might be in order, but it is inappropriate for the individual nurse to apologise, to admit to being at fault or to attempt to offer explanations to patients or relatives, as this might also expose the nurse, or the hospital, to prosecution for negligence in cases where the patient has suffered hurt or injury. In that sense, nurses are not accountable to their patients directly (although they may be held accountable by their patients, by prosecution or civil action through the courts).

The line of accountability in nursing must, in the first instance, be upwards to the line manager, then to the profession, as these authorities would be in a better position to decide whether a personal apology is due, or whether the issue should be dealt with through the appropriate complaints procedures. In some cases it will not be helpful (or wise) for nurses to give all the reasons for their actions to patients and relatives – at least not until demanded to do so by an enquiry. However, from the daily 'Kardex' (case review) meeting and meetings of the medical care team through to enquiries by the disciplinary committees of the NBS and UKCC and the courts, nurses are thus held professionally accountable.

Public accountability/civic duty

The nurse as a nurse does not act as a private citizen, but as someone who holds public office – and whether working in state or private hospital, in a community setting, or even as an agency nurse, is employed as a member of a public institution with corporate responsibilities. As such, nurses are held to be publicly accountable, in both a legal and a moral sense, for the standard of care they give to their patients and for responsible use of public resources. As qualified and accredited members of the nursing profession, and also as employees within the state health care system (or private institutions), nurses also have a duty of public accountability for maintaining the general standards of nursing. Nurses are public officers, even public servants, with both civic and political duties. For example, nurses have a civic duty to report or draw attention to specific examples of incompetence or negligence, where patients are being abused or where standards of patient care have become unacceptable. Nurses cannot avoid the 'political' responsibilities they carry as public officers, not only to seek to change bad practice or take action to improve standards of care, but also to address injustice or discrimination where it arises and to influence health policy and the allocation of resources – for the benefit of patients in general.

Power and authority

Public discussion of the ethical responsibilities of nurses tends to focus on the use and possible abuse of power which nurses exercise over patients who are entrusted into their care. However, from the nurses' point of view, some of the most painful practical dilemmas arise because they lack the authority to act on their own, e.g. to take their own initiative, to go against a doctor's orders, to give information to patients or relatives about the patient's medical diagnosis or prognosis, or to question the drug dosages prescribed by an inexperienced doctor. Here even the senior nurse can experience some of the classic problems of 'middle management' – of the person in the mediating or intermediate role between someone in authority and the client – namely of having power and responsibility, but without the necessary executive authority. In this regard, Bowden (1997) wrote:

Relations (of nurses) with patients are closely tied into relations with other members of the institution, and are importantly influenced by the terms of their place in the hierarchy. Nursing care thus occupies an 'in between' position in the organization of the public response to the patient's need, and is infused with the tensions of sustaining interdependent but differently focused relations with different levels of authority.

We have emphasised that ethics is about power-sharing and the responsible exercise of power, but we need perhaps to distinguish more clearly between the responsible exercise of *power over others* (whether power over patients or in managing other staff) and executive authority or *power to* initiate action, intervene, to direct policy or to issue orders. To have power over someone else either depends on one having the strength or ability to impress others to submit to your exercise of power over them – whether it be as a leader, expert or professional carer – or it may be the result of having been authorised to exercise some role or delegated power by some higher authority. In either case there is an assumption that if executive power is to be effective it must be based on actual strength, knowledge, skill, competence or experience of the kind required to give legitimacy to the exercise of that power. 'Power to act' relates to the concept of 'authority', whether that be the power to act on one's own authority based on one's position or acknowledged power, or on the basis of delegated authority from someone else with more power in the group or the institution.

Power relates to potential or actual ability to do something, authority relates to the conditions for actual exercise of power. Authority (from the Latin *augere* = to implement or augment) defines the moral conditions under which we exercise power – *to implement* actions or policies that serve to *augment the well-being* of those for whom we are responsible and over whom we have authority. These functions of implementing the policy in such a way that it is seen to augment the well-being of the institution or moral community legitimates the exercise of authority within it. Unless the exercise of authority can be seen to satisfy these conditions, it is without moral legitimacy and becomes the naked expression of the will to power or domination of others. These moral constraints apply to both established and delegated authority – where the power to execute orders or to ensure the implementation of the policies is given by higher authority.

When nurses are compelled to weigh their responsibility for individual patients against their institutional responsibilities for groups of patients, they may be faced with conflicts between their power to do things for individual patients and their lack of authority to deviate from ward routine or a doctor's orders. It may, for example, be as simple a matter as desiring to give a particular patient more time and attention than others, because the patient has confided in the nurse matters of a very distressing personal nature; or it may be feeling that the amount of pain relief prescribed by a doctor to a dying patient is inadequate and wanting to respond to the patient's request for more.

The actual authority vested in nurses, to serve the best interests of their patients, may contrast with the actual or relative lack of power which they have, depending on their position in the nursing hierarchy or their relationships with other professional staff. In reality, the culture of trust (or distrust) within a ward team may have a great deal to do with how much or how little power or scope nurses, individually or collectively, have to negotiate the routines on the ward or details of the management of specific patients. In the right climate of trust on the team, it may well be that an experienced staff nurse may be allowed to exercise some discretion or independent judgement. Alternatively, nurses may find both formal and informal ways to put pressure on doctors or to 'guide' inexperienced medical staff as to what 'ought to be done' and thus achieve increased influence over the management of 'their' patients. In the largely 'gendered' social order of hospital nursing (in contrast perhaps to community nursing services), nurses may find themselves having to resort to the stratagems commonly employed by people in subordinate positions of relative powerlessness, or under conditions of oppression, to achieve their ends. Some of these techniques (sometimes referred to disparagingly as the use of 'feminine wiles') may well be required, such as the use of flattery, ingratiating submissiveness and other devious means to subvert authority, or alternatively by more assertive means to embarrass those in power.

In keeping with the dominant norms of this (largely patriarchal) order, nursing care is encumbered with much of the social apparatus that operates to undermine both the value of women's

practices in general and the social possibilities of their practitioners (Bowden 1997).

What nurses are entitled to do by law, and what they are or are not allowed to do by their union or professional associations, may also have a bearing on the matter. Some of these dilemmas of responsibility and authority are among those to which we will return in Chapter 9.

FOUR MODELS FOR THE ETHICS OF CARER–CLIENT RELATIONSHIPS

In his now famous book, Illich (1977) put forward a wealth of historical evidence to demonstrate that over the past century and a half, the medical profession has come to exercise increasing power and control over our lives, from birth to death. This process of the so-called 'medicalisation of life' is reflected in several historical developments, described by Illich as expressions of 'medical imperialism':

● the increasing professionalisation of medicine, nursing and allied professions
● the 'colonisation' by medical services of areas of human life that have been, traditionally, the domain of lay care (e.g. antenatal care and obstetrics, care of the mentally ill, terminal care and bereavement counselling, sex 'therapy' and assisted reproduction)
● the growing dependence of lay people on medical or alternative medicine 'experts' for help, with the corresponding loss of skills and confidence among lay people
● the increasing institutionalisation of health care and consequent hospitalisation of mentally and physically handicapped people, of elderly people and those who are terminally ill.

Despite recent trends to de-institutionalise health care, the effects of this medicalisation of life in industrialised countries have been far-reaching. This is especially important if the effect of other general demographic trends is taken into account (such as declining birth rates and an increased proportion of elderly people in the populations of these countries). These developments also have profound implications for the way we understand the ethics of health care and choices about forms of service delivery.

Recognition of these world trends has already led in the past 15 years to major new initiatives such as the World Health Organization's Health for All 2000 programme (WHO 1978, 1979, 1981). This programme, driven by state-directed health education and health promotion services, has attempted to reverse the process, help develop the confidence and competence of lay people, and encourage them to take more responsibility for their own health. The programme has also sought to influence governments to shift resources from 'high-tech' intensive hospital care to primary care and prevention, for the sake of achieving greater equity in health care. However, medicalisation of human life and its *rites de passage* is still the dominant reality in most countries. The vast majority of mothers in Europe still have their babies delivered in hospital rather than at home; people with severe learning difficulties or who are mentally ill tend to be kept in special mental hospitals; people depend on specialist clinics to deal with problems of drug and alcohol abuse, obesity, family planning, sexual problems and stress management; and the great majority of people die in hospital or in special terminal care units, whereas a century ago these problems would have been dealt with at home or in the community. This medicalisation of life and institutionalisation of health care bring their own special complications to the discussion of nursing ethics.

First of all, it should be noted that there are subtle and important differences between the ethics of different situations and settings in health care. Professional ethics in primary care or community settings differs in important respects from that which governs relationships in hospitals or other institutions (Freidson 1970a, 1994, Bayles 1989, Windt et al 1989). Different rules and constraints operate in each case. Yet other rules govern hospital management, political roles in the health professions and the development of health policy, making the ethics of these domains different again. This is not to say that the fundamental principles and values are not the same, but the problems and constraints, rules and forms of accountability do vary considerably with the exercise of power and responsibility in each of these different kinds of setting.

In this and the preceding discussion we have made use of four key concepts which are derived from sociological analysis of caring relationships, but which are very important and useful in philosophical analysis of ethics too. These concepts are *situations*, *roles*, *rules* and *arbiters* (Emmett 1966, Thompson 1979a).

It may seem obvious that the nurse meets patients or clients in a variety of different kinds of *situations*, but we do not usually take account of how much these situations differ ethically, e.g.:

- the district nurse attending a patient in her own home
- the casualty nurse dealing with an unconscious patient
- a hospital nurse attending a distressed patient trussed up in bed in an open hospital ward
- a psychiatric nurse relating to a compulsorily detained patient in a locked ward
- a health visitor offering health education at a 'well woman' or 'well man' clinic
- a nurse manager relating to the staff and patients of a whole hospital.

While we may be aware of these different situations, it is not always so obvious that the nurse's *role* in each of these *situations* may be different, that the *rules* of practice defining ethical duties and responsibilities in each situation may be different, and that the nurse will be accountable to different people who act as *arbiters* of the nurse's performance in each different context.

It is the aim of the next two sections to explore a number of different models for direct care and management relationships, to demonstrate how roles, rules and arbiters change in different professional settings or situations. The significance of these concepts for analysing the social context of a moral decision is examined in detail in Chapter 9.

Code, contract, covenant and charter

Nurses work in a wide variety of contexts and each of these presents the nurse with different kinds of ethical demands and ethical responsibility. These may be grouped roughly into four types.

- *Crisis intervention* – in accident and emergency, intensive care, emergency obstetrics, or acute medical, surgical or psychiatric units.
- *Consulting role* – giving advice on family planning, antenatal or postnatal care, interviewing or assessing competent adult patients, and making domiciliary visits in a monitoring, advisory, supportive or clinical capacity.
- *Continuity of care* – assisting people with health maintenance or care with chronic conditions. The first is the situation where the nurse is being proactive, helping people who are well, but whose lifestyles put them at risk. The second is most commonly illustrated in terminal care, but it applies equally to situations of ongoing care of people with severe mental handicap, patients with chronic mental or physical illness, in geriatric nursing, and in support of the bereaved.
- *Competition for service delivery* – where nurses are part of a consortium tendering to supply certain services, within a purchaser/provider 'internal economy'. Here the institution may have to give certain undertakings, relative to its service delivery, to maintain certain standards of performance on the part of its staff, as part of its quality assurance to customers, e.g. to other hospitals, health centres, clinics, general practitioners or private patients.

In these four different situations – in crisis intervention; in a consultative role; in providing health maintenance or continuity of care in chronic illness; and in 'customer focused' service delivery – professional ethics tends to be governed by different kinds of ethical models, namely code-based, contractual, covenantal and charter-based ethics, respectively.

Let us examine each of these models, considering what ethical principles underlie them (Box 4.2).

The reactive *crisis intervention model* has tended to set the agenda for nursing ethics and the ethics of health care, rather than the model of proactive

---

Box 4.2   Code, contract, covenant and charter models for professional ethics

Code – the duty of advocacy, to care for the patient or client
- *Paradigm* – crisis intervention
- *Client* – very dependent, vulnerable
- *Professional* – in total control, acts *parens patriae* as parent for the state
- *Principle* – protective beneficence (or non-maleficence)

Contract – regard for mutual rights/duties of health professional and patient
- *Paradigm* – voluntary request for help
- *Client* – independent, competent, ambulant
- *Professional* – offers service, acts in client's interest (fiduciary responsibility)
- *Principle* – justice and equity (or universal fairness)

Covenant – professional seeks to enable and empower the patient
- *Paradigm* – befriending, mutual partnership
- *Client* – self-directed, seeking support, companionship, partnership
- *Professional* – promotes autonomy of client as equal partner, acts as equal among equals
- *Principle* – respect for a person's rights (unconditional regard)

Charter – professional gives assurance of quality and standard of service provided
- *Paradigm* – customer service and accountability to patients as customers or clients
- *Client* – seen as 'customer' or 'purchaser' of service
- *Professional* – professionals make themselves professionally/financially accountable
- *Principle* – contractual justice (professional responsibility and respect for client)

---

intervention (e.g. in screening, prevention and health education). It is important to be aware that the reactive and proactive stances involve different ethical rules, assumptions and responsibilities. For example, in crisis intervention and consulting roles that are mainly *reactive* to a presenting problem or crisis, the nurse is required to exercise a primary duty of care, i.e. one of protective beneficence and doing no harm. By contrast, the nurse is expected to be *proactive* in the different situations of screening, health promotion and health maintenance, for well persons, on the one hand, and in providing 'continuity of care' for the chronically ill or palliative care for the terminally ill, on the other. Here the nurse is required to show particular regard or respect for the rights and dignity of the patient or client. In these latter roles, the nurse seeks to anticipate problems, to identify available options, to actively suggest solutions and to continue to offer support when therapy is no longer effective and the patient is dying. Apart from the roles being different, namely in moving from a predominantly reactive to a proactive mode, the duties required of the nurse in health education and terminal care might be regarded as *supererogatory*, i.e. as duties to the patient that 'go beyond the call of duty'. As we shall see, these situations raise ethical issues of a quite different kind from those which arise for nurses in the exercise of their usual clinical roles.

Code

Historically, each of the caring professions, in formulating its professional ethics, has tended to do so first in terms of a *code of practice*. Such codes tend to be preoccupied with consideration of what duties professionals must exercise when they are required to intervene in a crisis, particularly where the client or patient (sufferer) is unconscious or unconsultable, or incompetent by virtue of youth, senility or mental disorder. On the one hand, codes tend to justify intervention in a crisis, by appeal to the protective duty to care which the carer has for the vulnerable and incompetent and to protect them from harm (the principle of beneficence or non-maleficence). On the other hand, because carers are in charge and have fiduciary responsibility for the well-being of the persons committed to their care, codes also seek to prevent malpractice or abuse of clients, and to protect the carers themselves from unfair claims or demands being made on them by those for whom they provide care (or their representatives) (Fig. 4.1).

The law and ethics may often speak of the carer as acting in such situations *'in loco parentis'* (in place of the parent) or *'parens patriae'* (as a parent on behalf of the state). This quasi-parental duty of care carries with it the risk of becoming patronising and of creating and perpetuating dependency in the patient or client, because professionals take it upon themselves to take decisions on behalf of the person dependent on them for help – exempli-

CODE — crisis intervention

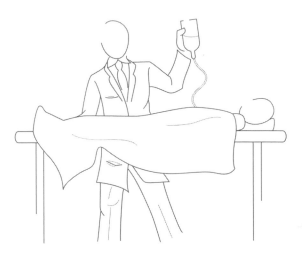

Patient	Health carer
• Very dependent and may be unconsultable, e.g. — unconscious — mentally disordered — infant or young child — incompetent or senile	• In position of power • Total responsibility • Acts *parens patriae* or *in loco parentis*

Key principle: BENEFICENCE or duty of care

Fig. 4.1

fied by the phrase 'doctor/nurse knows best'. Because of this, patronising professional attitudes and practices have been criticised for tending to 'infantilise' people, compromise their dignity and disregard their rights. However, we cannot dispense with protective beneficence for it remains an important professional value or personal virtue, because we are all extremely vulnerable at certain times in our lives and will always need others to help and protect us when we are weak or ill, and to defend our rights when we are unable to do so ourselves. (See Fig. 4.1.)

Contract

In the client-initiated consultation, the client voluntarily approaches the carer with some problem, seeking help. The carer is assumed to have the knowledge, expertise or access to resources to give the necessary help. The carer, in offering a service, is involved in direct negotiation with the client about the nature and scope of the help required and, in the process, establishes either a formal or informal *contract to care*. The client, by voluntarily entrusting herself into the care of the carer, accepts the responsibility to cooperate with the carer in the help or treatment given, e.g. by giving relevant personal details, allowing physical examination or other kinds of tests and assessments to be made. The carer accepts the duty to respect the trust shown by the client by providing a competent service, protecting the patient's dignity and observing the requirements of confidentiality. This contractual relationship, like other commercial and legal contracts, is governed by the demands of natural justice and recognition of mutual rights and duties. Although the relationship between the person with the problem

and the person with the power to help is an inherently unequal one, the same is likely to be true of our relationship with any service provider – accountant or lawyer, plumber or motor mechanic – from whom we seek help in a crisis (Fig. 4.2).

However, these situations are different from those where one is completely helpless and/or given help without being consulted. The fiduciary responsibility of the carer, as we have explained, is based on the fact that clients entrust themselves into the hands of their carers and agree to bear the cost of that commitment (and do not default on payment, where this is appropriate). Carers have a contractual moral and legal duty or responsibility to perform their service to the best of their ability, with knowledge, skill and consideration of the clients' rights and interests, and not to abuse or exploit their vulnerability. This is obviously a requirement of natural justice. (See Fig. 4.2.)

Covenant

In order to clarify what we mean by personal rights (particularly the rights of patients or clients), it is instructive to consider a third type of situation, which we may call a *covenantal relationship*. The need to recognise this different kind of relationship becomes poignantly necessary in situations where the patient is conscious and consultable, but chronically or terminally ill. In providing continuity of care in such situations, where there is no hope of cure but only amelioration of symptoms, a different kind of commitment is required on both sides. Here the contract to care may need to be renegotiated. Where the presuppositions of the original contract to care are based on therapeutic optimism, the expectation is that the carer has the necessary knowledge, skills and therapeutic resources to help. If this situation changes, so that the client's condition is chronic or deteriorating, and the carer can offer only palliative care or personal support, then the nature of the new situation ought to be acknowledged. The client has a particular moral right to know, to accept or refuse the new regimen of palliative care, and the right to appropriate privacy in

CONTRACT — request for help

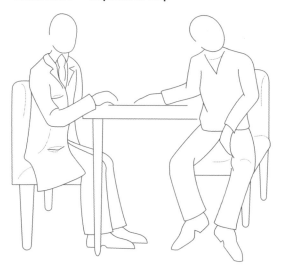

Patient

- Independent and able to negotiate terms of care, e.g.
  — lucid and competent
  — mobile and continent
  — voluntary request
  — cooperative

Health carer

- Offers expert help
- Contracts to care
- Acts on fiduciary responsibility

Key principle: JUSTICE — mutual rights/duties

Fig. 4.2

negotiations about these matters, because the terms of the 'contract' have changed. The carer, on the other hand, has a duty to make clear what is being offered. If this is emotional and spiritual support, counselling or just a commitment to 'care to the end', this should be understood on both sides as involving a change in the terms of the 'contract' and should not be imposed against the patient's will (Fig. 4.3).

The new kind of caring relationship which needs to be negotiated in such situations, and which requires a kind of supportive friendship or commitment of mutual fidelity, requires a different name. May (1983) suggested 'covenant', following the biblical meaning of an unconditional commitment and regard for the other. If care is not to be officiously given, or continued without due regard for the patient's views or personal rights,

COVENANT — terminal care

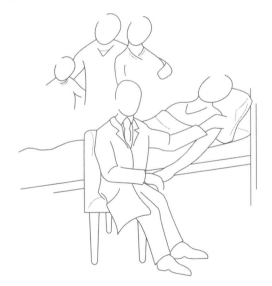

Patient

- Condition chronic or actually terminal,e.g.
  — lucid but very frail
  — mobility limited
  — needs much support
  — co operative

Health care

- Offers palliation, TLC (therapy not appropriate)
- Befriending and advocacy role
- Acts on supererogatory duty to promote patient's autonomy and dignity

Key principle: RESPECT— care for person

Fig. 4.3

and if the patient is to be prevented from becoming more dependent and either parasitic upon or exploitative of the care given, then despite the vulnerability of the patient, the scope and nature of the continuing caring relationship need to be reviewed and renegotiated. Another kind of situation to which covenantal ethics would seem to apply is that of non-directive counselling. Carl Rogers (1961) described one of the main ethical requirements for the counselling relationship as being a non-judgemental attitude of respect for the client or one of 'unconditional regard' (cf. Ramsey 1970).

The principle of respect for persons, which underlies this concept of covenantal ethics, is concerned with protecting not only the rights and dignity of the patient or client, but ultimately those of the carer as well. If the carer's exercise of these supererogatory duties is not to become a burden to the carer, or to be taken for granted by the patient, then they cannot be demanded, but have to be freely given by the carer on the basis of reciprocal trust and friendship.

The different principles of beneficence, justice and respect for persons, which underlie each of these three models, respectively, often stand in a relationship of tension to one another and we must address their competing demands. However, they are not usually mutually exclusive but often make complementary demands on us. Just as there are areas of overlap between the three different kinds of situations, so there are interconnections between beneficence, justice and respect for persons. In crisis intervention, beneficence has to be complemented by considerations of justice and respect for the rights of persons, if its exercise is not to lead to patronising attitudes to patients, and practices which create chronic dependency in them. In the voluntarily negotiated contract to care, the client may still need to be protected, as, for example, beneficence demands that the professional respects the patient's right to properly informed consent and does not exploit their vulnerability. In some situations, strict justice to groups of patients may have to be compromised when attention is required to address the special needs of individuals with acute conditions, resulting in less attention being given to the needs of other patients.

Conversely, regard for the rights of individuals may have to be balanced by consideration of the common good, as in the case where patients may have to be quarantined to protect others in an epidemic. Here, justice and respect for the rights of individuals may appear to be in conflict in the exercise of the general duty to care. (See Fig. 4.3.)

Client's charter

The fourth model we have mentioned is of a *client's charter*. Where hospitals, health care and other providers are expected to engage in competitive tendering for services, it has become popular to set out a charter of consumers' or clients' rights, and conditions for provider accountability and possible liability if the service offered were to fall below acceptable standards. The need for charters

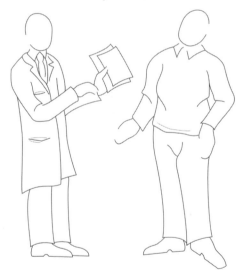

CHARTER — health promotion

Patient	Health care
• Healthy but at risk because of lifestyle, e.g. --- competent and lucid --- able to reject advice or accept need for help and freely co operate	• Pro active professional advice and training • Confidential counsellor and expert 'helper' • Acts on *supererogatory duty to promote patient's health and well-being*

Key principle: RESPECT— empowerment

Fig. 4.4

has arisen particularly with the attempt to operate health and social services provision on the principles of 'client choice' and 'customer focus' and more commercial models of 'quality assurance'. Issuing charters is supposed to assure consumers of greater public accountability on the part of health service providers for maintaining cost-efficient and effective services. However, the criteria for assessment tend to be determined by administrators rather than clinical staff, and whether or not they are in a better position to judge client needs can be debated.

The demand that health and social services should be operated on this kind of 'management ethic' or 'business ethic', rather than the more traditional 'service ethic' or 'caring ethic', is driven by several different kinds of moral demand. So far as the political rhetoric goes, the primary ethical demands, within this model, are for 'respect for consumers' rights' and 'justice to taxpayers' and to the 'purchasers of services', based on a guarantee from 'providers' of value for money. The first question to be asked is whether or not the interests of patients are best served in this way. The second is whether the role of 'beneficent protector of consumers' rights' sits comfortably on the shoulders of politicians, local or national, and whether, at the end of the day, it is not preferable that the health care staff who have direct care of patients should be responsible for decisions about the best use of scarce resources, based on their clinical expertise – provided that they can be held accountable for equitable, honest and economical use of public resources. (See Fig. 4.4.)

POWER RELATIONS IN INTERPROFESSIONAL TEAMWORK

Power structures and professional status

Few people, with the exception of a small number of self-employed practitioners, work on their own, and even the single-handed practitioner, doctor or nurse, as the workload increases is likely to require support staff. Most people in their working lives are employed in institutions of some kind and have to learn to work together, and make decisions together, with other people in teams. These teams would, almost of necessity, comprise people with a variety of professional backgrounds and expertise, this diversity, like that of a football or hockey team, being the basis of the strength of the team, but also a potential source of weakness. Our power is enhanced by participation in teams; we can do more together by cooperation, pooling our resources and a sensible division of labour, than we can do unassisted and on our own. However, lack of trust, non-cooperation, confusion of roles and inability to share power effectively can be a disaster – like a football team where a few 'stars' want to 'hog the ball'.

For the smooth and efficient functioning of a hospital, health centre or any other kind of health care institution employing a variety of medical, nursing, paramedical and administrative, technical and service staff, there has to be some clear division of labour, with a clearly understood hierarchy of power and authority, roles and responsibilities. In large hospitals, especially teaching hospitals, this can be further complicated by the involvement of part-time staff based in outside organisations – such as social workers or chaplains, hairdressers and podiatrists, counsellors and even entertainers. Like a stage cast for a play, or a symphony orchestra, there has to be some direction, some means of conducting and orchestrating the various functions and contributions of the various 'players' involved. Early work by the moral philosopher Dorothy Emmett (1966) drew attention to the four aspects of what she called *roles, rules, relations and arbiters* in the ethics of any functioning moral community.

Based on her pioneering work in social and corporate ethics, we suggest that if we are to do justice to the complexity of ethics in institutional life, then we must take account of what we call '*the four Rs*' – the diversity of *roles, rules, responsibilities, and lines of reporting*. These four dimensions serve to define the ethical aspects of our work in both multidisciplinary teams and complex institutions where there is a necessary division of labour and specialisation of roles and functions. As Emmett points out, the way that power is organised and shared, and responsibility and accountability determined, requires that we abandon simplistic models of individual ethical responsibility and decision-making.

In any formal institution there must be some people who, by virtue of their office, are responsible in the sense of being answerable for decisions, policies and their outcomes. This need not mean that they had a major share in making the decision (they may even have their own reservations about it, or may not have been able to prevent what happened). They have, however, to be prepared to take public responsibility without disclosing their private reservations or giving away confidential data on how the decision was taken (for some things must be discussed confidentially), and particularly they must be prepared to 'carry the can' if things go wrong. This is a feature of the nature of constitutional responsibility in institutional life (Emmett 1966, p. 201).

Using her analogy of a play, where actors are assigned different roles (and perhaps more than one role if the cast is small), it is necessary that each 'player' not only 'knows his lines', but understands and can enter into his role – be it king or beggar, scheming usurper, soldier, courtier, grand lady or flirtatious maid – for if he is to play the role properly and convincingly, he must be able to identify with the role and follow the rules of behaviour that apply to that role. There may even be, internal to the plot of the play, an established system of power relations between the players: the king has responsibility to rule and protect the interests of the country, the courtiers are responsible to (accountable to) the king and the court; the queen may in private 'rule' the king, but in public has to appear submissive; and while the flirtatious maid may have the king 'eating out of her hand', she may also be 'carrying on' with other members of court.

Many of the tensions and sources of conflict in hospital and primary care teams may well be due to lack of clarity about the scope of the responsibilities attaching to the roles performed by their various members, or lack of clarity about what rules apply and who is responsible to whom or for what. Research into teamwork in health care settings suggests that doctors, nurses, paramedics and administrative staff are generally ill-prepared to work in teams with other professionals – segregated as they are from one another in basic training.[3] Put another way, many professionals are trained as 'soloists' rather than as players in a symphony orchestra, and are ill-equipped or inexperienced in sharing power and responsibility. As in the production of a drama, or the training of a football team, the right kind of shared learning environment may be critical in building teamwork, as well as appreciation of the contributions or expertise which each 'player' can bring to the team.

Modern hospitals and health care institutions, especially in major cities, can be both very large and complex institutions. We may lament the fact that relations with patients or clients within such institutions tend to become impersonal and 'insti-tutionalised'. While the attempt to re-invent cot-tage hospitals and smaller nursing homes may help to restore a degree of intimacy to health care, we have to accept that the trend is towards the con-centration of health care facilities in ever larger institutions, or what WHO has called 'disease palaces'. The challenge is not only how to 'human-ise' such institutions, but also to ensure good work-ing relations between the increasingly mobile, and often part-time, professional staff working in them.

It may seem trite to say that one of the primary tasks in leadership of any team is to undertake role clarification, i.e. to clarify the structures of power, authority and responsibility in the team and to determine how power is to be shared in practice between members of the team. This means that the boundaries of roles and ground rules for their performance need to be carefully and explicitly negotiated, clarifying the scope of each player's responsibility and line of reporting or accountability to the other members of the team. As a means of preventing a lot of misunder-standing, tension and even conflict in a team, it may be useful as a team-building exercise for members to work together to complete a grid such as the one illustrated in Figure 4.5.

In the process of working through such a model, the areas of overlapping responsibility and of potential competition or conflict can be identified, and the team members can determine what ethical ground rules they would operate to resolve disagreements or conflict. In many cases, the confusions which give rise to misunderstand-ing or conflict within the team may be due to unusual or unexpected circumstances, or the arrival of a new member of the team who has not been through proper induction into the 'ward cul-ture' or the tacit or explicit ethical conventions operating within the team.

Consider Case History 4.1, which illustrates some of the complexities that may arise in a crisis

Player	Role or function	Rules that apply	Responsible for	Reporting to
Nurse manager or matron				
Other grades of nurses				
Consultant or other doctors				
Paramedics or therapists				
Manager or administrator				
Service staff, cleaners etc.				
Social worker or chaplain				

Fig. 4.5   Roles, rules, responsibilities and reporting – the four Rs.

case history 4.1

'David' – the boy with a broken neck. (From Thompson 1979a)

David, aged 13 years, was the only child of middle-aged parents. He was attending a local public school as a 'day boy'. Playing a 'banned' game – a special form of 'leap-frog' – another boy landed right on his neck, causing spinal cord transection, ischaemic, progressive and permanent damage.

Day 1. On admission to the paediatric neurosurgical unit, there was already very clear evidence of spinal cord damage: loss of movement and sensation in the lower limbs up as far as the lower abdomen. David was a handsome boy, large and obviously physically very fit, and was fully conscious and very anxious.

Over the next few hours, his condition deteriorated and the level of loss of function rose. A tracheostomy was performed under local anaesthetic, to enable a respirator to be used. David, responding to sedation and constant reassurance from the medical and nursing staff, coped extraordinarily well with this unpleasant procedure.

The consultant, who was pessimistic about the possibility of recovery of the cord from the damage, had a long session with David's parents. David was kept fairly heavily sedated and given 'constant care' nursing.

Day 2. David suffered total loss of all sensation and function of the upper limbs. The parents visited and asked if there was any hope of recovery. They were told as gently as possible by the consultant that he believed there was no hope. He discussed David's possible future as a quadriplegic. The ward sister was also present. The parents saw David and went out for lunch.

They returned after several hours and asked to speak to the consultant. They requested that no further efforts should be made to prolong David's life and asked that he should not be allowed to suffer. The consultant was surprised and disturbed by their response and suggested a second opinion. The parents did not feel this was necessary, but the consultant insisted. The second opinion confirmed the same diagnosis and prognosis.

A 'case conference' was convened by the consultant, involving the ward sister, staff nurse, registrar and the anaesthetist who operated the respirator. A decision was eventually reached to discontinue antibiotics, to provide suction to the tracheostomy only if the patient was distressed and to increase sedation.

Day 3. David was found wide awake, alert and very anxious. The night nurse had withheld two doses of sedation, because he was asleep (in spite of formal instruction that sedation be given 4–hourly). She said it was against her religion to give drugs unnecessarily. David asked to see the ward sister as soon as she appeared on duty. He asked her directly if he was dying. This she denied vehemently and spent some time with him talking to him.

The parents visited later in the day and when he was asleep they came to say goodbye. They never returned. David slept most of the day and sedation was given regularly. He had ice-cream and 'sherry and lemonade' to drink when he was awake, as this was his favourite tipple. That night there was a different night nurse on duty, because the consultant had intervened and had the other nurse removed.

Day 4. No sedation was needed. David died at approximately 13.00 h.

---

with unexpected developments in the case. In the 'wash-up' or debriefing with the staff involved in this case, which caused great distress to all 'players' in the drama, the following were some of the issues identified as causes of tension and conflict within 'the team':

● The unexpected reaction of the parents, which upset the whole team: doctors, nurses and support staff
● The lack of confidence of the consultant, upset by the reaction of the parents, and the resulting confusion caused by his apparent abrogation of responsibility to give decisive leadership
● The poor communication between the nurses, day staff and night nurses, over the agreed care plan, creating a crisis of conscience for the night nurse, lack of support for her, and resulting disarray on the team
● Lack of a clear focus to the case conference for members of the ward team (without including the parents), and whether it was a means of sharing responsibility or avoiding it
● Was the case conference designed to reach a consensus, or was it a device for the consultant to seek personal support and reinforcement for his decision?

Thus, many ethical problems, interprofessional tensions and even interpersonal conflicts may have their origin both in the traditional structure of power relations, between medical, nursing and other staff, and in the actual way in which power is exercised or shared within 'the team'. Understanding the ethics of such complex situations may have more to do with analysing the power relations involved than with analysing questions of disagreements of principle.

Power structures and gender roles

It is a remarkable fact of modern industrialised society that the services provided by the *caring professions*, e.g. nursing, physiotherapy, occupational therapy, radiotherapy, social work, counselling and primary school teaching, are provided mainly by women, while in these professions men still tend to predominate in senior positions and in management. Much attention has been given recently to the contribution of gender–role stereotyping to the social construction of the identity and character of nursing as a profession. This is reflected in both studies of the history of nursing[4] and sociological studies from a feminist perspective.[5] In her illuminating treatment of the ethics of caring and gender-sensitive ethics, Bowden (1997, p. 104) says about the position of nursing in health care:

The most outstanding feature of this functional organization and its hierarchical ranking is its sex-defined roles. Nursing practices are overwhelmingly carried out by women, and the activities, responsibilities and status associated with them call upon the kind of social capacities and standing that women have typically exercised in their traditional domestic roles. Accordingly the gendered social order is a crucial constitutive factor in the practice of nursing. In keeping with the dominant norms of this order, nursing is encumbered with much of the social apparatus that operated to undermine both the value of women's practices in general and the social possibilities of their practitioners.

It is sometimes claimed that the reason why women are attracted to these professions is that they are 'natural carers', and some feminist writers (notably Gilligan 1982) seem to suggest that an ethic of caring is distinctively feminine. While there is an increasing number of women medical practitioners, especially in primary care, in hospital medicine male doctors predominate and traditional male/female role stereotypes still influence typical doctor/nurse relationships. The assumption generally made is that doctors lead and nurses follow, that doctors have the power and authority to take decisions, and nurses are expected to be submissive, dutiful and obedient, like Victorian wives. These stereotypical roles in the division of labour in health care have greatly influenced the way power is exercised and shared (or not shared) in relationships between doctors and nurses in health care teams, and hence our understanding of nurses' ethical responsibilities to patients and their doctors within those roles. Bowden (1997, p. 104) continues:

[Nurses'] relations with patients are closely tied into relations with other members of the institution. Nursing care thus occupies an 'in between' position in the organisation of the public response to the patient's need, and is infused with the tensions of sustaining interdependent but differently focused relations with different levels of authority.

Many of the ethical problems which confront nurses in their daily practice are complicated by these underlying gender-related presuppositions which affect the way power and authority are traditionally exercised in hospitals as institutions, and also complicate the interpersonal relationships of nurses and medical staff as working colleagues. Growe's (1991) research illustrates that 'most doctors see the nurse "as provider of a conglomerate of insignificant services" e.g. "mother, child, secretary, wife, waitress, maid, machine and psychiatrist"!' While nurses sensitised to the sexual politics traditional in health care institutions are increasingly able to assert their professional independence and confront these issues with their medical and other colleagues, many still have to resort to informal ways to overcome the 'putdowns' and lack of respect for their expertise by the medical hierarchy. This is especially the case in old and established institutions, with entrenched rules and practices that can result in the oppression and exploitation of nurses.

Other analysts (notably Reverby 1987) have tried to avoid the idealised picture of women as archetypal 'carers' and pioneers of the 'caring professions', and have emphasised that they have been forced (often by economic necessity) to take up these forms of employment due to their exclusion from others where men have had a monopoly. Women have had to find niches for themselves in the male-dominated labour market – initially in domestic service, in child care, as governesses and teachers, and then as nurses etc. They have had to take advantage of opportunities for employment which did not necessarily require any special education or training (from which they were largely excluded anyway). The great attraction of nursing was that 'caring' gave respectable moral status to the role, while offering training on the job. This is summed up by Bowden (1997):

The key feature of [nursing] history is its profound entanglement with conventional social constructions of women's character and roles. Modern hospital nursing drew on the social virtues of caring as an act of love *and obligation* to the needs of family and friends, held to be embedded in the natural character of women, rather than a vital function of nurses' work, valuated by time, expertise and money.

In Chapter 6 we will have more to say about the 'ethics of caring'. But before we leave the issue of the gender-determined division of labour in health care, we will briefly comment on how this has affected the economics and organisation of nursing itself.

As Bowden points out (1997, pp. 129–130) the Victorian way of giving respectability to women's work was not to recognise either their need or their right to work, but to offer 'training' that was a 'disciplined process of honing womanly virtue'. Drawing on the work of Reverby, she observes that:

Two categories of nurses were to be trained: the 'gentlewomen' who would have the 'qualifications that will fit them to be superintendents', and those women 'used to household work' who would be the regular nurses . . . . The 'training programmes' at the heart of nursing's professional status offered the perfect forum for this co-opting of the womanly duty to care, turning it into obedience to external authority. Reverby explains that hospital administrators were quick to recognise that opening a 'nursing school' ensured a ready supply of low-cost and disciplined young labourers, who were eager to offer their services in exchange for the professional training offered. Frequently, however, the hospital's nursing school and its nursing service were identical.

Because nursing care has always been the major 'service' being offered or 'product' being marketed to potential 'consumers' by hospitals, the economics of providing nursing services at the lowest possible cost has driven the quest for profitability of private hospitals and cost reduction in the public sector. It can be argued that exploitation of nurses, in terms of relatively low wages, long hours and poor working conditions, has been rationalised in terms of their commitment to a service ethic based on a duty to care, and that this has not only been a feature of the political economy of hospitals and institutionalised health care from the beginning, but continues to be the case to a greater or lesser degree. It is only through collective bargaining and the unionisation of nursing labour that nurses have been able to achieve better pay and working conditions. However, they remain captive to a personalist ethic of dutiful care to patients and an ethos of subservience to authority that make it painful and difficult for nurses to go on strike.

The dilemmas faced by nurses over taking industrial action, which will be discussed in Chapter 9, strike at the very foundations of the identity which has been constructed for nurses by the health care system, the media and public opinion as 'self-sacrificing angels of mercy' dedicated above all else to 'tending the sick and alleviating suffering'. It goes against the grain for nurses to accept the role of employees in the workforce of a large service industry, rather than 'professionals'. However, issues of industrial relations, employee rights, fair pay and working conditions become increasingly important to nurses, as employees, with the industrialisation of health care.

FOUR MODELS FOR THE ETHICS OF MANAGEMENT

There is another group of situations in which nurses or other health professionals are involved when they move out of direct patient care into *management*, into *teaching and research*, in the exercise of *community leadership*, and in more 'political' roles in *corporate policy direction*. Here the models which are applicable become more complex and various, but we may discuss them under four different headings (see Box 4.3).

Command management

The exercise of power and responsibility in traditional management roles is tied up with the concept of authority. To exercise authority you must

---

Box 4.3   Models for management in delivery of health care

Command management – traditional model
(e.g. traditional hospital, preventive and health education services)
- *Style* – directive management based on power of office
- *Paradigm* – administration of medical or preventive services
- *Main ethic* – responsible duty to care (protective beneficence)

Critical expertise – research-driven model
(e.g. 'evidence-based' nursing, intersectoral 'new public health' approach)
- *Style* – authoritative advice based on scientific evidence and research
- *Paradigm* – medical or academic health research institute
- *Main ethic* – rational justice (concern for social equity and the common good)

Community development – facilitative leadership model
(basis of 'community health approach' and positive health promotion)
- *Style* – facilitative, participative and democratic
- *Paradigm* – promoting health through community self-help and skills transfer
- *Main ethic* – respect for personal and community rights (empowering people)

Corporate planning of health policy – strategic planning model
(e.g. 'purchaser/provider' internal market and economic management approach)
- *Style* – proactive engagement with politics of health care delivery
- *Paradigm* – business management and quality assurance
- *Main ethic* – economic justice for taxpayers through cost-efficiency savings

---

be authorised by some person or body of persons to hold some official post, or to carry out some official function. Authority in this sense means legitimate power – power legitimated by election, official selection or promotion, or direct appointment by higher authority – as might be exercised by a matron or nurse administrator. To exercise authority also means to exercise power in such a way that you work to promote the well-being of those over whom you have authority, and do not act just to promote your own interest or those of the institution. Thus the naked or dictatorial exercise of power offends against the duty to care, the

requirements of natural justice and respect for persons under your authority.

The traditional style of line management within medicine and nursing has been based on a combination of two types of authority – the authority of their supposed expert knowledge and skill and the power of office vested in the doctor/nurse manager, by virtue of their position of public responsibility within the hospital or health care system. Within this tradition, the emphasis has been on the personal responsibility and authority of the manager to take decisions under pressure and often in situations of crisis. It is often argued that the centralisation of authority in a single person is more efficient – where quick decisions are required. While such systems are not necessarily authoritarian, they can be, because they do not operate within consultative structures.

Management styles, even within the traditional line management model, can vary according to the personality and skills (or lack of skills) of the manager, and the models of management applied can also vary. Personal management styles can vary from a controlling style to a permissive one, from directive to democratic, from authoritarian to consensus-based. Line management, or a straight 'top-down' hierarchical chain of command, has tended to be the predominant pattern of management within nursing, and it has a long history in hospital organisation in most countries. This is hardly surprising given the historical associations of nursing with religious orders and military service, and the requirements of large institutions dealing with situations of crisis such as war or disaster, or medical, surgical and psychiatric emergencies. However, as the pattern of morbidity in the community is changing, new forms of team management, with shared authority and responsibility, are becoming accepted as more appropriate in other areas, such as primary care nursing, age care, rehabilitation and long-term nursing of medical and psychiatric patients.

Hierarchical line management in nursing and health care generally tends to have been associated with the predominant role of doctors in both clinical and administrative decision-making. This model serves well the patterns of management and administration appropriate to the delivery of clinical services and centrally directed public health and traditional health education. (Compare the discussion of the clinical and administrative models for resource allocation in Ch. 8.)

The ethical values which predominate in the exercise of responsibility within this model or system of management are ones predicated on the duty of protective and responsible care, particularly towards patients. Those in authority have not only great power, but also heavy responsibilities at both a practical and a legal level. In more democratic styles of management, both the authority and the responsibility can be shared. Instead of the most senior staff having to make all the decisions and carry all the responsibility, executive and clinical responsibility can be devolved downwards to less senior staff to a greater or lesser degree.

It is not our purpose to discuss the advantages or disadvantages of the different models or styles of management here, but rather to stress that each embodies certain values and is based on different formal and informal ethical conventions. Roles will be different within each system, as well as the formal and informal rules which obtain, and expectations about who is responsible ('who carries the can') and to whom officers are accountable ('who will blame me if things go wrong?'). From an ethical point of view, each kind of management may be exercised well or badly and needs to be assessed in context and on its own terms.

Thus traditional line management invests considerable power in those at the top, who, it is assumed, will exercise power responsibly in a just and beneficent way, for the good of patients and to maintain the quality of their care. When managers are employed with a specific mandate to improve efficiency and to make savings, whether they be health professionals or 'business' managers, the same ethical values are invoked. Appeal to the values of justice and beneficence is made in defence of the new managerialism ('Let the managers manage') and their application of the criteria of economic rationalism in determining priorities. Thus, for example, if there have to be staff cuts, it is implied that these will be justifiable on both ethical and economic grounds, that decisions will not be made capriciously but in a way that is fair, protects the wider interests of the service, puts the interests of patients first, does not discriminate against particular groups and has due regard for the statutory rights of employees. Whether these values are consistently applied may be disputed, but within this model they serve as its rationale.

Alternatively, in a more democratic style of team management on the ward or in the community, the values of respect for persons are likely to have higher priority. In principle, this should be apparent in the special respect and attention given to the rights of individual patients and their needs. It should also be reflected in the style of interaction between staff of different professional backgrounds, in showing respect for one another's expertise, power-sharing, fair distribution of work and responsibility, and exchange of information about patients or clients.

Critical expertise

Professional knowledge and skill have been commonly invoked as justifying the appointment of doctors or senior nurses to positions of management in hospitals and the administration of health services. This emphasis on the supposed critical expertise which would inform their contribution to management has worked together with the traditional hierarchical nature of the professions to influence the pattern of management in health services worldwide, for better or for worse.

In the 1980s and 1990s, politicians and health service planners and economists began to challenge the claims made by professionals that they were necessarily best equipped to administer costly health care resources – pointing out that few of the medical and nursing managers in positions of authority had any professional training in management or in the administration of public financial resources. However, whether the new generation of appointed 'business-style' managers has done a better job can be disputed and remains to be critically evaluated. Whatever the outcome of the debate, it cannot be a simple either/or (either health professionals or business-trained managers), but rather a case of health services needing input from both. There will always be a critical need for decision-making in health care to be informed by actual clinical experience in medicine and nursing.

All professions base their right to practise, their claim to special status and regard in the eyes of other professions and the public on their mastery of certain knowledge and skills. It is also on the basis of their expertise that they are given responsibility for the disposal and administration of certain public resources (Bayles 1989, Freidson 1994). Therefore, education and training play an important part in the preparation of professionals for their work, serving both as a basis for their claims to expertise, whether in helping others or in performing some other function, and as the means for legitimating their power and authority in the exercise of that service to the public. The responsibility of a profession to maintain the highest possible standards in education and training is not just about maintaining status and power, but perhaps more fundamentally it is a requirement of justice to ensure that they are competent to provide a skilled and efficient service for the benefit of their clients and society as a whole.

However, education and training are not of much value if they perpetuate bad practice, if they are never properly evaluated. Thus teaching and research must be integrally related, in the interests of ensuring the competence and efficiency of staff and the service as a whole, and the most effective and cost-efficient care for clients and patients. This is where 'evidence-based practice' becomes particularly relevant. Ability to provide objective evidence and sound research findings to justify specific interventions or general nursing practice is not only a demand of scientific integrity, but ultimately also an ethical demand. Incompetence or the use of ineffective measures is not only blameworthy in the individual, but is unjust to others who depend on one's expertise, and who may be paying as well. Not only the financial cost but also the human cost should be considered, thus raising questions of respect for persons and their rights as well. In comparative evaluation of the cost efficiency of different procedures or management practices, not only are considerations of an economic nature relevant, but so too is the common good of patients.

Specific ethical issues in teaching and research are discussed in Chapter 8, but the point of raising them here is that critical enquiry and proper evaluation are important ethical responsibilities of any profession. Competent and efficient care is a moral demand of the principle of beneficence, in the protection of clients from incompetence and malpractice, and it is not possible to prevent either without sound education and training, and scientific research to validate professional practice. Truthfulness is not only about honesty and sharing information with individual patients or clients, it is also about scientific integrity, rigour in enquiry, and honesty in the publication of research findings for the benefit of all. Use of sound knowledge and skills is essential for the training of professionals in the responsible care and rehabilitation of those who seek help. This is a requirement of beneficence and respect for their rights, and it is also a requirement of justice. Skills and knowledge acquired in training are meant to be shared with clients and used to assist them back to health and greater independence.

Community development

The traditional professions (clerical, legal, medical, nursing and teaching) have been shaped in their ethos and ethics by three factors: first that professionals claim a degree of autonomy in making decisions about their work, based on their expertise; secondly, that they have tended to deal with their 'clients' on a reactive, individual and one-to-one basis; and thirdly, that the profession itself has been self-regulating. However, the development of institutionalised and, to an increasing degree, commercialised and corporatised professional practice forces a reappraisal of the traditional image of the consulting professions. First, fewer and fewer are self-employed single-handed practitioners, but tend to be partners or employees in large businesses or public sector organisations. Secondly, they are increasingly forced to address the wider social context from which their clients come, and which influence their lifestyles and give rise to their problems.

Classically, as pointed out in the previous section, doctors and nurses have tended predominantly to provide a reactive service, responding to the obvious needs or symptoms presented by the patient, rather than actively seeking out undeclared pathology or hidden causes of the patient's illness. 'Health' professionals have been mainly employed in treating disease, rather than actively promoting health. With reductions in infant mortality, success in the control of infectious diseases, increased life expectancy of people in most countries (exclusive of those afflicted with HIV/AIDS) and a shift towards the greater bulk of morbidity being lifestyle-related, the demands being made on medicine and nursing are changing. Health professionals are being increasingly employed to undertake more preventive and screening functions, including positive health promotion, and as a consequence are having to move away from an individualistic model of health care provision to a greater involvement in community medicine.

However, professionals have never really been able to be simply a 'law unto themselves', for to be a professional, by definition, means that one exercises a public role, a public office. It is therefore impossible for professionals to ignore their duty of accountability to the wider community, without ceasing to be responsible professionals. In this sense all professionals have a public and political role in addition to the particular function which they perform within the division of labour. Nurses, especially those in senior positions, have to take on public and 'political' roles in many situations. Even within conventional hospital-based nursing, they are likely to be required to contribute to committees for a variety of purposes: administrative, planning, research and training. They may also be involved in professional associations, trade unions, government advisory and policy-making bodies, or interprofessional, interagency or international committees. They may also be professionally trained to be involved in community nursing and community health, where they are active in promoting self-help groups, community development projects and community action, or even in direct political action at local, regional or national level.

The relevance of the community development model for health care in the 21st century lies in the fact that it is increasingly obvious that people's health status is directly influenced by the socioeconomic conditions in which they live. These factors not only can contribute directly to increased morbidity or help promote better health for individuals, but social and economic conditions may increase or limit the freedom of groups of people to choose healthier diet or lifestyles, to change what may be a degraded or polluted environment or to influence the health behaviour of their society. Living under conditions of multiple deprivation, people often live in conditions of 'learned helplessness' (Seligman 1975, Peterson et al 1993), passive to the forces of their environment, the misleading influence of commercial advertising of products damaging to their health, and limited by the inadequacy of health and welfare provision by the state or voluntary organisations.

The more people are trapped in such conditions, the less effective traditional treatment-based health care tends to be in combating disease and disability, and the less able are people to make use of the opportunities that education and preventive services provide. It is here that a much more proactive approach has been seen to be necessary, and a community development approach shown to be effective. The example and success of community development initiatives pioneered in poor developing countries, in empowering people to improve the health of their communities, have led to these methods being applied in the industrialised world – where people have either become infantilised by dependence on institutionalised care, or where deprived communities, living on the fringes of affluent societies, suffer serious deprivation and lack of accessible services.

As a model for 'managing' health services, community development involves a radically different approach and a changed role for health professionals. Instead of administering health resources centrally, control of these has to be devolved to the local community and local people. Health professionals have to change their self-image and understanding of the contribution they can make. Instead of being providers of health services or health education, the health professional has to adopt the role of facilitator, information resource, skills trainer – encouraging people to take more control of their lives and health choices. The expertise of the health professional has to be put at the service of the people who are encouraged to identify their own health needs and to find the best means to deal with them. Doctors and nurses may have to surrender their controlling positions, to become involved in community action and community politics as resource persons rather than as patronising 'carers' always assuming the role of 'leaders'. They have to learn to work with a variety of people, both professionals and community leaders, to maximise the community's ability to help itself, rather than to depend either on paternalistic health or social service personnel, or on the 'nanny state'.

The skills required for effective facilitation of community development and participation in teamwork with what may be a very mixed bunch of people have to be learned, for they do not come naturally to health professionals who have been systematically trained to act as skilled soloists. While people are given management training and taught to teach and do research, most skills associated with the exercise of professional responsibility in these community-based roles have to be learned by experience, by a kind of 'baptism by immersion', living and working in the communities they serve, not living in comfortable suburbs and commuting to clinics in 'deprived areas'. However, community development cannot succeed without some reliance on and cooperation with more traditional health treatment and preventive services, and hence a 'mixed economy' of care may be required with a range of management styles appropriate to different aspects or functions.

Similarly, working on committees may be less glamorous than nursing patients. Campaigning for higher professional standards or better patient care, through professional bodies, unions or pressure groups, may seem remote from direct patient care. Community development and community action may seem to mix nursing and politics. But all these activities are relevant to nursing ethics. Ethics and politics are never totally separate or separable, but continuous with one another, as Aristotle recognised 2000 years ago (Thomson 1976). Personal responsibility and professional responsibility mix ethics and politics, for all professionals should be publicly accountable. Health care cannot be simply about the alleviation of individual distress. It also concerns the good of society and the promotion of the good of the commonwealth. Nursing ethics is about service which promotes the rights and dignity of individual patients, and also the common good, and it is also about local and individual health promotion as well as action to ensure global health for all in the 21st century.

Corporate planning

As long as the focus of medicine and nursing is on acute care, the tendency is for styles of management to be driven by presenting need and to fall into a kind of short-termism and crisis management. The strength of the caring ethic is its focus on the individual and the concrete needs of the present, and the personalist and individualistic values which go with direct involvement in the lives and crises of people have contributed to the particular character of the 'caring professions'. However, when it comes to managing resources for large hospitals or institutions, conducting scientific research in medicine or nursing, organising preventive and health promotion services, or health service planning, a more long-term and strategic approach is required. Whether traditionally trained health professionals are equipped to take on these responsibilities, without further specialised training, may be doubted. Another consequence of this bias towards a personalist and privatised ethics of health care is reflected in the reluctance of health professionals to engage in what they tend to refer to derogatively as 'politics'. However, to take on the responsibilities of management is necessarily to have to engage in 'politics' at several levels – internal hospital or institutional 'politics', health board or health authority politics, and perhaps at a wider level in relation to the national government health department. However, if the nexus between ethics, power and responsibility is recognised, then perhaps we can be liberated from the kind of 'bleeding heart' view of ethical responsibility and recognise that the ethics of management responsibility and public accountability requires a realistic understanding of power, politics and the relationships between them. The emphasis on corporate planning is a necessary consequence of moving onto the level where objective and transparent processes of accountability for staff and financial resources are required of those exercising management roles on behalf of society.

The emphasis on strategic planning, on models of organisational development based on continuous improvement of the quality and efficiency of services, and of corporate ethical responsibility and accountability are relatively recent developments in the history of health care. It is during the past 20 years, in particular, that the corporate planning model of management took hold. While it is often asserted that this was an import from the world of business and industry, in fact it is within the public sector, in the sphere of government planning and public administration that these concerns first emerged. The history of health services within the various welfare states around the world has been one of attempts to contain public expenditure on health and welfare services by centralised strategic planning and publicly accountable administration. However, before the advent of this kind of 'economic rationalism', there were serious attempts to base the administration of health services on a proactive public health model rather than to allow expenditure to be driven simply by reactive treatment-based services. A focus on epidemiology and scientifically based community medicine has contributed to a more strategic approach to the planning and administration of health and nursing services.

To evaluate any activity, it is necessary to have clear goals and set objectives so that achievements and failures can be measured against these objectives. The watch-cry 'management by objective' which became popular in the 1970s perhaps marked the beginning of a more systematic approach in the UK to strategic planning in health care, not simply at the macro level, but encouraged at all levels in the UK NHS. Since then, many philosophies of administration and styles of strategic management have been tried, each enjoying a period of fashionable influence under different government administrations. The 'quality movement' has perhaps been the most influential (see James 1996), including phases associated with 'quality control', 'quality assurance', 'quality improvement' and 'total quality management'! What is significant about the quality movement is that, while earlier approaches to strategic planning and management were essentially bureaucratic, the 'quality movement' insinuated values into the process, by emphasising the connection between corporate values and corporate goals and the critical role that values play in decision-making, whether implicitly or explicitly. The purpose of strategic ethical management is thus to combine the greater effectiveness and efficiency involved in applying the methods of strategic planning to corporate administration of human and financial resources and to improving production and / or the provision of services, with the development of a more coherent ethical culture and 'moral community' in a corporation driven by commitment to the same values.

Corporate planning thus does not simply involve the corporate executive writing a strategic plan and a detailed business plan which is then imposed on the organisation. While strategic planning is often attempted in that way, it is largely ineffective and its effects cosmetic rather than real. The objective of strategic planning is to change the behaviour of everyone in an organisation from the top down. By involving the whole organisation in the process, awareness of and commitment to the same goals and values should result, with associated movement of the organisation in the direction determined by the whole corporation. Strategic ethical management is essentially about an organisation setting a clear course, with defined milestones and realistic and achievable objectives within an agreed time-scale. It is a process of clarification of the primary *raison d'être* ('mission') of the organisation, and assessment of its strengths and weaknesses, of the challenges and opportunities it faces, as well as the threats to its continued existence. In this process, the 'vision' of what it is and where it is going emerges, and it becomes clearer what the whole organisation and its employees most desire to achieve, i.e. what their 'values' and 'goals' are. Values, as we have said before, are important, not only for individuals but also for corporations, for we stake our decisions on our values. They are the most important instrumental means by which we achieve our short- and long-term goals (see Ch. 1, 'Shared and changing values').

Within the framework of this process, if it is conducted thoroughly and well, it becomes clearer what is essential and what is non-essential business of the organisation, what problems need to be addressed, what opportunities there are for improvement and how best to deploy staff and financial resources. By determining clearly the priority values and goals of the organisation, it becomes possible to develop functional strategies to assess the resources required to achieve our goals, to set standards for performance and targets for achievement. Effective and efficient management is thus not driven simply by economic rationalism, important though cost reduction and

income generation may be, but also within a framework in which wider corporate and community values can be factored in to determine the real human and financial costs and benefits of our strategic plan. This is not possible unless ethical policy is developed alongside each aspect of the strategic plan and its application carefully monitored in practice.

The benefits of sound strategic ethical management do not accrue solely to the organisation itself, because such management also ensures that the organisation is able to be more fully accountable to all of its stakeholders for the administration of corporate and/or public resources (see Ch. 8 'Frameworks for policy-making on management of resources').

 further reading

History of nursing
Allan P, Jolley M 1982 Nursing, midwifery and health visiting, since 1900. Faber & Faber, London – *a comprehensive overview of the history of nursing, particularly in Britain*

Bullough V L, Bullough B 1984 History, trends and politics of nursing. Appleton-Century-Crofts, Norwalk, CT – *a more comprehensive global perspective on nursing from the USA*

Maggs C 1987 Nursing history: the state of the art. Croom Helm, London – *a critical review of the process and presuppositions behind constructing a history of nursing*

Teamwork
Barnett L, Abbatt F 1994 District action research and education: resource book for problem-solving in health systems. Macmillan, London – *an essentially practical guide for everyday use*

Clare A W, Corney R (eds) 1982 Social work and primary health care. Academic Press, London – *a critical overview of the reality of teamwork in primary care*

Mears P 1994 Health care teams: building continuous quality improvement. St Lucie Press, Delroy Beach, FL – *applying the methods of modern management theory to health care teams*

Pritchard P, Pritchard J 1992 Developing teamwork in primary health care: a practical workbook. Oxford University Press, London – *a useful resource for nurse teachers in primary care*

Robertson A, Thompson I E, Porter M 1992 Social policy and administration: certificate in health education

open learning project. Keele University, Staffordshire, vol 2, p 131–138 – *a critical review of some of the problems in 'teamwork' and what needs to be done about these*

Roe M 1995 Working together to improve health: a team handbook. Queensland Primary Health Care Reference Centre, Herston, Queensland – *an Australian view of the issues in PHC teamwork*

Thomas M 1990 Final report: development and improvement of primary health care teams. Centre for Medical Education, Dundee University Medical School, Dundee – *a revealing example of practical research*

The gender politics of nursing
Ashley J 1976 Hospitals, paternalism and the role of the nurse. Teachers' College Press, New York – *a critique of the built-in and institutionalised gender bias of traditional hospital structures*

Bishop A, Scudder J (eds) 1985 Caring, curing, coping: nurse, physician, patient relationships. University of Alabama Press, Alabama – *a critical examination of the price of gender politics in health care institutions and practice*

Bowden P 1997 Caring: gender sensitive ethics. Routledge, London, ch 3 – *a philosophical exploration of issues of caring in mothering, nursing, friendship and citizenship*

Davis C 1995 Gender and the professional predicament in nursing, Open University Press, Buckingham – *a sociological critique of gender as defining the scope and limitations of the nurse*

end notes

1 This section is adapted, with permission, from *Putting Ethics to Work*, by Thompson & Harries (1997).
2 Both these emphases can be found in Greek philosophy and in the Old Testament. Aristotle emphasises that ethics is concerned both with realisation of one's powers and the conditions for human flourishing (see Aristotle's *Nicomachean Ethics*; Thomson 1976). In particular, he emphasises that the 'good' for which individuals and societies strive is the fulfilment of their potential or power of being, and ethics is thus concerned above all with clarifying the conditions for human flourishing – in personal, family, business and political life. The biblical concept of Shalom, often translated as 'peace', means 'the tranquillity of right order' – where power is used responsibly and justly for the common good.
3 See recommended reading on research on teams.
4 See recommended reading on historical sources.
5 See recommended reading on social scientists.

some suggestions on method

Does everyone have different values?
Having first established clear ground rules for the exercise, one might begin by asking students to think about and write brief notes about a personal experience in which they became aware of the moral rules or boundaries within which they had to act. They could then be asked to share in confidential pairs the nature of the crisis they confronted. Each should listen to the others without interrupting for 3–5 minutes. Then they should be asked to discuss the similarities and differences between them and to report back in general terms to the class on their findings, without telling their confidential stories to the class.

Code, contract, covenant and charter
The class could be divided into four groups and each allocated a different model to think about. Next they should be asked to think of a case to illustrate the model they have been given. They could then be asked to explain the model to the whole class by:
● producing a group drawing to illustrate the case
● miming or role playing the scenario
● presenting the case to the group for discussion without giving away which model they are using.
Following discussion and feedback from the whole group, an overhead of the four models and table of comparison can be used to help consolidate their understanding and learning from the session.

Different models of management
If the class are already familiar with the four models for analysing the ethics of nurse–patient relations, you might introduce them to the command management, critical enquiry, community nursing and corporate planning models, and encourage discussion of the parallels and differences between the two sets of models. Then students might be set an assignment to go in small groups to interview nurses operating in these different roles and to report back to the class on what they have learned about the different kinds of ethical duty relating to each role. Alternatively, students can be set the task of finding articles in the nursing press which illustrate the ethical problems faced by nurses in these various roles, and then write up a report in essay form.

Sex discrimination in health care settings
Student nurses could first be sent out to do some research on the demography of nursing – to establish how many nurses there are in their country, how many are women and how many are men, and what proportion of senior posts are held by men. Alternatively, they could be encouraged to reflect on the relationship between medical staff and nurses and how much gender stereotyping there is in the way they relate to one another, both personally and in their professional roles.

The findings of either exercise could then serve as the basis of a useful and informed discussion of the ethical implications of the power relations between male and female staff. They could also be asked to discuss in small groups the degree to which power-sharing does or does not occur, and to what extent sex discrimination or sexual harassment is a problem in their day-to-day experience. (If the issue of sexual harassment is to be broached, clear guidelines should be set in advance about how the discussion will be handled and how feedback will occur, to ensure protection of individual confidentiality.)

Nursing ethics – practical applications

SECTION CONTENTS

5

Issues of life, death, madness and money

AIMS

This chapter has the following aims:
1. To explore the various meanings of 'care' and their relevance to understanding the ethics of 'nursing care'
2. To consider the moral issues of clinical nursing practice within the wider context of health as a personal and social value and the 'medicalisation' of life
3. To analyse some of the classic 'big issues' in biomedical ethics, and to illustrate the general ethical concerns which they raise from a nursing perspective.

LEARNING OUTCOMES

When you have read and worked through this chapter, you should be able to:
- Explain and illustrate what 'care' means in the context of professional and institutionalised nursing practice
- Explain and illustrate with concrete examples why nursing ethics must pay attention to the demands of specific cases

- Distinguish between the justification of particular decisions and giving reasons for a general rule or ethical policy
- Give an account of the relationship between 'health' and 'disease' as personal and social values and how we construct the 'problems' of nursing ethics
- Demonstrate ability to discuss the 'pros' and 'cons' of different approaches to at least one of the following classic issues: abortion, euthanasia, truth-telling, compulsory treatment, resource allocation
- Indicate what are some of the common ethical features of the classic 'dilemmas' and how they differ from one another.

THE CLASSIC ETHICAL DILEMMAS IN HEALTH CARE

In previous chapters we have explored the general nature of ethics, the social context of nursing values and the various kinds of professional relationships and institutional contexts in which we have to exercise moral responsibility and make ethical decisions. In this chapter we begin to examine what are perceived to be some of the classic 'big' ethical dilemmas in health care, such as the perennial issues of *abortion, euthanasia, truth-telling, prohibition of sexual relations with patients, compulsory psychiatric treatment* and *the allocation of scarce resources.*

While these issues demand proper treatment in any textbook on ethics in health care, it can be disputed, however, whether these are the most important issues for nurses to address. Judging from the nursing press, from discussion with student nurses, and looking at typical curricula in nursing ethics, it would appear that these *are* the 'big dilemmas' to be addressed. Why is this the case? There are two kinds of reason why these issues are perceived to be so important: the first is that there is a long history of debate about these issues in the literature of *medicolegal ethics* (four of these are even mentioned specifically in the Hippocratic oath,

c. 350 BC – see Appendix 1, p. 339). They obviously raise critical issues in the doctor–patient relationship, and perhaps the importance these issues have for doctors has determined the importance they are given by nurses. Secondly, these issues raise important questions of principle and policy that we must get clear if we are working in health care before we address the more specific responsibilities we have as nurses. For example, the Hippocratic oath gives classic expression to the three fundamental principles we discussed in Chapter 1, namely *beneficence* or the duty of protective and responsible care for patients, including the duty not to take advantage sexually or in any other way of the vulnerability of the patient; *respect for human life* and, in this context, the specific prohibitions against abortion and euthanasia, and respect for the patient's privacy and secrets; and *justice or fairness* to patients in not pretending to have expertise one does not have and in not discriminating against patients because of their status, gender or age (see Phillips 1988, p. 89f).

While these broad issues of principle are undoubtedly relevant to the nurse–patient relationship, as well as the doctor–patient relationship, most nurses are unlikely to be directly responsible for decisions to terminate a pregnancy, terminate treatment or assist a patient to die, or in the compulsory treatment of mentally ill patients, or the allocation of medical resources; but nurses do face the same questions and responsibilities about not abusing or exploiting vulnerable patients. The involvement of nurses with the ethics of the first group of problems is more indirect. They may have strong convictions about the issues and the principles involved, they may be consulted as members of the team about particular decisions, and they can certainly influence general policy on these matters, but the real moral dilemmas faced by nurses relate to their involvement in decision-making in specific cases in a subordinate role, where they may be instructed to do something with which they disagree. The issues are more about who has the power to determine ethical policy and who has ultimate responsibility for decisions, and about issues of authority and obedience.

Nurses should be alert to the differences between doctors' and nurses' responsibilities here. They need to attend to the specific issues that relate to their own particular roles and responsibilities, and be on their guard against medical preoccupations 'setting the agenda' for nursing ethics. Given the fact that the roles and responsibilities of nurses are different, it is the business of a book like this, on nursing ethics, to attempt to clarify these differences (see Melia 1989).

Therefore, before we address some of the classic 'big' ethical dilemmas in health care, we must first clarify some of the general ethical presuppositions underlying nursing ethics, and issues to which nurses have contributed insight from the distinctive perspective of nursing care:

- the general nature of the *concept of care*, in the context of *nursing care*
- the *use of 'typical cases'* – a 'casuistic' approach to ethics, based on cases and precedents
- the relationship between *general* rules and *particular* moral decisions.

CARING AND THE DUTY OF CARE IN NURSING ETHICS

First of all, what do we mean by 'care'? The meanings associated with this term go deep into the roots of Western culture. It is related first to the Latin term *carus* (= dear), designating something that is valued or expensive because it is scarce. By derivation it came to mean *loved*, *desired* or *esteemed* because of the intrinsic value of the object of care. The cooption of the term 'caritas' by Christian thinkers, such as St Augustine (354–430 AD), to express the meaning of the Greek term *agape* capitalises on these earlier associations of the word and enriches it by applying to it the meaning of unconditional love or selfless concern for the well-being, health and salvation of our neighbour. For Christians this love has its origin in God and is demonstrated in the redemptive forgiving love of Christ. More directly, the English word comes to us from the Old English and Teutonic *caru* meaning *sorrow*, or *to be anxious for*, or *solicitous for the welfare of someone*. The term 'care' therefore combines several meanings which make it peculiarly apt to express our deepest concern for our fellow human beings and their physical, emotional and spiritual well-being.

However, when we speak of nursing, we also have to take account of the moral and legal concept of 'a duty of care', namely the duty owed by all those with fiduciary responsibility for other people or their affairs, to protect their interests, health and safety. The moral aspects of one's 'duty of care' are likely to be spelled out in one's duty statement as a nurse, and also in the rules and procedures one is expected to follow in a hospital. The legal duty of care of nurses, social workers, teachers and lawyers, for example, derives from the nature of the implicit or actual contract between carers and those for whom they care, or into whose hands they have committed their lives, their children or their personal affairs and property. To fail in one's duty of care as a professional not only is to be morally blameworthy for a breach of trust, but may also be legally actionable for breach of contract and culpable negligence. Interpreted in this way, as a requirement of both natural justice and contract law, 'care' becomes a matter of the rules and obligations applying to contracts.

In the history of caring ethics, there has always been a tension between the demands of love and the demands of law. Care, in the context of nursing care, combines two different senses of caring:

- sensitive regard for the unique needs of individuals, as valued in themselves, and for the demands of their particular circumstances
- the general duty of care based on contractual and institutional duties and rules, designed to protect the vulnerability of those who depend on the care and protection of others.

The history of Christian ethics itself illustrates the problems of reconciling the demands of universal justice and moral rules that are applicable to everyone, with the demands of love, requiring that we address the particular needs of individuals in their unique circumstances. People have been exhorted to 'follow your conscience'; 'love your neighbour'; 'do to others as you would have them do to you'; and 'consider the effects of your actions on others'. On the other hand, people are charged 'to follow the Ten Commandments'; 'to obey the law of God and of the church'; and 'to respect the God-given and inalienable rights applicable to all human beings' (see Ramsey 1980, Gill 1985).

These tensions between the universal demands of moral laws and the specific claims of respect and care for individuals have their counterparts in the practical counsels of most other cultural and religious traditions too. In tension with the demands of the formulated moral laws of the society, we find emphasis in these different traditions on compassion, respect, tolerance and love which focuses on the needs and rights of the particular person. Their significance is that they attempt to ground ethical obligation in various ways that also give some direction for action.

In the attempt to do justice to the needs of specific people in particular circumstances, the Judaeo-Christian love ethic has emphasised the kinds of obligation that are rooted in caring for others, rather than a more legalistic approach. In fact, St Augustine, in his commentary on 1 John 7:8, summed up Christian ethics in the challenging phrase 'love, and do as you like' (Clark 1984). An ethics of caring (or agapeistic ethics) which strives to determine what is the most loving thing to do in the circumstances serves three different kinds of purpose:

● First, it offers an alternative to an impersonal rule-based ethics of duty, emphasising that the obligation to care for individuals, as we would want to be cared for ourselves, is more important than obedience to formal rules.
● Secondly, it emphasises that caring love demands that in decision-making we pay attention to the specific individual rather than society in general, to the particular circumstances rather than universal conditions and requirements.
● Thirdly, it underlines the fact that our actions have to be measured by their effects on particular people and situations rather than their conformity to general rules and duties.

Discussion of the possibility of an 'agapeistic ethics' or love-based ethics is not restricted to Christian moral theologians, but has been taken up by secular moral philosophy as well, for whether or not one is a believer, or has faith in a God of love, the challenge of love and mercy to legalism is a perennial theme of ethics. Modern debate about 'situation ethics' has focused on these issues, with philosophers like Fletcher (1967) advocating a love ethic, or ethics of caring which would do away with rules entirely, whereas Ramsey (1983) argues that love has its own rules, and that even as it directs us to the uniqueness of each situation and each existing individual, it is not arbitrary or capricious, but has to be consistent with the given structures and dynamics of being (see also Ch. 11).

More recent discussions of a caring ethics, and its particular relevance to nursing, have been dominated by feminist critique of patriarchal institutions and the masculinist ethics that supposedly supports them. Some of this arose out of the debate sparked by Kohlberg and Gilligan. Kohlberg (1973, 1976) claimed to have established in his research – on the stages of moral development in children – that the highest stage of moral development is a form of altruistic justice orientation or rational ethics based on universal principles. He also made the further highly controversial claim that women rarely reach this highest stage of moral development. Gilligan (1977), on the basis of her research, published empirical evidence to show that women express their understanding of ethics 'in a different voice'. This feminine ethic is not one that is inferior to Kohlberg's male idealisation of an organising and controlling ethic, but is rather an ethic concerned with conflict resolution, the acceptance of responsibility and caring – something, she argues, Kohlberg failed to do justice to in his categorisation of developmental stages.

Some nurses and other writers have seized upon Gilligan's work and attempted to claim that caring is a quality native to the make-up of women and is the basis of a different feminist ethic and approach to moral responsibility. Views on ethics have become polarised between 'the caring perspective' and the 'justice perspective', with some nurses attempting to appropriate the caring perspective as their own, claiming that it is what is different about the approach and values of nurses and nursing care. Bowden (1997, p. 6) sums up the difference between the two approaches:

The *caring perspective* is distinguished by a concern for care, responsiveness and taking responsibility in inter-personal relationships, and by a context-sensitive mode of deliberation that resists abstract formulations of moral problems. According to the *justice perspective*, emphasis is placed on rights, duties and general obligations, while moral reasoning is marked by schematic understandings of moral problems that allow previously ordered rules and principles to be applied to particular moral cases.

Useful though it may be to reappraise, from a feminist perspective, the presuppositions under-lying our public institutions, and health care institutions in particular, there is a risk that emphasising the distinctive character of the 'fem-inine voice' in ethics may simply reinforce male/female stereotypes and strengthen sexist prejudices rather than bring about appreciation of the contribution of women to broadening and deepening our understanding of ethics and the human condition. The spuriously 'scientific' attempts to mobilise 'phenomenological method' to prove that 'empathy', 'embodiedness', 'capa-city for tenderness' and 'listening skills' are dis-tinctively feminine traits is open to the same objection. While men may be conspicuously lack-ing in these qualities at times, the risk of adopting a determinist account of gender traits is that this implies that we can do nothing about these innate qualities of members of the different sexes. The value of moral education and ethics itself is undermined if we follow this course. Instead we should address the challenge of how we educate both sexes to repair the damaging effects of their social conditioning and thus make both capable of being more competent moral agents and more rounded human beings.

It is thus arguable that the polarisation of the 'caring perspective' and the 'justice perspective' not only risks entrenching male/female stereo-types and prejudices, but also is a distraction from the real task of ethics and moral education. This is admirably summed up by Bowden (1997, pp. 1–2): 'Caring expresses ethically significant ways in which we matter to each other, transform-ing inter-personal relatedness into something beyond ontological necessity or brute survival', and expresses her concern that attempts to 'pene-trate the essence of care' will distract us from the

'radical call to attend to the complex ethical possi-bilities of interpersonal relationships'. She further observes that while it has been the task of feminist criticism of conventional ethics and systems to draw attention to the way individuals disappear into the anonymous institutions which seek to base their ethics on universal rational rules, there is a risk that we may fall into the trap of 'grand theory-making' in attempting to construct a gen-eral 'feminist ethic' (cf. McAlpine 1996).

To set up caring and justice as antithetical to one another is dangerously misleading, for there can be no real care where the basic requirements of justice are not met, and no real justice where there is no care for the accused (or the victim), no due attention to the specific case, and no scope for mercy or recognition of excusing conditions or diminished responsibility. St Thomas Aquinas himself suggested that talk about care and indi-vidual rights is a luxury and somewhat meaning-less, unless the basic structures of justice are in place. This is equally true in the most intimate of our personal relationships as it is in society in gen-eral. Put very simply, we cannot say we care for someone if we treat that person unfairly, and infi-delity to one another is basically a violation of jus-tice rather than a failure of love.

THE VITAL IMPORTANCE OF THE PARTICULAR CASE

In applied ethics generally, and in nursing ethics in particular, we look at typical cases of moral problems and dilemmas in the hope that we may learn from the way others have thought about or dealt with similar problems. In ordinary life, it is important that we should be able to learn from our own past experience. Similarly, in nursing, the accumulated practical wisdom or common sense of the profession, our colleagues and wider soci-ety can give us some general guidance on how to act. However, this general knowledge, like the principles of the common law, does not tell us what precisely we should do in a particular situa-tion. Casuistry – or the ethical approach based on the study of cases and precedents – can be help-ful in ethics, as it is in law, but does not decide things for us, any more than does the ward sister's anecdote of how she dealt with a 'similar' case in the past, or her assurance that 'we've always done it this way'. We have to decide for ourselves, but knowing what others have thought or done prevents us from having to start from scratch.

Casuistry is an attempt to help us bridge the gulf between the universal and the particular, between moral absolutes and the relativities of everyday life, general moral rules and specific problems in concrete cases. Historically, casuistry developed as an approach to hard cases with attempts of confessors to deal with the problems presented to them by penitents in the confessional. Casuistry also evolved in the attempt to mediate between the seemingly absolute demands of Christian ethics and the canon law of the medieval Church, and the complex, contingent and often tragic circumstances of particular people, trying to live by the counsels of love and perfection.

The term 'casuistry' acquired a derogatory meaning at the time of the Reformation, as thinkers as different as Pascal and Luther criticised the Church for abandoning strict ethical principles, by appealing to precedents and particular cases and 'prudential ethics' to justify making all sorts of compromises with the absolute demands of the gospel. The Protestant churches in the 16th century claimed to be defending absolute moral principles against moral scepticism on the one hand and compromise on the other. Paradoxically, it is the Roman Catholic Church that appears rigid today in its defence of moral truths which it claims are absolute, and the Protestant churches which seem to have come round to advocating the need for flexibility and prudence. The debate about the need for casuistry has revived in the past decade, not merely in the domain of religious ethics, but in secular ethics as well. What this debate highlights is the need in applied ethics not for abstract and general discussion of moral theory, but for guidance on how to act in particular circumstances, how to deal with actual moral decision-making. Jonsen & Toulmin (1988) use the example of the abortion debate in the United States to illustrate the need to rediscover a practical, case-based approach to ethical decision-making as represented in the tradition of casuistry:

Behind the contemporary [abortion] debate, with all its topicality and newsworthiness, there lies a deeper intellectual conflict between two very different accounts of ethics and morality: one that seeks eternal, invariable principles, the practical implications of which can be free of exceptions or qualifications, and another, which pays closest attention to the specific details of particular moral cases and circumstances . . .

The public rhetoric of the abortion controversy has increasingly come, in recent years, to turn on 'matters of principle'. The more this has happened, the less temperate, less discriminating, and above all less resoluble the debate has been. Too often the resulting argument has boiled down to pure headbutting: an embryo's unqualified and unconditional 'right to life' being pitted against a woman's equally unqualified and unconditional 'right to choose'. Those who insist on arguing the abortion issue on the level of high theory and general principle thus guarantee that on the practical level the only possible outcome is deadlock.

Jonsen & Toulmin argue that neglect of practical and applied ethics, of training in ethical decision-making and problem-solving skills and practice in dealing with real cases has opened the way to what they call 'the tyranny of principles'. Pretending that all moral issues can be settled at the level of theoretical discussion of principles has encouraged debate to become polarised between antithetical and dogmatically held viewpoints, or dismissed as simply a matter of personal 'taste in morals'. This damaging view of ethics has been reinforced by the adversarial manner in which current moral issues are presented in the mass media. They describe three kinds of outcome resulting from this trend (Jonsen & Toulmin 1988, pp. 6 and 7):

- 'Much more widely, people at large tend to talk as though "ethical principles" or "moral rules" were exhaustive of ethics: that is, as though all that moral understanding requires is a commitment to some code of rules, which can be authoritative.'
- 'The central problem in philosophical ethics [has become] simply to explain what makes certain kinds of rules count as "moral" rules as contrasted with, say, the rules that govern sports or games, the rules for prudent investing, or the rules of social etiquette.'
- '[Principlism] leaves little room for honest conscientiously based differences of moral

opinion (on the interpretation of the rules or the facts).... Once we accept rules and principles as the heart and soul of ethics, it seems no middle way can be found between absolutism and relativism.'

However, as they point out: 'Taken by themselves, the general rules and maxims that play a part in people's ethical deliberations are only rarely matters of serious dispute... these things are typically "beyond dispute".' But what is more interesting, and what people do dispute about, is whether a given case falls under some general rule (e.g. is this a straightforward case of 'lying', 'murder', 'infidelity', etc.?) and whether one or more rules apply in the given case. In the case of two apparently conflicting duties, the debate is not generally about whether the duties are valid duties or not, but rather about the scope and priority of the conflicting duties involved. These are all matters that do vary from context to context and from case to case, even if the general principles are universal in nature (cf. Toulmin 1981).

In this and the following two chapters, we shall be discussing a number of cases in the attempt to clarify what some of the key ethical issues are in familiar cases and to discuss the merits and weaknesses of the decisions taken. In that sense we will be employing a kind of casuistic (or case-based) approach throughout, and, as we explained in the preface, we have deliberately left the discussion of general moral theory to the end. However, questions of moral theory arise from time to time and are dealt with as best we can in the context. We also return to 'casuistry' in another sense in Chapter 9, where we discuss practical methods and approaches to decision-making in ethics, and in particular a number of problem-solving models that may be of value to nurses in dealing with everyday problems.

GENERAL RULES AND PARTICULAR MORAL DECISIONS

Scientific knowledge is general and concerned with discovering universal laws. Ethics, however, like love, is concerned with particulars. Nurses, because they deal directly and intimately with individual patients, are only too well aware that rules are abstract and general, but decisions have to be made in concrete circumstances with reference to specific cases and particular people. There is a celebrated passage in Dostoevsky's novel *The Brothers Karamazov* where Fr. Zossima criticises a young revolutionary, saying of him that 'he loves everyone in general and no-one in particular'.[1] There is a similar risk that ethics can get lost in theory and 'head talk' and lose touch with reality, if it fails to address the fact that ethical decisions always relate to the specifics of particular cases and concrete situations. Moral rules and principles are of their nature general, while moral decisions are always particular. Moral rules are intended to apply universally – to human life in general and to all people – but decisions involve applying general rules to specific situations and can only be responsible decisions if they are a response to the actual needs and demands of a specific situation. We may take policy decisions about matters of a general nature, for ourselves, for a professional group or for an institution, but policy *decisions*, as decisions, are not general. They always relate to a specific context or to a specific professional group at a particular time in a particular country, or to a particular hospital or institution.

Paradoxically, in the study and teaching of ethics, we tend to start by examining general issues and typical cases. This is to illustrate general moral rules and to clarify the universal principles we use to guide us in everyday decision-making. However, discussing typical cases cannot help us decide what to do in a specific case, even if the case material may have once upon a time related to a specific situation (like all the cases discussed in this book). By discussing 'hypotheticals', 'typical cases', general situations or even specific past case histories (where we do not personally know all the relevant details), we can only reach general conclusions, not a specific conclusion relevant to a specific case.

In this chapter, we will discuss some of the general ethical issues raised by a number of typically recurrent human situations, where health care workers and nurses face conflicting moral duties and responsibilities. All of the following situations can give rise to moral quandaries for nurses:

- assisting with antenatal care and childbirth
- dealing with neonatal death and abortion
- advising parents on child and adolescent nurture and development
- helping people cope with physical and mental disability
- care and containment of mentally disordered people
- counselling related to sexual dysfunction
- assisted reproduction and infertility treatment
- coping with ageing and chronic dependency
- care of the dying and bereaved.

We will argue that the skills and experience we need to make sound ethical decisions, here as elsewhere, cannot be learned by discussion of 'dead' and 'past-tense' cases. To do so encourages the view that ethical decision-making is retrospective, i.e. about finding rationalisations after the event for what we or others have already done – *whereas, making ethical decisions is prospective, i.e. we must confront problems for which we do not have ready-made answers, and still have to find solutions in the future.* This is what makes decision-making challenging, difficult and sometime scary, even if we base our decisions partly on what we have learnt from past experience. The difficulty lies not in deciding *what* general rules or principles might apply, but rather *how* they should be applied in this particular case. If we think decision-making is about the former, then we are liable to get lost in theorising and 'head talk', whereas the practical challenge is to make a decision that leads to appropriate action in the actual situation.

So what practical use is the discussion of general ethical problems or typical cases in our moral formation and training in responsible ethical decision-making?

In order to orientate ourselves in life and the world of moral experience, we perhaps need tourist guides and maps to help us find our way. The information we can gain from a tour guide is indirect. It is the second-hand knowledge of someone who has been to the place before and has learned to find his way around. A map can also help us orientate ourselves by giving us general

bearings and directions, but it is no substitute for traversing the terrain and discovering its attractive and dangerous features for ourselves. Although a map is always a map of a particular place, the information it contains is general, abstracted from reality and represented in a different medium – say on paper – by means of formal conventions, techniques of projection, scales and colour codes, etc.

Approaching the subject of ethics by discussing general ethical problems and issues has the same kind of value to us that studying geography from textbooks has – namely, it gives us general knowledge of what kinds of things we are likely to encounter in that territory. Using typical cases or other people's case histories is more like relying on an experienced guide to show you around, but ultimately you only learn to find your own way about by venturing out on your own. Other people's experience can be no substitute for your own. With the best manual in the world, you cannot learn how to swim without getting into the water yourself!

These remarks need to be borne in mind as you read this chapter and the following three. You can learn some general knowledge of ethics from textbooks, but you cannot learn skills or wisdom in ethical decision-making from them. You may learn what is involved in making ethical decisions, and what is required to give a sound practical or theoretical justification for some course of action, but you can only learn how to become skilled in these areas by practising the skills, exercising practical responsibility and developing competence in applied ethics in real life and in relation to real-life moral problems.

WHAT ARE THE KEY MORAL ISSUES IN NURSING ETHICS?

In examining some of these classic dilemmas it is important to stress again, as we said in Chapter 1, that ethics is concerned not only with 'dilemmas', but also with how we learn to deal in a skilled and professional manner with those recurrent moral problems to which the bulk of our routine moral decisions relate. Further, it is important to stress that nursing ethics is not confined to dilemmas or problems of clinical nursing, but must include discussion of a much wider range of ethical issues, e.g.:

- examination of 'health' and 'disease' as personal and professional values
- managing conflict and cooperation in interprofessional relationships
- corporate ethical policy of hospitals and other health care institutions
- general ethical issues in the politics and economics of health care.

The Edinburgh Medical Group study of professional attitudes and values in the care of the dying and the bereaved (Thompson 1979a) set out to examine some of the classic moral problems in terminal care, such as 'to treat or not to treat', 'to tell or not to tell', and euthanasia and the right to die. What the study brought to light was the fact that,

---

Box 5.1 Micro, macho, meso and macro issues in the ethics of health care

Micro issues (clinical nursing ethics)
- Ethics of one-to-one nurse–patient relationship
- Ethics of clinical nursing in home or hospital
- Ethics of chronic and terminal care nursing
- Ethics of health screening/well person clinics

Macho issues (professional nursing ethics)
- Professional codes and professional dominance
- Nurse–doctor–nurse roles and responsibilities
- Teamwork – leadership and accountability
- Primary care/hospital team membership

Meso issues (ethics of managing nursing services)
- Nurse manager/nursing and general staff relationships
- Employment policies, work allocation, grievances
- Corporate ethical standards and quality assurance
- Human resource management and resource allocation

Macro issues (political ethics of general health policy)
- Health service policy, management and scarce resources
- Nursing research and health promotion strategies
- Political ethics of health authority/region cooperation
- 'Politics' and 'economics' of the National Health Service

---

in practice, these issues were less important (especially for nurses) than a host of other issues around care of the dying – interprofessional communication and conflict, 'buck passing' and institutional constraints on good practice – issues which tend to be neglected in most discussions of ethics.

In summary, we argue that there are at least four different levels at which we need to study nursing ethics: namely, what we shall call the micro, macho, meso and macro levels, or, collectively, the 'Russian dolls' model of ethics, for each level is nested within a more encompassing level (Box 5.1).

It is for these kinds of reasons that it is important not to restrict the scope of nursing ethics to examination of the *micro-ethical* issues involved in clinical nursing. We must examine the following range of questions around interprofessional relations and teamwork: questions of professional dominance and professional autonomy, individual roles and responsibilities, the accountability of teams, questions of leadership and who ultimately 'carries the can'. These are what we refer to as the *macho* issues. The third level at which important ethical issues arise, the *meso level*, is the level of internal management of health care institutions and the relationships of the various parties or 'internal stakeholders' who have a vested interest in the outcome of any management decisions. The fourth level, or *macro level*, relates to that of the political economy or political ethics of health care and applied social policy. These issues relate to differences between our personal philosophies of health and what values we invest in our health as a society; to the overall ethical culture and policies of institutions and hospitals, to standards policies and to quality assurance in both individual and corporate performance; and finally, to local and national health policy. These are what we refer to as macro issues (Campbell 1985, White 1985).

The tendency to focus first on the moral quandaries in clinical situations is probably sound, both because of their immediate appeal and because they focus directly on the nurse–patient relationship. They also illustrate the tensions experienced by nurses in accepting responsibility for the well-being of patients, between their personal feelings and moral beliefs, on the one hand, and their professional responsibilities on the other. These issues are important and cannot be avoided, but it should perhaps be emphasised that as a professional carer, paid to provide care, the nurse also has wider social responsibilities in this public role as a kind of public servant, hospital official or health service employee. The moral problems and dilemmas which arise in the exercise of the public office of 'nurse' are no less important and, in senior posts, often involve much heavier responsibility. Special ethical issues arise in the exercise of the wider responsibilities of nurses to groups of patients, relationships with colleagues, and in accountability to employers and the general public. These areas of responsibility are often regarded as more 'political', but are really continuous with the direct and intimate problems of patient care. Perhaps by regarding them as 'political' we implicitly recognise that they raise questions at the macro level about the basis of our social moral beliefs and ideological commitments, whereas the familiar dilemmas relate to the micro level, i.e. to specific problems or dilemmas raised by conflict within our personal systems of beliefs. Problems of cooperation and conflicts with other professions (doctors, social workers, chaplains and allied health professions) may not be merely problems of the pecking order of the various professions in the ranks of professional dominance, or who calls the shots. There may also be specific difficulties which arise because of the different theoretical perspectives from which each profession defines 'the problem', different 'diagnoses' and different kinds of interventions or 'treatment' of the problem, as well as different expected 'outcomes' (Downie 1971).

In dealing with a difficult case or complex situation, it may be useful to use the grid in Figure 5.1 with the parties involved, in order to clarify the conflicts of values and expectations involved.

HEALTH AND DISEASE AS PERSONAL AND SOCIAL VALUES

We cannot avoid making moral choices or debating matters of moral principle in health care since

Key player or STAKEHOLDER	Professional VIEW or VALUE BASE	Definition of THE PROBLEM	Proposed action or INTERVENTION	Hoped for result or OUTCOME
1.				
2.				
3.				
4.				
Areas of difference				
Areas of common ground				
Elements in possible joint action plan				

Fig. 5.1   Values clarification – distinguishing professional perspectives and value bases.

the whole question of our health – as individuals, in family life, in our work and in society – is not a matter of indifference to us. We all desire good health and seek to avoid pain and injury, disease and death. The illness or handicap of a parent or one family member can affect the well-being of all the others. Work-related accidents or absenteeism caused by illness affects the productivity of organisations and industry, often more seriously than do strikes. The cost of caring for the sick, injured, mentally disordered, severely handicapped, senile and dying is a burden on any society – a burden, first of all, in human terms on those in families who bear the brunt of most of the anxiety and direct care, and a burden, too, on the state, in providing primary care and hospital services, and on the professional staff who are paid to care (Wilson 1976, Downie & Calman 1987).

'Health' and 'disease' are terms with several meanings – scientific and medical meanings, and more popular meanings that relate to ideal states of personal and social well-being or states of personal and social disorder we wish to avoid. Even in physiology and pathology, 'health' and 'disease' are normative terms, i.e. they describe the state of an organism as approaching ideal or optimum functioning or varying degrees of malfunctioning or dysfunction – within a continuum, where health is at one pole and disease is at the other. At a more personal level, we do not have to be 'health freaks' in order to want to be healthy, because most of the things we do, most of the things that give us pleasure, are more fun and more enjoyable when we are fit and healthy than when we are unfit, ill or injured. Good health is something we value; it is an ideal and a goal we strive to realise for ourselves (and perhaps for others). And disease is an evil we try to avoid or prevent or, failing both, to cure. The classic WHO definition of health encompasses this sense of health and disease as personal and social values by stressing that health encompasses 'complete physical, mental and social well-being and not just the absence of disease, or infirmity' (WHO 1947).

In attempting to define health, we raise fundamental ethical, political and even religious questions about values and life choices, even before we get into specific questions about the personal and moral responsibilities of nurses and other health professionals in paid service to others (Seedhouse 1986). They also arise in wider policy debate about the nature of health services and the best systems for effective and efficient delivery of health care (Robertson et al 1992).

In making decisions about our personal health, we have to make both practical and moral choices about our behaviour and lifestyle, if we are to live healthy lives and avoid accidents, injury, disease or premature death. Alternatively, while we may tend to regard attempted suicide as a sign of mental disorder in an individual, the decision to end one's life prematurely, either by direct suicide or by taking risks that may result in death, is also a moral choice. We do not exist in splendid isolation and our lives touch and interlock with those of others in many different ways – in family life, in our friendships and love affairs, and in our work and recreation. Just as an attempted or actual suicide can cause intense pain and grief to many other people, so too, in a less dramatic way, illness, injury and personal distress can and do affect other people.

Society is, and has to be, interested in the health and well-being of its members: first, because we are part of one another; second, because the whole human family may suffer if we are unable to make or are prevented from making our own contribution to society; and third, because of the additional burden and cost of care and treatment that may result.

Public health education and public health measures, such as immunisation, screening, the imposition of quarantines and travel restrictions, compulsory notification of diseases, and general controls on sanitary supply of food and water, sewerage/waste disposal and environmental controls on housing, provision of public amenities and health services, are all undertaken by the state in order to prevent disease and to promote the health of society.

There is a potential conflict right here at the beginning between personal liberty to do what we want in pursuing the lifestyle of our choice and the well-intentioned but often officious and interfering attempts of family, friends, school and health professionals, mass media and political agencies to change or redirect our health behaviour. These issues involve basic ethical questions about personal rights and social responsibility and the wider good of society, and so have general relevance to the ethics of health care, but also in a more particular way to nursing ethics. Nurses are often involved in conflicts between what they preach and what they practise. As front-line health educators with a professional responsibility to prevent disease as well as to care for and treat those who are ill, nurses have to face the conflicts between their own health behaviour (e.g. with regard to smoking, drug or alcohol abuse, diet, fitness, responsible sex) and what they are advising their patients or clients to do. The issues are not only about the expectations relating to nurses or health professionals as role models, but also about their function as educators or agents of social control.

For example, health education can be presented in such a way as to encourage us to know more about healthy living, to make informed choices and to take responsibility for our own health and choice of lifestyle. Alternatively, health propaganda may seek to redirect our behaviour, either by persuasion or by subtle (or not so subtle) legal coercion. Aggressive promotion of healthy lifestyles by state agencies has to be justified by a kind of healthist ideology, whereas traditional preventive medicine simply sought to prevent disease. This is not necessarily to be condemned; rather we should understand what kind of values are being promoted and be willing to examine and challenge these. On the one hand, millions of pounds are spent annually by the tobacco, alcohol and junk food industries on advertising and sponsorship to promote the sale of products that are damaging to health; and on the other, we increasingly see the alliance of state propaganda with commercial interests in the marketing of health (sports equipment and clothing, public spectaculars and mass participation in spectator sports). The public fashion for jogging, health foods, diet and fitness is not just a product of individual people's desire to be fit and healthy. It is the result of many factors, including peer pressure, personal interest and raised awareness of health as an

issue in people's lives, but also of an orchestrated attempt of political and commercially controlled media advertising to 'market' health as an ideology and to change people's health behaviour and lifestyles accordingly (Ewles & Simnett 1985).

When 'health for all by the year 2000' was adopted at the Alma Ata International Conference of the World Health Organization as a policy objective (WHO 1978), this was dismissed by many cynics as wildly optimistic, impractical and unattainable. However, by setting such a goal, WHO has encouraged UN member states to formulate specific attainable objectives and action plans to achieve this target. As a result, member states have adopted and begun to implement programmes of health promotion, disease prevention and reorientation of resources to primary care that may well improve the health status of millions of people around the world and change the face of health care well into the 21st century (WHO 1981, 1999b). This has come about, and is coming about, through attention to the ethical and political implications of good health as something of personal and social value. If we start by recognising that 'health' and 'disease' are value terms, then we will be obliged to see that discussion of moral problems and responsibilities around direct patient care fall within the broader commitments we make as individuals, professionals and members of society to achieve good health. These may include individual and pressure-group activity either to promote good health for all and encourage people to help themselves to health, or to raise public awareness and mobilise public support for fiscal, legal and other controls on the advertising and marketing of products that will damage our health.

As nurses become more active as frontline agents of health education and health promotion, the ethics of this kind of activity requires more careful attention. State-initiated health promotion carries with it the risk that health professionals will be coopted to become 'health police', invading the privacy of households and intruding into the lives of ordinary people. Alternatively, major national health promotion campaigns or programmes are of the nature of experiments in health and social engineering, and should perhaps be subject to similar ethical constraints and controls as other forms of medical or nursing research, e.g. the World Medical Association's Declaration of Helsinki 1996 (see Appendix 1), or review by a public ethical review board. To prevent health promotion becoming authoritarian, officious and inclined to blame the victim, ethical guidelines are required. The WHO itself has sponsored workshops and issued discussion papers on the subject (WHO 1981, Robertson et al 1992).

THE 'MEDICALISATION OF LIFE' AND THE 'BIG DILEMMAS'

It is not the broader ethical issues related to public and community health that we think of first when medical or nursing ethics is discussed. Although the issues around prevention and positive health promotion are increasingly important in nursing, it is the ethical issues related to the treatment of injury, disease and death that have greater prominence in public debate and professional training. The popularity of hospital-based TV 'soap operas', including police dramas with a focus on forensic medicine, reflects perhaps a morbid preoccupation of a healthy population with the ever-present threat in life of suffering and death, but for whatever reason, the dramatic 'ethical dilemmas' of medical fiction grip us more than the ethics of healthy living! Further, the dramas of clinical medicine are perceived by medical students and trainee nurses to be important, because they are the issues which first challenge them when they enter the extraordinary world of hospitals and the crises they observe in acute medical and surgical wards, and in accident and emergency medicine.

The reasons for the focus on clinical medical ethics are complex and various, e.g. most health professionals are trained within the crisis-oriented treatment services rather than in prevention. The so-called 'health' services are in practice more concerned with the treatment of disease; and, indeed, with the bulk of the money and resources going into clinical research and therapeutic services, power and prestige tend to be concentrated there (cf. HMSO 1978b).

McKeown (1979), in his classic study, argued that diagnostic and treatment services have con-

tributed less to improving the health of society than improvements in housing, food supplies, income, clean water, hygienic sewerage disposal and general public health measures. However, the image of high-technology medicine and intensive care nursing remain more attractive to those drawn to working in health care, and the focus on individual patients and their problems has more human appeal. Similarly, although the majority of nurses will be employed in long-term care of the chronic sick, the mentally ill and the elderly, it is midwifery, neonatal and paediatric nursing, acute medical and surgical and terminal-care nursing which enjoy higher prestige and glamour. These factors influence our perception of what issues are ethically most important.

All the big ethical issues of common concern to health professionals relate to the way power (or control) is exercised over people, or power is shared with people – whether people seek their help voluntarily or are committed into their care by relatives or other authorities. Questions of respect for patient autonomy have become increasingly important as we have moved away from a position where medical and nursing authority were beyond question, and pressure has built from various special interest groups to defend patients' rights. While the division of responsibility and/or authority may differ in the ward or in the primary care team, and while many of the frustrations of nurses may focus on the fact that they often have responsibility without executive authority, it would be a mistake to overlook the very real and proper responsibilities of nurses as distinct from doctors.

The issues about which nurses probably bother most tend to be those which relate directly to their spheres of personal responsibility in either direct patient care or management roles, rather than the more general and intractable issues where they feel they can personally do very little or which are beyond their control. Issues around communication with patients (truth-telling and confidentiality) and conflicts with doctors, other carers and relatives over patient care tend to predominate. Nurses may well have an intellectual interest in, and need to be informed about, a wide range of current moral issues in health care, and some ave particular reasons to conscientiously object to assisting with abortions or be worried by requests from patients for euthanasia, but in practice they can also distance themselves from some of these issues as not being their responsibility but rather the doctor's.

In many cases, nurses may feel relatively powerless, in so far as others in more powerful positions (e.g. doctors or the competent legal authorities) take decisions which affect the admission or discharge of patients or the form of treatment they are to receive. In this sense nurses are not in control and inherit responsibilities which flow from decisions taken by others, and which they may feel powerless to change or influence. Most of the classic big dilemmas are problems in law or medical ethics before they become problems for nurses. However, this is not to say that these problems and dilemmas do not present in a different way in nursing, or that nurses do not have unique and distinctive responsibilities, or that nursing ethics does not have a unique contribution to make to the debate about these issues. In fact, if nurses were to focus their concern and frustration on their perceived powerlessness relative to doctors, and were to see nursing ethics only as a kind of commentary on or vicarious participation in medical ethics, then it would hardly be worth pursuing.

In reality, nurses do have considerable power over patients, and even influence over doctors. The way they organise staff time and ward or community resources can directly influence both the quantity and quality of care given to patients. They can influence the patient both directly and indirectly by the way they change or manipulate the patient's environment. They can influence the decisions of doctors, paramedics and other carers by their reported observations about patients and the appropriateness or inappropriateness of treatment, levels of pain control, compulsory detention in hospital or discharge. The nature and quality of their observations regarding the patient's physical, emotional and psychological state may be critical in the patient's management. They can also influence nurse and hospital management about necessary organisational and institutional change, or campaign for more resources, and in general have a responsibility to maintain the quality and standards of patient care.

While individual nurses may have reason to object to carrying out a doctor's orders, whether in administering drugs with potentially fatal side-effects, assisting with abortions, offering euthanasia or administering electroconvulsive therapy (ECT), the real focus of concern in nursing ethics should be, rather, on those areas where nurses have specific responsibilities which are different from those of other health professionals or social workers. These areas relate to such matters as the organisation of the patient's day, observation and communication skills, skilled attention to the patient's physical, psychological and spiritual needs, making the environment more patient-friendly, and counteracting institutionalisation and dependency. These nursing issues are often overlooked while more attention is given to the big dilemmas of medical ethics.

One way of looking at the big dilemmas of direct patient care – namely, abortion, euthanasia, truth-telling, compulsory psychiatric treatment and the allocation of scarce resources – is to see them as having become issues of importance in medicine and nursing in modern life through an historical process, which Illich (1977) first called 'the medicalisation of life'. According to his analysis, the concentration of human populations in cities, the loss of extended family support and the increasing isolation of the nuclear family have led to the de-skilling of ordinary people in their ability to deal with suffering, illness, injury and death in the community. We have all become more dependent on doctors and other health professionals to cope with the problems of life, and they have effectively become the priests of modern society, presiding over and controlling all the crucial rites of passage from birth to death. The treatment of health and disease, injury, mental disorder, death and bereavement have come to embrace the whole of life and all its stages.

Health professionals and health care delivery systems are now directly involved in providing some or all of the following range of services to the public:

- advice on fertility control or assistance with reproduction
- antenatal preparation or termination of pregnancy
- assistance with childbirth and neonatal death
- supervision of postnatal care and/or screening for genetic abnormalities
- monitoring the growth and physical and psychological health of children
- providing treatment for the physical and mental disorders of adolescence
- giving advice and treatment for nutritional disorders
- dealing with drug dependency, sexual and marital problems
- overseeing sport, leisure and recreational activity
- supervision, custodial care and treatment of the mentally disordered
- caring for the severely handicapped and senile
- pre-death counselling, terminal care and post-death follow-up of the bereaved.

The 'medicalisation of life' has meant that health professionals have inherited some of the power and control over matters of life and death which in more traditional society were the domain of lay-carers, priests and religious healers. Faith in religion and in divine judgement or providential care has to a large degree been replaced by faith in secular science and the 'miracles' of modern medicine. As health professionals have come to supervise and control the rites of passage 'from the cradle to the grave', so too have they acquired awesome, even god-like, responsibility for making life-and-death decisions. Some of the ethical problems are self-generated, by institutionalisation of people and their life-problems. Problems in the division of labour in this vast and growing 'health industry' have also complicated interprofessional relations and competition for clients. At the macro level, major fiscal problems have been created for governments by the expectations of total care of society by health care services.

Illich (1977) offers us a critique of the dominance which doctors have come to exercise over our lives and the temptations they face to 'play God'.

Nurses often use his arguments to reinforce many of their criticisms of the arrogance and assumed moral superiority of doctors. However, the implications of Illich's analysis go much further and relate to the role of nurses too – whether in the traditional role of 'doctors' handmaidens' or as modern self-consciously independent health professionals with distinctive roles and responsibilities of their own. In both cases, nurses are part of the process and the system which has resulted in this medicalisation of life, with its corresponding removal from ordinary people of the power of decision-making and responsibility for their own lives. It is arguable, too, that while the power of priests and religious healers was limited by acknowledgement of a transcendent divine power and authority to which they felt ultimately accountable, secular health care is subject to no such limitations.

Some of the big dilemmas arise as a direct consequence of the responsibilities health professionals have acquired in this process of the medicalisation of life, and the expectations they have created in people that there is a 'magic bullet', technological 'fix' or medical solution to every human problem. The high risk and high cost of many of these life-saving interventions, and attempts to deal with human distress and unhappiness, have created their own crop of unprecedented ethical quandaries. This is particularly the case in areas such as genetic screening and gene 'therapy', assisted reproduction, in vitro fertilisation and surrogacy, organ 'donation' and replacement, and chemotherapy for human distress and mental disorder. Discovering that a subject of routine screening is a carrier for a serious disease such as Huntington's chorea not only presents the health care worker with the dilemma of whether or not to tell the person involved, but also presents the subject with terrible dilemmas about whether or not to marry and attempt to have children. While assisted reproduction techniques such as in vitro fertilisation of previously harvested ova or intracytoplasmic sperm injection in severe cases of male infertility may result, after several attempts, in a successful live birth, there is also a high failure rate for these expensive procedures. They not only involve serious additional risks to women in the 'harvesting' of sufficient numbers of their ova for experimental purposes, but also raise serious questions about the long-term genetic and health consequences, and costs relative to benefits, of such interventions. In addition, there are the questions that arise about the propriety of the long-term storage of fertilised ova, to whom they belong, and who pays for the costs of storage – perhaps even beyond the life span of the donors.

Another consequence of the medicalisation of life, to which Illich drew attention, was the increasing volume of medically induced pathology or *iatrogenic disease*. Examples where medical treatment has itself created health problems are multiplying. These include unnecessary surgery; indiscriminate use of antibiotics (creating pathogens that are immune to all available drugs); vast numbers of patients addicted to prescribed drugs (particularly stimulants, antidepressants and major tranquillisers); the risks of ovarian hyperstimulation in the 'harvesting' of ova in the treatment of infertility; the risks of multiple births and cerebral palsy in low-weight babies associated with IVF; and the risk of unscrupulous pharmaceutical research on vulnerable patients in the attempt to be the first to market new 'wonder' drugs.

Obviously, we need to look at the specific issues raised by each of the big dilemmas, but it may be useful to bear in mind this more general historical perspective and be prepared to consider its broader implications too.

INDIVIDUAL 'HEALTH CAREERS' AND PROFESSIONAL CONTROL

Because ethical decisions usually relate to concrete cases, it is tempting to address the fundamental questions of ethics from a consideration of particular cases. Such an approach gives rise to difficulties when we try to generalise to other cases what can be learned from one specific case. However, there is another difficulty involved in looking at illustrative cases. This relates to the question of *what defines a 'case'* – how much background information, contextual detail, family and social history is relevant? What we may call a case from a medical or nursing perspective can be eas-

ily caricatured by phrases like 'the case of the burst appendix in bed number 6' or 'the hysterectomy patient in side ward 3'. What the caricatures illustrate is not only that 'being a case' from the patient's point of view means something rather different from the concerns of health professionals, but also that the aspects of reality that are considered important to illustrate a medical or ethical point constitute an abstraction from life for the person involved, a person with a past and an ongoing history.

A 'case' may appear to be relatively self-contained too from the medical or nursing perspective – an example of a particular problem or pathology. From the patient's point of view, the crisis which gives rise to the need for medical treatment or nursing care is just one episode in the ongoing drama of his life. It is too easy to forget the whole human and social context in which the health crisis or illness episode occurs, and perhaps to forget the real person in the process and the fact that the health crisis may be of life-shattering importance to him, affecting his whole future life and prospects. To achieve a balanced ethical judgement about a specific situation it may be just as important to understand the background of the person involved, as it may be important from a nursing perspective to know not only the patient's medical but also his personal and social history.

The concept of a 'health career' – a concept derived from developmental psychology – may be useful here, for each 'case' or 'incident' has to be seen in the context of the person's health career. As we grow from infancy through childhood to maturity and decline into old age and die, our life passes through a series of ups and downs which comprise our particular life or health career. From a medical or nursing perspective, episodes of illness or health crises need to be located in this dynamic context of 'before' and 'after' if their full significance is to be grasped. Listening to the patient's story, however, is not just useful but essential if we are to acknowledge and respect the dignity of the individual in genuinely 'patient-centred' nursing. The concept of a health career has proved very important in health education, particularly in understanding patterns of both health promoting and dysfunctional health behaviour (Baric 1974,

Dorn & Nortoft 1982). For example, the acquisition of a smoking habit, of heavy drinking or drug addiction involves a 'career' of initiation or introduction to the practice, repeated reinforcement of the habit through practice and then developed dependency, attempts to cut down or quit, and so on. Such a dynamic view of human life crises can be as illuminating for ethical decision-making as it is in arriving at clinical judgements, whereas the 'typical case' tends to be frozen in time, abstracted from the context.

If we represent the whole of our life career by a parabolic curve, starting with conception, rising to the peak of our physical and mental development and curving down to meet the horizontal axis again at death, then along that line, our progress is not necessarily smooth; it has its 'ups' when we are healthy and things are going well for us, and its 'downs' when we are sick, suffer injury or external factors limit and arrest our development. As we get better, or get over a crisis in our lives, so we regain some of the lost ground and our development continues. As we get past middle age or suffer severe illness or disabling injury, so our capacity for recovery becomes more limited and our general condition may decline, until we finally succumb to the disintegrating effect of disease, injury and the wear-and-tear of old age, and die. Some people may live a long time with a very steady rhythm, other people's lives may be marked by numerous crises, and others may be cut short tragically by sudden, accidental or violent death. It is possible to examine the medicalisation of life across the whole span of an individual's health career, but it is also illuminating to apply it to the specific analysis of smaller sections of people's lives or individual episodes of illness, injury or mental disorder.

If we map the course of an episode in a person's life career – from a state of relative health and independence through some health crisis where he becomes relatively or completely dependent on help from others and on to recovery and a gradual return to something like his former state of health and independence – this process can be illustrated on a simple graph by an inverted

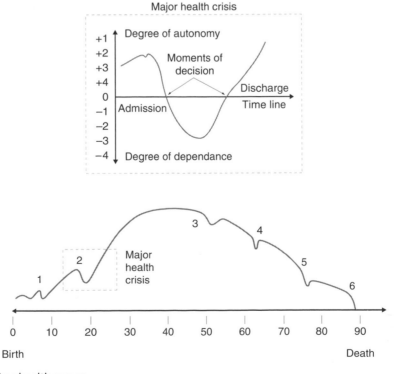

Fig. 5.2 Overall lifetime health career.

parabolic curve. On such a graph the horizontal axis would represent the continuous time-line. On the vertical axis we could represent various degrees of autonomy above the line and various degrees of dependency below it. Such an episode relative to one's life career could be illustrated as in Figure 5.2.

What is ethically significant about health and illness for the person involved is that normal physical and mental health means growth towards greater autonomy. Illness and injury usually involve loss of autonomy and greater dependence on other people. 'Making a good recovery' usually means recovering more control over our lives and being able 'to stand on our own feet again'.

When a healthy person, who is, say, lucid, mobile, continent and independent, experiences some health crisis (through injury, disease or environmental insult) he may rapidly decline into a state of relative or deep dependency on others, from which he has to be assisted to recover. The process of assisting people to get back onto their feet we call 'rehabilitation'. *The deeper the downward curve, the more total will be the carer's responsibility for the person entrusted into her care*, but as that person is assisted to recovery, or recovers spontaneously, then the carer has to assist him back to recovery and independence, not keep him in a state of perpetual dependence. There are at least two points of 'crisis' in this process ('moments of decision'; from Greek *krino* – to judge or decide): first, when the individual hands over responsibility, or is handed over, to the carer; and secondly, when responsibility is handed back to the patient or client. The crossing of the horizontal axis by the downward and upward movement of the line illustrates these points in the episode, making these crisis points on the boundary line between autonomy and dependency on the parabolic curve.

What is important about this model for illustrating a person's health career is that it emphasises that there is a dynamic process, or movement, or a *shift in responsibility from the patient to the carer, and back again*. This is clearest in cases such as emergency admissions for major injury or severe mental disorder, but even in the minor illnesses or ups and downs in life there are considerable fluctuations in our need for help and support and our capacity to stand on our own feet. The problems arise for patients and clients when professionals are either reluctant or too eager to take on responsibility for them when they are in a crisis or need help. Alternatively, professionals may be slow to give up the control over people's lives which they acquire, or may too readily abandon them before they are able to take control of their own lives again.

The effects of institutionalisation in reducing the capacity of people to cope with responsibility for themselves and their health, and in reinforcing the dependency-creating attitudes and behaviour of carers, have been well studied from a psychological point of view but not always from an ethical one (Goffman 1968). This particularly applies to the often unwanted moral responsibilities which carers inherit as a result of taking on people in need. Where the health crisis requires emergency treatment, the pressures on the carers to take urgent life-and-death decisions may be considerable. They may well find it emotionally costly and physically exhausting. Without respite or adequate support they may risk 'burn-out'. Alternatively, they may soldier on, but resent being left to carry the can, and they may then experience exaggerated guilt if things go wrong.

Ethical codes in the caring professions have focused mainly on the responsibility the carer accepts for the client; few have stressed the importance of the commitment the carer must make to return control to the client as soon as he is capable of being independent again. None of the existing medical codes stresses that the doctor has a primary moral duty to assist (where possible) the rehabilitation of the patient. It is significant, however, that both the International Council of Nurses and the Royal College of Nursing have emphasised the responsibility of the nurse to work to restore autonomy to the individual who has lost it as a result of illness, injury or mental disorder. These statements emphasise a value fundamental to nursing ethics which appears to arise out of reflection on the distinctive nature of nursing care.

ABORTION AND THE 'RIGHT TO LIFE'

From the dawn of time women have sought assistance to terminate unwanted pregnancies, whether or not this has been permitted by law or morality. If help has been refused or unavailable, women have attempted by an infinite variety of means to effect an abortion themselves, or have resorted to infanticide. Some societies have tolerated abortion, but it has generally been prohibited and those seeking to procure or assist with abortions have been severely punished. In a sense, it is only with liberal legislation decriminalising abortion that the issue has, strictly speaking, become a matter of clinical and moral responsibility for nurses. Of course, nurses in Britain had to grapple with the problem before the Abortion Act 1967 and they will have had views on the morality or immorality of abortion before this time, but it is only since then that nurses as nurses in Britain, and particularly in the National Health Service, have had to face the issues as a direct challenge to nursing ethics. For the nurse, or more specifically the midwife, it might be argued that there is an immediate and apparent contradiction between the responsibility to protect, nurture and save the life of the child and the responsibility for the wider care of the woman for whom an unwanted pregnancy is a personal disaster.

The issue of *abortion* is usually debated from the pro-life point of view in terms of the sanctity of life or the rights of the unborn child. From the point of view of those who favour further liberalisation of the law and moral attitudes on abortion, the issue is about women's rights and in particular their right to control their own fertility, including recourse to termination of pregnancy. Relatives and wider society tend to enter the debate in an attempt either to protect the rights of the unborn child or to defend the rights of the woman. Here the issues tend to be discussed in terms of the tensions between popular morality (represented by different pressure groups) on the one hand, and the law and social policy on the other. The passionately held and opposing moral beliefs of those representing, say, the Catholic Church or other faith communities and those representing women's rights are not necessarily in disagreement about fundamental values, but rather about which values, as a matter of policy, are to be given priority. It is not generally the case that one group believes abortion is an absolute wrong and the

other that it is absolutely right, for both groups would probably regard termination of pregnancy as neither a good nor an ideal solution in general. Where the differences arise is in relation to what discretion may be allowed in dealing with specific cases, which may be devastating for the specific individual woman.

It is important to distinguish two very different levels of moral argument in relation to abortion:

● debate about the right or best (or least harmful) thing to do in a specific case, given the circumstances
● debate about how abortion should be dealt with in society in general, as a matter of law and social policy, given the widely differing cultural and religious attitudes to these matters.

Of course, religious and other specific interest groups have a right in a democratic society to campaign to have their views more widely accepted and to influence social policy and the law. However, it cannot simply be assumed that the morality of a particular faith community can be legitimately imposed on the whole community, even in societies where they represent the majority. Considerations of justice and equity, as well as respect for the rights and freedom of conscience of individuals, make it necessary that there is scope for dissent, otherwise the society is on course to becoming authoritarian, whether the position entrenched in law and social policy is an extreme libertarian one or strictly anti-abortion.

The health professionals may get left out of the abortion debate, except where they are called in as expert witnesses, but in reality they are often left playing 'piggy in the middle'. The duty to care for both mother and child leaves them in an impossible situation, e.g. where they have to choose between the life of the one or the other. The conflicting demands of such a situation cannot be resolved by carers by consulting the law (which may be a convenient 'cop-out') or their personal consciences about which individual (mother or baby) is owed a greater duty of care. Other considerations of personal rights and justice have to be taken into account, and the tension between these conflicting values in real life is what makes these problems so painful and presents us with apparently unsolvable dilemmas (cf. Davis & Aroskar 1983, Johnstone 1994).

The sanctity of life argument that so easily leads on to claims that abortion is murder raises both fundamental issues and insuperable problems in ethics. If all life is sacred, where do you draw the line – with the newborn, the fetus, the conceptus, the ovum or the individual sperm? Is it only human life that is sacred, or is animal and vegetable life sacred as well? If we say human life, when does life become human in the continuum between individual cell and adult person? Attempts to legislate that human life begins at conception do not solve the problem; nor did the position adopted by St Thomas Aquinas in the 13th century that the fetus acquires legal and moral rights at 'quickening' (when ensoulment was supposed to take place); nor does the modern legal limit of 28 weeks' gestation. Why not at birth, or at puberty, or at age 21 years? What all these attempts to find a secure biological foundation for the definition of a 'person' fail to recognise is that they beg the question: 'What is a person?' This is essentially *a moral question* and a matter of value judgement, namely, a judgement about what in particular is to be valued about human persons as such. The debate about what we mean by 'a human person' is not a scientific question but an ethical one, and the various ways in which different societies and religions define personhood directly influence how we give a concrete meaning to the legal concept of a person as 'a bearer of rights and duties' and how we define the scope and limits of membership of the 'moral community' (Gill 1985).

What is distinctive about the Judaeo-Christian and Muslim faiths is the high value placed in these traditions on fetal life, and on the 'right to life' as a God-given natural right. In European philosophy, since the Protestant Reformation and the Enlightenment, the emphasis has been placed on the exercise of individual moral responsibility and rational choice as essential prerequisites for any claims to moral rights. As a result, liberal humanists have tended to regard our entitlements to rights and our obligations as increasing with our growth in maturity and responsibility, with the exercise of personal moral autonomy. So within this tradition, neither rights nor duties would be attributed to prenatal life. In complete contrast with both of these European traditions, traditional Hinduism and animistic religions around the world regard all life as sacred – respect for the rights of animals and even plant life means that the moral community is expanded to include all living things. Taken together with the doctrines of reincarnation and Karma, all living things are bound together in one chain of being, one moral community of reciprocal rights and responsibilities, and one's progress up or down the hierarchy of more or less complex forms of life is dependent on one's Karma – on how well or badly one fulfils the responsibilities of one's fate or station in life.

Dogmatic definitions simply foreclose rational debate and exploration of these complex questions to which fundamentally different answers have been given in different societies and cultures. In Hinduism, where all living things are regarded as sacred, and strict vegans would not kill any animal or eat animal products, the moral community is so broad as to include all living things as having rights. At the other extreme, the Nazis sought to restrict the moral community to pure Aryans, and other 'lesser' races were denied fundamental moral rights or even the protection of the law. In Western culture we tend to have regarded only human beings as having moral rights or qualifying as members of the moral community, and have extended protection to animals on the grounds that cruelty or abuse of animals is inhuman, not that animals as such have rights. The animal liberation movements have sought to challenge this view. Furthermore, within our own culture, we have been very confused about whether all human beings – including women and children, slaves, and the mentally and physically handicapped – should enjoy the same rights. The present legal debate about in vitro fertilisation is bedevilled by confusion in many countries about the legal status of the unborn, and where we draw the line in experiments with embryos or the storage of embryos. English law, for example, acknowledges, on the one hand, the right of the unborn child to inherit property or to recover damages for injury suffered *in utero*, but on the other abrogates the unborn child's right to life by permitting abortion under specific conditions.

This analysis is not meant to decide the abortion issue one way or the other, but rather to raise a fundamental series of questions in ethics (Glover 1977): what do we mean by a 'person'; what do we mean by respect for personal dignity and rights; what is the scope of the 'moral community'; what criteria do we apply to determine membership of this community; what rights and responsibilities does membership entail?

Ironically, those who campaign for women's rights and the 'right' to termination of pregnancy on demand rest their claims upon similar presuppositions about the nature of the rights of members of the moral community to those raised in defence of the moral and legal status of prenatal life. The dispute is not so much about the nature of rights, but rather to whom they apply and the boundaries of the moral community. Whether the unborn child and the mother's rights are equal and apply in the same way and on the same level are questions about the scope and limits of our definitions of personhood and the terms for full membership of the moral community. These are all issues which relate back fundamentally to the Principle of Respect for Persons and how we define the rights and responsibilities of members of the moral community (Campbell 1972, Rumbold 1993).

Consider some of the conflicting rights of the different parties in Case History 5.1.

Issues surrounding euthanasia and compulsory psychiatric treatment relate to extremes in the balance of power between carer and client and the tensions that such situations generate – between the requirements of the duty to care for and protect the vulnerable and incompetent, on the one hand, and respect for the autonomy and personal rights of the patient or client, on the other.

EUTHANASIA AND THE 'RIGHT TO DIE'

Euthanasia is a term that is used rather loosely. It comes from two Greek words: *eu* meaning good and *thanatos* meaning death. The term 'euthanasia' is sometimes used to describe both the situation in which a carer, on her own initiative, assists a patient to a good death – which may involve withholding treatment (passive euthanasia) – and the intentional killing of a patient by administering a drug or treatment which hastens his death (active euthanasia). In both situations, the carer would probably justify the action in terms of an extension of the duty to care, e.g. to prevent unnecessary suffering. However, the term 'euthanasia' is also used in cases where the patient requests assistance to put an end to his suffering (assisted suicide) or where he has stated in advance (perhaps in a sworn statement or 'living will') that he does not wish his life to be artificially prolonged if his condition is terminal. This kind of 'voluntary euthanasia' involves the patient or client insisting on respect for his personal wishes and claiming the 'right' to die or at least to be consulted about the scope and limits of what we euphemistically call 'terminal care'.

The prohibition of murder, intentional killing or assisted suicide, with or without the instructions of the victim, is proscribed in almost every jurisdiction around the world. Therefore, the legal definition of euthanasia as 'the intentional

case history 5.1

The question of termination of pregnancy for a mother with AIDS

Vicky is an 18–year-old student with a boyfriend, Jack, who has been using drugs. She is very fond of him and they have been living together for some months. Vicky misses a period and goes to her local health centre for a pregnancy test. She is shocked to discover that she is pregnant, but after a few days makes up her mind that she wants to keep the baby at all costs. She does not initially tell either her boyfriend or parents. When she goes to the maternity hospital for an antenatal examination, routine blood tests reveal that Vicky is HIV-positive. Her boyfriend is worried and insists that she should have an abortion. Vicky is upset, mainly because she says her parents 'will go berserk' if they know she is pregnant. However, she still wants to keep the child regardless. Her boyfriend's argument for her having an abortion is that 'there is a risk the baby will be born with AIDS and then die', and he 'wants to protect her from that'.

Were you the community midwife caring for Vicki, how would you support Vicki and try to assist her in reaching a responsible decision about her pregnancy?

termination of a patient's life, by act or omission, in the course of medical care' makes the practice morally and legally problematic regardless of what may be an overwhelming desire on the part of the carer to see someone who is suffering a painful death put out of his misery. Where the carer feels compelled to act to put an end to the hopeless suffering of a patient, there is also an inevitable clash between the ethical duty of protective care owed to the patient by the nurse – to do good (beneficence) and to avoid doing harm (non-maleficence) – and respect for the patient's autonomy and right to choose.

Alternatively, nurses may feel pressurised by patients who demand respect for their 'right' to die, while they, as nurses, feel that nursing care is about sustaining life, not about assisting patients to kill themselves or about hastening their death. The question is whether we do in fact have a 'right to die', and nurses generally feel that no patient has any entitlement to impose on them the duty to assist in the termination of a life. This raises a crucial philosophical question about the difference between liberties and rights.

The UK Voluntary Euthanasia Society has long campaigned for the legalisation of voluntary euthanasia, but there seemed to be insuperable legal obstacles as long as attempted suicide was illegal. When the Suicide Act of 1961 was passed, suicide ceased to be a criminal act in England (it had never been so regarded in Scotland). Supporters of the Voluntary Euthanasia Society claimed a moral victory and argued that the Suicide Act created a legal 'right to die'. This argument was based on a misunderstanding of the permissive nature of this particular piece of legislation, as a permissive or 'enabling' Act. What the legislation did was to decriminalise suicide and attempted suicide; it conceded that people may be *allowed the liberty* to take their own lives without suffering the penalties of the criminal law. But did the Act create a positive legal right to die?

Generally speaking, *moral and legal rights are justified claims that entitle us to demand that other people act, or desist from acting, in certain ways – i.e. our 'rights' impose either positive or negative duties on others* (see Box 5.2). Although we argue passionately about our moral rights, they may be

---

Box 5.2   Rights and duties

What do we mean by 'rights'?
Generally speaking, moral and legal rights are justified claims that entitle us to demand that other people act, or desist from acting, in certain ways – i.e. our 'rights' impose either positive or negative duties on others.
- *Negative rights* – the right to demand that a person desist from doing something to you is generally stronger than the positive right to have something given to you or done for you.
- *Positive rights* – your right to some personal or social benefit will depend on the generosity of others as well as on the available resources or benefits.

Rights may also be particular or universal, depending on their moral and legal foundations.
- *Particular rights* – these arise where we make promises, bets, vows or enter into contracts with particular people, where only the contracting parties have rights and duties to one another.
- *Universal rights* – these rights which we claim are applicable to all human beings regardless of race, sex, creed or age (e.g. the UNO Declaration of Universal Human Rights) and are based in claims that we all share a common species (e.g. rationality, sociability or freedom) which makes the possession of these rights essential if we are to lead a recognisably human life.

'Rights' and 'duties' relate to one another
My rights impose duties on you, and your rights impose duties on me, so my rights are relative to your rights and your rights limit mine. Thus, no rights can be absolute, while they may nevertheless be inalienable to me as a human being.
- *Moral rights* – these only have such force as the accepted rules and consensus of the moral community give them, may depend on available resources, and are often not enforceable.
- *Legal rights* – these may be enforceable through civil or criminal courts, in the case of both particular contractual rights and fundamental human rights, such as the right to privacy or freedom from assault, with the sanctions of fines or imprisonment applying in some cases.

Rights and responsibilities
On what basis do we praise or blame people for their actions? Or hold them responsible for their actions?
- If they knew what they were doing (i.e. are not ignorant or insane)
- If they acted voluntarily (i.e. are not acting under compulsion)
- If they had other options (i.e. are not powerless to act otherwise).
Persons can only be said to have rights and duties in the strict sense if they are responsible for their actions and thus capable of being responsible to other people. Other 'rights' are rights by analogy (e.g. rights of animals) or 'rights' by proxy (e.g. rights of children).

unenforceable, because they only have the strength which existing social consensus and convention give them, and impose only moral rather than enforceable legal obligations on others. We can, in some cases, seek the assistance of the courts to uphold our legal rights, e.g. where there is a breach in our contract of employment or invasion of our privacy, but the enforceability of our moral rights involves persuading enough people to support us and act in our interest.

In the strong sense of 'right', the UK Suicide Act 1961 does not create a right to die, or one which is legally enforceable, in the sense of imposing on one person a legal duty to assist someone else to die, nor could the law impose a duty not to intervene to prevent a person from taking his own life. In fact, the Homicide Act of 1957 specifically precludes the former by making assisted suicide a form of criminal homicide, and some mental health legislation imposes on professionals who are directly responsible for patients a legal duty to act to prevent patients from committing suicide. The various provisions of both English and Scottish Mental Health Acts make it possible for both health professionals and lay people to take action to have persons detained in hospital compulsorily if they are considered a serious suicide risk.

In the weaker sense of 'right', where the individual is allowed the liberty in law to attempt suicide, it may be argued that in cases of patients dying in extreme pain or undignified circumstances, nurses or other health care staff may *feel an obligation* to assist the patient to an easy or good death. However, feeling obligated would not be sufficient grounds to make such an action legal (or ethical), as most societies would argue. The action would have to be taken at great personal risk and as a lonely, individual and ambiguous act of compassion. Although there has been growing public support and sympathy for such acts in individual cases, e.g. of spouses assisting one another to 'an easy death', and the courts have tended to take a lenient line on charges brought against doctors and nurses who have practised active euthanasia, the recent murder conviction in the United States of Dr Kevorkian, who openly practised euthanasia, and the overturning by the Federal Court of

Australia of the Rights of the Terminally Ill Act 1995 introduced in the Northern Territories may indicate a swing towards a more conservative position on euthanasia. This attempt in the Australian Northern Territories to legalise euthanasia on demand may have failed, as much as anything, because it attempted to create a legal *right* to die, rather than simply introducing a permissive act that would allow people the *liberty* to seek assistance to terminate their lives under specified conditions (Kerridge et al 1998).

In general, neither law nor public morality concedes that anyone has a right to demand the assistance of another person to terminate his life. In practice, some nurses (or doctors) may feel moved to stop treatment or life support, or may actively intervene to terminate the life of someone in extreme suffering by the administration of drugs or by other means. However, such action would be illegal, whatever the circumstances, and in most cases would not be morally sanctioned either, because carers are expected to sustain life not end it, and most societies have moral principles forbidding suicide except in the most extreme circumstances (Beauchamp & Veatch 1996). (Similarly the 'legalisation' of abortion in Britain and many other countries has not, with the possible exception of Hungary and Western Australia, created a legal 'right' to termination on demand – at least not in the sense of an enforceable right or a duty which can be imposed on individual doctors and nurses.)

The provisions of the law and the constraints of public morality may or may not suffice to help the nurse in a particular case to decide whether to refuse the desperate request from a patient for deliverance from a living death. The 'legalisation' of euthanasia in Holland is a case in point. Like the 1967 UK Abortion Act, it is permissive legislation intended to formally decriminalise acts of euthanasia under certain defined conditions. No law permitting voluntary euthanasia can impose on doctors or nurses the duty to perform euthanasia against their will or conscience, and neither can legislation remove the painful tension, for both doctors and nurses, between the duty to care and respect for the dignity of the suffering patient in a particular situation. Neither could such legislation adequately prevent the misuse of euthanasia by unscrupulous individuals who might benefit from another's death. Arthur Clough's ironic wisdom remains relevant: 'Thou shalt not kill, but needst not strive officiously to keep alive'.[2]

There have been several attempts to legalise euthanasia in the UK, but the arguments which have invariably prevailed are: (a) that it is impossible to build in adequate safeguards to prevent the misuse of euthanasia by unscrupulous doctors or relatives, or both in collusion with one another, to take advantage of someone in a situation of extremity; (b) that introducing permissive legislation to permit 'voluntary euthanasia' will inevitably lead 'down the slippery slope' to 'nonvoluntary euthanasia' or intentional killing of the terminally ill. Evidence over a period of 15 years from Holland, based on official statistics, two large-scale surveys and critical analyses of both specific cases and interviews with practitioners, suggests that these fears may indeed be well grounded.

In the first survey in 1991 there were 2300 officially notified 'euthanasia deaths', 4000 cases of 'physician assisted suicide' and 1000 cases where euthanasia was performed without evidence of a specific request from the patient. All in all, there were 10 500 cases where withdrawal of treatment or increased use of drugs had 'shortened life'.

Given the specific conditions prescribed in Holland that were to be fulfilled if euthanasia was to be performed legally, there was less than 25% compliance with one or other of the following requirements (Keown 1995):

- the patient must have made an explicit and voluntary request for euthanasia
- the patient must be suffering unbearably and euthanasia should in such cases be a last resort
- the physician must have consulted with another medial practitioner regarding the case
- The doctor must submit an official report that he/she had complied with the law.

Another line of approach to the question is illustrated by the Council of Europe Working Party on Euthanasia (1999), which identified the following rights of the terminally ill:

- the right to adequate and competent palliative care
- the right to self-determination of the dying, rooted in their human dignity
- the right to be protected from involuntary euthanasia, or intentional killing by any person.

In order to ensure these rights are protected, the Council of Europe Working Party identified areas of need where action is necessary by member states if the rights and autonomy of the dying are to be properly respected and protected from neglect or abuse (Box 5.3).

The detailed and specific recommendations to member states of the Council of Europe are classified in the report under the headings of the basic rights listed above. These include requirements

---

Box 5.3   Measures required to protect the rights of the terminally ill

- To ensure adequate access of all people to expert palliative care and good pain management
- To ensure skilled treatment of physical suffering, and care for the psychological, social and spiritual needs of dying patients
- To avoid artificial prolongation of the dying process either by using disproportionate medical measures or by continuing treatment without a patient's consent
- To ensure adequate funds and training facilities for the continuing education and psychological support for health professionals working in palliative care medicine
- To provide means for the care and support of relatives and friends of terminally ill or dying patients, both for their own sake, but especially to alleviate the suffering of the dying patient
- To help alleviate the fear of patients of losing control of themselves and becoming a burden to or totally dependent upon relatives or institutional care
- To provide a suitably quiet and private space, within institutional environments, where a dying person can take leave of relatives or friends
- To ensure adequate allocation of funds and resources for the care and support of the terminally ill or dying
- To educate people, including health care staff, to overcome the social stigma of weakness, terminal illness, death and bereavement, and the associated discrimination against the dying

that member states should ensure legal protection for the following rights of the terminally ill:

● the right of access to appropriate and skilled palliative and terminal care
● the right to truthful, comprehensive yet compassionately delivered health information
● reaffirmation of the right enshrined in Article 2 of the European Convention for the Protection of Human Rights and Fundamental Freedoms, namely 'everyone's right to life shall be protected by law and no one shall be deprived of his life intentionally'.

In addition, the Council of Europe recognises that there are very practical things that need to be done to ensure the improvement of the general standards of terminal care, such as ensuring adequate funding for terminal care facilities, both institutional and mobile home care services, training and supportive services. In addition, it emphasises the importance of formal recognition of palliative care as a proper area of specialisation in medicine and nursing, of skilled training of health care staff and evidence-based research in the area. Finally, it recognises that with increased life expectancy, dying has become increasingly unfamiliar to the majority of people and that the public requires to be educated about the needs of those who are dying, be it from degenerative diseases or old age.

One of the most commonly expressed fears of the terminally ill is the fear of losing control – of their bodily functions, of their lives and personal affairs, and of the process of dying itself. It has been suggested, therefore, that death itself might be defined in terms of progressive loss of control. Being alive means having some degree of control over one's life and decisions; bodily functions are maintained in a balance, albeit precarious, of homeostasis, and one has some control over one's finances, property and relationships. Part of the pain of death is that it is something that happens to us, that is beyond our control – bodily systems disintegrate or 'self-destruct', our bodies corrupt and dissolve, and we lose control over our futures and fortunes. There is even a paradox in suicide, as Sartre (1969) pointed out, in the fact that by attempting to remain in control, to assert our autonomy by taking our own lives, we put an end

case history 5.2

A time to die?

The difficulty is to know when it is 'time'. Consider the following case.

Kenneth Bergstedt was 31. A quadriplegic with injuries to vertebrae C1 and C2, he had been on a respirator for 20 years. He spent his days lying on a hospital bed, watching television and writing poetry on a computer by blowing into a special device. He was cared for by his father, who was 65 and in failing health himself. Through the agency of his father, Kenneth Bergstedt applied to the courts to have his respirator turned off so that he could die. An affidavit filed with the court said '[he] has no happy or encouraging expectations to look for from life, receives no enjoyment from life, lives with constant fears and apprehensions, and is tired of suffering'.

A psychiatrist interviewed Kenneth and found him 'alert and intelligent'. The psychiatrist further found that Kenneth's 'quality of life' was 'very poor' and that his future 'offered no relief'. Kenneth's judgement was considered good and not unduly influenced 'by impulse or emotion'.

Faced with this evidence, the judge ruled that Kenneth Bergstedt's life support could be turned off and he could be allowed to die. Further, this action would not constitute suicide and thus no laws would be broken. The judge then ordered the case sent to a higher court, so that a legal precedent might be set to assist other disabled people who sought to end their lives. One reporter suggested that Kenneth Bergstedt's wish to die, and his father's desire to help him do so, 'probably are the greatest gifts of love either man could give the other'. Example used by Karen Lebacqz (Berkeley).[3]

to our autonomy! We all wish to retain control over our lives for as long as possible.

Glaser & Strauss's (1965) research showed that the health care team do not like to feel that they are losing control of the process and have difficulty giving in to the inevitable. From this perspective, voluntary euthanasia may appear to help the patient and the health professional to maintain the illusion of being in control in the face of death. In the end it may be a form of collusion to avoid facing the fact that death itself ultimately means loss of control (Sartre 1969). This is not to make light of the painful issues faced by carers and their patients in situations of terminal illness. Some of these anxieties would appear to be present in Case History 5.2.

Commenting on this case, Karen Lebacqz (1999) stated that the most remarkable and disturbing thing about it was the absence of controversy or protest about the judge's decision and the fact that this may indicate that popular opinion in the United States is moving towards acceptance of the concept of 'a time to die', without examining critically the position of the patient and the contribution to the suffering of the patient of his circumstances of inadequate social support. She quotes Carol Gill, a disability psychologist, who says: 'In the vast majority of cases, when a severely disabled person persists in wanting to die, there is an identifiable problem in the support system'. She continues:

Social structures are crucial to the meaning and purpose that people find in their lives. Kenneth was taken care of almost exclusively by his father. Two consequences of this care-giving arrangement are significant. First, Robert Bergstedt had recently lost his spouse and was ruminating on his own death. The father's grief and preoccupation with death undoubtedly influenced the son to seek his own death. Second, and more important, all his future possibilities came from his father. Robert Bergstedt painted a bleak picture of what would happen to Kenneth if Robert were hospitalised or died. Kenneth believed that if his father died, he would die from lack of care, or be placed in a nursing home. He was never told that people with his severe level of quadriplegia and need of respirator support can live active and productive lives. His entire view of the world – and of its possibilities for someone with his disability – was filtered to him through his father's eyes. At no time did anyone from a disability rights movement have access to Kenneth, whose friends and outside contacts were controlled by his father. The social structures that might have made a difference to Kenneth's understanding of the meaning of his life were not provided.

However, in hospice care, another kind of irony emerges in the ethics of terminal care. The more staff seek to respect the autonomy of dying patients, to discuss the implications of their imminent death with them, to support them through the anticipatory grief and distress, to consult them and respect their wishes regarding how, when and where they are to die, the more that good terminal care, which was supposed to be an alternative to voluntary euthanasia, actually approximates to it. If terminal care is not 'assisting patients to a good death', what is it? The pain and the dilemmas do not go away, although each case may be sensitively handled in a quite different way. In the case of a major disaster or where, for example, a person is crushed and trapped in a burning motor vehicle, the doctor or nurse may feel there is no alternative but to end the victim's misery; but where the patient has been so well maintained by 'good' terminal care that his death has become unduly protracted, where he has outlived his death sentence, it may be much more difficult not to press on regardless with care and treatment. What should be done, how it should be done and by whom can all be agonising questions, but something may need to be done. No universal prescriptions are possible in such situations, nor would they be appropriate (Doyle 1984).

DILEMMAS OF TRUTH-TELLING AND CONFIDENTIALITY

Francis Bacon once remarked that 'knowledge itself is power'.[4] The doctor's or nurse's knowledge of health matters gives them *power to help* people in distress, but also gives them *power over* such people. People give or withhold information about themselves in communication with health professionals depending on whether they trust the professionals involved and believe the information will be used for their benefit, for the better diagnosis and management of their problems. While people are generally willing to disclose sensitive and private information about themselves to doctors and nurses, they also realise that they make themselves vulnerable by doing so, and are aware that possession of this information gives health professionals further power over them. Legal safeguards for confidentiality of patient records and information are required to protect the vulnerability of patients and to ensure that possession of secret information about people is not abused by those caring for them, and that such information is not inappropriately disclosed.

On the other hand, the amount of information about a patient's medical condition, diagnosis, treatment and prognosis that is or should be disclosed to the patient is also a matter of sensible and responsible judgement. The control of information and its selective disclosure are part of the power exercised by doctors and nurses over patients, and can be used as a tool to secure their compliance with treatment. It is also a grave responsibility for nurses and doctors to decide when, how much and by whom information should be disclosed to patients. Refusal to disclose relevant information may deprive people of the power to make important decisions affecting their lives – if 'knowledge is power' then to be kept in a state of ignorance is to be kept in a state of impotence, infantilised and controlled. However, callous imparting of a fatal diagnosis would not only be insensitive and irresponsible, but could constitute a form of abuse – an inappropriate expression of professional power and expertise.

Dilemmas of truth-telling and confidentiality arise because of apparent or actual conflicts between the patient's right to know and the carer's duty to care. The classic situation of whether and when to tell dying patients that their condition is terminal illustrates the tension between two opposing moral concerns:

- respect for patients' autonomy and right to know their condition
- the feeling of carers that they should protect patients from news which might shock and distress them, perhaps causing them to give up in despair.

It may seem simplistic to say that what such situations require is honesty, but if we interpret honesty as demanding that we *honour*, i.e. show sensitive respect for the particular patient's needs and capacity to assimilate the information at the time, then maybe we can learn to 'titrate' the truth to the pain and needs of the individual. Responsible and compassionate truth-telling requires maturity, experience and sensitive counselling skills on the part of the nurse or doctor.

The situation may be further complicated in practice by the intervention of relatives demanding to know or forbidding communication with the dying, or by the unexpressed hopes or anxiety of the staff that a fatal diagnosis might be wrong in this case. The various parties involved may not be willing to acknowledge failure or to relinquish control. They may simply wish to protect themselves from the emotional burden of the

dying patient's grief. It is difficult to discuss these subtle problems of communication with the dying. They require great sensitivity, trust and confidence in the relationships of carers, patients and relatives. They are not susceptible to universal prescriptions and the predicament of nurses may be that, in practice, they are caught in the middle and prevented by 'doctor's orders' from doing what they believe to be the best in the circumstances. What makes these issues perennial dilemmas is that they bring opposing rights and duties into painful conflict. Whether priority will be given to the patient's right to know or to the professional's duty to protect the vulnerability of the dying patient cannot be decided by mere appeal to principle but has to be worked out in the complexity of each unique situation, in the way that seems most caring and responsible at the time (Thompson 1984).

Respect for the patient's secrets, his right to privacy, is again complicated by the often overriding duty to care and to do what is in the best interests of the patient. This may involve the carer in passing on confidential information to another professional in the hope that it will assist in the better care of the patient. Ideally, carers have a duty to seek the consent of persons who have confided in them before sharing their secrets, but if it is not possible to get it, then the dilemma arises: which is to take precedence – the patient's right to privacy or the professional's duty to provide the best possible care for the patient? Dilemmas of confidentiality generally do not arise out of careless disclosures of patients' secrets, but rather when the responsibilities of nurses to their patients, for example, come into conflict with the requirements of team management of patient care or in sharing information with relatives. They are further complicated by the problems of shift work and lack of continuity in care, while the need remains for carers to have crucial information.

Responsibility for sensitive confidential information about clients or patients is often both a burden and a privilege for carers, but it also gives them a special relationship with those in their care and subtle power over them. It can be a burden where it is difficult to set limits to the process of self-disclosure in a patient with a compulsive need to 'tell all'. Here the nurse may have to negotiate clear boundaries about what information is relevant and what is not, what information is strictly secret and what can be passed on to the rest of the care team. Doctors and nurses are sometimes inclined to guard jealously 'confidential information' about patients and are reluctant to share it with other members of the team because it means compromising the special relationship they have with 'their' patients/clients. Situations also change within the carer–client relationship, for example, as the client enters a crisis and becomes increasingly dependent, so the carer acquires greater power and control over the life of the client. Part of this control consists in management of the flow of information to the client, from the client and about the client. Giving or withholding information is a powerful way of encouraging cooperation or compliance and maintaining control in the caring relationship. Because knowledge is power and to be kept in ignorance is to be kept in a state of dependence, the manner in which the information and confidences are shared is a sensitive indicator of whether professional attitudes are creating dependency or are being used to assist clients towards autonomy, to enable them to take control of their own lives again (Thompson 1979b).

COMPULSORY PSYCHIATRIC TREATMENT – FOR WHOSE BENEFIT?

The dilemmas of confidentiality and truth-telling, as well as general conflicts between protective beneficence and respect for a person's rights, arise in the most acute form where the patient or client has become incompetent. This is particularly the case where the patient is psychotic and rendered practically and legally incompetent by virtue of mental disorder.

Treatment of people who are suffering from what political correctness demands we call 'mental disorder' has varied dramatically in the UK and Europe from the Middle Ages to the present day. Some of these changes are reflected in the range of terms we have historically applied to those whose mental states have resulted in bizarre and often dysfunctional behaviour. In the Middle Ages, the mentally ill were treated as 'holy innocents' or 'possessed of devils', depending on whether their condition seemed socially benign or evil. In the Enlightenment, people were deemed to have 'lost their reason' and were subjected to floggings and other indignities to help them 'regain their senses'. Other terms, e.g. 'lunatic', 'nutter', 'crazy', 'cuckoo', 'mad', 'insane', 'imbecile' and 'mentally ill', reflect the history of changing attitudes to people suffering from different kinds of mental disorder. Significantly, all these terms originally had neutral meanings, but have tended to acquire derogatory meanings and stigmatising effect over time. These examples illustrate clearly Wittgenstein's (1958) observation that 'language shift' usually signals both a shift in social values and explanatory paradigms. For example, 'lunatic' implies that insanity is caused by the moon; 'nutter', from the Latin word 'to nod, stagger', suggests a diagnostic sign of some forms of disorder; 'crazy' originally meant 'broken or shattered'; 'cuckoo' meant that one's reason had been usurped by some other power; 'insane' simply meant 'not whole'; and 'imbecile' meant 'weak'. What all these terms illustrate is our deep ambivalence about disordered or deranged mental states – both fear of the strange and unknown, and awe in the presence of something extraordinary or paranormal.

The treatment of mentally disordered people has also varied dramatically around the world from the compassionate tolerance of some societies to persecution and execution in others. There have even in modern times been wide divergences between psychiatrists themselves in the classification and definition of types of mental disease. Most striking in the recent past have been differences in the definition of schizophrenia by American and European psychiatrists. One of the great achievements of psychiatric epidemiology in the past decade, sponsored by the World Health Organization, has been research evidence of broadly similar distribution of the classic psychotic disorders around the world, and the achievement of a remarkable degree of consensus in the universal classification of psychiatric disorders (Scull 1992, WHO 1992).

Definition, as Aristotle noted 2500 years ago, is not only an essential tool of scientific method, but it is also a means by which we gain control over the world, other people and our subject matter. Precise names help to define people and things as individuals and of distinct kinds. The word 'definition' comes from the Latin word 'finiens' for a fence or *boundary*. By naming and defining things, we draw boundaries around them so as to order our knowledge and thus control reality better, both conceptually and practically. Thus knowledge gives power. Stokeley Carmichael, the American Black Power leader, said of white racism: 'Definition is the primary instrument of the white man's will-to-power over blacks'.[5] By the same token, we establish boundaries to intimacy with people by determining what names, titles or forms they are permitted to use in addressing us. Clinical labels, as observed in Chapter 2, have value both to the health care worker in defining the problem and to the patient in legitimising the treatment and being off work etc. However, these same labels, such as 'schizophrenic', 'HIV positive', etc., can be seriously stigmatising and affect people's status and rights in society. Exercise of the power of definition is a serious ethical responsibility for all professionals, namely to exercise it for the benefit of those in their care (Scull 1992, Boudreau & Lambert 1993).

The legal power of definition may be illustrated in the fact that given a psychiatric diagnosis of serious mental disorder or mental incapacity, society may require that the affected individual be taken into hospital against his will and even subjected to compulsory treatment. Deciding whether an individual should be compulsorily detained in hospital may be relatively easy in cases of severe dementia or florid mental illness, but the vast majority of psychiatric cases are not so clear-cut. The general legal requirement in most jurisdictions, that individuals must be 'a danger to themselves or others', leaves the mental health officer in an extremely difficult situation, for 'dangerousness' is notoriously difficult to determine in practice. To avoid public criticism or legal action for negligence, caring staff may tend to err on the side of caution and thus compromise the rights of individuals when the degree of danger would be virtually impossible to assess. Furthermore, the individual who is admitted in a severely disturbed state may recover without treatment or may have periods of reasonable normality and periods where he is clearly incompetent. Whether the system is sensitive enough to respond to these fluctuating changes in the moral status of the detained patient, and to respect his right to information or to be consulted about his treatment, is doubtful. The disabling effect of mental disorders, in affecting the patient's competence to exercise responsibility to control and/or direct his life, makes it peculiarly difficult to decide at what stage in the rehabilitation process it is appropriate for the carer to relinquish control. Conservatively, protective and defensive practice on the part of carers may seem to be common sense, but it may keep patients in a state of chronic dependency.

There are several peculiar features of the medical treatment of mental illness which create moral difficulties or dilemmas for nurses. These problems arise because of ambiguities in the diagnosis, treatment and rehabilitation of people with mental illness (including senile dementia and severe mental handicap). These ambiguities are to be found in all of the following:

- the moral/legal status of the patient
- the scope of definitions and diagnosis of 'mental illness'
- the variety of activities which count as 'treatment' in psychiatry and rehabilitation
- the definition of which patients are the carer's responsibility.

The status of the 'patient'

The ambiguous moral/legal status of someone suffering from a mental disorder is reflected in the fact that health professionals have unique legal powers to detain and treat patients who are regarded as 'incompetent' because they are mentally ill. The central moral paradox of psychiatry is that people may have to be deprived of their liberty and treated against their will in the hope that this will make it possible to restore their autonomy and enable them to take control of their lives again. To legitimate the use of these extraordinary legal powers by professionals, most legal systems require proof that a person is either a danger to others or a risk to himself. Assessment of these risks is necessary to justify detention of a patient for treatment, and this action is justified morally as both a duty of protective beneficence towards the patient (in protecting his health and safety, and ultimately his rights as well) and a requirement of justice to wider society (in maintaining lawful order, preventing others from harm and defending the common good). Ensuring adequate safeguards for patients' rights becomes the key ethical issue.

Mental health legislation varies considerably around the world, from the most libertarian, such as in Italian experiments with community psychiatry, to the most authoritarian and repressive, such as in the old Soviet Union and some traditional societies. These differences are reflected both in the stringency or laxity of requirements for proof of 'mental disorder' or 'dangerousness', and in the controls placed on compulsory detention and treatment of patients against their will. Concerns about the abuse of psychiatry, not only in the USSR during the Cold War period, but also in the USA during the Vietnam War, to control political dissidents by having them certified insane, led the UN World Psychiatric Association in 1977 to introduce the Declaration of Hawaii on the ethics of psychiatric practice and protection of the rights of psychiatric patients (Boyd et al 1997).

To protect the rights of the patient, various legal safeguards and rights of appeal tend to be built into mental health legislation and there is generally some kind of recourse to the courts or mental health tribunals for independent review of patients and their care. But serious questions may be asked about whose good the system serves, whether (with a few exceptions) the mentally ill are really a danger to others and whether legal action is justified to restrain attempted suicide by 'mentally ill' patients, if attempted suicide is not a proscribed course for 'normal' people.

National concern for the protection of mental health rights in the UK led to campaigns by MIND and the Scottish Association for Mental Health demanding reform of mental health legislation.

The provisions of the new Mental Health Scotland Act 1964 were considered at the time to be very progressive in protecting the rights of patients. The Act required that apart from short-term emergency orders, requiring only a second medical opinion or endorsement by a registered Mental Health Officer, compulsory detention orders should be subject to confirmation before a court and subject to periodic review by an independent Mental Welfare Commission. Patients were given the legal right to appeal directly to the Mental Welfare Commission, but the Commission was also legally obligated to review all patients detained in hospital on long-term orders on a regular basis. The Commission comprised an independent panel of expert psychiatrists, nurses, social workers, lawyers and lay advocates with quasi-legal powers to investigate and to discharge patients judged to be inappropriately detained. While this model appeared to be a great step forward and was copied in a number of other jurisdictions around the world, after a period of 20 years its operation was judged, on the basis of research, to provide inadequate protection for patients' rights. This was mainly because emergency detention orders (for up to a week) were being applied without these safeguards. The system was being abused, either by discharging patients prematurely or by simply applying successive 'emergency orders' to circumvent the need for court appearances and mandatory visits and reporting on cases.

Ironically these developments were made possible partly by the success of new pharmacological treatments for schizophrenia and bipolar affective disorders, which allowed patients on long-acting depot drugs to return home in what was described by some nurses as a 'chemical straitjacket', rather than be detained for more labour-intensive and expensive treatment in hospital. What came to be called an 'open-door' policy in mental hospitals (or 'revolving door policy' as it became) also suited the prevailing mood of economic rationalism in government, which favoured quicker bed turnover and 'community care', as this was thought to be a cheaper way of delivering mental health services. A decade of experiment with the de-institutionalisation of people with mental illness has resulted in serious problems in many countries adopting this approach, because resources to support community-based services have nowhere been adequate and psychiatric patients have tended to simply be recycled through prisons and the criminal justice system. Criticism of 'community care' as a solution to the problem of mental health treatment services and the protection of the rights of patients, in Italy, the UK and Australia, has led to renewed demands for adequate mental hospital services and 'the right to asylum'.[6] In North America and Canada, there have been considerable variations between different states in views regarding compulsory community treatment or community commitment. These are critically reviewed by Boudreau & Lambert (1993).

The definition of mental illness

The notorious imprecision of definitions of 'mental illness', and even serious disagreement as to whether mental illness actually exists – as distinct from physiological disorders, or emotional distress and problems of living – led to considerable debate in the 1960s about whether we should refer to 'mental illness' at all. Laing & Esterson (1970), in *Sanity, Madness and the Family*, argued that 'mental illness' is a response to dysfunctional parenting and Thomas Szasz (1974), in *The Myth of Mental Illness*, argued that mental illness is a social construct to categorise a range of maladaptive behaviours causing people to deal ineffectively with problems of living. These approaches contrasted sharply with the current attempts to explain mental illness in terms of disturbances in the biochemistry of the brain or malfunctioning brain metabolism. There may be more agreement today about the causes of different types of mental disorder and about the methods of classifying types of psychiatric disorder, which may make the furious debates about the definition of mental illness in the 1960s and 1970s seem somewhat passé. Nevertheless, there remains a considerable degree of medical and scientific uncertainty about the predisposing conditions and aetiology of mental illness.

This uncertainty makes it at least questionable whether individuals who are diagnosed as suffering from some kind of 'mental' disorder should be singled out for special legal sanctions, deprivation of liberty and the denial of their fundamental rights. Examples of the rights of 'mental patients' which may be compromised are (Szasz 1987):

- the right to be adequately informed and to give voluntary consent to treatment
- the right to privacy and confidentiality (which may be compromised in group therapy and team management)
- the right to refuse treatment and/or to discharge themselves from hospital (where even voluntary patients may fear imposition of a compulsory order if they do not comply)
- the right to vote in general elections, to emigrate or, in some cases, even to go on holiday abroad.

Western Australia, which, well into the 1990s, had some of the most conservative mental health legislation, might serve to illustrate how concern for patients' rights over the past 30 years has resulted in greater caution being exercised over the involuntary admission of people to a mental hospital and the provision of safeguards to protect the rights of psychiatric patients. For example, the West Australian Mental Health Act 1996 sets much more stringent conditions which must be fulfilled before a patient can be deprived of his liberty and treated without his consent. In *A Clinician's Guide to the Mental Health Act 1996* (Health Department of Western Australia 1997), the criteria justifying compulsory admission are set out as follows:

- The individual must have a mental illness, as described by the Act, requiring treatment
- The treatment can be provided through detention in an authorised hospital, or through a Community Treatment Order and is necessary in order to:
  - protect the health and safety of that person or any other person
  - protect the person from self-inflicted harm, which includes financial harm, and lasting or irreparable harm to any important personal

relationship caused by damage to the reputation of any of the parties

– prevent the person doing serious damage to property

● The person has refused or is unable to give consent to treatment

● The treatment cannot be adequately provided in a way that would involve less restriction.

What is significant is that the Act does not attempt to define different forms of mental illness or syndromes in clinical terms, but rather in terms of observable behaviour and the extent to which the person's behaviour would be seen to be bizarre, even within his unique cultural milieu (Health Department of Western Australia 1997).

The 'benefits' of a psychiatric diagnosis (asylum, access to care and treatment, relief from the burden of family or work responsibility) have to be counterbalanced against the 'costs' of the disabling and stigmatising effect of being labelled 'mentally ill' or a 'psychiatric patient' and the denial of some fundamental human rights – even if one is no longer called a 'lunatic' or imprisoned.

The limits of 'treatment'

In psychiatry, there is a further irony related to interpretation of 'consent to treatment' even for the 'voluntary patient', for this consent amounts to almost 'writing a blank cheque'. What counts as 'treatment' in psychiatry possibly covers a wider range and is perhaps more inclusive than in any other area of medicine – ranging from protective asylum to being 'straitjacketed' in a locked and padded cell, from one-to-one psychotherapy to group therapy of various kinds. Also included is an enormous range of other 'therapies', including occupational therapy (art, music, dance, sheltered employment), physiotherapy, behaviour therapy, chemotherapy, ECT and psychosurgery. It is by no means clear to the average patient (or nurse for that matter) what he is consenting to or what will be included in the scope and limits of 'treatment'. There is a risk that health professionals will arrogate to themselves the right to simply decide what therapies are in the best interests of the patient without consulting the patient or relatives. For the compulsorily detained patient,

cooperation and compliance can be elicited by the mere hint of the extension of compulsory powers or their re-imposition. Nurses are intimately involved in the whole complex of relationships which operate and sustain these systems of social control in psychiatric and psychogeriatric institutions. Since the publication of Goffman's (1968) *Asylums* and his research on 'total institutions', we have been more aware of the effects of 'institutionalisation' on both patients and staff in, for example, mental hospitals. While much can be done to 'humanise' the environment of institutions, the fact remains that in the sphere of mental health in particular, nurses perform a dual role, as carers and as agents of social control. Popular films such as *One Flew over the Cuckoo's Nest*, while possibly exaggerating the punitive and repressive nature of mental institutions, nevertheless bring out the unavoidable conflict there is for nurses between a caring ethic and their role in policing the behaviour of people compulsorily detained in hospital.

Community psychiatry, which involves not only the supervision of psychiatric patients in the community, but also the investigation of the 'social supports' or family background of the patient, raises serious new ethical questions for the nurse in dealing with the family. Who is the patient? How many family members are included within the scope of the responsibility of the community psychiatric nurse? Has the nurse the right to intervene in the family life of the patient – to draw other family members into the therapeutic net? Again, the situation is without parallel in nursing (except perhaps in contact tracing in HIV or venereal disease). Do health professionals have a right to seek out undisclosed pathology or undeclared 'patients' who have not recognised that they have a problem? Because the legal powers taken in psychiatry are extraordinary, they raise all sorts of difficult ethical questions about the scope and limits of professional responsibility and the rights and status of patients and their families (Reed & Lomas 1984).

MANAGEMENT AND ALLOCATION OF RESOURCES

All the previous examples discussed tend to occur within one-to-one relationships in patient care, where the primary tension is between the professional's duty to care for and protect the patient, and the demand that the carer respects the dignity and rights of the patient/client as a person. There is a whole class of other ethical problems and dilemmas which arise for nurses when they move from simple one-on-one clinical nursing responsibility into ward or hospital management, or teaching and research roles. In these situations, they are responsible not only for groups of patients and staff, but also for the allocation of staff time, administration of drugs and equipment, and general allocation of resources and the well-being of a whole institution. While we will discuss other examples of these kinds of one-to-many ethical responsibilities in Chapters 7 and 8, the ethical issues which are raised most frequently in discussion are on the borderline between problems of direct patient care and management.

The critical decisions which doctors face when there are scarce resources have been the subject of much attention, from television dramas and discussions in the popular media to more serious academic debate. Such crises are often illustrated by situations where there are two or more patients urgently requiring kidney dialysis and only one machine, or where there is a patient needing a heart transplant and a shortage of donor organs. While the crises over limited resources in nursing may not be so dramatic, they are certainly more common, such as a staff nurse having to decide between keeping to the agreed ward routine for staff and mobilising more staff to deal with an emergency or the needs of one particular patient. In more prosperous countries where hospitals are reasonably well funded, the ethical crises for nurse managers over allocation of scarce resources may not be of major proportions, but in developing countries these problems and dilemmas may be acute: there may not be enough routinely prescribed drugs to go around; disposable hypodermic syringes and scalpels may be unknown, requiring regular sterilisation of non-disposable ones, and even bandages may have to be boiled and reused; and there may be a shortage of beds. Determining who gets the treatment or resources may not be so simple as the application of 'triage' methods in an urban road traffic acci-

dent. The sheer volume of need may be so overwhelming that the ethical question is whether the nurse should perhaps give up her job in the field and return to the USA or Europe to campaign for resources for 'her patients'. A moving example of this was a British nurse working in Uganda appealing at a World AIDS Conference 'not for facilities to test for HIV, not for AZT, but for calamine lotion and means to palliate the suffering of AIDS victims, where the cost of treating 100 of the 1 000 000 AIDS victims with AZT would consume the entire national health budget'.

In more prosperous societies, the resource allocation 'dilemmas' may have more to do with the possible diversion of resources from the 'hi-tech' expensive treatment of a few patients to the treatment of larger groups of patients with chronic disorders, mental illness or the growing number of elderly people. Here, even in dealing with chronic disease conditions or the multiple pathologies of geriatric patients, while technical clinical considerations may be relevant to determining what may be done, and might in some cases help to decide the issues, the fundamental moral question remains one of justice. The ethical problems concerning the allocation of resources have less to do with the traditionally opposing moral demands of the professional duty of care versus the rights of the patient. Here the problems concern the tensions between equality of opportunity in access to the best available health care and equality of outcome for all groups in society. Applying a simple utilitarian calculus to determine 'the greatest happiness for the greatest number' will inevitably mean that minorities are disadvantaged, whether it is those marginalised in society by intellectual disability or mental illness, or ethnic minorities. This is not only a problem in the UK, where studies have shown the relative disadvantage suffered by immigrant populations, but also in Australia where whites enjoy one of the highest standards of health care in the world, yet where the Aboriginal people have been described in one WHO report as enjoying Fourth World standards of health and health care services.

The ethics of resource allocation concerns the right of everyone to equal access to appropriate care and treatment, particularly in a system of health care to which all contribute by taxation directly or indirectly. The claims of certain individuals, because they are wealthier, more powerful or just more attractive human beings, have to be balanced against the common good. The priorities determined by professionals on their own criteria for giving certain clients preference over others because they are 'in need of greater care' may also have to be challenged or questioned in the name of justice, if others suffer neglect as a result (Boyd 1979, Ch. 3).

The dilemmas of responsibility and accountability in nurse management roles are not restricted to dilemmas in the allocation of limited resources or reconciling conflicting needs of different patients. There are some prosaic problems about the management and deployment of staff, the management of time and resources in the routine care of large groups of patients, and the rational ethical choices which have to be made between the balance of time spent on patient care and/or patient education, teaching or research and evaluation. Current concern with quality assurance and individual and corporate performance review and assessment is, at its best, the application of research criteria and principles of rational justice to the responsible management of resources. While nurses may feel passionately about the care of individual patients and feel that 'research-driven' or 'evidence-based' practice is impersonal and ignores the needs of the individual, they have to resolve, even in particular cases, the difficult tension between the competing demands of care and justice, while in management the tensions between the demands of beneficence, justice and respect for the rights of individuals are at the very centre of routine administrative responsibility.

Even the economic thinking which gave rise to the 'internal market', where hospitals and health care staff become part of the purchaser–provider 'contract culture', is driven by ethical concerns with the most fair and cost-efficient use of public resources and protection of the common good. But, given the culture in which nurses begin their careers in a clinical context, these issues all raise important new ethical problems for the management of staff and resources. Some of these issues will be further addressed in Chapter 8, but suffice

it to say at this point that the tensions between a very individualistic, personalist, even 'privatised' morality based on one-to-one relations in clinical settings does not translate very well into dealing with these broader issues relating to the well-being of groups of patients or to management and service of the common good of wider society. The former 'privatised' perspective tends to see all moral issues in personalist terms within the tensions between the duty to care for patients and respect for patients' rights. The wider issues of distributive justice and equity in health care, of effectiveness and efficiency in the responsible administration of public resources, require not only a different perspective on things, but different kinds of skills in management, team-building and teamwork, committee procedure and 'political' action.

We have stressed earlier that to be a professional is to exercise a public office and carries 'political' responsibilities. This is all the more true of management and administration. These roles are inherently political, in the sense that they involve balancing interests and powers of various kinds. This may be within the institution or it may involve negotiating with a higher authority outside the institution about policy, staffing, wages and resources. It may involve using collective action through professional or union organisations to seek better working conditions for nurses or to maintain or achieve better standards of patient care. Such 'political' action may generate new moral conflicts, e.g. issues of the rights of patients versus the rights of nurses; of the duties of nurses and the duties of patients; of justice in the sense of non-discrimination against individuals and equality of opportunity and outcome for groups; of the duty to care for vulnerable patients and the duty to care for staff. These all involve the same fundamental moral principles and require skills in balancing or resolving the tensions and conflicts between them. The demands of justice and the common good may limit the liberty of doctors and nurses in the exercise of unlimited clinical autonomy (e.g. not just which drugs they may prescribe, but on larger matters of where patients may be referred for treatment). Similarly, the rights and autonomy of patients may have to be compromised in the interests of public health, not only in circumstances of emergency or life-threatening epidemics, such as cholera or AIDS, but also where scarce medical resources do not permit priority to be given to procedures such as cosmetic surgery, assisted reproduction or transplant surgery (White 1985).

The moral problems in the remainder of this book will be examined within a structure where we move, in ever widening circles of responsibility, from consideration of the personal moral issues in direct nurse–patient relationships to consideration of problems in managing groups of patients and, finally, to the wider responsibilities of nurses in institutional settings, in relation to society and in the national and international political order.

 ## further reading

Exploring the nature of 'care'
Bowden P 1997 Caring: gender-sensitive ethics. Routledge, London, chs 1, 3 – *a sympathetic but critical appraisal of feminist and other treatments of caring in mothering and nursing*

Brown J, Kitson A, McKnight T J 1992 Challenges in caring: explorations in nursing and ethics. Chapman and Hall, London – *a more advanced philosophical discussion of ethics in caring relationships*

Stevenson J, Tripp-Reimer T (eds) 1990 Knowledge about care and caring: state of the art and future developments. American Academy of Nursing, Kansas City, MO – *a useful overview which includes discussion of the ethical dimensions of caring*

Clarifying different professional values
Bok S 1995 Common values. University of Missouri Press, Columbia, MO – *a sensitive discussion of common values with helpful analysis of their practical applications*

Downie R S, Calman K C 1987 Healthy respect: ethics in health care. Faber, London – *a discussion of a wide range of value-related questions which arise in health care*

Rokeach M 1976 Beliefs, attitudes and values: a theory of organisation and change. Jossey-Bass, San Francisco, CA – *a classical study of values in organisations and as affecting behaviour change*

Simon S B, Howe L W, Kirchenbaum H 1995 Values clarification. Warner Books, New York – *an advanced study and overview of the values clarification debate*

Steele S M, Harmon V M 1983 Values clarification in nursing, 2nd edn. Appleton-Century-Crofts, Norwalk, CT – *a practical guide with useful introductory material on value theory*

Lay and professional concepts of 'health'
Armstrong D 1983 An outline of sociology as applied to medicine. Wright, Bristol – *an illuminating general introduction to the concepts of health and disease as social constructs*

Benner P 1984 From novice to expert: excellence, and power in clinical nursing practice. Addison-Wesley,

Menlo Park, CA – *a critical and empirically grounded study of caring interactions in nursing*

Cousins N 1979 Anatomy of an illness – as perceived by the patient. WW Norton, New York – *an important view of medicine and nursing from the patient's point of view*

Kitson A 1987 An analysis of lay-caring and professional [nursing] caring relationships. International Journal of Nursing Studies 24: 160–161 – *a brief paper analysing lay and nursing perspectives*

Melia K M 1988 Learning and working: the occupational socialisation of nurses. Tavistock, London – *an analysis of the findings of detailed research undertaken on the changes occurring in nurse students*

Decisions of general principle and specific cases (see Ch. 10)
Johnstone M J 1994 Bioethics: a nursing perspective. Saunders/Baillière Tindall, London, ch 6 – *a helpful discussion of systematic and experiential approaches to dealing with moral problems*

Thompson J, Thompson H 1985 Bioethical decision-making for nurses. Appleton-Century-Crofts, Norwalk, CT – *a critical discussion of ethical decision making for nurses with examples*

Toulmin S 1986 The place of reason in ethics (reprint). University of Chicago Press, Chicago – *a re-issue of a well-respected discussion of justification of both ethical policies and specific judgements*

Euthanasia and the 'right to die'
Doyle D 1984 Palliative care: the management of far advanced illness. Croom Helm, London

Glover J 1977 Causing death and saving lives. Penguin Books, Harmondsworth

Keown J 1995 Euthanasia examined: ethical, clinical and legal aspects. Cambridge University Press, Cambridge

Kerridge I, Lowe M, McPhee J 1998 Ethics and law for the health professions. Social Science Press, Katoomba, NSW

Ramsey P 1978 Ethics at the edges of life. Yale University Press, New Haven

Thompson I E 1979 Dilemmas of dying – a study in the ethics of terminal care. Edinburgh University Press, Edinburgh

end notes

1 Dostoevsky F (Garnett C, tr), 1927 *The Brothers Karamazov*. Everyman Library, Dent, London
2 Clough A H 1974 *The Latest Decalogue*. From: Mulhauser F L (ed) *Poems*.Oxford University Press, Oxford
3 Quoted with permission from *Biomedical Ethics* 4(1): 16, 1999.
4 Francis Bacon (1561–1626) *Religious Meditations, 'Of Heresies'*.
5 Stokeley Carmichael, in his address to the World Council of Churches Consultation on Racism, held in Notting Hill, London in 1969.
6 Typical would be the critical Burdekin report (Burdekin et al 1993) on the inadequacy of the mental health services provided in Western Australia, a society with a very high per capita income and one which prides itself on its general standard of health care, but where community mental health services were considered unacceptably low.

some suggestions on method

Exploring the nature of 'care'
This topic lends itself to treatment at two levels: the personal and the sociological. Learning exercises should include both if the connection is to be made between them by students. First, subject to agreed ground rules for sharing in confidential pairs, students could be asked to explore in personal terms the meaning of caring for one another as nurses, and what relationship this has to ability for self-care. Second, in groups of six to eight students, each group could be asked to explore the concept of 'care' in one of the following kinds of relationship: 'mothering', 'friendship', 'nursing', 'teaching' and 'counselling'. During feedback from the groups, the task would be to clarify similarities and differences between personal and professional dimensions of caring.

Clarifying different professional values
Using a real-life case (involving say a ward team or primary health care team) and using the pro forma in Figure 5.1 (p. **102**), the tutor might get the class to work in small groups to identify the various professional stakeholders, their roles and value bases, their different ways of defining 'the problem', likely interventions and expected outcomes. This can be done by discussion or, more effectively, by role-playing the parts of the various 'actors' in the 'drama'. Whichever method is used for the first part, the groups should be required to address the task of clarifying the points of agreement and disagreement between the 'players' and what basis there is for common agreement about a joint action plan.

Lay and professional concepts of 'health'
To start with, students could be asked to draw a 'map' of their own 'health career' so far, and how they see it developing – using a diagram such as that Figure 5.2 (p. **109**). This should illustrate the various 'ups' and 'downs' of their lives, as well as periods of growth and development, major life events and cases of loss of autonomy and permanent disability.

Having done this, the class could be encouraged to discuss their respective 'health career maps' in small groups of three or four and to report back on common features and major differences between them.

Decisions of general principle and specific cases
To bring out the difference between arguing a point of general principle (e.g. about abortion or not-to-resuscitate procedures) and making decisions in particular cases, it may be helpful to set up a class debate in which one team argues the issue in general terms and the other entirely in terms of what is demanded in particular cases. It should then be possible to clarify the difference between policies or rules designed to apply to *classes* of situations, and decisions which apply only in a particular case with a specific patient at a given time and place.

This should help students to recognise the need to distinguish between policy debate and making ethical decisions and the complementary relationship between the two in our practical moral life, discussions and decision-making.

6

Direct responsibility in nurse–patient relationships

AIMS

This chapter has the following aims:
1. To explore the reciprocal nature of rights and duties within any moral community, in relationships between nurses and patients, and in determining the nature of patients' rights
2. To clarify the difference between liberties and rights, positive and negative rights, institutional, legal and moral rights, and particular and universal rights
3. To explore the value and limitations of 'rights talk' as a basis for deciding in difficult cases: disclosure of information, resuscitation, sedation and involuntary treatment of patients in crisis situations.

LEARNING OUTCOMES

When you have read and worked through this chapter, you should be able to:
■ Give a coherent account of the particular rights arising from your contractual commitments and acceptance of the rules which apply in the community where you work

■ Explain the nature of and the basis for 'universal human rights', demonstrating ability to discuss specific examples and their justification

■ Illustrate the nature of patients' rights by discussing examples of particular cases from your own experience of nursing where issues of patients' rights arise

■ Demonstrate ability to tease out the conflicting rights and duties of patients, staff and other stakeholders in analysing work-related case histories

■ Demonstrate ability to discuss the general policy issues involved in the protection of patients' records and personal confidences

■ Demonstrate ability to recognise how changes in the level of dependency of the patient and the power relations of nurse and patient impact on human rights

In the previous chapter, before discussing some of the classic ethical dilemmas in health care, we examined the difference between the ethics of caring for a specific individual in a particular case and the question of developing general ethical policies to deal with types or classes of problems. Part of the chapter was devoted to discussing a number of preliminary questions relating to the moral environment within which we make ethical decisions in health care. These were: the different ways we construe 'health' and 'disease'; the different levels at which we encounter ethical problems (personal, team, institution, health service); the issues raised by the 'medicalisation of life'; and the need to consider the whole 'health career' of individuals (and not just isolated episodes or health crises) when making decisions about them in the real world. Having considered these prior general and methodological questions, we can now proceed to look at how ethics bears directly on specific cases in the one-to-one relationship of the nurse with the patient, in hospital or community. We will begin with some remarks on the concepts of 'rights' and 'duties' and consider how these apply in a variety of different situations in nursing.

THE RECIPROCAL RIGHTS AND DUTIES OF PATIENT AND NURSE

Given the power nurses have over people when they are at their most dependent and vulnerable, and the privileged and intimate access nurses have to people, both to their bodies and to their private lives, the 'duty of care' and other general 'duties' of nurses have rightly been emphasised in nurse training since the beginning. Talk of patients' rights in the context of such relationships is a relatively new phenomenon. Several factors have contributed to this emphasis on patients' rights.

The movement was undoubtedly given impetus by publication of the Universal Declaration of Human Rights (UNO 1947). Also, popular demand for rights of more equitable access to health and social services after World War II led to the establishment of welfare states in a variety of countries around the world. However, it was probably the increase in litigation over cases of alleged medical malpractice, and campaigns by consumer rights and patient advocacy groups that did most to raise awareness of 'patients' rights'. A typical response to this was the American Hospital Association's attempt to codify a bill of rights for patients (AHA 1992 – Appendix 3).

Clamorous demands for rights on behalf of one group often lead to counter demands from those from whom recognition of rights is being demanded. Pope John XXIII (1963) stressed that we should always pay attention when people start demanding their rights, because this usually signals deeply felt injustice for which people are demanding redress. Not surprisingly, demands by patient advocacy groups for patients' rights have been met by counter demands from nurses for recognition of the 'rights of nurses' as well. Expected to be 'always dutiful', nurses have found themselves becoming more militant in campaigning for their rights, e.g. as their wages and working conditions have often failed keep up with the general standard of living and improvements in the economic and social conditions of other workers. The unionisation of nurses and their willingness to take industrial action are due to this growing awareness of their rights.

Legally and morally, nurses clearly share the individual and industrial rights of other employees, but they also have specific rights and duties in the context of health care where they work, in relation to doctors, nurse managers and patients. Rumbold (1993) devotes a whole chapter of his book to the discussion of the rights of nurses, and clearly this area of ethical debate is becoming of increasing importance to nurses. However, we must pause and ask whether 'rights talk' gets us very far and whether it is an adequate basis from which to examine nursing ethics (Johnstone 1994, Ch. 13).

In Chapter 4 we distinguished between four kinds of situations in which nurses deal with patients, namely *crisis intervention*, *voluntary requests for help*, *nursing chronic and terminal illness* and *proactive screening and health promotion*. In each of these situations the degree of independence or powerlessness of the patient affects the ethics of the situation and the weight given to the duties of the nurse relative to the rights of the patient and vice versa. Just as in family life the balance of duties and rights changes as children grow from infancy to adulthood, so in nursing the balance of rights and duties will change with the degree of dependency or autonomy of the patient.

For example, the patient's right to know will be differently interpreted if the patient is unconscious, insane, very distressed or anxious, than if she is conscious and in possession of her faculties. In accident and emergency (A&E), the nurse's first duty to a vulnerable patient relates immediately to the patient's right to adequate care and treatment. Because 'rights talk' has to be interpreted in relation to different and changing situational demands, it is necessary, before we can proceed to discuss ethical decision-making in specific cases, that we clarify what we mean by 'rights' and 'duties,' how are they related and distinguished, and how they apply in nursing contexts.

THE MEANING OF 'RIGHTS' AND 'DUTIES'

In the previous chapter, in discussing abortion and euthanasia, we briefly distinguished between liber-

ties and rights and introduced a number of preliminary distinctions between positive and negative, particular and universal, moral and legal rights (see Box 5.2, p. 114). In that context we said *moral and legal rights are justified claims that entitle us to demand that other people act, or desist from acting, in certain ways – i.e. our 'rights' impose either positive or negative duties on others*. Rights and duties are thus connected, but what is the nature of this connection?

The literal meaning of the word 'right' – from the German *recht* for rule – has to do with what a rule entitles us to expect or allows us to do. The word 'duty' – from the French *deu* for what is owed – relates to what obligations we owe to others or have under the rule in question.

If rights are 'justified entitlements', the first question to ask is how are our rights to be justified? This immediately raises some difficult theoretical questions about the nature of human rights and their philosophical justification. We will return to discuss 'rights theory' in the final chapter, but here we need to simply clarify the use of the terms 'rights' and 'duties' in everyday usage.

Most simply, particular rights and duties exist where we are subject to rules or agreements with other people. This applies in every kind of moral community to which we belong and in which we act as responsible members. For example, the rules of a sports club impose certain *duties* on members (e.g. to pay subscriptions, to support the club's aims, to participate in club competitions, to dress and behave appropriately, etc.), but they also give members certain *rights* or *entitlements* (e.g. to gain access to club amenities, to be included in club competitions, to represent oneself as a member of the club, to bring guests, under specified conditions, etc.). Similarly, if I wish to drive a motor car in the UK, I am required by the Highway Code to drive on the left. It is my *moral and legal duty* to do so, to prevent accidents which might be caused by uncertainty on the part of other drivers, who would otherwise be unable to predict my behaviour. On the other hand, I have a *legal right*, or justified entitlement, to expect that you will drive on the opposite side of the road and will not collide with me because you decide to drive towards me on 'my' side of the road!

The rights and duties of members of a sports club do not apply to non-members. The rights and duties that we enjoy as motorists in the UK do not apply in other countries where the rules of the road may be different. These rights and duties are first of all *particular rights and duties* in the sense that they are peculiar to those who are participating members of a particular society. The rights and duties involved do not apply to everyone, but only to those who agree to abide by the rules of that particular community.

These specific agreements give rise to specific obligations and justified entitlements for those involved in the agreement, and not to outside parties. *Particular rights* – as opposed to universal rights – arise as a result of a number of different kinds of agreement between individuals or groups of people. Some philosophers have suggested that *promises* and *promising* are the foundation of all rights and duties. If Jack promises to take Jill out to dinner and does not turn up as arranged, Jill has a right to be annoyed because Jack has a moral obligation to keep his promises – on pain of never being trusted again. Here, only Jack and Jill have rights or obligations to one another related to the promise. They are particular to them and no other party is involved. However, if Jack fails to keep his promise, because of some overriding duty (say to go to his mother's bedside if she has had a stroke), or if he had a motor accident on the way to meet Jill, then we might say that he could be excused from his obligation to meet Jill. Other types of agreements where we acquire particular rights and obligations are *vows*, *bets* and *contracts*. The obligation to pay up if you lose a bet could be enforced through the courts, provided there were witnesses to the bet having taken place. Solemn vows, such as those sealing a contract of marriage, create both moral and legal obligations, breaches of which give rise to much conflict and litigation in the divorce court, and often high legal costs! Contracts of employment and business contracts with suppliers of goods and services again give rise to moral and legal duties and entitlements, where breach of a contract can lead to civil court action – either to enforce the right or to seek compensation for the breach.

Claims that we enjoy certain universal and inalienable rights as human beings cannot be justified by appeal to social agreements or conventions, or they would not be universal or inalienable. These *fundamental human rights* or *universal human rights* form a different class of 'rights' or 'entitlements', which have to be justified in a different way. The ancient Greeks, and particularly Stoic philosophers and lawyers, argued that we all share a common human nature and common needs as rational beings or members of the species *homo sapiens*. They, as well as modern rights theorists, argue that universal human rights exist on the basis that certain conditions must obtain if we are to achieve our full potential as members of our species, and that all human societies must recognise this. Universal human rights purport to express necessary conditions without which we cannot flourish or develop as human beings, or lead anything like recognisably human lives.

The claim, expressed in the preamble to the United States Constitution, that all human beings are created equal and independent, and from that inherent equality possess the inalienable rights to 'the preservation of life, and liberty and the pursuit of happiness' is rooted in this tradition. The ancient belief and moral claim that because we all share certain characteristics and needs in common as rational human beings, we are therefore entitled to fundamental 'human' rights – like freedom of speech, conscience and association – rests on certain general metaphysical assumptions about the unique nature or essence of human beings, as well as specific beliefs about what particular characteristics and needs are definitive of our species and distinguish it from other animals.

While there is an interesting range of theories, and much debate, about what is the most essential defining characteristic of the human species, there would not be much disagreement about the fact that we are really different, for example, from crocodiles and giraffes (which are visibly different from us) but that we are also distinguishable from the higher apes (or hominids) which we resemble in so many amusing ways.

How we understand human rights and duties will depend on how we define a 'human person'. The terms 'person' and 'personality' serve to define what we mean by humans, both as members of our species and as individuals. The term 'person' comes from *persona*, the Latin word for a mask, and signifies the role or identity we assume in life. Kant (1724-1804), in his *Groundwork to the Metaphysic of Morals*, argued that the term 'person' is foundational for ethics and that without it ethics cannot get off the ground. Why is this? There are two kinds of reason:

- The 'mask' we assume in the drama of life defines both our role or identity and also public expectations of the normal rights and obligations that go with that role
- The way we define a 'person', or specify the defining characteristics of 'personhood', sets the boundaries for the 'moral community' and determines who qualifies for membership.

In its most general and abstract sense, the term 'person' has been interpreted in law from the earliest times as simply 'a bearer of rights and duties'. Individuals who are 'bearers of rights and duties' may not only be individual people, but also, as in Roman law, individual partnerships, clubs, businesses or public associations. In this sense, the term 'person' is a formal and empty concept until we fill it with some meaning. It is like a 'blank cheque' until we 'cash' it, by filling in some value in the blank space, by defining what we mean.

How we define personhood will determine what we regard as 'universal human rights'. The emphasis we place on certain essential attributes in our definition of human nature, or the way we specify the defining characteristics of our species, will profoundly affect how we interpret and apply concepts of universal human rights. Thus different human rights will be given priority depending on which characteristics we value most and regard as definitive of human nature. Different traditions have emphasised different characteristics as definitive of human nature. Greek philosophy emphasised that 'man is a rational animal' (Aristotle); the Bible, that 'we are made in the image of God, who is love'; Marx, that 'man is *homo faber* – man is man the worker or manufacturer'; existentialist philosophers, that 'to be human is to be condemned to be free' (Sartre). When 'cashed out', each of these definitions has

different practical implications, because each embodies different social and moral values, leading to different rights being given priority.

If we invest 'rationality' or 'critical intelligence' with ultimate importance and value in human life, as we have done in modern Western society, then this has considerable impact on our view of what education is about, the priority given to science and technology in society, and the value given to IQ scores and academic grades in defining who and what we are. This affects us both positively and negatively. Intellectual ability and academic achievement have enormous positive value, and intellectual disability and mental illness a corresponding negative dis-value. This is reflected in the priority given in the allocation of

---

Box 6.1 Universal human rights derived from universal human attributes

If to be human is to be a **rational animal**, then certain conditions or rights must be satisfied before we can become fully rational beings, e.g.:

- the right to know, to information
- the right to freedom of conscience
- the right to freedom of speech
- the right of access to education and training.

If to be human is to be a **social being**, characterised by the capacity to love, for social intercourse and social cooperation, then other requirements have priority:

- the right to be nurtured in a human community
- the right to freedom of association
- the right to freedom of movement
- the right to marry and found a family.

If to be human is to be a **worker**, defined by the capacity for creative work, and to be able to transform the world and humanise it, key rights would be:

- the right to work, to contribute to society
- the right to profit from one's labour
- the right to own land and property
- the right to emigrate to seek employment.

If to be human is to enjoy **freedom** or **autonomy**, then in order to be able to realise one's freedom and express it in one's life and work one would require the following rights:

- the right to freedom from oppression or discrimination
- the right to freedom of opportunity for self-development
- the right to freedom of cultural self-expression
- the right to participate in political activity.

funding to the former and the marginalisation of people with mental disorder or handicap and fewer resources for psychiatric medicine. Similarly, if we overemphasise a capacity for sociability, productive work or autonomy, then we will devalue people who have difficulty relating to others, those who are unemployed and those who do not have the education, resources or opportunities to exercise any meaningful kind of autonomy. The variety of claimed universal human rights based on these definitions can be illustrated as in Box 6.1.

While these definitions of human nature and the corresponding human rights derived from them appear to differ considerably from one another, they are not mutually inconsistent or incompatible with one another – unless interpreted as exhaustive definitions in themselves. Thus the 1947 UNO Universal Declaration of Human Rights represented to some extent a combination of several complementary views of what is fundamentally important to us in defining what it is to be human.

In distinguishing 'liberties' and 'rights' we pointed out that if we concede that other people have certain 'rights', then recognition of their rights imposes certain 'duties' or 'obligations' on us, but the same is not true of our freedom or liberty to do something. For example, smokers frequently claim that they have a right to smoke. If this were the case then other people would have a duty or obligation to enable them to indulge their habit. Here it is incorrect to speak of having a 'right to smoke,' for no-one is obliged, if they do not want to, to provide us with cigarettes or smoking breaks or rooms in which to smoke. If, however, we are over the legal age, we do have the liberty to purchase and smoke cigarettes (and damage our health) without being interfered with or prevented by others (unless our habit is irritating or harming them). While there is a reciprocal and complementary relationship between rights and obligations, there is no positive reciprocal relation between liberties and duties. A liberty is something we are permitted to do without being subject to sanctions or physically prevented from doing it – provided it does not interfere with the liberties of others. As we saw in Chapter 5, for example, if abortion is permitted, or has been de-

criminalised, then a woman has the liberty to procure an abortion and to request others to assist her, without being prosecuted or physically prevented from doing so. However, such 'permissive' legislation does not create a 'right' or entitlement of a woman to demand that anyone provide termination services as a duty.

Here it is important to stress the difference between positive and negative rights. In general, our negative rights are stronger than our positive rights, and most negative rights are secured by law.

A negative right is an entitlement to demand that someone *not do* something to you, or desist from doing something to you. In a sense negative rights do not cost other people anything, for they do not have to do anything to observe your negative rights. The rights involved, e.g. demanding not to be tortured, not to be assaulted, not to be raped, not to be abused and not to have one's privacy invaded, are all *negative rights* and are all rights protected by law.

We all regard the negative rights listed above as fundamental human rights and express outrage when these rights are violated. Yet, hospital patients are constantly at risk of having these rights compromised or abused, because of their 'captive' state as inmates of institutions of various kinds. The doctors and nurses who performed experiments on prisoners in Nazi concentration camps were rightly condemned by the Nuremberg War Crimes Tribunal. There have been highly publicised cases of assaults on patients in psychiatric and mental handicap hospitals (and no less serious assaults on staff by patients). Examples of the rape or sexual abuse of patients by staff, their physical and emotional abuse, and invasion of their privacy, have all been reported in the press in the past decade. Not surprisingly, the courts take a very serious view of crimes of this kind because nurses and other health care staff are expected to exercise a protective duty of care or fiduciary responsibility towards patients committed into their care.

However, there are other important negative rights of patients where doctors and nurses may sometimes feel that in the interests of the patient these rights may have to be compromised. Such rights are the right to refuse treatment (or the right not to be treated without one's consent) and the right to not have private information shared with a doctor or nurse divulged to anyone else without one's permission. These negative rights of patients are also subject to legal safeguards, in so far as treatment without consent is treated in law as a form of criminal assault, regardless of the good intentions of the nurse, and breach of a patient's confidences may be subject to claims for damages in a civil court. Nevertheless, there are borderline and difficult situations where doctors and nurses may have to decide to treat a patient against her will or to pass on confidential information where a patient's competence is in doubt, where there is grave risk to her life, or where sharing the information with a colleague is essential for the patient's proper care and treatment.

A positive right is an entitlement to demand that someone *do something for you* or *give you something*. Such rights are weaker than negative rights, because they depend on the ability, generosity or willingness of others to do what you ask, and also on available resources. While some positive rights may become entrenched in law, such as the right to free health care for UK citizens on the National Health Service and the right to education and welfare, other positive rights are unenforceable, such as 'the right to a job'.

Even within the UK and other wealthier nations these are not unlimited rights, and, some would argue, even these rights are being progressively circumscribed. The entitlements to free dental and optical treatment were removed some years ago, and many more exotic medical treatments may not be available on the NHS because of the cost and the scarcity of medical resources to deal with more essential matters of life and death. Debate about whether cosmetic surgery and IVF for infertile couples are essential treatments and should be available on the NHS will depend not only on available resources, but also on the seriousness of the condition and how much it is seen to affect the person's ability to lead a normal life in society. What is possible in Europe may be quite unimaginable in Africa, so how much leverage we have in claiming our positive rights, even those listed in the Universal Declaration of Human Rights, will depend on where one is living and the resources available. This, in turn, is a reason why people are

often motivated to migrate to better provided countries, in an attempt to secure adequate education, employment or health care.

Finally, although some people claim that there are some rights which are absolute, this seems to us to be a difficult position to sustain, for two reasons: first, because my rights impose both direct and indirect duties on you, and my rights impact upon your rights and limit them; and secondly, because human generosity and resources are limited, entitlement to claim our positive rights will always be relative to what is available. My negative right not to be assaulted restricts your freedom to assault me and imposes on you a duty to respect my right (even if you want to assault me), because I can seek redress if you do. My right to education is not unlimited, but limited by what free education the state can afford to provide. While most countries attempt to guarantee primary education for all, and some secondary, virtually none guarantees access to tertiary education, but may provide some assistance to deserving candidates. Thus, it follows that all rights are relative because my rights limit your rights and yours mine. We work within a world of compromise.

INSTITUTIONAL, LEGAL AND MORAL RIGHTS

Broadly speaking, we may distinguish between institutional and legal rights, on the one hand, and moral rights on the other. Consider the example in Case History 6.1, summarised from a 1987 report of the child abuse controversy in Cleveland. In this case, several parties claimed that their rights, or those of others, had been violated or infringed. However, if we look carefully at each use of the term 'right' or 'rights', we will see that they do not all mean the same thing. In the first instance, the term clearly has a legal meaning, referring to the legal authority of the social services to issue care orders and to have children taken into care. This also applies to the authority of the paediatricians to examine the children. Here it is the legitimacy of their authority which is being questioned.

With reference to the parents' 'rights', the term is being used in a double sense – both a legal and a

case history 6.1

Whose rights are being abused?

In Cleveland Health Authority, between January and July 1987, 110 children were taken into care by the social services, on the advice of two paediatricians, because of suspicions that these children were subject to sexual abuse at home. Legal representatives of the parents contested the right of the social services to take these children into care. In seeking leave to appeal to the High Court, it was claimed that the rights of the parents had been infringed. Furthermore, it was claimed in evidence that the children had been subjected to several painful and humiliating examinations of their genitalia and other private parts, that repeated examinations involved violation of the children's rights (to privacy and respect for their persons) and that the doctors had not shown due care for these vulnerable patients. The local police surgeon complained that the right of the police to be consulted by the paediatricians before care orders were signed had not been respected. Also at issue were the rights of the paediatricians – their right to examine the children and recommend they be taken into care and their right to a fair hearing in the public enquiry.

moral sense. The legal sense relates to whether their proper entitlements to a second medical opinion, or appeal to the High Court, had been taken into account. However, public interest in this case and the enquiry which followed was stimulated by the insinuation in the press that the general moral rights of parents were at risk, such as their right of access to their own children. The rights of the children which it was claimed were not respected were fundamental moral rights, based on the principle of respect for persons – in particular their rights to privacy, dignity and proper care and treatment. What is of particular interest here is that the doctors and social workers claimed that they were exercising a proper duty to care in having the children medically examined and placed under care orders, to protect their rights, i.e. to protect them from further sexual exploitation or abuse. What we have here is two different parties taking up the defence of the children and basing their arguments on appeal to different rights.

Finally, the right appealed to by the police surgeon is what may be called an institutional right, i.e. an accepted protocol or courtesy exercised in

the relationships of doctors, social workers and police. The rights of the paediatricians to a fair hearing would ordinarily be protected by institutional provisions for their legal representation by their employing authority, failing which they would be defended by the Medical Defence Union. However, their 'right' to a fair hearing could be said to be a right to which we are all entitled as a matter of natural justice, a fundamental moral right, but it is a right which may also be guaranteed in law, as a legal right as well.

Each of these different kinds of 'rights' and 'duties' has a different kind of justification. Like our positive and negative rights, positive and negative duties may be legally enforceable or may depend simply on the agent recognising the moral duty to act or to desist from acting in a particular way. Because of this important practical connection between rights and duties and the fact that we often have reciprocal rights and duties to others, it is important to understand that different kinds of rights will be subject to different kinds of justification (Waldron 1984).

Institutional rights are created, and can be abolished, by decisions of people with competent authority. For example, the rule that only members of the Marylebone Cricket Club have the right to use the club facilities or to introduce visitors to the members' bar is decided by the elected and life members of the governing body of the MCC. While some women cricketers argued on legal grounds that their exclusion from membership of the MCC constituted sex discrimination, this did not succeed because the Act did not apply to private clubs. However, women did succeed in gaining access by an appeal to broad moral rights and by mobilising the media to support their cause!

Legal rights must either be enacted by competent legal authorities, such as Parliament, regional or local authorities, or be based on bills of rights such as the United Nations Universal Declaration of Human Rights or the American Constitution. Alternatively, they must be based on common or natural law, i.e. the body of principle and precedent embodied in the legal tradition of the country.

The first kind of legal rights, statutory rights, are explicitly enacted in law, and in most cases are legally enforceable – in the sense that individuals can claim their rights or seek redress for the violation of their rights through the courts. The second kind, based on bills of rights, may be enforceable through appeal to an international agency such as the International Court of Human Rights, provided the country of the person making the appeal respects the authority of the higher court. However, these rights may be expressed in general terms and it would be the task of constitutional or international lawyers to interpret the constitution, or bill of rights, to see if the particular claim of the individual was justified in terms of the principles embodied in these statements of general rights. Claims based on common law, or principles of natural law, may also have to be interpreted in this way, as both embody general statements of a moral rather than a legal kind. Their application in specific cases may have to be a matter of appeal to precedent, or some specific legislation may have to be introduced to make the principles applicable to the type of case in question.

In fact, if we consider the way that the term 'rights' is used in political life, in the general rhetoric of politicians and in the activity of pressure groups, it is significant that both are seeking as a rule to clarify or extend the scope of the law, or mobilise public opinion to change the law. Thus debate about the 'woman's right to choose' (to terminate a pregnancy on demand), or the 'right to employment', or the 'right to a living wage', or the 'right to free health care', or the 'rights of the unborn child', or the 'right to die', are all concerned with the actual or possible reform of the law in the light of what people believe are their moral rights.

On what basis, then, do we justify moral rights? Generally, people appeal to their 'rights' when outraged by some injustice, or are protecting their human dignity when faced by degrading social conditions. In fact, appeal to moral rights presupposes the existence of fundamental moral principles, or at least a common intuition or consensus about fundamental moral principles. Thus appeal to 'the right to adequate care and treatment' or 'the right to protection' (for children, the old, the mentally and physically handicapped) is based on

the assumption that society and the law will recognise the fundamental *principle of beneficence* (or the duty to care). The appeal to the 'right to equality before the law', the 'right to freedom from discrimination on the basis of sex, class, religion or political affiliation', and the claimed 'right to equality of opportunity' or 'equal rights of access to health care' is based in each case on appeal to the fundamental *principle of justice*. Similarly, appeal to individual rights, such as the 'right to know', the 'right to privacy' and the 'right to refuse treatment', is based in these cases on appeal to the fundamental *principle of respect for persons*.

As we have pointed out, the argument about human rights, particularly universal moral rights, rests on appeal to some general concept of human dignity, i.e. to some concept of what it means to be human and what minimum conditions would have to be satisfied. Alternatively, if we argue that universal moral principles are decided by society on the basis of a kind of social contract or consensus, moral rights would be derivable, as practical implications, of these social contracts for the lives of ordinary people as moral agents. Whether human rights are 'inalienable', and in what sense, will depend on whether you believe that fundamental moral principles are God-given, grounded in the nature of things or determined by social convention. Whether human rights can ever be regarded as 'absolute' is debatable, but it is more plausible to argue that the fundamental moral principles from which rights are derived, rather than the moral rights themselves, can be treated as absolute or unconditional moral demands. Thus, in the interests of justice and public health, our rights may have to be subject to limitation to protect the common good, e.g. the freedom of movement or association of people may have to be limited in times of epidemic, natural disaster or war. People may also have to be subjected to compulsory immunisation in similar circumstances.

RIGHTS AND DUTIES OF NURSES IN DEALING WITH PATIENTS

If we consider practical examples of recurrent moral dilemmas in nurse–patient relationships, we shall see that many of these raise fundamental questions about the rights of patients and the scope and limits of the responsibilities of nurses. Quandaries such as 'to tell or not to tell?', 'to treat or not to treat?', 'to limit the patient's freedom in her best interests?' and 'which patient's interests or needs take precedence?' all raise questions of this kind.

Patients' rights form a subclass of general human rights, but how do we derive the rights of people as patients from their general human rights? How do patients' rights relate to the fundamental moral principles of beneficence, justice and respect for persons? It is to these questions that we must now turn.

One approach would be to attempt to derive patient's rights from their general human rights (e.g. from The UNO Universal Declaration of Human Rights). The UNO Declaration now includes certain health rights, but more specific rights of people as patients would have to be derived from these general rights. However, another approach might be to start with the contract-to-care between the carer and client, nurse and patient, to examine the implicit assumptions involved in such 'contracts' and to analyse their moral and legal implications. In what follows, we shall adopt this approach, looking first at the way contractual obligations arise in consulting relationships and then considering the rights and duties that flow from these formal and informal contracts between people in need and their professional carers.

In general, when people with health problems seek help, they go first to a doctor. If the doctor agrees to take someone on as a patient, then that general agreement is first formalised by the patient registering with the doctor's practice. The boundaries of another kind of contract become the subject of the initial consultation – taking down the patient's details, her medical (and perhaps family) history, followed by a physical examination and perhaps a series of tests. All this is essential to, but preliminary to, the 'contract-to-care'. The contract-to-care only comes into operation once the doctor has offered a diagnosis and suggested a possible course of treatment, and the patient has accepted the doctor's medical opin-

ion. The (informed) consent to treatment by the patient is an essential part of the contract. The patient 'entrusts herself into the doctor's hands'. The doctor then assumes responsibility for the care and treatment of the patient and decides what form this should take. The doctor may prescribe treatment directly, refer the 'patient' to hospital or to a specialist, or refer the patient to a nurse for continuing care. Although it is increasingly common for patients to consult directly with nurses, particularly in well-person clinics and community settings, nevertheless the contract-to-care is usually made with the doctor, and the nurse usually has derived rather than direct duties following from the 'contract' with the 'patient'.

Despite these considerations, it may be useful to think through the process by which a person negotiates the help she requires from a specific carer, and what assumptions underlie the agreements made. In general, the specific rights of people as 'patients' flow from the kind of relationship into which they enter with health care staff. When a patient is lucid, ambulant, continent and able to approach the health services independently for help, there is a kind of contract set up in which the patient agrees to cooperate in investigations, treatment and rehabilitation, in return for appropriate therapy and supportive care. The situation is rather different if the patient is brought in unconscious, or is unconsultable because of the specific nature of her disease or injury or by reason of mental disorder. Here the health professionals have to assume total responsibility for the patient and must fall back on their own and their professional moral code for guidance. A third situation is where the carer is involved with the patient as a friend – either through previous association, special circumstances of shared confidences, or because the person is dying and needs care and support rather than further therapy. Here the relationship may take on a more intimate form and the moral commitment in the contractual relationship may need to be renegotiated as something more personal and informal.

In Chapter 4 we described four possible models for carer–client relationships: code, contract, covenant and charter. The relationships between the rights and duties of client and carer vary in each type of situation. The *first type* of situation – which has traditionally been taken to define the relationship between carer and patient – is one of crisis intervention, where the person is incompetent and the professional carer is expected to exercise a quasi-parental and protective duty to care towards the vulnerable patient, governed by the *code of practice* of the profession. The *second type* of situation, where a person independently approaches the health services for help with a health problem, is one in which an implicit or explicit *contract-to-care* is established by negotiation. In such a contract there will be rights and duties on the part of the patient and corresponding duties and rights on the part of the carer. In the *third type* of situation, which we have suggested is *governed by a covenant* of friendship, special consideration may be given to the rights of the patient as a person, and the patient may feel able to make unusual demands on the carer in the knowledge that he is prepared to act over and beyond the call of duty. Likewise, in the *fourth type*, where services are ostensibly based on 'customer focus', *priority is given to the rights of the 'customer' or 'client'* – her right to choose, her right to guaranteed quality control in services and her right to value for money.

When a person approaches a doctor or nurse for help, the health professional has the right to refuse to help that particular person. Such a refusal might legitimately be made for several kinds of reasons, e.g.:

- if the doctor or nurse has such a heavy caseload already that adequate care and support could not be provided to the particular person
- if the doctor or nurse does not believe he possesses the necessary competence
- if the person is being abusive and unpleasant, and the doctor or nurse does not wish to have that person as a client.

If carers refuse clients on such grounds, they would be exercising their ordinary moral rights, but they would also have a professional duty at least to refer them on to someone else who might be willing and able to help them with their problem.

Refusal in the first case would be justified on the grounds that carers have the right not to be exploited or to have heavier demands imposed on them than they could reasonably be expected to cope with. Furthermore, carers have a duty, in justice to their clients, not to take on more clients than they could possibly provide with adequate care. So, too, in the case of difficult clients, refusal to take them on may be in the clients' best interests as well as the best interests of the carers. In these examples, the rights in question would appear to be derivable mainly from considerations of justice, although respect for persons comes into it as well.

Once the carer agrees to take on the person seeking help, he acquires fiduciary responsibility for the client, i.e. a responsibility to look after the client's interests and to protect her rights. This responsibility of the carer follows from the trust the client shows in the carer, but the client also has responsibilities towards the carer. This is shown as soon as the carer proceeds to interview the client or patient.

In a medical consultation, a doctor would not only ask the patient a well-rehearsed checklist of questions about her health and any adverse symptoms, and take down a medical history, but would probably proceed to physical examination as well, if necessary. Carrying out a psychiatric assessment and taking a social history may also be indicated. A nurse, in making an assessment of a patient in order to develop a proper care plan, would quite likely follow a similar series of steps. The general assumptions underlying the exercise of these rights by the carers are that they are *entitled* to these privileges of intimacy because they are exercising a beneficent *duty to care*, in the best interests of the patient. The patient has a corresponding *obligation* to answer truthfully the questions asked by the doctor or the nurse about herself and her problems, and a duty to cooperate in treatment, if she is to be *entitled to* assistance.

Doctors and nurses have a fundamental fiduciary duty not only to protect the interests of and to care for people who have entrusted themselves into their care, but they also have an obligation to give patients relevant information in return for their cooperation (concerning the diagnosis of their problem and the proposed methods of care and treatment), to enable them to make an informed choice about whether they wish to continue with treatment. In this, health professionals have a fundamental duty to ensure that the consent to treatment given by patients is both 'fully informed' and 'voluntary'.

This means that the information must be given in a simple and intelligible form, preferably both verbally and in writing, and written material should be tested for readability for people of average reading age, not that of professionals. Patients' consent must not be obtained under pressure, when they are confused, or when they are subject to extreme stress or anxiety, as they are unlikely to be able to assimilate the necessary information, even if they are capable of understanding it. Health professionals have a duty to give clients all the information they require to make an informed decision about their treatment options, or the drugs or procedures involved in their treatment, including the degree of risk and possible complications involved.

On both counts it may be difficult to determine in practice whether the consent obtained is truly voluntary or fully informed. On the one hand, it can be argued that to be under the duress of pain or anxiety, or trussed up in a hospital bed, may place considerable limitations on your liberty to dissent from what the doctor or nurse proposes by way of treatment for you. On the other hand, who decides how much information is enough? And how fully must all the possible risks of treatment or side-effects of treatment be discussed with a patient? And when would failure to meet these criteria amount to culpable negligence?

For some time, within the sphere of jurisdiction of English law, the Bolam principle has been applied to determine whether or not a health professional is negligent in the discharge of his or her duty to a patient. The principle (discussed by Kerridge et al 1998) was enunciated to the jury by McNair J in the English case of *Bolam v Friern Hospital Management Committee [1957]*, namely:

A doctor is not guilty of negligence if he [sic] has acted in accordance with a practice accepted as proper by a responsible body of medical men skilled in that particular art.

What this means is that in the past it has generally been assumed that the courts would follow the guidance of responsible members of the medical or nursing profession in deciding whether a particular doctor or nurse acted responsibly or not. This principle was further reinforced by the judgment of Lord Scarman in the Sidaway case in which he stated that:

a doctor is not negligent if he acts in accordance with a practice accepted at the time as proper by a responsible body of medical opinion, even though other doctors may accept a different practice. In short, the law imposes the duty of care: but the standard of care is a matter of medical judgement.

As Kerridge et al (1998, p. 110f) have pointed out, the Bolam principle has been challenged repeatedly in the Australian courts where the 'courts have tended to opt for standards of care that are defined by the courts, rather than the profession itself'. However, what has had a considerable influence in confirming this trend and changing legal policy on the rights of patients to fully informed consent, as determined for them by the courts rather than by the professional group involved, is the 1992 case of *Rogers v Whitaker*, 175 CLR 479. The issue was that Mrs Whitaker, who was nearly blind in her right eye, had developed an extremely rare condition of her remaining good eye. She was referred to Dr Rodgers for advice on possible surgery. She was told that he could operate to remove scar tissue from her right eye, probably improve her sight in that eye, improve its appearance and help prevent the development of glaucoma. Following successful surgery, Mrs Whitaker developed an inflammation in the treated right eye which infected her left eye as well, resulting in the total loss of sight in her good eye and virtually total loss of vision. Because Mrs Whitaker had specifically requested reliable advice about the risks of the operation and had not been told that there was a risk of cross-infection between the two eyes, she sued for damages for not having been properly informed, and won. In his defence the doctor argued that the known risk of this complication was 1:14 000 cases and he had not considered it significant, and appealed to the Bolam principle in his defence. Commenting on their verdict, the learned judges remarked however:

Further, and more importantly, particularly in the non-disclosure of risk and the provision of advice and information, the Bolam principle has been discarded, and, instead, the courts have adopted the principle that, while evidence of acceptable medical practice is a useful guide for the courts, it is for the courts to adjudicate on what is the appropriate standard of care after giving weight to 'the paramount consideration that a person is entitled to make his own decisions about his life'.

Kerridge et al observe that while the judges in this case reaffirmed that doctors have a duty to disclose and warn patients of material risks to their health and well-being, they rejected the use of the expression 'informed consent', arguing that it was misleading, and suggested the use instead of the phrase 'duty of disclosure'. Kerridge et al point out that given the broad terms in which the principle was expressed by the court it was clearly intended to cover other professions besides medicine, and hence is of relevance to nurses as well. They proceed to describe the fundamental elements enabling informed and valid consent as consisting in (a) competence and (b) voluntariness, whereas elements that enable a person to be informed are (i) disclosure of relevant information, and (ii) understanding and acceptance of the information by the patient. In communicating information to patients about their care and treatment, nurses would do well to note these criteria, and apply them. Kerridge et al (1998, p. 145) give a helpful checklist, which is shown in Box 6.2.

THE RIGHTS OF PEOPLE AS PATIENTS

Although rather belatedly recognised, patients also have rights within these contracts-to-care. The Bill of Rights for Patients put forward by the American Hospital Association (AHA 1992) lists 12 rights of patients. The list is quite helpful in that it indicates areas where patients experience problems in dealing with health professionals. Attempts have been made to derive a simpler list from consideration of general contractual and moral rights. For example, the Edinburgh Medical Group Working Party on the Care of the Dying and the Bereaved (Thompson 1979a)

| Box 6.2   Requirements for information transfer in clinical practice |

1. Diagnosis (including degree of uncertainty about this)
2. Prognosis (including degree of uncertainty about this)
3. Options for investigations/treatments
4. Burdens and benefits of investigations/treatments
5. Whether the intervention is conventional/experimental
6. Who will perform the intervention
7. Consequences of choosing or not choosing treatment
8. Significant expected short-term and long-term outcomes
9. Time involved
10. Cost involved

Information given may have to be modified by considering:
● the seriousness of the patient's condition
● the nature of the intervention
● the degree of possible harm
● the likelihood of risk
● the patient's needs, attitude, understanding, etc.

---

suggested three fundamental rights of people as patients:
● the right to know
● the right to privacy
● the right to treatment.

The right to know

People generally do not readily disclose information about themselves of an intimate or private nature, unless they expect some benefit from doing so. Although some people make a nuisance of themselves by pouring out their hearts to anyone and everyone whom they can get to listen to them, or use self-disclosure as a means of attention-getting or of manipulating the carer, this is not generally the case. Patients, it has been argued, do not disinterestedly give doctors or nurses access to private information about themselves, nor allow intimate physical, psychological or social investigations, without the expectation that the carers will give them some indication of their diagnosis, tell them what they propose to do by way of treatment, and give them sufficient information to enable them to make an informed decision.

The normal expectation of clients is that carers will discuss their problem with them and give an opinion as to its nature; that they will discuss the proposed course of treatment or management of the problem; and that they will discuss the possible options and outcomes. Thus it can be argued that the right to know is implicit in the contract with the carer who is being consulted by the patient and is predicated on the trust shown in the carer. Similarly, the requirement in law and medical ethics of informed and voluntary consent to treatment (unless the patient is incompetent) presupposes the patient's right to know. However, in this case the right to know tends to be based on wider considerations of the rights of the individual as a person (in the legal sense), i.e. as someone who can be held responsible for her actions since she is capable of making informed and voluntary choices for herself.

When a patient is recruited to be a 'volunteer' in a clinical or drug trial, especially if that patient is unlikely to benefit directly from the experiment, or there is a significant element of risk involved, the requirements for obtaining properly informed and voluntary consent are more stringent than in the case where the direct treatment of the patient is involved. This is not only because of the specific ethical requirements for medical research involving human subjects (Declaration of Helsinki 1996 – see Appendix 1), but also because the nature of the contract is different.

When a patient is dying or when news of a bad prognosis has to be communicated to a patient, a health professional may feel that he has a duty to protect the patient from knowledge which may be too painful to bear or which she is not yet ready to receive. In such cases, there is a tension between the patient's right to know and the professional's duty to care. How this tension is resolved in practice may vary from case to case. It may be further complicated by relatives who demand that the patient should not be told. In such cases, whose rights are to be given priority?

However, the question of the patient's right to know has been given new poignancy and practical urgency for health professionals, because of the court finding, in the case of *Rogers v Whitaker*, that Dr Rogers was negligent in failing to give full disclosure to his patient of the risks entailed in her operation. Writing in the *Journal of Medical Ethics*, Australian judge Michael Kirby (1995), commenting on the significance of the *Rogers v Whitaker* case, argues that times have changed and greater weight should be given in English and American law to the rights of patients, rather than retaining the 1958 Bolam principle and defending the entrenched privilege of doctors:

We must see the moves towards . . . the provision of greater information to patients in the context of the wider social developments that affect society and the law. All professions, including the judges, are now more accountable . . . . The difference between the standards expected in England and in the other countries is not large. But it is significant. And at the heart of the difference is an attitude to the fundamental rights of the particular patient. Those rights should take primacy both in legal formulae and in medical practice.

What is at stake here is not only the question of the relative importance of the rights of doctors versus the rights of patients, but the question of how far we can go with the concept of rights in determining moral choices in particular situations. The strength of the justice perspective, reflected in law and in the moral theory of rights and duties, is that it purports to be objective, but in any particular case, like that of the unfortunate Mrs Whitaker, the question of sensitivity to the needs of a particularly vulnerable but intelligent woman might have resulted in a more honest disclosure of information and less reliance on medical judgement and formal procedural rules.

The right to privacy

The right to privacy covers both the right to respect for the dignity of the person (physical privacy) and respect for the person's secrets (confidentiality). The right to privacy does not mean the right to have a private ward or the right to private medicine, although in some circumstances it may include that. For example, an elderly lady who has never shared a room with another person may be emotionally distressed at having to be nursed in a public ward, and might prefer to pay extra health insurance to ensure that she can get the privacy that is so important to her. While most people entering hospital may expect some general loss of privacy, it often comes as a shock to people to realise how little privacy they have. Hospital staff often show scant consideration for people's sensitivities or need for privacy, particularly the needs of those who are dying.

Generally, people are prepared to expose their secrets, expose their bodies and reveal their vulnerabilities when they need help and when they feel they can trust the person from whom they are seeking help. In such a situation, sensitive carers will respect the patient's confidences and privacy. The carers will also recognise that the information is to be used only for the benefit of the patient, and that they thus acquire duties of advocacy, to protect the rights and interests of the persons in their care, in the light of what they have learned about them.

The right to privacy, to have confidences kept, is not an unlimited right (UKCC 1992, clause 10). When the interests of justice require that evidence is brought before a court to establish the guilt or innocence of an accused, it is generally assumed that the principle of justice and the common good takes precedence over the individual's right to privacy. In the UK, only lawyers enjoy professional privilege, i.e. the right to refuse to disclose information in court (e.g. information which may compromise the defence of a client). Priests, journalists, doctors and nurses do not enjoy this privilege, and if they refuse to divulge secrets of patients or penitents, because they may feel obliged to protect their confidences, they may have to suffer the penalties for being 'in contempt of court'. In practice, the court may not insist if the confidant is adamant, but as the law stands, it is entitled to impose fines or send a person to prison for refusing to give evidence.

Similarly, when the public interest is threatened, for example by a serious epidemic, the nurse may be expected to divulge information to the responsible authorities if a patient's condition is likely to put the lives of other people at risk. In the context of the AIDS epidemic, if a nurse learns that a patient is having a sexual relationship with a person who is HIV-positive but is not prepared to disclose this to her doctor, what is the nurse to do? The patient's personal right to privacy may have to be compromised to protect the right to life of others. Many other cases could be considered to illustrate the same moral quandaries in less dramatic circumstances, e.g. the epileptic who discloses to the nurse that she is a long-distance lorry driver, or the unemployed and disabled patient who reveals to the district nurse that she is falsely claiming benefits when she is actually making a good living on the side.

The disclosure of information by a nurse to another health professional involved in a patient's care may be expressly forbidden by the patient. In such circumstances, especially where the patient's safety or welfare is at stake, the nurse may have to decide, on the principle of beneficence, that his duty to care takes precedence over the patient's right to prohibit disclosure of vital facts (UKCC 1984a).

A different kind of problem can arise for the nurse when people use the sharing of secrets or self-disclosure as a device to establish a kind of intimacy with the nurse, and thus to create a kind of obligation on the part of the nurse towards them, which they manipulate. Being at the receiving end of people's secrets can create burdensome problems for carers, e.g. when the intimacies shared are irrelevant to the management of the patient's health problems. Similarly, health visitors can be faced with a conflict of duties when they discover on domiciliary visits that patients/clients are concealing the true nature of their problems, or that they, or someone living with them, are breaking the law or have some contagious disease. Setting boundaries in advance may be helpful, or limits to information sharing with patients, and may be in the interests of both the patient and the nurse.

The guidance given by the British Association of Social Workers to their members, namely that social workers should seek to establish explicit 'confidentiality contracts' with clients, remains fundamentally good advice for all professionals in consulting professions (BASW 1971). This may not be easy in practice, although it is particularly important on domiciliary visits. The extent to which this is possible, and the nature of the confidentiality contracts involved, will vary with the context and setting. In a public hospital ward, confidentiality means one thing; in the privacy of a consulting room or a patient's home, another. Here, as with many other moral rules, the context may be very important in determining the scope and applicability of the rule (cf. BASW 1996).

While patients may share secrets in an attempt to gain some influence over their carers, it is also true that knowledge of their secrets gives professionals great power over patients. This power can be used for the patient's benefit, but it can also be abused, e.g. as a means to get a patient to cooperate in treatment. Direct blackmail and breach of confidentiality are both serious offences and can lead to heavy penalties against professionals. However, the use of confidences as leverage to get patient compliance is more difficult to prove, and in some cases the carer may feel that the action is justified. Doctors and nurses are given great power to help or hurt people by the secrets people share with them, and with this power goes a great responsibility on the part of all those in the consulting professions (Thompson 1979b, Windt et al 1989).

The right to care and treatment

The right to adequate care and treatment can again be argued as a fundamental human right, as it is in the UN Universal Declaration of Human Rights, Article 25, where it is implied that without basic health protection people cannot survive, let alone lead a full human life or exercise any of their other human rights. In the UK, the National Health Service Act of 1947 also created the legal right for citizens to claim medical treatment, which should be free at the point of delivery (although financed by general taxation).

However, the right to adequate care and treatment can be argued on different grounds, namely, as a direct consequence and implication of the contract-to-care negotiated with the doctor or health professional. Every person who has been taken on by a doctor or nurse as a patient has a right to expect proper care and treatment. The doctor or nurse is employed to provide a service, or offers a service on a fee-for-service basis, and patients are entitled to treatment in fulfilment of the deal made with the carer to whom they have

entrusted themselves. Malpractice and negligence are not confined to incompetent, dishonest or faulty practice. They also apply to the failure to provide due care in fulfilment of the contract-to-care.

In reality, the right to treatment is based, for all practical purposes, on the contract, formal or informal, between the particular doctor or nurse and a specific patient. This right is not absolute, however. Patients cannot demand whatever drugs or treatment they fancy – even if they are in a position to pay for it. It is for the doctor or nurse to decide whether the treatment requested is appropriate. It also may not be possible to give particular patients the special treatments which they request without detriment to the interests of other patients. Furthermore, while the patient has a fundamental moral right to adequate care and treatment, that 'treatment' may in certain circumstances be neither drug therapy nor surgery, nor any other active intervention. In the case of the dying patient, 'treatment' may simply mean tender loving care and settling for comfort rather than therapy. The fact that the term 'treatment' covers both palliative care and therapy can be a source of confusion in discussions about stopping treatment. While it may be appropriate to stop therapy, it would never be right to stop palliative care, such as the alleviation of pain or treatment of distressing symptoms. In summary, there are three points which should be emphasised about patients' rights, as with human rights in general, namely:

- having rights does not mean that one is bound to exercise them
- having rights does not mean that their exercise is unlimited
- patients' negative rights are in general stronger than positive ones.

Thus having the right to know does not mean that one has to exercise it. One may not wish to know that one is dying, for example; or, even if one suspects that one is dying, one may not wish to discuss it; or one may not wish to discuss it with a particular doctor or nurse. One has a right to be asked, but one is not obliged to accept unwanted information or 'counselling'. The right to privacy is not an unlimited right, because the demands of caring for others in similar need with limited staff and resources may require that patients sacrifice some of their privacy and consent to be nursed in public wards. While doctors and nurses are encouraged to regard confidentiality as an important moral duty, it is generally recognised by hospital staff (and often by patients themselves) that team management necessitates the operation of a kind of 'extended confidentiality', which includes other members of the caring team. While the right to treatment is a fundamental right of patients, it does not include the right to demand particular therapies. However, the negative right to refuse treatment is a much stronger right – in law it is virtually an absolute right, unless the patient is mentally disordered. The treatment of a patient against her will, as we have already said, is technically a criminal assault and is actionable in law.

TELLING THE TRUTH TO PATIENTS OR RELATIVES

Consider the situation faced by a staff nurse in a paediatric hospital, as outlined in Case History 6.2. The staff nurse in this case recognised that knowing the truth that Mary was dying imposed certain responsibilities on her, to protect Mary's vulnerability (a feeling she shared with Mary's parents), but she also recognised that Mary had a right to know the truth. The dilemma she faced was the conflict between loyalty to Mary and loyalty to her parents, because of the trust and understanding that had grown up between her and Mary, on the one hand, and her and Mary's parents on the other. The problem was made more difficult by her uncertainty that it was right to tell Mary, and her sense of guilt at going against the wishes of Mary's parents. She may also have been aware of having been specially chosen by Mary as the one to ask this momentous question. Was it not possible that the distraught parents, faced with the loss of their daughter, were using the staff nurse in a vain attempt to reassert their rights over their daughter? In such a situation, which does the nurse put first: the rights of the parents or the rights of the patient?

It is questionable whether doctors, nurses or relatives ever have a right to keep information

case history 6.2

When is a child not a child any longer?

Mary, aged 13 years, was admitted with acute myeloid leukemia. Over the next three years she was in and out of hospital at increasingly frequent intervals. The permanent ward staff established a good relationship with Mary and her family during this period. Initially her parents did not accept the diagnosis, but with much support and reassurance they eventually accepted the situation fairly well.

Two and a half years after her first admission, Mary was admitted for terminal care. Throughout the course of her illness her parents had been adamant that Mary should not be told what was wrong with her. This was still the situation when Mary was admitted for the last time. We tried to point out to her parents that Mary was no longer a child and that if the question of her condition arose, it might help her to know the truth, but they still refused to let her be told.

Three days before she died, Mary asked outright if she was going to die. She said she felt she was getting worse rather than better, and she asked directly what it was like to die.

In spite of her parents' views, I felt that I had to be truthful with Mary as she was no longer a child, but 15 years old. We talked about death and I explained to her that everyone had to die sooner or later. I was with her when she died, as were her parents, and she died peacefully and calmly. I felt I had done the right thing in telling her, but felt that I had betrayed the trust of her parents, which had been built up over nearly 3 years.

from a dying patient. Whose death is it anyway? If the dying patient does not have a fundamental right to know that she is dying, then who has? However, in this case the patient was a child, 12 years old when myeloid leukemia was first diagnosed, and only 15 when she died. Both the nurse and the parents assumed that they had a duty to protect Mary from the knowledge of her impending death, because she was a child. But did they have the right to deny her this knowledge? Because Mary was so young, at first the staff nurse felt that the parents were right to protect her from the painful truth, but as Mary grew older and asked more searching questions, the staff nurse's attitude changed. However, did Mary have any more right to know at age 15 than at the age of 12? Are parents or relatives of dying patients entitled to withhold the truth from them, however young or old they are?

In general, the right to know is derived from the principle of respect for persons. If people are to be treated as persons with rights – for example the right to make informed choices, the right to autonomy, i.e. to be in control of their own lives – then they cannot be denied the knowledge or information which will enable them to make important life choices. We say glibly that 'ignorance is bliss', but many studies show that dying patients are often frightened because they do not know what is going on, are aware of the conspiracy of silence around them, and are too afraid to ask. More than 20 years ago, research by Parkes (1966) and Hinton (1979) showed that, contrary to common belief, dying patients are often reassured by knowing their prognosis, as the anxiety based on doubt and uncertainty is ended, and there is evidence that the condition of patients may improve, and they may enjoy remission of their symptoms, once they 'know the score' (see Parkes & Markus 1998).

The policy of openness adopted by hospices for the dying is based not only on the belief that the patient has a right to know (particularly if she asks), but that good terminal care presupposes the knowing cooperation of the patient. The conspiracy of silence around the dying patient deceives no-one – except perhaps the conspirators themselves. Several studies involving terminally ill patients have shown that, in units where it is the policy not to tell, more than 75% of patients nevertheless do know that they are dying (Hinton 1979). Not surprisingly, patients pick up this information from various sources: by comparing their symptoms and treatment with other patients, by what they learn indirectly from conversation with other patients and hospital staff (including cleaners and porters), by observation of their own deteriorating condition and by what they infer from the body language (non-verbal communication) of nurses and medical staff (hushed voices, telling looks, silent passing of the bed, over-solicitous care). The available evidence suggests that when told that their condition is terminal, patients do not 'give up', 'turn their faces to the wall' or 'go to pieces', provided they are given adequate emotional support and time to come to terms with dying.

However, it is not such pragmatic considerations that are of fundamental importance in this argument, but rather the fact that knowledge is power. Deliberately keeping another person in a state of ignorance is to deprive that person of power, which results in a state of dependency and powerlessness. The attitude of Mary's parents had the effect of infantilising her, depriving her of the opportunity to discuss with them her grief and anxiety at facing death. Their protective paternalism mirrors the attitudes often adopted by doctors and nurses – in being more concerned to protect patients than to respect their rights as persons to know and choose for themselves.

Consider another case, taken from an obstetric ward, where a mother has to be told that her baby, born by caesarian section, was stillborn (see Case History 6.3). Here, the mother not only has a right to know, but is bound to know sooner or later. The grief cannot be avoided. However, the nurse cannot simply 'tell facts as they are' without considering the consequences for the mother (and father). Truthfulness carries with it the burdensome responsibility of deciding how much truth a person can take at a given time, how full disclosure must be in the circumstances. The questions are: can the nurse cope with being the one who tells; who shares the mother's grief and the mother's likely sense of her own failure; and who is available to provide ongoing support afterwards? The inhibition the nurse feels about sharing the truth in this situation, particularly if there is no convenient way out of facing the challenge, probably has more to do with her fear of accepting the responsibility for telling the truth, than with any uncertainty about the mother's rights. Sharing the truth can be a costly business. Once the midwife accepts the responsibility to tell the mother, she implicitly commits herself to share her grief (and perhaps the partner's). If she knows anything about loss and bereavement she will also know that telling parents that a longed-for baby has died will not only cause them immediate grief but will initiate a process which may take many months to work through. She will also know that she has a duty to continue with support for as long as possible, while they deal with their bereavement.

Truth-sharing means accepting responsibility to share the pain and grief, anger and despair, shock and depression which knowing the truth

case history 6.3

Death in the obstetric ward

A nurse midwife is caring for a mother who has had a stillborn baby, by caesarean section, and who is just recovering consciousness and asking to see her baby. How, when and where does the nurse tell the mother that her baby is dead? Should she call for the doctor and get around the difficulty that way? Should she tell the absent father first? Should she avoid telling the mother until the father is present and can comfort his wife? Should she arrange for the couple to see the baby? How does she cope with her own grief, her own feelings of failure, her need to appear strong in order to comfort the parents and to continue providing care for the mother?

may cause. If there is not well-established understanding, trust and caring, if there is no possibility that the nurse can provide continuing support to the individual concerned, then 'telling the truth' may be cruel and irresponsible (Doyle 1984, 1994).

Sharing painful truth requires great sensitivity and skill in judging how, when and where it is appropriate to tell. Once the midwife accepts the responsibility to tell the mother, she also has to face the difficult practical decisions, requiring tact and judgement, about whether the mother will be most helped by being allowed to cuddle her dead baby, or whether she needs to be protected from an experience which may be too painful for her to bear or for which she is not yet ready. Being *honest* with other people is a measure of how much we honour them – how much we trust and respect them as persons. Honesty, or truthfulness, is about being sensitive to 'where other people are at', in their own present experience and ability to cope. In making an assessment of a patient, nurses will have to rely not only on their own common sense, but also on the opinions of their colleagues and perhaps the relatives. But nurses can never shelve their responsibility by relying on, or being tied by, the opinions of others. Sooner or later all nurses have to face situations where they have to accept responsibility for sharing the painful truth with patients, and this means becoming as skilled at 'titration' of the truth to the needs of the patient as they are at administering appropriate doses of painkilling drugs.

A different but related problem about sharing information arises when patients know the truth yet refuse to let the medical or nursing staff tell their partner or family. Here, in no direct sense do the relatives have a right to know since it is not their death that is at issue; but as people who are intimately involved and likely to be affected by the patient's death, the nurse may feel that they ought to be told. As we do not exist in isolation from other people, least of all our families, family members, in an extended sense, have a right to know – based both on considerations of compassion and on the reciprocal responsibilities which obtain in families and close communities.

Faced with such a situation, nurses may be helped by discussing the matter with the persons prohibiting the disclosure of information, to make them aware of how the interests of others are involved and to help them see what comfort may be gained by sharing the truth and the grief together. For example, Mary's parents might have been persuaded to tell Mary themselves (with or without the support of the medical and nursing staff); the husband might be persuaded and assisted to tell his wife about the stillborn baby himself, with the midwife providing support; and dying patients might need to be encouraged and assisted to share their anxieties about dying with their partner and family and to set their affairs in order. However, if they still refuse, nurses may be able to gain moral support from discussion with other members of staff. But in the end, nurses may have to make their own painful decisions about whether or not to tell. Here they have to balance several conflicting interests and duties: their responsibility to their patient against their wider responsibilities to the family and other concerned parties.

In the cases considered, it can readily be seen that dilemmas about truth-telling relate to the rights of patients (e.g. the right to know and the right to privacy) and to the tensions between these rights and the duties of nurses (e.g. the duty to protect the vulnerable patient from knowledge too painful to bear, or the duty, in fairness to others, to share information that may affect them). Here we see that considerations other than respect for persons and their individual rights come into play.

The principles of beneficence and justice are also involved, and it is precisely this actual or apparent conflict of principles which makes these present as moral dilemmas and which makes decisions in these areas difficult, painful and uncertain.

DECIDING BETWEEN THERAPEUTIC CARE AND PALLIATIVE CARE

As already indicated, the right to treatment is a fundamental right of people as patients, regardless of their age and whether or not they can speak for themselves. Problems arise in interpreting this right, because of the varying degrees of competence of patients to make decisions for themselves. Not only do different patients differ in the degree of competence that can be attributed to them, but depending on the severity of their illness, injury or mental disorder, their degree of competence may vary from one stage of their illness to another.

The least problematic situation is where an independent adult, in full possession of her senses, enters into a contract for treatment with a doctor, or the caring team, when she becomes their patient. In principle, infants, mentally handicapped people and elderly patients have the same rights and are entitled to the same standards of medical and nursing care as anyone else. When, by reason of physical or mental illness, a patient is in a very dependent and vulnerable condition, decisions have to be taken about her care and treatment by others. The lucid, independent and ambulant patient can actively claim her right to treatment or refuse treatment. The confused or unconscious, bed-bound or unconsultable patient is in a different situation, depending entirely on others to protect her rights and dignity, to ensure that she gets adequate medical treatment and proper nursing care. Infants born with serious physical or mental defects also need to have their interests safeguarded. Just as special tribunals are set up to oversee the care and management of compulsory psychiatric patients, so the courts have a special responsibility to protect the rights of others who are not competent to defend themselves, owing to physical or mental infirmity, old age or infancy.

These safeguards are required not because health care workers cannot be trusted to care for their patients in a responsible fashion, but because they need protection as much as their vulnerable patients do, from criticism and litigation or worse. The patient who is not consultable needs an independent advocate to represent her interests, where there may be doubt and uncertainty about the right course of treatment or conflict between doctors and nurses, e.g. about whether the patient's rights have been protected.

Part of the difficulty centres around the ambiguity of the word 'treatment', when we speak of the 'right to treatment'. Treatment can be taken to embrace every kind of medical intervention and every form of nursing care. So it is important to be clear, in negotiations with patients, about what 'treatment' is being referred to in a particular context, as there are important ethical differences between the justification for therapeutic measures and palliative care, compulsory hospitalisation and asylum. In certain contexts, the purpose of an operation may be to cure, by repairing injury, removing diseased tissue or preventing the spread of infection. In another context, surgery may be purely palliative, to relieve pain or to delay the spread of malignant disease. Alternatively, the operation may be strictly unnecessary for medical reasons, but indicated for psychological or social reasons, as, for example, in cosmetic surgery, sterilisation or sex change. In each case, the 'right to treatment' will have a different ethical significance.

Because 'treatment' is often taken to include both 'cure' and 'care', it may in practice be difficult to separate the one from the other. When a patient has a potentially fatal disease, which might be curable or at least treatable, it may be extremely difficult for the ward team to decide when further therapeutic measures are no longer justifiable and it is time to 'settle for comfort'. For the caring team to be clear about when a patient has reached the pre-death stage is vitally important for good terminal care. But if a change of management from a therapeutic regime to palliative care is indicated, the patient has a right to be consulted about this step. The contract with the patient to provide therapy may not cover 'palliative care' and may need to be renegotiated. A conspiracy of silence about the true condition of the patient may also lead to conflict between nursing staff and doctors about which type of 'treatment' is appropriate. This may be particularly difficult if the patient or relatives are desperately demanding that everything possible should be done, or that all treatment should be stopped (Ramsey 1978, Doyle 1994).

In what follows we consider three different kinds of problems or dilemmas relating to the 'right to treatment': (1) resuscitation of a baby with a severe heart defect; (2) struggles between nurses and doctors over sedation; and (3) treatment without consent.

Resuscitation of a baby with a severe heart defect (Case History 6.4)

There are broadly speaking two schools of thought in this case – the one that emphasises the rights of the baby and the one that emphasises the responsibility of the medical team. In principle, the baby has the same right to life and right to treatment that any adult has, and the law should safeguard these rights as it does those of other vulnerable individuals. An outside party (e.g. a social worker) should have the right to appeal to the courts to ensure that the child's rights are protected. Although all citizens have a moral duty to protect the rights of others – thus protecting their own rights – certain professionals, such as social workers and hospital chaplains, have special responsibility to act as advocates for those whose rights

may be compromised or neglected. The parents do not have a moral right to refuse the treatment that their child requires for survival, but nor can they be forced to care for the child. If, as a society, we recognise that the child has a right to treatment, then we must also recognise that society has an obligation to provide adequate care and support for the child (and possibly for the parents as well).

In practice, the situation is more complicated. The social provision for the care of severely handicapped children in most societies is inadequate, and support for affected families is insufficient to prevent hardship and distress. Compassion for the parents, who, understandably, may feel unable to cope, and compassion for the medical and nursing staff, who are faced with immediate decisions about care and treatment for the child, may point to letting nature take its course and allowing the child to die. In reality, the hospital team and the parents have to try to resolve the situation in the most responsible way. The risks of medical intervention are that the child would still be left severely handicapped for life and would require constant nursing care and medical attention. The parents would almost inevitably have to carry the main burden of caring for the child because of the lack of practical alternatives.

Issues of social justice are involved as well, because the painful reality is that the child's right to treatment and the medical team's duty to care have to be reconciled in most cases where there is inadequate social provision for the care and support of such children and their families. This places unjust pressure on the family to accept responsibilities greater than they may be able to cope with themselves, and pressure on the medical team who may not feel free to do what is in the child's best interests. This illustrates how issues of rights cannot be separated from considerations of justice relating to the equitable distribution of resources in society generally.

Clinical decisions in such cases are not unambiguous. Past experience may show that there is little hope for such children or that particular interventions can be successful in ensuring survival and reasonable quality of life. However, medical evidence will not be enough to resolve the moral dilemmas. How objective are assessments

case history 6.4

Birth of a Down's syndrome baby with a congenital heart defect

When I was a student midwife, a baby with Down's syndrome and a severe heart defect was born to a 38-year-old mother and a 42-year-old father. Both parents were unable to accept the baby. The father expressed the wish that the baby should not be resuscitated if a crisis occurred. This happened soon afterwards and a junior member of the medical team initiated resuscitation. The baby died, however, several weeks later.

of 'quality of life'? How does one judge that a life of severe physical or mental handicap is better or worse than no life at all? We might set up criteria and tests of competence and capacity for independent living, but they may palpably fail to take account of the patient's own view of things – even if this is possible. A survey of adults with mental handicap in Scotland found, contrary to prevailing opinion among medical policymakers and managers of large institutions for the mentally handicapped, that over 75% of those in long-stay care wished to live, and would be capable of doing so, in the community with minimal support (Baker & Urquhart 1987). There are considerable risks in depending on one group of professionals to define what 'quality of life' means for other people. Where the political will to provide adequate community care is lacking, there is the additional risk that medical opinion will be used to rationalise the detention of mentally handicapped people in special asylums for life.

The infant with Down's syndrome in Case History 6.4 certainly had a right to treatment, but it does not follow that everything possible has to be tried, including the most expensive, untried or dangerous treatments. Treatment may mean direct interventions which aim to cure, or it may mean simply the provision of good nursing care and control of symptoms. Deciding which is appropriate in such a case may be difficult and morally ambiguous. It may be tempting to simply 'treat' the parents' distress or the ward team's anxiety by removing the object that is the cause, but that would not represent the kind of moral initiative the situation demands – the courage to act in spite of the practical uncertainty and moral ambiguity and to live with the consequences.

The distinction drawn by moral theologians between 'ordinary' and 'extraordinary' means is often invoked to deal with such situations. The health care team are obliged to give the child in such a case the 'ordinary' means of assistance but are not obliged to employ 'extraordinary' means in an attempt to save its life. However, it is doubtful that this distinction solves the moral dilemma in such cases, but points to the need for decisions to be based on common sense and due regard for the circumstances and needs of the patient and all

parties with a responsibility to care. 'Leaving nature to take its course' seldom means doing nothing more for the affected infant; it would normally mean continuing to give fluids (and possibly food or drugs to suppress hunger) and keeping the infant comfortable and pain-free. But it could also mean not intervening actively to give antibiotics, not performing an operation with a poor record of success and not resuscitating the infant should it suffer cardiac arrest (Glover 1977).

In the case we are considering, the houseman acted decisively to resuscitate the child, but she died anyway. His action was a perfectly understandable one. It was one possible response to a distressing situation, one possible attempt to resolve the painful dilemma. It was an action which had its own possible medical and moral justification. The child did, after all, survive for several weeks, and this may have been of some help to the parents in coming to terms with their bereavement. However, it might have been no less morally courageous, and possibly more difficult in the face of the pressure to 'do something!', to have left the child to die. Such situations are called dilemmas precisely because there is no way one can know with certainty, or unambiguously, what is the right thing to do in the circumstances (Stinson & Stinson 1981).

Not taking any action to resuscitate a patient who has suffered cardiac arrest, or choked, is sometimes referred to as 'passive euthanasia', in contrast to 'active euthanasia' when someone takes direct action to end the life of a patient. Some philosophers argue that there is an important moral distinction between active killing and letting someone die, in terms of the different intentions of the agent, and that while active euthanasia is not morally acceptable, in some circumstances passive euthanasia may be. Others argue that if the doctor or nurse knows that the patient will die as a result of discontinuing life support, this amounts to the same thing. The consequences are identical: the patient dies; the intentions 'to kill' or 'to deprive of life support' are virtually indistinguishable. There are complex and important arguments on both sides, but medical and nursing staff faced with decisions to stop treatment or not to intervene tend to maintain that there is a valid common-sense distinction between actively killing a patient (with or without the patient's consent) and taking no action to save her life when she is dying.

This so-called common-sense distinction between 'active' and 'passive' euthanasia, as well as the distinction between 'ordinary' and 'extraordinary' means, is put under strain when we consider what has been made possible by the development of modern drugs, new anaesthetics and life-support machines. To some extent, the boundaries between 'ordinary' and 'extraordinary' means are changing all the time with the development of more sophisticated techniques and knowledge (e.g. the definition of 'viability' has had to be changed from 28 weeks for neonates as it has proved possible to keep younger babies alive). These changes in the boundaries do not make decisions in these cases any easier. The presence or absence of sophisticated resuscitative equipment can make all the difference to how a case is viewed. Is actively switching off a life-support system to a brain-dead patient being kept 'alive' for transplant purposes active or passive euthanasia? Or neither? With more precise medical and legal criteria for defining death, this particular dilemma may be removed, but with live and conscious patients who are dying, the problems remain (Harris 1981).

Struggles over sedation (see Case History 6.5)

In the conflict between the nurses and the doctors over the level of pain control to be given to Margaret, we encounter a common problem in doctor–nurse relationships in terminal care. The problem relates to the different functions of the nurse and the doctor, and their perceived roles in relation to the severely ill patient – the nurse being more concerned with the comfort and well-being of the patient, and the doctor being more concerned with sorting out the medical problems. However, conflicts also tend to arise in the preterminal stage when it is as yet unclear whether the patient is dying or whether her life could be saved. While there is hope, curative measures are appropriate, even to the point of denying painkillers if these may jeopardise the possibility

case history 6.5

Pain control in a severely ill patient

In my second year of nursing, during my second spell of night duty as a staff nurse, Margaret was admitted to our ward. She was 23 years old and recently married. She was suffering from oesophageal varices, and the consultant surgeon had used a new technique of portacaval shunt in an attempt to treat her condition. Margaret's condition deteriorated after the operation and she was in considerable pain. The surgeon insisted she be kept completely drug-free to rest her liver, and the resident doctor consequently refused to sign her up for any painkilling drugs and instructed me to give a placebo only (whether intravenous or intramuscular). Margaret was in considerable pain and had more and more distressing nights. She was a most charming person and the staff were very fond of her. This made it very difficult for us, feeling we could not help. In the mornings the ward sister would come on duty, often very early, and would demand to know whether Margaret had been sedated. When I told her that I had not been allowed to give her any sedation, she would become very angry with me and would (to my relief) instruct me to give her sedation. Each day the same battle would go on between the consultant, resident, ward sister and myself – with the nurses concerned to make Margaret as comfortable as possible and the consultant concerned that his operation should be a success. The battle continued until very close to her death, when the consultant surgeon finally conceded that she should be given adequate sedation.

of a cure. Once the situation is recognised to be hopeless in therapeutic terms, then appropriate palliative care should be given. Deciding when it is appropriate to switch from therapeutic to palliative measures may be difficult and fraught with uncertainty for the doctor faced with possible charges of negligence if he misses something. The anxiety of the medical staff not to be found wanting drives them to do all they can, while the anxiety of the nursing staff at having to cope with the distress of the patient (and relatives) may drive them to demand that they should 'settle for comfort'. The doctor's experience that patients (especially young patients) may sometimes be 'snatched from the jaws of death' has to be balanced by the insight of experienced nurses that patients have 'turned the corner never to return'. Decisions about the type of management appropriate may have to be taken under pressure from rebellious nurses, or by the doctor asserting his medical authority. But decisions do have to be taken by someone, and that is usually the doctor, because of his ultimate legal responsibility.

A common dilemma in such circumstances relates to the use of powerful pain-controlling drugs such as diamorphine, which nevertheless can have dangerous side-effects – such as suppressing respiration – which may hasten the patient's death or make her more susceptible to infections which may kill her. Some nurses object to giving diamorphine to dying patients even if they are in great pain, because they regard this as a form of euthanasia. Even more nurses are afraid of being the one to administer the last injection, thereby appearing to be responsible for the death of the patient. Clearly, nurses have a moral right to refuse to do something which violates their conscience, but they may not have a legal right to refuse to carry out a doctor's orders.

The *principle of double effect* has sometimes been invoked to help provide common-sense guidance for action in such circumstances. When nurses are confronted with a situation demanding action which they can foresee will have two effects, one good (such as relieving a patient's pain) and the other bad (putting the patient at risk of earlier death), they would be justified in performing the action subject to the conditions listed in Box 6.3 (O'Keeffe 1984).

It may be doubted whether these conditions entirely solve the dilemma, but they may help some people to cope with the painful responsibility involved. Better knowledge of pain control and experience gained in terminal care units have shown that the proper use of diamorphine and other drugs not only greatly improves the quality of life of dying patients, but can actually give them the determination to live longer.

Treatment without consent

Case History 6.6, which concerns Jehovah's Witness parents refusing blood transfusions for their child, raises in an acute form the questions of whether parents have the right to decide for their children in such vital matters as those affecting their right to life, and whether the parents' authority can override the ordinary human rights of the child. Leaving aside the merits of the theological and scientific arguments adduced by Jehovah's Witnesses to justify their position, the case is discussed here in order to illustrate some of the issues of parental 'rights' versus the 'rights' of the child. (Another type of case which could have been used to illustrate the problems for professional staff would be where serious physical or sexual abuse of a child is suspected.)

So far as the law is concerned, a child does have the same right to life as an adult, and in most societies the courts can overrule the authority of parents – where the life or even the mental health of the child is believed to be at risk. In this sense the courts exercise a protective duty of care towards minors and people who are incompetent by virtue of mental illness or mental disability. Those concerned about the well-being of a child can appeal to the court to intervene. However, they would have a duty to prepare an appropriate case

---

Box 6.3	Criteria for applying the principle of double effect

1. The action must itself be a good action, or at least morally neutral.
2. The performance of the action must bring about at least as much good as evil.
3. The evil effect must not be a means to achieving the good effect.
4. The agent must have a justifying and sufficient reason for acting rather than refraining from acting.

---

 case history 6.6

A child whose parents refuse treatment

While nursing in A&E, a child victim of a road traffic accident was brought in by ambulance with severe injuries and loss of blood. The child's parents were Jehovah's Witnesses and insisted that the child should not be given blood transfusions. The parents were asked to wait while X-rays were taken and other tests made. While these were being done, it became apparent that the child would not survive without immediate blood transfusions. The child was given the necessary transfusion. The parents were not informed. The child survived.

for making such an appeal, and the parents would have the right to be heard in their defence.

In this case, the medical and nursing staff, whether for the best of intentions or not, acted as a law unto themselves, and in seeking to protect the rights of the child could be said to have failed to show due regard for the moral and legal rights of the parents. They colluded in deceiving the parents so as to ensure that the child was given the necessary life-saving blood transfusions. They might have applied to a judge and had the child made a ward of court, and this might have been a more proper procedure, not least to protect themselves from litigation. (Although proxy consent to treatment by parents is often accepted on behalf of a child, the law is not clear on whether proxy consent, as exercised here by hospital staff, is legally adequate, let alone morally acceptable (McCormick 1976, Ramsey 1976, 1977).)

However, even if the ward team had obtained the proper legal authority, the action of the doctor and nurses in this case leaves much to be desired. They made assumptions about Jehovah's Witnesses which might in this case have been un-founded, and they failed to address the issue of what the parents might do if they discovered what had been done. A more sensible course would have been to attempt to persuade and negotiate with the parents about the available options, and only failing all attempts to persuade them would recourse to the courts have been justified.

Where parents and professionals do not share the same beliefs or value system, the interpretation of rights and responsibilities can become a matter of great difficulty. Common examples in work with people of different ethnic and cultural backgrounds may relate to dietary or dress taboos or particular sensitivity about issues related to sexual health or reproduction. The value of institutions such as the courts is that they remove the problem from the domain of private professional responsibility and enable discussion to take place in a public arena, where the parties involved in the disagreement both have the right to legal representation and the responsibility to present arguments and evidence to enable the court to make a reasonable decision in the public interest.

 # further reading

Exploring the nature of 'rights' and 'duties'
Dworkin R 1977 Taking rights seriously. Harvard University Press, Cambridge, MA – *a discussion of natural law and natural rights by a distinguished jurist and legal philosopher*

Finnis J 1999 Natural law and natural rights. Clarendon Press, Oxford – *a defence of the theory of natural law against the claims that it cannot deliver practical guidance*

Macintyre A 1988 Whose justice? Whose rationality? University of Notre Dame, Indiana – *a critical view of rights theories from a postmodern Christian standpoint*

Waldron J (ed) 1984 Theories of rights. Oxford University Press, Oxford – *a useful collection of essays on rights and rights theories*

The rights and duties of nurses
International Council of Nurses (ICN) 1973 Code for nurses: ethical concepts applied to nursing. ICN, Geneva

Johnstone M-J 1994 Bioethics: a nursing perspective. WB Saunders/Baillière Tindall, Sydney – *good chapters on nurses' and patients' rights: Chapters 13 and 5, respectively*

Staunton P, Whyburn B 1997 Nursing and the law, 4th edn. Harcourt Brace, New York – *a more technical discussion of the rights and duties of nurses, from a legal perspective; helpful though*

UKCC 1992 Code of professional conduct for the nurse, midwife and health visitor, 3rd edn. UKCC, London

Patients' rights (and duties)
American Hospital Association 1973 A patient's bill of rights (revised in 1992). American Hospital Association, Chicago

Beauchamp T L, Childress J F 1994 Principles of biomedical ethics, 4th edn. Oxford University Press, Oxford – *a useful range of comments on patients' rights throughout the text, particularly in Chapters 6 and 7*

Charlesworth M 1993 Bioethics in a liberal society. Cambridge University Press, Cambridge – *a liberal and communitarian defence of autonomy and personal rights in a modern secular society*

Selective disclosure of information
Beauchamp T L, Childress J F 1994 Principles of biomedical ethics, 4th edn. Oxford University Press,

Oxford, chs 3, 7 – *this familiar textbook has updated material on informed consent, confidentiality and security of information*

Kirby M 1995 Patients' rights – why the Australian courts have rejected Bolam. Journal of Medical Ethics 21: 5–8 – *a provocative discussion of legal and ethical considerations in the vexed question of informed patient consent*

UKCC 1984 Guidelines on confidentiality. UKCC, London

Windt P Y, Appleby P C, Battin M P, Francis L P, Landesman B M 1989 Ethical issues in the professions. Prentice Hall, Englewood Cliffs, NJ – *a collection of classic essays on topics in professional ethics, and chapters on confidentiality in particular*

Scope of 'treatment', 'control' and 'care'
Beauchamp T L, Childress J F 1994 Principles of biomedical ethics, 4th edn. Oxford University Press, Oxford, chs 3, 6 – *the right to informed consent to treatment, to refuse treatment and issues of entitlement to treatment discussed*

Kerridge I, Lowe M, McPhee J 1998 Ethics and law for the health professions. Social Science Press, Katoomba, NSW, ch 12 – *issues related to the limits of medical 'treatment' discussed from an ethical and legal perspective*

Reed J, Lomas G 1984 Psychiatric services in the community: developments and innovations. Croom Helm, London – *popular discussion of the scope and limits of treatment and the right to treatment, discussed in a psychiatric context*

some suggestions on method

Exploring the nature of 'rights' and 'duties'
In order to introduce the nature of rights, it is perhaps most helpful to begin with the specific rights and obligations arising out of promises, bets, vows and contracts. Small groups could each be assigned the task of clarifying what is involved in promising, betting, etc. and asked to clarify why the parties to these commitments acquire both entitlements and obligations. The whole group can then be asked to clarify what these kinds of rights and duties have in common. Another related exercise would involve taking the written rules of the ward/hospital and discussing what rights and duties arise out of commitment to observe the rules.

The rights and duties of nurses
The class could be set the task of studying the UNO Universal Declaration of Human Rights and thinking about how these might be justified. Next they should be asked to apply these to themselves as nurses. Then, in small groups, the students can be asked to brainstorm lists of 'universal rights for nurses' and to discuss how they would justify these to the rest of the class/hospital management. The exercise could be extended by role-playing a delegation of student nurses approaching management to make the case for the rights they believe they should have.

Patients' rights (and duties)
Students should familiarise themselves with the AHA Charter of Patients' Rights and the contents of this chapter, and then clarify for themselves what

obligations they believe patients have on accepting hospital care. Having done this preparation, the class then might be set the task of interviewing a number of patients in order to determine what patients perceive to be their primary rights and whether they feel these are being respected, and if not, why not. (This would mean that they would have to obtain the appropriate approval from management, or ethics committee, and consent from patients, before starting – itself an exercise in clarifying rights and obligations.)

Selective disclosure of information
Small group discussion of either a given case or their own anecdotal experience should explore the issues involved in breach of confidentiality or disclosure of information in patients' notes, and the ethical basis of confidentiality clarified in terms of the duty of protective beneficence and the patient's right to privacy. Each group should then discuss what conditions a contract of confidentiality should have.

Scope of 'treatment', 'control' and 'care'
The cases given in the text (or others like them) can be used in group discussion, to explore the systematic ambiguity that the terms 'treatment', 'control' and 'care' have in nursing contexts. Further, students should be encouraged to explore the fuzziness of the 'rights' and 'duties' that arises when there is lack of clear definition of the scope of responsibility to provide treatment with or without consent, and the nature of the contract with the patient.

7

Conflicting demands in nursing groups of patients

AIMS

This chapter has the following aims:
1. To explore the positive meaning of 'moral autonomy' and to distinguish this from the 'absence of external constraint' or mere personal freedom 'to do your own thing'
2. To explore the meaning of the 'common good' and the role this concept plays in our thinking about social justice and the responsibilities of the state for health and welfare
3. To apply these concepts to the analysis of a range of moral choices we face in deciding on the scope and limits of our responsibility for patients, and to intervene in their lives, namely in preventing suicide, behaviour modification, health screening and prevention of illness, and 'counselling'
4. To explore the ethics of those situations where nurses have to exercise authority to refuse admission or 'persuade' patients to cooperate, or make difficult decisions about the allocation of scarce resources, in the interests of others.

LEARNING OUTCOMES

When you have read and worked through this chapter, you should be able to:

- Distinguish theoretically and in practice between the right to freedom of action and one's responsibility as an autonomous moral agent to demonstrate commitment to a clear set of values
- Demonstrate understanding of the nature of our commitments within any moral community to promote the health and well-being of others and to protect their interests for the common good
- Demonstrate insight into the nature of issues of social justice in health care, by ability to give examples at ward or community, state and international level, and explain the issues
- Demonstrate ability to analyse and critically evaluate the competing 'rights' of various 'stakeholders' in given situations, with a view to reaching fair appraisals of their relative priority in making decisions
- Demonstrate sensitivity and understanding of the conflicts between the responsible exercise of power and authority and patients' rights.

The previous chapter discussed two classes of moral difficulty in direct nurse–patient encounters; these centred on moral problems related to truth-telling and confidentiality, on the one hand, and the problematic area of deciding between therapeutic and palliative treatment on the other. While cases of these types could be discussed without particular reference to the rights of other patients and relatives, the moral difficulties examined in this chapter cannot be discussed without taking into account the rights of other people, or the good of society. The moral problems we propose to examine relate to setting limits to the 'management' of patients, i.e. the control and direction of their lives, and balancing the rights of individual patients with those of

other patients, or third parties. It may be useful in this connection to remind ourselves of the four different, but related, senses of responsibility that we discussed in Chapter 4:

- Responsibility *for* one's own actions – personal responsibility
- Responsibility *for* the care of someone – fiduciary responsibility
- Responsibility *to* higher authority – professional accountability
- Responsibility *to* wider society – public accountability/civic duty.

When nurses are compelled to weigh their responsibility for individual patients against their responsibilities for groups of patients, conflicts may arise between these different types of responsibility which the nurse exercises as an individual and as a professional. The authority vested in her, to serve the best interests of her patients, may contrast with the actual or relative lack of power which she has, depending on her position in the nursing hierarchy or her relationships with other professional staff. What she is entitled to do by law and what she is or is not allowed to do by her union or professional associations may also have a bearing on the matter. Some of these complex issues of responsibility and authority are examined in this chapter.

PERSONAL AUTONOMY VERSUS THE COMMON GOOD

Championing of individual autonomy and 'the individual's right to choose' has become a hallmark of much contemporary ethical debate. This is evident in changing models of family life where there has been a reaction against traditional models of parental authority and overprotective care. It is evident in skepticism towards forms of religious ethics based on appeal to divine authority, rather than reason (e.g. to justify policies on contraception, abortion or euthanasia), and in feminist critiques of male-dominated 'patriarchal' society and its moral norms. In both the public and private sectors of the economy and service provision, there has been a shift of emphasis from the authority and duties of the service provider to the rights of the 'customer' and issues of 'client choice'. The adoption in health care of models of management and client relations taken from business and professional life has also given impetus to a change in our discourse from talk about 'patients' to talk about 'consumers', 'customers' and 'clients', and, with these, a renewed emphasis in ethics on the issue of 'client autonomy' and the 'client's right to choose' (Murley 1995).[1]

Traditional models of care in the health and human services (medicine, nursing, ministry, school teaching and social work) tend to have given priority to the principle of beneficence – to the professional's duty of responsible care for the person being cared for. The very term 'patient' suggests that the person is the *passive* recipient of active care or treatment given by another (agent/patient); the term 'patient' from the Latin *patior* (to suffer) also suggests that the person being cared for is in a dependent state due to their pain or suffering. Within this model there is little scope for talk of the 'patient's right to choose', for the 'patient' is regarded as relatively helpless and the doctor or nurse is presumed to know what is good for him. As we have already remarked, the emphasis on patients' rights is a relatively recent development in health care, even within the 20th century. But it is also true that emphasis on the autonomy of the moral agent is a relatively late development in the history of philosophy as well, i.e. since the Enlightenment.

The classical philosophers, from Plato and Aristotle to the Mediaeval Scholastics, treat autonomy not as given or innate, but as a capacity that has to be developed and which grows with wisdom, experience and maturity. In radical contrast to many modern thinkers who regard 'the right to autonomy' or the 'principle of autonomy' as something given with human nature itself, one could say that for traditional Graeco-Roman and Judaeo-Christian thought, autonomy is something we have to earn by proving ourselves to be responsible and capable moral beings. Virtue ethics, as we shall see, emphasises that by cultivating the intellectual and moral virtues, sound habits and competence in the areas of knowledge and human action, we gain greater control over ourselves, and hence both greater freedom and greater capacity to act responsibly. By the same

token, we are not born free, but become progressively more free as we develop the capacities required to control and direct our own lives. A baby is almost totally subject to the determining forces of its heredity and environment. Even to learn to walk, it has first to be assisted onto its feet by other people, before it becomes capable of walking on its own and determining which direction it will take on life's journey. For the classical philosophers (Aristotle in particular), to say that 'man is a rational being' does not mean that we are born with fully developed rational capacities; on the contrary, 'rationality' (and 'autonomy') is a capacity that requires to be developed through habit and practice. In other words they are not concepts with a fixed meaning, but *developmental concepts* which would apply to different people to differing degrees, depending on their knowledge, experience and maturity (cf. Hill 1991, Mele 1995).

The term 'autonomy' came into prominence in modern philosophy with Kant (1724–1804), who stressed that in order to be held a fully rational, responsible moral agent, one must be an autonomous person – one must demonstrate personal commitment to the moral law, and not just mechanically obey external authority. An 'heteronomous' law is one imposed on me by someone else; this may be my parents, the Church or the state, or any other moral authority. Autonomy is the state of moral maturity where one is able to personally acknowledge the validity of the moral law, choose by oneself to live by it and commit oneself to uphold it – not because one is told to do so, but because one chooses to do so of one's own free will. 'Autonomy', for Kant, stands in opposition to 'heteronomy' as an attitude to the demands of morality, the latter of unthinking and uncritical obedience, the former of fully adult understanding of one's responsibilities as a moral agent. In this sense, we cannot treat a person as a fully responsible moral agent unless he fulfils the requirement of being an autonomous agent. This means that he must act both freely and without compulsion, and also with insight into and personal commitment to the requirements of the moral law (Paton 1969).

The current tendency in North American bioethics to treat 'autonomy' as an inherent *right* of human beings, or even as a fundamental ethical *principle*, as do Beauchamp & Childress (1994, Ch. 3) when they include 'respect for personal autonomy' along with non-maleficence, beneficence and justice as fundamental ethical principles, presents us with some philosophical difficulties. This classification seems to involve a category mistake – for autonomy is surely not a principle but a *precondition* for one to be able to affirm principles as your own, or the liberty to claim one's rights or the freedom to act as a fully responsible person. Alternatively, it is a *capacity to apply moral principles* with insight and discrimination, not a moral principle as such. Respect for the rights of others would seem to include *respect for their need to act freely* and to make their own moral choices, making autonomy the ground for the principle, rather than a principle itself. If we follow Kant in saying that we should always treat persons as 'ends in themselves' and never simply as 'means to an end', this means that 'respect for persons and their rights' really means 'treating other persons *as if* they were fully autonomous moral agents', even if they are not.

Our Western concept of the 'self' has come under critical scrutiny in the past 100 years, from Eastern philosophies such as Buddhism, which regards the self at best as a provisional construct and, in the end, as 'unreal'. It has also been subject to 'deconstruction' in recent postmodernism, where the presumed ontological foundations of selfhood, i.e. its foundations in reality, have been subject to radical criticism. While some may be puzzled why this is of such concern to philosophers, in particular feminist philosophers, the debate raises fundamental questions about our nature as moral agents. Is our nature something determined, fixed or given, which we cannot change, or is our nature something we can shape by our choices and projects (Berlin 1969, Taylor 1992)?[2]

Jean-Paul Sartre (1956, 1973), French atheist philosopher and existentialist, maintained that if the Creator does not exist, to give us a predetermined nature and purpose for living, then we are totally responsible for ourselves and 'must make ourselves by our decisions'.[3] Feminist writers, including Sartre's companion Simone de Beauvoir, have argued that *essentialist* philosophers and theologians who contend that human nature is given and predetermined all too easily use

essentialist arguments to justify sex-role stereotyping and male dominance as 'natural'. In criticising patriarchal structures in society (and perhaps particularly in the world of medicine and health care), feminist philosophers like de Beauvoir and others have been concerned not only to address questions of sex discrimination against women, but also to encourage women to see that by the exercise of their own autonomy they can mould and change their identity, both as individuals and as an oppressed group in society (de Beauvoir 1988, Bowden 1997).

In defence of the traditional view of human nature or species being as something given, while we can (and ought) to take control of and direct our lives, shaping our destiny as best we can, nevertheless there is a fundamental sense in which I cannot choose to become something other than what I am (e.g. a shark or a baboon). While we might say the behavior of some lawyers or money lenders justifies us in calling them 'sharks' or 'loan sharks', and otherwise civilised men can behave like baboons under the influence of alcohol, we would not deny that we can never actually change our species being, however much we may seek to transcend its limitations or may abuse ourselves. Furthermore, postmodernism tends to caricature the traditional view, because Aristotle, for example, does not presuppose a static and unchanging human essence, but speaks of our nature in terms of potentiality and its developmental possibilities (which may be unending). Indeed, we can get stuck with fixed stereotypes, and these have done great damage in the past. The real challenge is whether or not we actually develop our full potentialities, including our autonomy, through participation with others in a moral community, for we certainly cannot do it on our own.

'Personal autonomy' always stands in tension with the 'common good', for we do not spring ready-made out of nothing, either biologically or psychologically. We are the products of the sexual activity and love (or lack of love) of our parents, and of generations before them. We are moulded and nurtured by our families, communities, schools, religious and political associations, and our emergence and maturation as individuals, with an identity of our own, are products of the interaction of our growing capacities for self-determination with these forces of social determinism, as we grow and mature as human beings. In seeking to express ourselves and to realise our autonomy, we do not do this in isolation, but in action and reaction within both our given and the chosen moral communities in which we live and work. For this reason, my good can never be intelligibly discussed apart from the common good of others in society, who are responsible for me and to whom I am responsible. The cult of 'personal autonomy' above all else fails to do justice to the other side of the equation.

When we speak of health care, we are concerned with services provided by society, in principle at least, for all its members. While most health care systems in fact discriminate positively in favour of the rich and powerful, and negatively against the weak, poor, elderly, mentally incapacitated and insane (and perhaps against ethnic minorities in some societies), nevertheless the public resources which are spent on health care (and other public services) are meant to contribute to the common good. As it was said in the 18th century, 'the common wealth of the Commonwealth should be used for the common weal' (where 'weal' meant welfare, suffering or need).

Our modern state-funded or state-subsidised health care systems, and in particular modern welfare states, are intended to achieve a greater degree of equity for all, both in access to health services and in distribution of health resources. The source of inspiration for these models can perhaps be traced back to the development of the concepts of 'commonwealth' and 'commonweal' in the Enlightenment. They also present us with the practical political and ethical challenge of how we develop systems of health care delivery that will serve the urgent needs of individuals, and ensure some measure of distributive justice for all in society.

We have pointed out before that there is always a tension in any society between the competing demands of the principles of beneficence, justice and respect for persons, for while the protective duty of care and respect for persons tend to focus on individuals, justice concerns how we share power and social benefits fairly and equitably in society, for the common good. In many respects, popular 'medical ethics' and 'nursing ethics' tend to focus undue attention on the 'dilemmas' that arise between the competing duties of beneficence and respect for persons: on the one hand, to promote the well-being of the individual and protect him from harm; and on the other to respect the rights of the individual. This 'bed face' clinical mentality finds it uncomfortable to address the further demands of social justice – when it becomes a matter of choosing between more or less 'deserving' patients, managing limited staff and resources, undertaking randomised control trials, or dealing with the demands of public health, public screening and health education of the masses.

In discussing the 'common good', it is important to draw attention to two related but different notions of distributive justice, apart from the more commonly understood retributive sense of the word 'justice'. To the extent that 'justice' is understood in its connection with the civil or criminal courts or the criminal justice system, we tend to think of justice in primarily negative and punitive terms, as exacting retribution, compensation or punishment from those who have infringed our civil or personal rights. However, even the courts can be seen as institutions of last resort in which people seek to achieve fairness in terms of distributive justice (e.g. over breach of contract). Nevertheless our main concern is with distributive justice in the sense of fair and equitable distribution of benefits and burdens, resources and responsibilities, and with power-sharing in society. The two types of distributive justice that need to be distinguished here are (Woozley 1981):

- fairness in the sense of *equality of opportunity* for individuals
- fairness in terms of equity, or *equality of outcome* for groups of people.

In a culture which emphasises 'the right to personal autonomy' (usually prosperous conservative societies) there is a tendency to focus on the right to equality of opportunity for individuals, and to ignore the question of whether or not the circumstances in which individuals find themselves make it actually possible to claim their rights. The fact is that one requires a certain level of education, financial self-sufficiency and social leverage to be able to claim and exercise the 'right to equality of opportunity'. Poverty, lack of parents, social and racial discrimination may so disempower you that you are actually prevented from exercising these rights. Shifting the emphasis from 'justice' to 'equity' involves a shift of emphasis to the means to achieve 'equality of outcome for groups'. The impetus to set up 'welfare states', and, in the UK, the National Health Service, systems of universal and compulsory health insurance, and state provision of health care in socialist states are all driven by concern about social inequalities in health and access to health care. Each represents an attempt to ensure greater equity in the sharing of health care services and resources across the whole of society, so as to achieve equal outcomes or benefits for all groups in society.

Similarly, 'affirmative action' and 'positive discrimination' have been adopted as strategies which attempt to compensate for the inherited circumstances of social disadvantage in which people find themselves and over which they have no control. These strategies have been applied in education and training, and employment in particular. In England, for example, where a large proportion of hospital nurses are black, but few have gained promotion to positions of seniority within the nursing hierarchy, adopting a policy of 'affirmative action' would mean giving preference to a black nurse over a white nurse, with equivalent qualifications and experience, in making appointments until the balance is more equitable. Alternatively, positive discrimination might involve giving preference to a woman rather than a man in making senior appointments to nurse management, in an institution where men predominate, even if the man might appear better qualified. In the heady 1960s, these strategies enjoyed popular political support in many countries, but in the 1990s there was a backlash against these measures, because it has been argued that they are not in fact fair (to the individual involved). The argument is that affirmative action discriminates against the best candidate in favour of achieving some ideal ethnic or gender balance in organisations, and it is questioned whether this

achieves the desired benefits intended. While there is considerable evidence that policies of reverse discrimination have achieved the social goal of greater equity (in access to education, health and social services) in many countries, the arguments based on 'merit first' and 'equality of opportunity for the individual' have some degree of popular ascendancy at the moment – possibly connected with economic recession and unemployment affecting the middle classes and economically privileged.

David Thomson, in his incisive paper *Welfare States and the Problem of the Common* (1992) and his more controversial book *Selfish Generations? The Ageing of New Zealand's Welfare State* (1991), points out that the generation which has grown up with the rights and benefits of the welfare state has become more concerned about protecting their own entitlements than extending the benefits of the welfare state to the younger generation. While the postwar older generation were willing to make sacrifices to ensure that the younger generation had access to education, health care and welfare (particularly protection against unemployment), he argues that the beneficiaries of this generosity have not been prepared to show the same altruism to the new generation, that the welfare states have become welfare states for the elderly, at the expense of the young. While his general thesis is hotly contested, he marshals sufficient historical evidence to give us pause for thought (cf. Mishra 1990).

In facing up to the ethical responsibilities of dealing with groups of patients rather than simply with individuals, and the responsibilities of management and administration, public health and research, it should be obvious that nurses should grapple with the tensions between autonomy and the common good, between respect for the rights of individuals and social justice.

Lars Reuter (1999) argues, in a paper to the Council of Europe symposium on protection of the human rights and dignity of the terminally ill, that the public attention given to the ethical debates about the issues of abortion and euthanasia is related to the current preoccupation with 'the right to personal autonomy'. He further points to some of the inherent contradictions in the kinds of arguments advanced, from a post-modernist point of view, in favour of 'the woman's right to choose' or the 'patient's right to die'. His point is that if the self is a construct in Sartre's sense then it is difficult to argue from the necessary relativity of different chosen forms or expressions of selfhood to any kind of universal right to abortion or voluntary euthanasia. If we adopt the traditional view that all human beings, as members of the wider moral community, share a common species being, then our claims to universal human rights only make sense on the basis of what serves the common good. In other words 'rights' cannot be decided on the basis of subjective choices, but our rights are circumscribed by the rights of others and the duties we owe to them besides ourselves.

Thus, the woman claiming to exercise her 'right to choose' to terminate a pregnancy is denying any actual or potential right to autonomy to the child. This begins to sound like Humpty Dumpty speaking to Alice: 'When I use a word [like 'autonomy'] it means just what I choose it to mean, neither more nor less'.[4] Similarly, to insist that one has an unconditional 'right' to be helped to terminate one's life ignores the question of whether one is entitled to impose duties on others that they would find morally unacceptable. So, we may ask whether it really helps to talk about 'rights' in these contexts, for what are one's corresponding obligations to the moral community?

SETTING LIMITS TO THE CONTROL AND DIRECTION OF PATIENTS

The management of patients is a complex art, ranging from subtle persuasion to the use of force to subdue violent patients. What gives the nurse the authority to control other people in this way?

In psychiatric wards, in accident and emergency departments and in working with people with mental handicaps, nurses often encounter violent patients who have to be restrained by physical means, by the use of drugs or by invoking the law. In such cases it may appear that the nursing staff are justified in using 'reasonable force' to control patients simply in order to defend themselves, other patients and staff. They may also be acting to protect the patient from injury, self-mutilation or suicide, or, less dramatically, 'acting in the patient's own best interests' (COHSE 1977, UNISON 1997).

The fact is that the nurse is not responsible only for the individual patient and his needs, nor is the nurse simply concerned with his rights. The nurse also has to protect the interests of other patients and, as a public officer who is accountable to society at large, to consider the public good. The rights of individual patients may have to be restricted where the rights and safety of other people are put at risk. In addition, the nurse has a responsibility to protect the interests of the patient who is incapable of understanding what his own best interests are, e.g. if he is mentally ill, under the influence of drugs, intoxicated or intellectually impaired. The nurse has to decide what is in the best interests of the patient and good patient care. Depending on whether the patient is competent and the circumstances in which the patient comes into care or is referred to the nurse for appropriate care, nurses may have to interpret their responsibilities differently (see Ch. 4, pp. 71–76, for a discussion of models of care based on code, contract, covenant and charter). In general, nurses exercise fiduciary responsibility for patients entrusted to their care, and they must be guided in their decisions by training and experience, professional code and personal conscience, acting always in such a way as to 'safeguard and promote the well-being and interests of patients/clients' (UKCC 1984b, 1992).

Concern with the 'best interests of the patient' means that the nurse has to exercise both clinical and moral responsibilities towards her patients. These responsibilities are determined not only by consideration of the patients' rights and respect for their freedom, but also by consideration of the wider health needs of the individual and the community. 'Management' of patients (including those who cooperate fully in treatment) can involve various degrees of control, ranging from physical restraint, or legal measures, to behaviour modification through health education or just directive managerial communication. Skill in nursing means, in part at least, learning to control people in the nicest possible way.

case history 7.1

'Half in love with easeful death?'

On our ward we had a 70-year-old woman who was described as an alcoholic and had taken several overdoses over a period of 2 years. The staff feared that if she were to be discharged, she would return home to her alcoholic husband and sooner or later would be found dead. However, when she was sober she appeared completely rational and demanded to be allowed home. Her compulsory detention in hospital on the grounds that she might commit suicide seemed to me a flagrant violation of her freedom when there did not appear to be adequate evidence that she was mentally ill.

Preventing suicide and the 'right to die'

In Case History 7.1, a psychiatric nurse is faced with the possible discharge of a patient thought by the doctor to be a suicide risk. The nurse's concern was whether she had a moral or legal duty to prevent someone from committing suicide if she wanted to do so.

In this case, the moral ambiguity of the situation for the nurse arises because of uncertainty about the elderly woman's mental state. Was the woman capable of making rational decisions about her life? The action of the hospital in protecting her might appear paternalistic and restrictive of her liberty, but it could be said to be a natural extension of her right to treatment and the contract of the staff to care for and protect her (as well as to offer her such therapy as might be appropriate). Here the nurse has to exercise fiduciary responsibility on behalf of the patient, which may involve restricting her movements 'in her own best interests' – this is a demand of protective beneficence and may even be construed as required as a defence of the patient's rights where the patient appears unable to take responsible decisions for herself. Of course, this argument presupposes that suicide is never in the best interests of the patient. The moving play, *Whose Life Is It Anyway?*, about a young quadriplegic who is being kept alive against his will, by artificial means, challenges this assumption – at least as far

as the young man is exercising his right to refuse further treatment and wants to be left to die (Clark 1978).

Unlike the questions previously discussed in Chapter 5 relating to voluntary euthanasia and assisted suicide, this case is less concerned with the question of the rights and autonomy of patients than with the scope of the nurse's responsibility to prevent patients from committing suicide, and whether or not the nurse, in this case, should use the legal powers available under the law to detain the elderly lady in hospital against her will, for her own protection. However, while there are important differences here that we wish to discuss relating to social attitudes to suicide, there are some aspects of our discussion of Case History 5.2 (p. 117) that are relevant. First, there is overwhelming evidence that people who commit suicide are clinically depressed or suffering from some form of mental illness, so there is a factual foundation to the common-sense view that people do not commit suicide unless 'the balance of their mind is disturbed' as the coroner's court expresses it. Second, there is important research evidence, from both the field of geriatric medicine and the study of people with severe disabilities, that people who request assistance to commit suicide or euthanasia generally lack adequate family or social support systems and tend to be very pessimistic about the future and anxious that they will be a burden to their families (Sommers & Shields 1987, Thompson 1993, Shaw 1994, Lebacqz 1999,). Because of this evidence and prevailing social attitudes to suicide, there is still an expectation that nurses and other professional carers will take action to prevent people committing suicide.

A less generous construction which could be placed on the action of the hospital in this case is that the staff were acting less to protect the old lady than to protect themselves against the charge of negligence and the guilt which might result if the patient succeeded in killing herself. The fact is that no matter what precautions are taken, some patients do succeed in committing suicide and that does cause great distress to the staff responsible for their care. Nevertheless, defensive action and conservative measures, although somewhat repressive at times, are morally justifiable. Staff are entitled to protect themselves and their professional reputations from allegations of culpable neglect of patients in their care. The courage to take the risk of discharging a potentially suicidal patient may show admirable regard for that person's autonomy but can always be attacked as irresponsibility. Achieving a balance between both caring for and protecting patients, and respecting their freedom, between defensive medicine and attempted rehabilitation, is always difficult, a matter of risk and often complicated by the threat of legal action.

Throughout history, most societies have condemned suicide, unless in extreme circumstances, e.g. to avoid capture by one's enemies or to avoid being sold into slavery. Many societies have applied extremely severe penalties to those who attempt suicide, and in Europe those who committed 'self-murder' could not be buried in 'Christian' cemeteries or in 'hallowed ground' but were buried at the crossroads. Although we tend to be more compassionate today towards suicides, and seek to explain or excuse their actions as due to psychiatric causes, nevertheless we still react with involuntary horror at the news that an acquaintance has ended his own life. G. K. Chesterton's (1927) comment that 'the suicide refuses to take the oath of loyalty to life' or the belief that the suicide acts in a way that 'contradicts our natural instinct for self-preservation' might partly explain the reason for popular disapproval of suicide.[5] In Roman times, for a man to commit suicide was regarded as a crime against the state, depriving it of a potential soldier. In a somewhat similar vein, Lenin argued that suicide was a crime because it deprived the state of a worker! While we might not want to endorse such simplistic views, we may recognise that there is more than a grain of truth in these ideas, for we do not exist in isolation but are involved in and are part of the extended human family, and only have rights as members of a moral community.

There have been attempts to justify acts of suicide or even to regard them as heroic acts of defiance in the face of overwhelming fate. The Roman Stoics maintained that a person was justified in taking his own life, not only as a soldier in war

might do to prevent his being tortured for information, or taken prisoner and sold into slavery, but also if circumstances were such as to totally overwhelm one's ability to make rational choices. Stoics were encouraged to cultivate their freedom and power of self-determination by developing an attitude of *apatheia*, i.e. of emotional detachment and indifference to pain, suffering and desire, in order to achieve self-mastery and a life that could be lived in conformity with nature, ruled by purely rational principles. Our modern ideal of personal freedom and moral autonomy might be said to have its roots in this Stoic philosophy. Regarding suicide, the cultivation of an attitude of indifference or apatheia to both life and death was supposed to enable the Stoic philosopher to choose with complete freedom between them, as Seneca suggested, 'like a man calmly leaving a smoke-filled room'. Or, as Tillich (1952, pp. 9–17) emphasises: 'suicide as an escape from life, dictated by fear, contradicts the Stoic courage to be'. As the Lutheran theologian, Bonhoeffer (1955), says (cf. Aldridge 1998):

Suicide is a specifically human action, and it is not surprising if it has on this account repeatedly been applauded and justified by noble human minds. If this action is performed in freedom it is raised high above any petty moralizing accusation of cowardice and weakness. Suicide is the ultimate and extreme self-justification of man as man, and it is therefore, from a purely human standpoint, in a certain sense even, the self-accomplished expiation for a life that has failed .... Suicide is a man's attempt to give a final human meaning to a life which has become humanly meaningless. The involuntary sense of horror which seizes us when we are faced with the fact of a suicide is not to be attributed to the iniquity of such a deed but to the terrible loneliness and freedom in which this deed is performed, as a deed in which the positive attitude to life is reflected only in the destruction of life.

Paradoxically, however, the atheist philosopher Jean-Paul Sartre, who believed that existence is freedom, argued that a person must be deluded to think that to take one's life is a supreme act of freedom in which one can triumph over fate, for it is the ultimate absurdity to use one's freedom to end one's freedom (Sartre 1957).

Thus, our attitudes to suicide are ambivalent, and this is reflected in the fact that there is generally no legal obligation on people as citizens to prevent someone attempting suicide, although they may feel that they are duty-bound to do so if they can, for a variety of moral reasons. However, the law takes a different view of the responsibilities of doctors, nurses and other health professionals who have charge of patients. As long as a person is in a nurse's care, the law requires the nurse to protect the patient from harm, including self-inflicted harm. In fact, a nurse can be charged with negligence if a patient succeeds in killing himself. The nurse has this legal duty towards patients in her care in spite of the fact that suicide is no longer illegal in Britain. Because the law assumes that those who attempt suicide are mentally unbalanced, they are no longer prosecuted for attempting to take their lives, but nevertheless health professionals are expected to protect them from suicide. The fact that the law allows people the licence or liberty to attempt suicide without prosecution does not mean that the law or morality recognises that persons have a right to kill themselves. We ordinarily understand by a 'right' (as discussed in Ch. 5, pp. 110–118) the entitlement to demand that other people either assist us in particular ways or desist from acting towards us in particular ways. In this sense of 'right', the so-called 'right to suicide' is not a right. There is no way we can appeal to the law or to morality to compel others to assist us to end our lives. Whether we can extend the use of the term 'right' to cover personal entitlement to act in a particular way, e.g. to attempt suicide, will depend on our understanding of the reciprocal obligations we owe one another as members of the moral community.

Behaviour modification

Another type of control which raises ethical problems is the use of rewards and punishments to reinforce behaviour modification in long-term psychiatric patients. For example, money or cigarettes may be given as rewards to encourage better self-care among institutionalised patients – for washing, shaving, dressing, bed-making, care of living area, etc. Alternatively, sanctions may be applied – by the removal of privileges such as access to television, opportunities for exercise or

recreation. Is it ethically justifiable to extend the definition of treatment to include the retraining and rehabilitation of patients by these means?

Health care staff, trained to standards of cleanliness, order and tidiness, may find the slovenliness of some patients intolerable. (In the same way that community nurses may find offensive the behaviour of elderly people with Diogenes syndrome, who accumulate rubbish and live in a mess.) It is easy to rationalise the use of retraining measures for such patients on the grounds that it is necessary, for reasons of hygiene, to avoid fire hazards and to protect other patients' interests. 'Retraining' patients to care for themselves and their environment may also ease the burden on the nursing staff and make the institutional management of such individuals easier and more pleasant for everyone. The use of aversion therapy in the treatment of some phobias and to help people, for example, to give up smoking, stop abusing drugs or alcohol, can be justified reasonably easily in practice because the patient generally wants to overcome the phobia or dependence on addictive substances and, as a rule, can be consulted about treatment and can give informed and voluntary consent. Each of these kinds of reason may carry some weight in justifying the use of behaviour modification techniques, but unless balanced by respect for the patient's right to non-cooperation, they can lead to abuse (Matthies et al 1997).

When the patient is competent to give consent, these cases are reasonably straightforward. However, the situation is much more complicated when the patient is intellectualy impaired, mentally ill, senile or suffering the consequences of long-term institutionalisation. Here there may be serious doubts about whether consent can be either informed or voluntary in any true sense. It becomes a matter of interpreting what the 'duty to care' means in these circumstances for the health care staff. They have to fall back on other kinds of justification: arguments that such measures are ultimately in the best interests of the patient (in the attempt to restore some degree of autonomy to the patient), or that the retraining is necessary to protect the rights (health and safety) of others, or that the staff cannot be expected to work in intolerable conditions (Ross 1981, Hamberger et al 1997, UNISON 1997).

The argument that something is in the best interests of the patient is acceptable if, and only if, it is informed by a proper respect for the dignity of individual patients, by a concern to rehabilitate them, improve their quality of life or environment, or at least to improve the general standards of patient care. Respect for the dignity of persons will obviously set limits to the degree or forms of coercion which are employed, and even the use of cigarettes as inducements may be ruled out on the grounds that they may damage the health of patients. There is always a risk that the assumption of fiduciary responsibility may lead to paternalism and even to abuse of patients if it is not limited by respect for persons. Mildly demented elderly people are often assumed by neighbours and anxious caring professionals to be at risk from house fires – a common argument for their being put in 'sheltered accommodation'. Studies of the extent of the actual risk have shown that it is in fact much lower than it is imagined to be and that the use of alternative forms of heating can sometimes circumvent the need for institutionalisation.[6]

It is far too easy for health professionals to rationalise their prejudices against people who adopt different lifestyles or standards of cleanliness and to impose a regime on patients for their own convenience rather than the real benefit of patients. If this risk is recognised, then the use of behaviour modification techniques for the rehabilitation of those whose standards of self-care have deteriorated through illness or institutionalisation may sometimes be justified on the kinds of grounds already discussed. The rights of nursing staff members to decent working conditions are important, but not so important as to justify coercion of patients to conform to staff demands, when perhaps collective action by nurses may be required to ensure better staffing levels, modernisation of equipment and the provision of adequate resources.

Health education

Health education itself, in so far as it seeks to change people's attitudes and behaviour, raises ethical questions as well. Are nurses entitled to tell people that they should stop smoking, reduce their alcohol intake or go on a diet? Or, more controversially, are nurses morally justified in advising people to practise contraception or to seek sterilisation? If so, how directive should this advice be? Should people just be given the facts and left to decide for themselves? Should nurses actively try to change people's attitudes and lifestyles? Should they be campaigning for legislation to control advertising of alcohol and tobacco? Should they support campaigns, e.g. for seat belt legislation, laws against driving under the influence of drugs or alcohol, or compulsory fluoridation of water? Should they be involved directly in community development in areas of high unemployment and social deprivation (GNC 1980, Coutts & Hardy 1985, Downie et al 1996)?

One of the main difficulties presented to doctors and nurses by their becoming involved in health education, screening and immunisation is that *proactive* preventive health initiatives involve a change of mind-set for the average health professional. Trained to react to crises of various kinds and the presenting symptoms, they are generally loath to seek out undisclosed pathology. To shift from a *reactive mode* of interaction with patients to a *proactive mode* involves not only a change in attitude and practice, but some subtle changes in ethical orientation as well. Crisis intervention and treatment of the symptoms identified by the patient fit comfortably with a service ethic based on responsible care or protective beneficence. Actively seeking out undeclared morbidity, e.g. in screening for breast or cervical cancer in women and prostate cancer in men, requires a different kind of ethical justification. Recruitment of people for screening, or suggesting to patients that they undergo screening, may cause people a great deal of anxiety. If the tests involve biopsies, these can be more painful and inconvenient than is generally indicated, and people can experience considerable fear and anxiety until the results are known. Given the doubts which have been raised about the effectiveness of some forms of screening, e.g. for prostate cancer, it can be seriously questioned whether it is ethically justifiable to put people through all this and the inconvenience involved. The costs of some methods of screening, relative to their benefits for patients, can be seriously questioned on both ethical and medical grounds. The justification for such public health measures is generally a utilitarian one, namely that they contribute to improved health for the majority of the population, even if they cause distress or health complications for individuals (e.g. untypical reactions to vaccines, or anaesthetics used for biopsies, or painful screening procedures). Here the principles of protective beneficence and justice may be invoked to justify interventions which it is claimed will contribute to the common good, but individual interest and individual rights may be compromised. Trained to care for individuals, nurses may hesitate to get involved.

Health education, if it is to be relevant, must be related to the patterns of morbidity and mortality in society. In the past, the infectious diseases and diseases associated with poverty were responsible for high infant mortality and the deaths of young people. These diseases have been largely controlled by general improvements in the standards of living (better housing and diet), public health measures (better sewage disposal, cleaner water supplies) and medical measures (immunisation and the development of effective drugs). Today in the developed countries, the pattern of morbidity and mortality is quite different. Infant mortality rates have been dramatically reduced and most dying is done by the elderly. There has been a vast increase in the proportion of the population over the age of 50 years, and most illness in this group is lifestyle-related. Apart from accidental and violent deaths (a small proportion) the vast majority of deaths and morbidity in the population are associated with smoking, alcohol abuse, inappropriate diet and lack of exercise, and here the contribution of alcohol and drug abuse to accidents, domestic violence and suicide is considerable. While poverty and social deprivation can be aggravating factors contributing to poor health status, the epidemic of chronic and disabling diseases of middle and later life is clearly lifestyle-related. If the major causes of premature death are to be eliminated, then people's attitudes, values and lifestyles have to be changed (McKeown 1976, Ewles & Simnett 1985, WHO 1984, 1985, 1999b).

The key ethical questions about health education concern the *question of means and methods*: how are people's attitudes, values and lifestyles to be changed, and what methods, inducements or sanctions is it ethically permissible to use to achieve the long-term goal of reduced morbidity and mortality in the general population? Is it legitimate to exploit our knowledge of psychology and of people's vulnerability, to play on their anxieties, to use subliminal advertising, to actively promote alternative lifestyles in conjunction with commercial marketing of 'health products'? More subtle, but just as important, is the question of the style of education. Is it to be authoritarian and guilt-inducing; take-it-or-leave-it 'scientific' information-giving; focused on developing individual knowledge and life skills for more competent living; or about community development and mobilising the resources in local communities to help themselves (Downie et al 1996)?

Obviously, the major ethical justification for health education is the same as that which was invoked in the 19th century to justify compulsory immunisation, notification of infectious diseases and compulsory public health measures. This was based on an appeal to both the principles of beneficence (to protect the health and safety of people) and justice or the common good. Such action was felt to be justified even if it meant restricting the rights of some individuals and dissenting minorities (compulsory seat belt legislation and fluoridation raise similar questions today).

The problem is that legal and fiscal measures cannot be forced on a community entirely without their consent, even in a totalitarian state. Public opinion has to be informed and persuaded, a consensus created – and that is a task of health education. If health educators are not to give offence, they have to respect the rights and autonomy of individuals, their right to decide on their own values and lifestyle. People cannot be forced to take responsibility for their health. They may be given inducements to do so or be subjected to various forms of sanctions if they do not do so.

If health education is to be effective, it may be necessary to use a wide variety of health education measures. It will not be sufficient just to give people the facts and leave them to make up their own minds. Other forces come into play, influencing people's health choices, such as peer group pressure and mass media advertising of products damaging to people's health (such as tobacco, alcohol and junk foods). It will not be sufficient to promote the value of positive health and healthy lifestyles through the education of individuals when people's social conditions mean that health has low priority in their scale of survival values – where housing, food, clothing and employment are more urgently needed. It will not be sufficient to try to influence health behaviour through taxation and legal measures when huge vested interests are at stake in the tobacco, alcohol and food industries. Advertising may need to be controlled, funds may have to be allocated for community development and the combating of social deprivation and poverty. State subsidies and tax incentives may need to be given to companies to diversify and phase out the production of things damaging health (Thompson 1987a, Robertson et al 1992, Tones et al 1994).

If we are to define health, as WHO does, as 'complete physical, mental and social well-being, and not merely the absence of disease or infirmity', then all health professionals have a fundamental responsibility for the prevention of disease, as well as for its treatment (for 'prevention is better than cure'). The UK National Health Service, for example, was not intended to be simply a national disease service, but to improve the nation's health (Wilson 1976). So-called 'health professionals' have both a moral and a professional duty to be health educators. Nurses, in particular, whether on the ward or in the community should be committed, as nurses, not only to the treatment of disease but also to active health promotion. Nurses and other health professionals therefore have a special responsibility to act as role models. Doctors or nurses who are heavy smokers or abuse alcohol cannot expect their advice to be taken seriously. Their credibility as health professionals is called into question. The tobacco industry regard them as the best possible advertisers of their products – 'one doctor or nurse who is a smoker is worth 100 advertisements elsewhere'!

This does not mean that all nurses have to be angels, but their example in taking responsibility for their own health is important, because it is closely observed by their patients. The high cigarette consumption among nurses as a profession may have many explanations, including the alternating periods of stress and boredom which characterise their work. However, the example of doctors in giving up smoking has not only had a dramatic effect on reducing the incidence of heart disease and lung cancer in their ranks, but has obviously impressed their patients, who have given up smoking in large numbers (Coutts & Hardy 1985, Pender 1996).

Health professionals, as a body of people with public responsibility for maintaining the health services, cannot simply rest content with passive implementation of health policies decided by other people. As those who see the casualties on the wards and in the community every day, they have a responsibility to try to use their political influence actively to shape health policies. Through their professional associations and unions, nurses have the power to influence public opinion and so achieve by political, legislative and fiscal means what cannot be achieved simply by counselling individuals, important and effective though that may be for individual patients. However, respect for the rights of individuals must be maintained when pressure is being exerted on individuals and nations to change their lifestyle. The ultimate justification for health education is that the rights of patients demand it – especially the right to know and the right to treatment – for good health empowers people to claim and exercise their other rights.

Communication and 'counselling'

Communication with patients is not only important as a means of discovering or conveying information, and as a means of expressing sympathy, encouragement and personal interest, it is also the single most important way of securing cooperation and compliance. In other words, communication plays a vital role in the management and control of patients (Bradley & Edinberg 1990, Porritt 1990, Balzer-Riley & Smith 1996).

It has become fashionable to talk about the importance of communication in medicine and nursing, and to explain the failures in relationships with patients as being due to 'poor communication'. This explanation is misleading if it implies that health professionals are poor communicators. Experienced doctors and nurses are highly skilled at certain forms of directive managerial communication – using language and the selective disclosure of information as a means of securing patient compliance and as a means of control. However, they may be much less skilled than their junior colleagues at listening to patients, communicating with patients as persons, understanding their personal needs and responding to their different levels of comprehension of information.

Early research in health education showed up major problems in the attempts of health professionals to communicate with ordinary people. Several reasons emerged: their use of specialist jargon, their different educational level and level of literacy, and their quite different life expectations. Simple tests for readability and comprehensibility can now be applied to written material, such as patient information sheets and consent forms. It is both a professional and a moral duty of nurses to ensure that patients can in fact read the information they are given, particularly when informed consent is required for treatment or participation in a clinical control trial (Fletcher 1971, Bennett 1976, Baric 1982, Church 1982).

Research at the same time into communication with patients in hospital, regarding their treatment or the likely effects of surgery, showed wide discrepancies between the levels of actual comprehension and recall by patients and that attributed to them by nurses and doctors (in particular) (Ley 1976, Faulkner 1984). The form of training to which health professionals are subjected, the demands of institutional life and the need to 'manage' large numbers of patients may make nurses and doctors less sensitive, with the passage of time, to the way manipulative communication can offend patients and create mistrust. (Patients often remark that they learn more from porters and cleaners than from medical and nursing staff. Nurses and doctors would do well to recognise that these hospital workers have an important role to play in communication with patients, and to consider why this is the case.)

First and foremost, all health professionals need to enlarge their repertoire of communication skills. In some circumstances, 'controlling' and 'managerial' communication may be required and appropriate, particularly in a crisis, but the other more sensitive communication skills, associated with 'counselling' and 'helping' patients to sort out their own problems and take their own decisions, require quite different training and the development of quite different skills. On the whole, the traditional forms of education and training for health professions, as well as clinical experience, do not equip health professionals with these skills – if anything, the available evidence suggests that, in the process of their training in patient care, there is 'serial desensitisation' of nurses and doctors to the need for these skills (Porritt 1990, Horne & Cowan 1992).

For more than a decade nurses have shown a growing interest in learning counselling skills, and in-service training in counselling has become a veritable growth industry (Dryden et al 1989).

While some psychiatric nurses have undergone specialised training in techniques of psychotherapy and group therapy, and as nurses have long been familiar with the methods of 'client-centred' and 'non-directive' counselling, the wide application of these methods in other areas of nursing is relatively recent. However, skills in these approaches are increasingly being required of nurses working in areas such as terminal care, midwifery, genitourinary medicine, family planning, screening for cancer or genetic disorders, and in dealing with people with HIV/AIDS. (In the case of 'safe sex' counselling and counselling people with HIV/AIDS, there are particular legal issues that need to be addressed by counsellors – McCall-Smith 1991). The ethics of the counselling relationship could be the subject of a special chapter on its own, because it involves a very different orientation from that most commonly practised in nursing. Much communication between nurses and patients is necessarily directive and often involves giving specific advice or warnings, and it is generally legitimised in terms of the nurse's duty of protective care. 'Counselling', as used in its more specialised and professional sense, is the antithesis of 'advice-giving' or the 'counselling' or 'formal cautioning' which is part of the disciplinary process.

Within the classic schools of psychological counselling associated particularly with the names of Carl Rogers and Gerald Egan (Rogers 1961, Egan 1986), 'counselling' is a term that has come to be applied to the process whereby a helper facilitates clients to communicate more effectively about their concerns, so as to enable them to first clarify the nature of their problem(s), to spell out what options they have, and to assist them to find their own solutions to their problems. 'Client-centred' counselling requires the nurse to restrain herself from giving advice or trying to 'help' the patient by solving his problems for him, and rather, by attentive listening, focusing and clarifying, challenging and presenting of options, and possibly by teaching the patient problem-solving skills, to address his own life problems and empower him to exercise more control over his own decision-making.

As an intimate exchange of often very sensitive private information, the first ethical requirement for the counselling relationship is one of clear and agreed boundaries of confidentiality. Secondly, the counsellor is bound to exercise a protective duty of care towards the client, both in terms of protecting the client's vulnerability and privacy, and in terms of the counsellor recognising the limits of her own competence and being prepared to refer the client to a psychiatrist or other appropriate specialist, if necessary. Thirdly, the counsellor has a fundamental duty to respect the individuality and opinions of the client, even if the client disagrees with what the counsellor is saying. This non-judgemental attitude (what Carl Rogers calls 'unconditional positive regard') is essential if the client is to feel free to explore his feelings and conflicts without fear of disapproval or subsequent discrimination. The requirement of empathy (the ability to put yourself in the other's shoes) is often cited as another ethical, as well as functional, requirement of counselling. This is not equivalent to sympathy, which can often be condescending, but rather an attempt to put oneself professionally in the client's position.

Several counselling organisations have developed codes of ethics and practice for counsellors, and the latest nursing codes include terms that relate to the counselling role of the nurse (UKCC 1992). In particular, we would recommend the British Association for Counselling's *Codes of Ethics For Counselling and Practice* (1999) as being of wide general relevance to nurse–patient communication as well.

In general, communication between nurses and patients can raise two kinds of ethical problem: first, when communication fails to express respect for the patient as a person; and, second, when the patient's right to know is ignored. The first kind of problem arises when hospital staff members talk over the heads of patients or, more seriously, fail to respect confidences. The power relationship between patient and health professional is an unequal one, and communication can be used to control the patient rather than to relate to him as a person. The sick or injured patient is often anxious and distressed because he does not understand what is happening to him or why it is happening. He is vulnerable and dependent. Not only does he need the reassurance which the expert can give him, but he needs information to be able to exercise any degree of control over his life. Medical and nursing staff have a responsibility to share their knowledge and their specific information about the patient with him, and to share it in the most helpful and caring way.

BALANCING THE RIGHTS OF PATIENTS WITH THE INTERESTS OF THIRD PARTIES

In general, and for very good reasons, the focus of training in nursing and medicine is on direct patient care, on the one-to-one relationship between carer and patient in the clinical situation. Less attention is given to the wider responsibilities in management, research and health promotion. Clinical practice is grounded on the more individual, or 'personalist', values of beneficence and respect for persons. The values on which the other functions of health care are based are the more universal values derivable from principles of justice. In practice, nurses – like doctors and paramedical staff – usually have obligations to several patients at the same time. Because each nurse has 'only one pair of hands' and 'cannot be in two places at once', she has to make decisions about which patients should be given priority while doing the best for all her patients. These more universal considerations of justice and the common good may suggest different responses to the charge nurse than if she were only responsible for one patient. The same could be said of doctors: the demands of teaching, administration, research and public health all introduce more universal obligations to be balanced against their duties to individual patients.

Health professionals often feel most comfortable at the level of ethical decisions of a personal kind relating to individual patients and their health needs. Their expertise and clinical experience relate best to the treatment of individual patients and decisions about their management. A personalist ethic, based on 'caring', appears most appropriate to such situations. Doctors may well feel that their expertise (unless they are epidemiologists or trained administrators) is not applicable to decisions about the general allocation of manpower and resources. Nurses, on the other hand, while sharing the same personalist ethic, may have more experience in management of large groups of patients and feel less uneasy about making decisions based on the general good. The conflict between these different kinds of values, personalist and universal, comes out most clearly in cases where the rights of individual patients have to be balanced against the interests of third parties. The situations that may serve to illustrate some of the problems and dilemmas are:

- decisions to refuse admission to a patient, either because of risk to other patients or because of lack of a bed
- persuading patients to 'volunteer' as research subjects in clinical trials and/or non-therapeutic research
- the use of patients as teaching material for the instruction of nurses

- decisions about allocation of resources within the hospital or in the community.

It is to the discussion of these that we now turn, before looking at some of the wider 'political' responsibilities of nurses, both as individuals and as a profession.

Refusing to admit a patient

A classic dilemma facing a charge nurse may be whether she can accept responsibility for another patient when there is an acute shortage of staff or resources, where the patient is too disturbed and likely to be disruptive or where there are too few staff to ensure management of the patient. The conflict here is between her straightforward duty to care for the patient who has been brought to the ward and her duty to provide adequate care for the other patients on the ward (and perhaps to consider her staff and what it may be reasonable or unreasonable to expect of them in such a situation). An alternative way of viewing the problem is to see it as a conflict between the right to treatment of the patient seeking admission and the rights of those in the ward already receiving treatment. Either way there is a dilemma to be faced.

Referring to Case History 7.2, the issues faced by the charge nurse in that situation concerned the relative weight to be given to the rights of the various patients in her care and the conflict between her responsibility to a whole ward of acutely ill patients and her duty to help a particular woman who clearly needs urgent psychiatric attention. At one level, the decision taken by the charge nurse might appear sensible and possibly the only thing to do in the circumstances. She did not perceive it as a moral dilemma in the strict sense, but rather as a moral problem which she solved by giving priority to the demands of justice to her staff and the 10 patients on the ward. The young doctor clearly saw the problem differently and gave greater weight to the needs of the suicidal woman, perhaps because he felt responsible for taking the legal decision to have her admitted on an emergency order and perhaps because he felt he could do something about her problem. The tense and difficult situation gave it the proportions of a 'cri-

case history 7.2

'I've only got one pair of hands'

Recently, when I was doing night duty as charge nurse in the acute admissions ward of the local psychiatric hospital, I was faced with a very painful decision. We were short of staff. This was due to the freeze on vacant posts – seemingly part of the policy of 'cuts' imposed by the local health authority, but also aggravated by an epidemic of flu which had affected several nurses and medical staff. We had been operating for several days below what I would regard as safe staffing levels. The duty doctor was a young trainee psychiatrist with little experience of the application of the Mental Health Act, but we managed because we had most of the patients well under control and had not had a new admission for several days.

On the night in question, one of the patients on the ward, Mrs M, was upset by an accidental injury caused to her by another patient and became very disturbed and violent towards other patients and staff. I called for help from the duty doctor, as I had only one staff nurse and an auxiliary to deal with the demands of 10 disturbed patients. We had difficulty subduing Mrs M and persuading her to take some medication – a powerful tranquilliser – and were trying to calm down the other patients, who had become very agitated, when we were informed that the police were at reception with a woman who was hysterical, who had attempted to slash her wrists and was being abusive and violent towards the police. They were demanding that she be admitted under the relevant section of the Mental Health Act which gives police the authority to detain people who, in their opinion, are mentally disordered.

The young doctor was undecided about whether we could cope with the new admission, but felt we ought to accept the woman because she was in a bad way and needed immediate medical treatment. In the circumstances I felt I had to refuse, as I knew we could not cope and that the care of the other patients might be put at risk. The doctor was angry, although he later admitted that he thought I was right to refuse. The suicidal woman was given the necessary first aid and some medication and taken to the police cells for the night, until other arrangements could be made for her care.

sis' for the overstretched staff, and this atmosphere of crisis was aggravated by the differences between the charge nurse and the doctor. In such circumstances, it becomes difficult to make sensible and responsible moral choices, and the moral issues may in fact be secondary to other agendas between the nursing and medical staff or hospital administration. However, it is important to tease out what moral issues are involved and to develop models for sensible decision-making in such circumstances (see Ch. 9).

Some of the most critical decisions faced by health care staff occur in situations where there are numerous people in need of urgent attention and limited staff and resources to deal with the emergency. Part of the problem may again relate to factors of a non-moral nature, such as the youth and inexperience of the doctor, or the sense of helplessness of the charge nurse faced with staff shortages and an unsympathetic health authority, and the arrival of another patient being 'the last straw'.

The moral questions raised by this case are of various kinds. There are the questions which relate to the rights of the various patients involved, the apparent conflict between the rights of one acutely disturbed patient and the rights of others. Clearly, here, no one patient's rights are paramount. As indicated in Chapter 6, our rights are not absolute or unlimited. Provision of treatment or a bed for one patient, for example, may mean that another patient is deprived or that there are fewer resources to go around for others. Sensible decisions have to be made in the best interests of all. In some cases, this demand of distributive justice may mean that a patient cannot be given treatment at a particular time, because all available resources are committed. Alternatively, in some situations of extreme emergency, where the life of a patient is at risk, less ill patients may have to suffer a degree of neglect for the sake of saving the life of another.

In the one case, the demands of justice for the common good prevail, and in the other, the right of a particular person to treatment. Both cases could be said to arise from competing demands for justice to individuals and a fair outcome for the group. In theory we may derive most personal rights from the principle of respect for persons, but we may not be able to resolve conflicts of rights between different parties without other considerations based on justice and beneficence.

There are also questions raised by this case about the moral and legal entitlement of nurses and doctors to administer compulsory treatment in an emergency without fulfilling the procedural requirements of the relevant Mental Health Act. Forced administration of tranquillisers in order to subdue a violent patient may be necessary even if the patient has not given consent to treatment. (Some of these questions were covered in Ch. 5 when discussing the ambiguous status of the mentally disordered patient. Other questions raised by this type of case relate to the nurse's right to object, on conscientious grounds, to assist in treatments ordered by the doctor – a subject discussed in Ch. 3.)

Another area of concern, on which the health service trade union COHSE and the Royal College of Psychiatrists have pronounced, is the matter of the legal responsibility of staff in dealing with violent patients, both with respect to their own safety and in protecting themselves from subsequent litigation if charges of negligence or physical abuse are brought against staff (COHSE 1977, Royal College of Psychiatrists 1977, UNISON 1997). The issues here relate, on the one hand, to the rights of nurses or doctors – their own entitlement to justice, to fair conditions of service and protection from mischievous prosecution when coping with difficult and dangerous patients – and, on the other hand, to their duty of public accountability in situations where the very legal powers and circumstances of compulsory detention which are necessary to control disturbed and vulnerable patients give rise to fears that 'captive' patients may be abused or maltreated by staff. The provision of legal safeguards for the rights of psychiatric patients, in particular their rights of access to a mental health tribunal/mental welfare commission in the UK, are necessary because of the extraordinary legal powers exercised by health professionals in the case of psychiatric patients. These relate both to their power to deprive them of their liberty and administer compulsory treatment; and to the special vulnerability of patients who are 'incompetent' by virtue of mental disorder.

Finally, there is a whole series of ethical questions to be raised about the marginalisation of psychiatric services and the inadequate resources provided, compared with the acute medical and surgical services, despite the large proportion of patients requiring psychiatric treatment. In spite of official recommendations to the contrary, the low priority accorded to mental health services generally raises questions about the rationality of health service planning and justice in health care. The kind of crisis which makes a charge nurse refuse to admit a patient demands more of the nurse than merely a gesture of non-cooperation. The wider 'political' responsibilities of nurses are painfully illustrated in such situations, and their protests (to the hospital, health authority or even the press) may be the most effective and successful way of drawing attention to the inadequacy of the service for these particularly vulnerable patients, who by and large are unable to defend their own rights to have proper care and treatment.

Persuading patients to 'volunteer' as research subjects

Nursing practice, like medical science, can only advance through properly controlled scientific research. The controls required are both scientific and ethical. Research which is not conducted according to rigorous scientific methods is valueless, and research which is not conducted with proper respect for the rights of patients may become inhuman. The World Medical Association's Declaration of Helsinki (1964, amended 1996) on the ethical and scientific requirements for sound research involving human subjects is of general value in discussing issues related to research in which a nurse may be involved, whether as responsible investigator or merely in an auxiliary role (Appendix 1).

In order to be scientific, nursing research must be based on sound scientific knowledge and proper scientific methods. This means that the research must satisfy several conditions, namely:

- Initial investigations (e.g. by data collection or literature survey) must establish what has already been done in the field, to avoid unnecessary repetition and waste of public resources.
- New research instruments must be properly pre-tested to establish their reliability and validity, or, alternatively, well-tried methods should be used.

- The project must be based on sound research design, approved by one's professional peers and independent assessors, and undertaken by properly qualified research staff.

These requirements are both scientific and ethical. The researcher has an obligation in justice not to engage in research which is valueless and a waste of time and resources. This is not only because most research is funded by public money and involves the use of public resources, but also to protect research subjects from unnecessary investigations of no benefit to them or to anyone else. Here nurses have particular responsibilities to patients in their care, whether they are conducting the research themselves or assisting in someone else's project.

In order to be ethical, nursing research must be based on prior critical consideration of the ethical basis and implications of the research:

- Consideration should be given to whether the proposed research satisfies the demands of beneficence, justice and respect for persons.
- The duty of protective beneficence demands careful prior assessment of the potential risks to patients from participation in the project, and clarification as to what benefits the research may bring directly to research subjects or to the wider community. No research is ethically acceptable when the risks outweigh the benefits. If clinical research involves potential risk to research subjects, then prior laboratory tests and animal experiments are demanded to satisfy the researcher's duty to care for her research subjects, and protection of their rights.
- The principle of justice demands that no research should involve abuse of or discrimination against particular patients, or groups of patients (whether on grounds of race, gender, social class, captive status or the medically 'interesting' nature of the complaint being investigated); and further, that it should potentially benefit the whole population.
- The principle of respect for persons means that for research to be ethical, it must ensure the patient's right to know, right to privacy and right to treatment are respected:
  - Patients should not be involved without a fully informed understanding of the nature of the research, and without their free and voluntary participation in the research. Where the patient is not competent to give consent, special safeguards must be established to protect his rights (e.g. proxy consent or tribunals to monitor research in the patient's interest).
  - The physical privacy and confidentiality of the research subjects must be protected by appropriate procedures and protocols, preferably scrutinised and approved by a competent multidisciplinary ethics of research committee.
  - The patient's right to proper care and treatment should not be compromised or his health put at risk by participation in research (e.g. involving placebo or in randomised control trials).

Clinical research may be therapeutic or non-therapeutic. Therapeutic research is directly related to the patient's complaint and the patient stands to benefit directly from the treatments or procedures used. Non-therapeutic nursing research is where patients participate in general investigations, e.g. research aimed at improving patient care, techniques of management, nurse–patient communication, or general knowledge of the physiology or pathology of particular complaints, where the investigations are of a general nature and neither have a specific therapeutic purpose nor are of any direct benefit to the research subject. In practice, the distinction may not be so clear-cut, for patients may stand to benefit in the long run from even the most academic studies of sociology or psychology, as they may from laboratory studies of the composition of the blood or the biochemistry of the brain. Furthermore, in randomised control trials using placebos, some patients may receive potentially therapeutic drugs or treatment and others no effective treatment at all, and yet no progress can be made without such trials. The claimed effectiveness of drugs cannot be proved by mere accumulation of evidence without testing the 'evidence' in rigorously controlled experiments, in order to exclude other possible explanations of why the health of some patients appears to improve with their use (Buchanan & Brock 1989).

However, in broad principle the distinction between therapeutic and non-therapeutic research is a useful one even if only to emphasise that the ethical safeguards in the latter type have to be more stringent. In general the greater risks taken in clinical research are justified on two grounds: first, that there may be direct benefit for the patient; and secondly, that the research may contribute to the benefit of humanity even if it does not directly benefit the patient. The right of the patients to treatment includes the implicit assumption that they will cooperate in the trial of various procedures but have the right to withdraw if they believe they are suffering harm, or that the responsible researcher will withdraw them from the study if they are at risk of harm.

It has been argued that the right of the patient to benefit from research carries with it a corresponding duty to assist in research which may be of benefit to other patients too. On the other hand, the patient's right to care and treatment cannot rest solely on this premise. Our entitlement to treatment cannot depend on our capacity to barter for it by payment in time served as a research subject. Our entitlement to adequate care and treatment must rest on some more fundamental right – related to our right to life and membership of a moral community, caring not only for the strong, but the weak and vulnerable too. The 'duty' to assist medical research by participation in clinical trials, if it is a moral duty, is so in an extended sense of the word 'duty' and may or may not be recognised as such by the patient. It is not a duty which can be forced on anyone (McCormick 1976, Hellman 1995). The patient has a right to be properly informed and to give his consent without coercion or moral blackmail. He also has a right to be informed of the risks and possible benefits, and to withdraw from any trial or research project without prejudice to his treatment.

The nurse or doctor in charge of patients in research trials has a special responsibility to protect the interests of the individual patients, to act as their advocate, advising them about the conditions of participation and their right to withdraw

from experiments. Because patients in hospital are to some degree captive, it is important to ensure that they feel quite happy about participation in a trial, particularly if it is not one from which they stand to benefit directly or where there is a significant degree of risk or inconvenience involved. Ethics of research committees are increasingly requiring of investigators that independent assessment is made of the quality of consent given by patients, by a competent professional not involved in the research project. However, medical and/or nursing staff involved in the research may also have to persuade patients to cooperate, and here the personal values of clinical practice and the more universal ones justifying research may come into conflict. These may be particularly acute in justifying clinical research involving children, prisoners, mentally disordered or mentally and physically handicapped people. In such cases, legal and institutional safeguards (such as proxy consent) are particularly important, to protect the wider interests of those not competent to give informed and voluntary consent – whether they stand to benefit or will merely be contributing to the welfare of others (Kerridge et al 1998, Ch. 21).

The issue of whether it is ethical to use children as subjects of clinical research has been hotly debated. On the one hand, it has been argued that children cannot be said to give consent that is either informed or voluntary in any proper sense. Children's lack of knowledge and understanding of the implications of medical procedures, and even of the legal significance of consent, may be said to invalidate any attempt to justify their use as research subjects on moral grounds. Children's dependency on adults for protection and advice makes them peculiarly vulnerable to moral pressures, and it is doubtful whether their consent could really be voluntary. This case was classically argued by Ramsey (1976, 1977). On the other hand, it has been counter-argued that this issue cannot be settled by simply appealing to the rights of the individual child – for advances in the treatment of paediatric disorders often cannot be made without research or clinical trials involving children. Against Ramsey, McCormick (1976) argued that the right to benefit from new discoveries in the clinical sciences carries with it the corresponding indirect moral duty to contribute to the advance of clinical research, and this correspondence between rights and duties applies to children as much as to anyone else. This argument was advanced in the Belmont report (DHEW 1978). However, in both sources it is emphasised that the researcher has a fundamental duty to protect the rights of children and incompetent adults, to avoid their being put at risk and to prevent their exploitation. Furthermore, the researcher has an obligation to avoid subjecting human subjects to hazardous procedures where other procedures involving competent adults or animals as subjects would do just as well, or where the risk outweighs the possible benefits.

Those people who are contemplating research involving children (or mentally disordered individuals) sometimes fall back on the proxy consent of the parents or a relative. This can be an attempt to safeguard the interests of vulnerable individuals, but the question can be raised, too, whether the insistence on proxy consent is not more to protect the doctor or institution from legal action. Ramsey (1976, 1977) maintained that it is never permissible to use children as research subjects in non-therapeutic research and that proxy consent does not make it ethical either. McCormick (1974) argued, on the other hand, that since the ultimate justification for clinical research is that it contributes to the common good, and justice requires that we are prepared to accept risks ourselves if we wish to benefit from medical discoveries (in either the short or the long term), then we ought to be able to understand the principle of this exchange if we have the capacity. Even if we did not have the capacity, it can be argued by analogy that we would give our consent if we could understand, and should therefore not be deprived of the right to contribute to the common good merely because we are not competent to give fully informed and voluntary consent. In fact, it can be doubted whether even the consent of normal adult patients can ever be fully informed or completely voluntary, and with children it is just a difference of degree.

This line of argument was used in the past in the United States to justify experiments using institutionalised psychiatric patients, patients with men-

tal handicaps and prisoners (Hornblum 1997). It would seem a dangerous line of argument to pursue, not significantly different from arguments used to justify the infamous Nazi medical 'experiments' with captive patients. There are, of course, particular problems about whether the consent given by captive patients can ever be voluntary in an ethically satisfactory way, and this is where the argument from analogy becomes suspect and tendentious. Research involving children and people of borderline competence is a highly controversial area in the ethics of clinical research, and while, more often than not, doctors have to take the key decisions, nevertheless nurses may have to cope with the enquiries of both children and their parents, and will therefore be required to have a clear view on where they stand on these issues – especially if it is the nurse who is required to seek the 'consent' of the child, psychiatric patient or person with learning difficulties (see Goodare & Smith 1995, Kerridge et al 1998).

In reality, the health professional has to exercise discretion about how much to tell and to judge whether consent is being given under duress. Respect for persons and the duty to care stand in a relationship of tension to one another here. A degree of beneficent paternalism is necessary to interpret the needs of the individual, to judge his competence and to decide what is in his best interests. But paternalism can become officious and arrogantly indifferent to individuals if it is not based on sensitive regard for their condition and respect for their rights as persons.

The establishment of ethics of research committees in the UK and elsewhere (institutional review boards in the United States) has been hailed as a major step forward in the attempt to monitor research involving human subjects. This came about in the first instance as the result of public concern in the late 1960s over the possible abuse of patients as 'human guinea pigs' and, more seriously, the abuse of captive subjects such as prisoners and the mentally ill in research, not only for clinical purposes, but also by pharmaceutical companies for merely commercial ends (Pappworth 1967, DHEW 1978, McNeill 1993). Researchers are required to submit research protocols for scrutiny by these committees, to ensure that they fulfil the requirements of sound scientific and ethical research. In some cases these committees may insist on direct monitoring of the ongoing research or may require periodic reports to ensure that the general guidelines are being adhered to by all concerned. Nurses are increasingly taking a significant part in the work of these multidisciplinary committees. In their role as nurses, they have important professional and moral responsibilities, not just to ensure the proper vetting of nursing research but to provide a considered nursing viewpoint on the implications of the research proposed on patient care and well-being, as well as the implications for staffing and resources. Nurses also arguably have a responsibility to ensure that ethics of research committees actually work and do their business in a conscientious way. Surveys of some such committees suggest that there is a lot of room for improvement (Lock 1990, McNeill et al 1990, 1994, NH&MRC 1995, 1999).

Use of patients as teaching material

Should patients be used as teaching material for the training of doctors and nurses? Should patients with rare or exotic disorders or unusual complications be expected to put up with the additional inconvenience, embarrassment and even discomfort of being examined by students? In a major teaching centre, where the population does not have the opportunity of being treated in non-teaching hospitals, should patients be given the choice of consent or refusal to act as demonstration material for clinical tutorials without suffering prejudice in treatment? And what about the right to privacy of psychiatric patients and the dying, as subjects of research?

Clinical training without the opportunity to work on real patients would be like learning to swim on dry land. Here the justification for compromising the right to privacy of individual patients is that they stand to benefit by having highly trained staff to care for them. Alternatively, the common good of all patients is served by having properly trained staff. However, this does not give medical or nursing instructors an unlimited right to do as they like with patients.

The requirements for the provision of sound clinical training for nurses (like the demands of medical research, health care planning and public health measures) are such that they tend to give greater importance to considerations of the common good than to the specific needs or interests of individual patients. The nurse on the ward and the junior medical resident with a particular interest in and clinical responsibility for the individual patient may feel protective towards 'their' patients and critical of the insensitivity of those passing through on a 'teaching round'. The tension between universal and personal values in health care is well illustrated here. Neither view is exclusively right. Each needs to be tempered by the other. Institutionalised health care imposes some limitations on personal rights, including the right to privacy, but teaching and research institutions and hospitals generally need to be humanised as well (Johnstone 1991).

Justice demands that patients with unusual or 'exotic' disorders should not be unduly exposed to students, with or without their consent. Even unconscious patients deserve to have their privacy respected and dignity protected. Lack of respect tends to breed insensitivity, callousness and lack of consideration in trainees. Some patients, or patient populations, may be at risk of being over-investigated and overscrutinised because they are 'interesting teaching material'. Some reasonable and just limits have to be set to the demands made on such patients. The 'duty' of patients to participate in clinical teaching cannot be an unlimited demand and has to be secondary to their own treatment and general well-being. Apart from the need to preserve the trust and goodwill of patients by not exploiting them or trying their patience beyond endurance, professionals also have a duty to protect the dignity and privacy of those in their care. This is particularly important if the complaint makes them vulnerable (as in cases of mental illness) or liable to embarrassment (as in cases of pregnancy, disfiguring injury and handicap, or venereal disease) (Goodare & Smith 1995).

It may be questioned whether it can be morally justified to place additional stress on anxious and distressed patients (e.g. disturbed psychiatric patients) by exposure to a group of nursing or medical students, even with the patient's 'consent'. The tutor may have to decide against using particular patients, however interesting, because of their vulnerability. On the other hand, it needs to be stressed that the expectations of people with regard to their privacy vary according to their situation. People tend to expect the greatest degree of privacy and strictest confidentiality to be observed when they are visited in their own homes or when they see health professionals in a private consultation. However, when people enter public institutions, they recognise the implicit restrictions on their rights, for in order to benefit from institutional care they may be obliged to surrender some degree of their privacy. In an institutional setting, the health professionals may be more anxious about privacy and confidentiality than are the patients (where, for example, much intimate information about patients may be common knowledge on the ward). Nevertheless, professionals cannot ignore the need of individuals for privacy, and they have a primary moral duty to protect the rights of the patients entrusted to their care.

Because nurses are in the front line in dealing with patients, whether it be in hospital or in a clinic, they have a particular moral responsibility to protect their patients, or to advocate on their behalf, when they believe the treatment of patients may be compromised or they may be put to serious inconvenience, if not risk, by participation in a research study, whether being conducted by a doctor, an outside researcher or another nurse. For example, it may be awkward but necessary for a duty nurse to challenge the research methods of a nursing colleague if that colleague is upsetting patients by her approach.

Allocation of resources

Although the ethical problems related to the allocation of humans and material in health care are discussed more fully in the next chapter, there are some issues which arise here in the context of having to balance the rights of individuals against the interests of third parties. Let us consider a few examples. Should elderly patients be discharged from hospital to make way for more acute cases if there is a doubt that they will be able to cope on their own, even with domiciliary services and support? Should nursing staff be allocated according to need or according to the number of patients? Should more effort be put into nursing those who might show real improvement, or should all patients get equal treatment even if their state is chronic? What role do nurses have in decisions to ration drugs and medical equipment where these are in short supply (Gross 1985, Cummings 1994, Johnstone 1994, Ch. 7)?

In real life, decisions have to be taken and these may be both painful and subsequently found to be mistaken or based on inadequate knowledge. All decisions where the rights of one patient have to be balanced against those of other patients or third parties may involve agonising choices. In formal terms it may be a choice between the demands of personal care for the individual patient and justice for a larger group of patients or society. In practical terms, it may be a matter of responding to external pressures and the internal guilt and anxiety generated by an unresolvable tension between conflicting duties. The extreme case may be a medical emergency such as an air crash or train disaster in which many people are injured or dying and there are limited medical supplies and perhaps only one qualified doctor or nurse available. As in wartime, the responsible health professional may have to adopt a policy of *triage* – dividing the victims into three groups: those who must be left to die because they are beyond help, those who can wait for treatment later, and those who must be attended to first because they need treatment urgently and stand to benefit from it most. (How do we reconcile the conflicting demands of the principles of beneficence, justice and respect for persons here?)

Faced with the problem of having several patients with renal failure who need urgent dialysis but only one dialysis machine, who is to be given priority? Generally, the decision will be the doctor's, but if there are no obvious clinical criteria which would decide the issue in favour of one patient rather than another, other criteria might have to be considered, and nurses might get drawn into discussion of the available options.

Would the decision be made most fairly by drawing lots or by adhering to a first-come-first-served basis? Would attempts to assess the usefulness/value/importance of individuals be reasonable or invidious? Attempts to involve patients in group decisions about the allocation of a dialysis machine would seem to be unfair. In such circumstances, a decision by team consensus or by outside assessors might be justified if there were objective grounds on which the choice might be made. However, the judgements would tend in practice to be based either on the assessment of probabilities on the basis of the personal experience of staff, or on the subjective judgement of professionals. In the case of a real moral dilemma, where there are no practical strategies to avoid the problem of choice, the responsible health professionals have to be prepared to take a decision and to live with the guilt and anxiety which that responsibility entails. (It has been remarked that doctors are paid well 'to pad their shoulders' in carrying the burden of decision-making responsibility. Perhaps the difficulty experienced by the nurse is that, faced with having clinical responsibility for decisions in similar situations, she does not have the necessary padding!)

In making decisions affecting the lives and well-being of individuals in their care, health professionals act as guardians and advocates of the rights of their patients. They have to make decisions based on their knowledge, expertise and available resources. They will have to exercise courageous initiative and be willing to take risks as they try to effect the best compromise between the demands of justice, beneficence and respect for the rights of individual patients.

While fit today, we may be ill or in desperate need of treatment tomorrow. Thus all of us are potential patients (including doctors and nurses), so we all should have an interest in protecting patients' rights. The right to know, the right to privacy and the right to treatment are all better understood by health professionals who have experienced the impotence and vulnerability of patienthood. Health professionals who take their duties seriously will also be willing to act as advocates, defending the rights and dignity of patients. They will also be aware that as public officers they have a responsibility to uphold the common good and to promote the health of the whole community. These competing duties may indeed give rise to painful and difficult choices.

 further reading

Autonomy
Berlin I 1969 Four essays on liberty. Oxford University Press, Oxford – *a classic and accessible analysis of the foundations of the liberal doctrine of autonomy*

Clement G 1996 Care, autonomy and justice: feminism and the ethic of care. Westview Press, Boulder, CO – *a feminist critique of the way 'autonomy' has been interpreted in society*

Lindley R 1986 Autonomy. Macmillan, Basingstoke – *an older but still useful general discussion of autonomy*

Mishra R 1990 The welfare state in capitalist society. Harvester Wheatsheaf, London – *a critical view of the tensions between liberal and social justice models of human services*

Thomson D 1991 Selfish generations? The ageing of New Zealand's welfare state. Bridget Williams Books, Wellington – *a conservative critique of the liberal 'right to autonomy'*

Behaviour modification
Braun J V, Lipson S 1993 Toward a restraint-free environment. Health Professionals' Press, Baltimore, MD – *raises important issues about physical and pharmacological restraint*

Erwin E 1978 Behavior therapy: scientific, philosophical and moral foundations. Cambridge University Press, Cambridge – *advanced philosophical discussion of ethics of behaviour change*

Häring B 1975 Ethics of manipulation: issues in medicine, behaviour control and genetics. Seabury Press, New York – *an early discussion of some of the issues which still has general validity*

Matthies B K, Kreutzer J S, West D D 1997 The behaviour management handbook. Therapy Skill Builders, San Antonio, TX – *a practical but humane discussion of the requirements of practice*

Suicide
Aldridge D 1998 Suicide: the tragedy of hopelessness. Jessica Kingsley, London – *an exploration of the contemporary significance of suicide for modern society*

Bonhoeffer D 1955 *Ethics*. SCM Press, London, ch 3, p 122–128 – *a compassionate Christian view of suicide by a theologian executed by the Nazis*

Chesterton G K 1927 Orthodoxy. John Lane, Bodley Head, England – *a forceful statement of a traditional view critical of 'rational suicide' or its justification*

Durkheim E 1952 Suicide: a study in sociology. Routledge and Kegan Paul, London – *the great classical study of the sociological significance of suicide in the modern world*

Health education and health promotion
Gold R S, Greenberg J S 1992 The health education ethics book. Wm C Brown, Dubuque, IA – *a practical guide to ethical issues in health education*

Hill L, Smith N 1990 Self-care nursing: promotion of health. Appleton-Century-Crofts, Norwalk, CT – *a valuable examination of practical skills required by patients to care for themselves*

Lipson J G, Steiger N J 1996 Self-care nursing in a multi-cultural context. Sage, Thousand Oaks, CA – *a timely examination of some of the practical and moral problems that arise in health-promoting activity in nursing in a multicultural society*

Murray R B, Zilner J P 1989 Nursing concepts for health promotion. Prentice Hall, London – *an illuminating discussion of the potential contribution of nurses in health promotion*

Pender N 1996 Health promotion in nursing practice. Prentice Hall International, London – *an exploration of the scope of the responsibility of nurses for the promotion of health*

Sidell M 1997 Debates and dilemmas in promoting health: a reader. Macmillan (with The Open University), Basingstoke – *an important exploration of the ethical issue in health promotion, of relevance for nurses, particularly those working in the community*

Tones K, Telford S, Keeley-Robinson Y 1994 Health education: efficiency, effectiveness and equity. Chapman & Hall, London – *a critical discussion of the practical and ethical reasons for proper evaluation of health education and health promotion activity*

Violence and nurses
Hamberger L K, Burge S K, Graham A V, Costa A J 1997 Violence issues for health care educators and providers. Haworth Maltreatment and Trauma Press, New York – *the North American experience*

UNISON 1997 Violence at work: a guide to risk prevention for UNISON branches and safety representatives. UNISON, London – *practical advice from UNISON*

Communication
Balzer-Riley J, Smith S 1996 Communication in nursing. Mosby, St Louis, MO – *an overview of research and practice in nurse/patient communication*

Bradley J C, Edinberg M A 1990 Communication in a nursing context, Appleton & Lange, CA – *a broad examination of the issues of nurse/patient and nurse/doctor communication*

Horne E M, Cowan T 1992 Effective communication: some nursing perspectives. Wolfe, London – *a practical guide to communicating more effectively with patients*

Kagan K, Evans J 1995 Professional and inter-personal skills for nurses, Chapman & Hall, London – *another perspective on improving communication and interpersonal skills in nursing*

Nursing research
Burnard P, Morrison P 1994 Nursing research in action: developing basic skills. Macmillan, Basingstoke – *a practical guide to nurses on skills required for good nursing research*

Burns N, Grove S K 1999 Understanding nursing research. WB Saunders, Philadelphia – *explores the specific scope and issues raised by conducting sound ethical nursing research*

Eggland E T, Heineman D S 1994 Nursing documentation: charting, recording and reporting. JB Lippincott, Philadelphia – *a reminder that all nursing research depends on accurate recording of data and skilled application of methods of recording these*

Goldman J 1982 Inconsistency and institutional review boards. Journal of the American Medical Association 248(2): 197–202 – *a timely reminder that without more standardised procedures and protocols decision-making of IRBs can be arbitrarty*

Hellman S 1995 The patient and the public good. Nature Medicine 1(5): 400–402 – *a look at patients as 'research material' and the justification for using them in nursing research*

Johnstone M-J 1991 Ethical issues in nursing research: a broad overview. Faculty of Nursing, RMIT, Bundoora, Victoria – *a helpful overview of ethics in nursing research by an experienced nurse*

McNeill P M 1993 The ethics and politics of human experimentation. Cambridge University Press, Cambridge – *encourages one to look at 'research' in the wider context of social trends*

Royal College of Nursing 1977 Ethics related to research in nursing. Royal College of Nursing, London – *practical ethical guidance and discussion of ethics in nursing research*

Nursing dependent elderly people
Benson S, Carr P 1994 The care assistant's guide to working with elderly mentally infirm people. Hawker, London – *a very practical and helpful resource for both nurses and care assistants*

Copp L A 1981 Care of the ageing. Churchill Livingstone, Edinburgh – *an earlier but still illuminating text on care of the ageing*

Couglan P B 1993 Facing Altzheimer's: family care givers speak. Ballantine, New York – *an important reminder of the care needs, and rights of the carers of dependent relatives at home*

McClymont A, Thomas S E, Denham M J 1991 Health visiting and elderly people. Churchill Livingstone, Edinburgh – *an examination of practical ethical issues arising in the care of elderly people*

Rathbone-McCuan E, Fabian D R 1992 Self-neglecting elders: a clinical dilemma. Auburn House, New York – *raises some of the practical and ethical dilemmas of intervention with elderly people*

Tice C J, Perkins K 1996 Mental health issues and ageing: building on the strengths of older persons. Brookes/Cole, Pacific Grove, CA – *a reminder of the importance of ongoing support for skills training in work with older people*

Informed consent
Buchanan A E, Brock D W 1989 Deciding for others: the ethics of surrogate decision-making. Cambridge University Press, Cambridge – *a careful examination of the vexed issue of proxy consent for minors*

Faden R R, Beauchamp T L 1981 A history and theory of informed consent. Oxford University Press, New York – *a useful overview of the debate about the ethics of informed consent*

Kerridge I, Lowe M, McPhee J 1998 Ethics and law for the health professions. Social Science Press, Katoomba, NSW – *an important up-to-date account of the legal and ethical aspects of informed consent, criteria for assessing competence, and decision-making for incompetent people.*

end notes

1 Here, as elsewhere, we should take special note of the phenomenon of 'language shift' for, as Wittgenstein pointed out in his *Philosophical Investigations*, 1958 (Blackwells, Oxford), shifts in terminology often signal changes of paradigms and theoretical perspectives, and embody important value changes as well.

2 Taylor (1992) presents a most helpful survey of trends in the discussion of self-hood and autonomy.

3 Jean-Paul Sartre gave popular expression to this idea in his play *No Exit* (1956), and in his essay *Existentialism as a Humanism* (1948), but his detailed analysis of the phenomenology of the self and selfhood is to be found in his *Being and Nothingness*, 1957 (Methuen, London).

4 Carroll L 1954 *Alice's Adventures in Wonderland, Through the Looking Glass and Other Writings*. Collins, London, ch 6, Humpty Dumpty, p. 209.

5 Chesterton G K 1927 *Orthodoxy*. John Lane, Bodley Head, ch 5, 'The flag of the world'.

6 Research by the Department of Geriatric Medicine at the University of Edinburgh does not support the common view that demented people living at home constitute a serious fire risk to themselves and others. On the contrary, available evidence from the Chief Fire Officer for Lothian and Borders points to most domestic fires being associated with alcohol abuse; and, over a period of 10 years up to 1982, not a single fire in the region occurred in houses or flats occupied by patients known to the psychiatric services as demented.

some suggestions on method

Personal freedom and moral autonomy

In exploring the relationship between personal freedom and moral autonomy, like the issue of individual liberty and individual rights, students need to understand the relevance of these concepts to their own lives before applying them to patients. One might begin by getting students to share in confidential pairs the nature of a conflict with their parents or authority, where they felt obliged to take a stand on a matter of principle important to them. Next they might be encouraged either to role-play the admission of a patient for elective cosmetic surgery or to observe the conflict for patients between required submission to the routine and discipline of the hospital, and ability to assert their own rights.

Individual rights and the common good

If it is possible to arrange for students to observe a meeting of a hospital management team, local health authority or local health consumer council, then they could be given the task of giving a careful report of proceedings in which they discuss the way in which the rights of individuals (or groups with 'special' needs) are reconciled with the public duty to use resources equitably for the common good.

Exercising power over patients for their good

Before discussing nurses' relations with patients, it may be as well to explore in small groups how nurses themselves feel when subject to pressure to give up smoking, to diet or to change their lifestyles for the sake of their health. The groups can then be asked to develop a rationale for proactive intervention in other people's lives 'for their good'.

The conflicts which arise for nurses in balancing their duty of care for patients with respect for their rights can be explored initially by discussing Case History 7.1 (p. 162) or by getting students to prepare their own case studies on the moral conflicts involved in initiating deliberate strategies to modify patient behaviour, or demanding compliance with compulsory immunisation or health screening, or 'counselling' patients to change their diet, lifestyle or to give up smoking.

Balancing the rights of different patients

While student nurses may not have experience in making management decisions or exercising responsibility in making investigations or doing research on patients, it is important that they consider the ethical issues involved in practice. Case History 7.2 (p. 171) might well be used as the basis for a group discussion to identify and discuss the issues involved for the patient, other patients and the staff.

To make the remaining issues 'real' for students, they could be asked to either role-play or write about the issues involved, from the patient's standpoint, in being asked to participate in some form of medical or nursing research which may not benefit them directly, or in being 'asked' to allow medical students or nursing students to practise history-taking or physical examination on them. The issues involved where there is competition for scarce resources might be explored from the personal angle considering access to physiotherapy for backache.

Ethics in nursing administration

SECTION CONTENTS

8

Nurses and society: responsibility for managing resources

AIMS

This chapter has the following aims:
1. To assist nurses to grasp the fact that ethics is relevant at the personal, team, institutional and state levels of practice
2. To examine the tensions between various types of professional values in the work of nurses, and the way these impact on ethical decision-making in nursing
3. To identify five different theoretical approaches which influence planning and resource allocation decisions in health
4. To use epidemiological and other research data to illustrate the importance of evidence-based decision-making in nursing.

LEARNING OUTCOMES

When you have read and worked through this chapter, you should be able to:
■ Give an account of the scope of political ethics in nursing and health care and the various levels at which this applies

■ Apply the conceptual distinctions between competing values in the work environment of nurses so as to identify areas of conflict and possible consensus

■ Demonstrate understanding and ability to apply the different frameworks to the analysis of issues of resource allocation

■ Demonstrate knowledge of major trends in morbidity and mortality in your region and the relevance of this to planning nursing services and training

■ Source local and global demographic and health data relevant to nursing practice.

THE POLITICAL ETHICS OF CARING FOR PATIENTS

The two previous chapters attempted to clarify some of the moral issues that arise in direct nurse–patient encounters, either in one-to-one relationships or in nursing groups of patients. However, this was done without examining the broader and more impersonal issues faced by the nurse involved in management, administrative and public responsibility. Attention was confined to moral difficulties in interpersonal relationships between nurses and their patients in order to bring out the nature of patients' rights and the professional duties of nurses, and to clarify the difference between institutional, legal and moral rights, within the contractual relationship between them. In so doing we have skirted around the larger issues of social justice in health care, but could not avoid mentioning them altogether. This is because the interpersonal moral questions in nursing arise within a broader social and political context. The answers to questions about patients' rights and the duties of nurses depend on broader principles and beliefs about the role of nurses in society and in Britain the nature of the National Health Service (NHS).

Chapter 4 began with the assertion that ethics is concerned in a fundamental way with power and power-sharing. This connection between ethics and power relationships was affirmed in order to challenge a popular view of professional ethics that can be expressed as a series of interconnected beliefs as follows: that ethics is just about caring for people; that caring is about feelings; that feelings are personal and subjective; and, therefore, that ethics is a matter of personal and subjective judgement.

Of course, caring is of fundamental importance in human relationships. No one could deny this. However, caring can be patronising, it can be sentimental, and it can be selective. For care without proper recognition of the individual's objective needs and of the duty to preserve the patient's independence can be intrusive and unwanted, or dependency-inducing. People who need help want competent help to deal with their problems, and efficient delivery and management of the services provided. They are not necessarily looking for 'a meaningful relationship'.

In any case, caring cannot be simply a matter of feeling or sentiment if it is to be an adequate basis for nursing, or nursing ethics in particular. The concept of 'care' in Judaeo-Christian thought has more practical origins. *Caritas* in the Latin tradition, or *agape* in Greek, is not primarily concerned with how you *feel* about someone, but rather how you *deal* with someone. Caring for people means that you act for their good – help restore their autonomy, assist them to achieve their full potential, attain their goals in life and reach personal fulfilment. In theological language, the ultimate goal of *caritas* or *agape* is the salvation of the other person, and the word 'salvation' means 'to be made whole'. In that sense, the goal of caring is always to help others to achieve their optimum fulfilment as human beings. For the person who has been injured (and are we not all injured in one way or another?), the need is for healing, to be made whole. For the person who is sick, the need is to be restored to health. Patients need to be 'put back on their feet', to recover their independence (if possible), to feel that they are in control of their lives again – a point stressed as a primary objective of nursing in the Royal College's first code of ethics discussion document (RCN 1977a).

Obviously, we are all vulnerable, and we may even be afflicted by the same problems as the patients we care for. This is not necessarily a bad thing. In fact, the experience of suffering may not only make us more sympathetic (from Greek *sum* = with; and *patheo* = to suffer) but it may also help us to empathise with our patients, i.e. to view the world as they see it, from the inside. While sympathy is a spontaneous feeling we either have or do not have for people, empathy, the ability to put ourselves 'in someone else's shoes', is an art that can be learned, an exercise of imagination that can be practised. Furthermore, we need to develop insight into the desires and feelings which attract us into nursing and other caring professions in the first place. While these feelings (and needs) may be powerful motivators, they can also get in the way of doing our professional duty. This is because we may be determined more by our own unconscious agendas, our own need for help, our own fear of illness or death, than by motivation to do a skilled and professional job (Feifel et al 1967, Feifel 1977). Studies of the helping personality show that personal experiences in childhood, or suffering and bereavement in adolescence, may be powerful motivators in the type of person attracted to 'caring' for other people. If we choose nursing to fulfil a personal need, or just as an unconscious form of autotherapy, to deal with our own problems or anxieties, then patients will suffer as we work out on them our own agendas, or 'act out' our own 'scripts' (Eadie 1975, Smithson et al 1983, Mackay 1989, Lawler 1991, Green & Green 1992, Laschinger & Goldenberg 1993, Branmer 1993) (see Box 8.1).

'Caring' can be damaging to others if we do not understand its true dynamics, i.e. the complex psychological forces which come into operation when we are in the powerful position of 'helpers', relative to weak and dependent 'patients' or 'clients'. This is why psychiatrists in training and psychiatric nurses are encouraged to undergo personal psychoanalysis or to participate in group therapy, as this process obliges carers to explore their deeper feelings and often hidden ulterior motives. While the care and attention of a good nurse can do one a power of good, overprotective, intrusive or overbearing and infantilising care, like the corresponding forms of bad parenting, can be very destructive too. It is well said that our greatest virtues are also the potential sources of our greatest weaknesses and vices. Just as paternal strength and authority can be used in a protectively beneficent way, it can and has been used to justify all types of subtle oppression of women and children – as feminist critics of patriarchal systems have shown. Feminist writers such as Sara Ruddick (1989) celebrate the maternal virtues such as women's often heroic protection of vulnerable life, feeding, care and nurturing of their dependants and training them for acceptance by the wider society. However, these virtues can all find perverse expression in overprotective attitudes that are dependency-creating, and induce fearful conformism to group norms. In a nursing context this can mean turning people into perpetual patients, in need of ongoing professional support, less able to cope on their own, passively conforming with ward routines and uncritically accepting of what may be bad practice. Here, too, some conservative nursing attitudes and practices can bring them into direct conflict with health professionals concerned with assertive action to achieve rehabilitation of patients, with physiotherapists and occupational therapists. Conflict here is not just due to interprofessional rivalry or blurred boundaries of work responsibility, but also to differences in work

---

Box 8.1 The wounded surgeon and the dying nurse. (Extract from *The Four Quartets* by T. S. Eliot)

The wounded surgeon plies the steel
That questions the distempered part;
Beneath the bleeding hands we feel
The sharp compassion of the healer's art
Resolving the enigma of the fever chart.

Our only health is our disease
If we obey the dying nurse
Whose constant care is not to please
But to remind of our, and Adam's curse
And that, to be restored, our sickness must grow worse.

The whole world is our hospital
Endowed by the ruined millionaire,
Wherein, if we do well, we shall
Die of the absolute paternal care
That will not leave us, but prevents us everywhere.

practices and interpretations of 'care' (Creek 1997, Ch. 20).

From a more prosaic point of view, nurses are also employed to get certain work done as efficiently and effectively as possible. As a result, considerable limitations and practical constraints may be placed on the time available for 'caring relationships' and attention to the needs of particular patients. This means that, in practice, 'care' has to be more impersonal and altruistic. Furthermore, as Campbell (1985) points out in *Paid to Care*, the care provided by nurses and other caring professions is not based entirely on disinterested altruism. Nurses enter nursing to care for people, but they also nurse to earn a living. Like any other employees, they will have concerns about their own pay, shifts and working conditions, as well as being concerned about the well-being of their patients. As we shall see in the following chapter, many of the issues raised about the nurse's 'right to strike' revolve around the ambiguities that arise because the nurse is supposed to be, first and foremost, a carer bound by the duties of caring, and perhaps only secondarily a paid health service employee. In Chapter 2, we discussed some of the differences between lay care and the professionalisation of caring services. 'Care' takes on new meaning and subtly different nuances in the context of paid-for services – whether paid for directly by the patient or indirectly through state-provided health care services. Peta Bowden (1997, Ch. 3), as we have already pointed out in Chapter 5, explores both the value and limitations of 'caring' as a model for the interpretation of professional nursing practice.

Preceding chapters have explored the moral implications of the complex dynamics of nurse–patient relationships and the responsibilities within such caring relationships. If we remember that the term 'dynamics' means power (from Greek *dynamis* = power), then we may understand that in such expressions as 'interpersonal dynamics', 'group dynamics' and 'psychodynamics', we are actually dealing with different kinds of power relationships and forms of power-sharing. *The ethics of such relationships is intimately tied up with the power issues – of domination and control, or facilitation and empowerment, of helping or enabling, of the exercise of authority and compliance or submission.*

The experience of nurses in dealing with the reality of power/dependency relations in working with both patients and doctors means that they recognise that ethics has to do with power and power-sharing in direct interpersonal relationships. However, the challenge is to understand the nature of power relations and the ethics of power-sharing, in teaching, in management, in research and health education, in lobbying for resources, and in the politics of health locally and nationally. Nurses need not only to learn to *care for their patients,* but also to *care about the well-being of patients generally.* This means caring about the standard and management of services, competence of staff, effectiveness and efficiency of procedures used, improvement of hospitals and the health service, and public health. If 'caring' about health care is understood from this wider perspective, nurses quickly discover that nursing ethics and nursing politics are continuous with one another, that caring and sharing, respect for persons and justice, values and power relationships are all interconnected, and impose wider 'political' responsibilities on them. Ultimately, the struggles for better and more equitable conditions for patients, and better and more equitable conditions for nurses and other health care employees, are inseparable.

The virtues of altruistic care for others, of selfless devotion to duty and of self-sacrificing service tend to have been given priority in the formation of nurses. Thus there may appear to be a conflict for them between the demands of a caring altruism and the demands of getting involved in the more impersonal tasks of management or trade union activity, or in becoming directly involved in local or national politics. However, it is not impossible to combine the personal qualities of sensitivity and caring with competence and efficiency in management, or empathy for others with toughness in staff or union negotiations. Here the personal circumstances of nurses, as a predominantly female profession, often means that for many nurses their work has to be combined with the demands of running a home and often raising a family, or caring for elderly relatives. These practical and economic constraints, as they affect women in particular, as well as society's expectations about women's roles, may inhibit the participation of female nurses in the politics of the profession or the wider politics of health care. While men represent only a small proportion of all nurses, they are disproportionately represented in nursing management and political leadership in nursing unions and public sector administration of health care and nursing (WHO 1999a).

The historical reluctance of some nurses 'to get involved in politics' – evidenced by the past opposition of the RCN to support industrial action by nurses – is reflected in the ambivalent attitudes of members of many other 'caring professions' as well. There may be many reasons for this, but one on which sociologists are generally agreed is that the emphasis on an individualistic ethics of caring reflects a tendency within the wider *embourgeoisement* of society. As people aspire to become members of the 'professional middle classes', they tend to adopt *bourgeois* (middle class) values. In contrast to the emphasis on social solidarity in the working class struggle for social justice and civil rights, the new *bourgeoisie* tend to be more concerned about their individual rights, professional autonomy, status and earning capacity. Going with middle class aspirations and its emphasis on personal fulfilment and autonomy, there is also a tendency, already remarked upon, to 'privatise' or 'psychologise' ethics, and treat it as confined to the private sphere, leading to a divorce between ethics and politics, ethics and science, and ethics and business. This not only has unfortunate consequences for our understanding of ethics at the level of our personal rights and responsibilities, but it also creates the impression that being concerned with economics or politics is somehow socially inferior or morally questionable – described as 'money grubbing', or meddling in 'dirty politics'.

In the remainder of this chapter we will consider a number of issues which bear on the *political ethics of health care*, and the *political responsibilities of the nurse*. The political ethics of health care is the area where the personal values of caring come into abrasive contact with the realities of power and economic rationalism. The areas to be considered are as follows: power relations within the nursing hierarchy; conflict and cooperation between nurses and other professionals; competition between different departments for limited staff or resources; and employer/employee relations in the struggle to achieve better pay and working conditions. We must also examine the moral issues related to the vested commercial and political interests which determine the proportion of national resources allocated by governments to health services, compared with, say, social services, education, or defence.[1]

Nurse tutors do their students a disservice if they do not address these real-life issues in nursing. If the only values examined or professed are those based on a personalist ethic of caring, then the nurses produced will be ill-prepared to deal with the harsh economic and political realities of nursing. It will be a training for frustration without the basic knowledge or skills to cope with the problems of 'caring' effectively for patients in difficult times of budget cuts, 'down-sizing' and 'contracting out' of services. Ethics in our terms means, among other things, that nurses themselves must have enough influence to command respect in the corridors of power when it comes to decision-making about resources and health policy, and being financially accountable (Caplan & Callahan 1981).

DIFFERENT CONTEMPORARY MODELS FOR PROFESSIONAL ETHICS

There is a difficulty in reconciling a personalist ethic of caring with the type of ethics required for management of complex modern health delivery systems. This arises because of tensions between different kinds of competing ethics in professional life – differences between 'the caring ethic', 'the service ethic', 'the public office ethic' and 'the business ethic'. Some of the relationships between the competing ethics of different professional groups are illustrated in Box 8.2.

Recently, governments have imposed the financial disciplines of economic rationalism on hospitals and health care systems. A real tension has emerged between the service ethic and/or the caring ethic of the traditional caring professions,

---

Box 8.2   Competing 'ethics' in working and professional life[2]

Caring ethic – individualistic helping role
Primacy given to values of caring for others:
● the role of advocacy
● protecting the rights of the weak.
(*Personalist ethic – one-to-one relationships – protective beneficence*)

Service ethic – private fiduciary relationship
Primacy given to contractual relationship in service:
● recognition of reciprocal rights and duties
● based on private accountability/confidentiality.
(*Privatised two-party ethics – respect for persons/justice*)

Public office ethic – universalistic and cooperative
Primacy given to service of the common good:
● recognition of reciprocal rights and duties
● acceptance of public accountability.
(*Community participation and welfare focus – justice and equity*)

Business ethic – self-assertive and competitive
Primacy given to liberty to pursue personal well-being, fulfilment and commercial gain:
● assertion of personal right to equal opportunities
● assertion of right to the fruits of personal success, wealth and power
● exercise of personal autonomy as a primary value.
(*Empowers the powerful, is tough on the weak – personal rights and autonomy*)

---

and the business ethic of the new-style business management and contract culture of the purchaser–provider internal market. Nurses, doctors and other health professionals who have been attracted to working in the health service may well find the new 'values' antithetical to their own primary professional values (Robertson et al 1992).

However, it is not so much that those who endorse a service or caring ethic are moral and the 'hard-nosed' business managers are not. It is rather the case that these different ethics are constructed (as all are) on the principles of beneficence, justice and respect for persons, with a quite different priority given in each case to different principles within this trinity. Instead of maintaining a balance between them, one kind of principle tends to be given exaggerated importance or priority over others. An exaggerated emphasis in the past on the doctor's duty of care to his patients

and his right to professional autonomy has led to pressure for recognition of patients' (or consumers') rights and for greater professional and financial accountability of doctors. An exaggerated emphasis in the ethic of public office on the duties of public servants to protect the common good leads to conflict with those operating services on a caring or service ethic. This is because the bureaucratic demands for efficiency and cost-effectiveness are seen to compromise 'patient care' by emphasising more abstract 'common goods' rather than ability to respond to the needs of the patient. Nurses and other health professionals often face a conflict within themselves between the different sets of values that go with the changes of role and responsibility involved in moving from the more personal 'hands-on' clinical work to the more impersonal roles of management, administration and policy-making. Unlike medicine, promotion upwards into the ranks of nursing management often involves loss of ongoing clinical involvement with patients and a distancing effect from the 'bed face'.

The rhetoric of neoconservative politics suggests an antithesis between 'the bleeding hearts' and 'the economically hard-nosed', between an 'ethic of caring' and 'business ethics', but these are false antitheses. They are like the spurious contrast drawn between a 'Christian' ethic based on caring and selfless service of others and a 'secular' ethic based on seeking one's own fulfilment, developing one's potential, and striving for prosperity, success and power. In reality, our Western heritage has always tried to synthesise both these two approaches to human fulfilment – as in the WHO definition of health that includes the physical and mental, personal and economic well-being or 'salvation' of people (from the Latin *salus*, whole). A caring ethic based on love alone is naive, unless it gives serious attention to the dynamics of social, political and economic power or has the necessary structures or checks and balances of justice built into the system. Likewise, the business ethic, with its faith in the inevitable benefits of free-market capitalism and its ability to achieve success and prosperity for all, is naive about human nature and the regulatory effect of the market to deal with the realities of power and vested interests. What is required is a robust understanding of the necessary interdependence of love, power and justice in the structures and actual dynamics of human life and society (Tillich 1954).

Thomas Aquinas suggested that the first demand of charity (care) must be justice, otherwise it degenerates into sentimentality, but also that the object or goal of care or charity is not the common good, but the highest good for the other. He emphasised that it is rather meaningless, and perhaps dangerous, to speak of care for others or to speak of one's personal rights as primary, unless a proper balance of power and the basic structures of justice are in place in a relationship or in society (Gilby 1964).[3]

Traditionally, the caring and consulting professions have been characterised by a self-professed altruism – 'selfless service on behalf of others'. A leading member of the legal profession has described his profession, without apparent irony, as 'one of the caring professions'! Those who aspire to the status of professionals have to persuade the public that they are a responsible and trustworthy body of people. This is why one of the first steps in seeking recognition and formal statutory registration as a profession is often to formulate a code of ethics (Freidson 1970a, 1994). The difficulty with this stand is that it seems to be incompatible with the values on which other industrial and public utility workers base their claims to take strike action in pursuance of just settlements of their grievances. The demands for some degree of professional autonomy, respect for nursing knowledge and expertise, recognised status and appropriate financial reward depend upon nurses fulfilling the other criteria which the public expects of caring professionals. These are objectivity, non-discrimination in the treatment of clients, altruism and dedication to duty, and commitment to care (often over and beyond the call of duty). These values are often incompatible, and are seen to be so, with strategies of industrial action. In a sense, nurses may have to choose between being regarded as professionals (and enjoying the ambiguous privileges of that status) and accepting the status of health workers along with the rest and being subject to the same kinds of employment legislation and negotiating rights, including the right to strike, as other workers and public servants.

The problem facing both doctors and nurses in a nationalised health service is that it is difficult for them to act as autonomous or self-employed professionals might. The position adopted by the RCN on strike action by nurses (RCN 1977a, UKCC 1992) to some extent turns on the status of nurses, i.e. whether they are 'health workers' or 'health professionals'. Nearly 40 years after the founding of the UK NHS, the Black report (DHSS 1980) showed that the greater equality in the distribution of health care, which the nationalised system of health care in the UK was supposed to deliver, had to some extent been achieved. Health professionals sacrificing some of their economic privileges and autonomy helped to bring this about. This was supposed to correct a situation where doctors and other specialists might profit from the nation's ill health. Today, moves to reintroduce private medicine in health services around the world are, it is claimed, designed to allow a greater degree of choice to the public; however, it is probably more accurate to say that policies of privatisation have been driven by the demand to reduce public expenditure. The rhetoric of the political argument for increased privatisation gives the right to choose and individual autonomy higher priority (for those who can afford it) than considerations of equality of opportunity in access to health care or equality of outcome for all groups in society. Part of the argument is based on the need to cut the escalating cost of health services, and the need to make health services more cost-effective and profitable, where possible, in order to be able to divert more of our limited resources into direct patient care. Whether the profit motive and the provision of good health services and social services for all citizens are compatible is a matter of the greatest moment in the current debate about the ethics and politics of health care.

However, there is considerable confusion in the international political debate about the right of nurses or other essential health workers to go on strike, and whether in a nationalised system of health care (e.g. the UK) or a profit-making private sector, the problems are essentially the same.

These 'industrial relations problems' require urgent attention, and in particular there is a need for better negotiation and conciliation machinery to deal with the pay and working conditions of health workers in many countries. Nurses in a number of countries where there have been moves towards greater privatisation and commercialisation of health care are already expressing concern. There has been an increased trend to employ unqualified or underqualified staff in responsible positions, to save costs, and the pay and working conditions of nurses have not improved. In many cases, workloads and stress have increased to intolerable levels in pursuit of 'greater productivity'. Changes will only be brought about once again by pressure from the nursing unions. The unionisation of nursing labour has many advantages and has achieved many improvements in general health care and in protecting the rights and promoting the entitlements of nurses. It gives considerable power to nurses, but it is a power which has to be seen to be used responsibly, within the limits of professional morality, if nurses are to command the respect of society and society's attention to the justice of their cause. However, 'justice' is not some perfect or ideal state, but will, in practice, inevitably be whatever can be negotiated in the social context and what is politically and economically possible. These issues are discussed in more detail in Chapter 9.

SOME PROBLEMS OF RESOURCE ALLOCATION IN HEALTH CARE

Headlines such as that quoted in the caption of Box 8.3 highlight the problems facing health care staff in dealing with the ethics of resource allocation. Similarly, emotive reports have dramatically highlighted the life-saving character of heart transplant surgery, in spite of high costs and poor survival rates with these still experimental procedures. Dr Peter Draper, from the Unit for the Study of Health Policy, Guy's Hospital, London, argued forcefully some 20 years ago that the money spent on heart transplant surgery would be better spent on health education. This was because most of the heart conditions being treated by transplant surgery were preventable, and there was disturbing evidence that unless the lifestyles of recipients of heart transplants were changed (e.g. smoking), their problems would simply recur (Draper & Popay 1980, Davey & Popay 1992).

Consider two other kinds of problem: first, the justifiability of assisting couples otherwise unable to have children to have a child by in vitro fertilisation (IVF); and second, the justifiability of life-saving surgery and long-term intensive care for seriously defective newborns.

In Australia, where IVF-assisted reproduction was pioneered and much research has been done by medical entrepreneurs, there are women's support and pressure groups (often set up by IVF doctors) who claim that IVF is every woman's right. One, in particular, has even claimed that all women have the 'right' to 'compassionate IVF surrogacy' (Yovich & Grudzinskas 1990). On the other hand, an eminent Australian woman child health research specialist has argued that the cost of such assisted reproduction is not justified in the face of other maternal and child health priorities, such as the evidence of birth complications among IVF babies (notably prematurity, low birthweight and a high incidence of birth-related cerebral palsy) (Stanley 1992).[4] Feminist social scientists

---

Box 8.3 'Costs "killing" kidney children: lack of money and donors deny the young vital treatment.' (Extract from *The Guardian*, 15 January 1982)

'Funds for kidney units are running seriously short. About half the 2200 people whose kidneys fail, die because there are no facilities to save them,' Professor Cyril Chantler of Guy's Hospital said yesterday. 'Most are over 45, but only 61 children under 15 were treated in 1980, while an estimated 90 suffered fatal kidney failure.'

'If there was enough money to treat every kidney failure, we would be treating 1000 more patients a year and would save hundreds of lives. It costs £10 000 a year to keep someone on a kidney machine. A transplant costs £5000 a year for five years. So prevention not only saves lives, it makes economic sense,' said Professor Chantler. 'Britain is sixteenth in the European league for kidney treatment. The Swiss do more, and both Spain and Cyprus treat more patients per head of population.'

have also argued that the commercialisation of assisted reproduction, including IVF, intracyto-plasmic sperm injection (ICSI) and surrogacy arrangements, is degrading and risky to the health of women. Their ethical objections are of two kinds: the first is that male chauvinist culture has made reproduction an imperative of sexual 'partnership' and women who may well have had children in earlier partnerships cooperate with IVF (often to 'treat' male infertility) and are turned, in the process, into 'baby machines', at the service of men's need to prove their virility; the second is that the process tends to treat children simply as a means to an end, to satisfy parental reproductive ambitions, regardless of the risks to mother and/or child (Grayson 1993).[5]

On the other hand, the dilemmas about commencing and terminating assisted life support to defective newborns raise some of the most difficult medical decisions for obstetricians and very painful problems for nurses involved in their ongoing care. The painful nature of the clinical moral dilemmas was perhaps most graphically illustrated in the historic case of Dr Arthur. He was committed for trial, and convicted, on a charge of infanticide, because he took action to terminate the life of a child on life support whom he believed had a very poor prognosis. However, in the Dr Arthur case, the problem was not discussed from the point of view of dilemmas of resource allocation, but rather on the definition of 'treatment' required by continuing care for the child. In this chapter we are concerned not with clinical dilemmas or moral problems, but ones which are more specifically about the management of resources. The Dr Arthur case could be discussed from that perspective, but in fact the case was decided and appealed on other grounds. (Brahams & Brahams 1983).

The pros and cons of decisions about IVF or life support for defective newborns can be debated at two different levels – the clinical level and the policy level. At the clinical level, specific decisions have to be made about particular patients. Here nurses may not have much power to influence medical decision-making, but they more than likely have to deal with the disappointment of the infertile couple or grief of the parents with a defect-ive child, and have to cope with their own feelings about the child's death. At the policy level, however, where the practice of IVF and intensive care for defective newborns raises important questions about the responsible allocation of scarce resources, nurses have both a right and a duty to contribute their knowledge and expertise to public debate on matters of such general public interest. The making of public health policy cannot be the exclusive preserve of doctors or bureaucrats, politicians or any particular class of 'experts'. Nurses have the same right to participate in public debate about the ethical implications of these procedures as any other citizens, but they also have a duty to do so, in view of their own frontline experience and professional expertise. In fact, the objectivity of the judgement of doctors in these matters may be questioned because they often have a vested interest in defending the prestige and budgets of their units and their related research programmes. Nurses, both as citizens and as professionals with an inside knowledge of the working of health services and of the practicalities and costs of day-to-day health care, have a particular responsibility to speak out on issues of resource allocation.

The issues of resource allocation in health care do not refer solely to the expenditure of money on life-saving medical or surgical procedures and high-technology equipment such as whole-body scanners or kidney dialysis machines. They also refer to expenditure on staff salaries, to the cost of building and equipping new hospitals or rebuilding and refurbishing old hospitals, to the cost of medical research, to expenditure on drugs and disposable medical supplies and expenditure on such homely things as furniture, fittings, decor and the quality of hospital food. They also relate to the debate about the use of public and teaching hospital resources for private medicine and private patients, and the tendency of private hospitals to concentrate on those areas of health care where bed turnover and profits are highest. Moral arguments in these areas cannot be based simply on ideological dogma or unquestioned moral assumptions, but require practical wisdom and political judgement as to how best to balance emphasis on different values and to reconcile competing interests. Here again, the use of practical methods for analysing the value conflicts involved may be helpful in bringing to light the complexities involved, clarifying the choices to be made and helping to develop a consensus (cf. stakeholder analysis model, p. 278).

Responsible decisions, especially by nurses involved as managers and administrators, cannot be simple matters of right or wrong, black or white, but require the ability to make sound value judgements based on proper assessment of the facts. Those making decisions must be properly informed, and the decisions grounded in research into the clinical and epidemiological facts and in sound financial accounting. To put the 'expense' of controversial new medical procedures or life-saving medical intervention into perspective, it is necessary for nurses in general, and nurse managers in particular, to be well informed about the actual costs of these procedures relative to the priority needs of their own region, as well as nationally and internationally. Below, some of the salient facts for health services in Scotland and the UK are outlined, as perhaps being typical of trends in developed countries, in order to illustrate some of the other areas of potential conflict in decision-making with regard to resources in health services (see p. 195).

When Professor Chantler complains of the risks to children of inadequate resources for the treatment of victims of kidney disease (see Box 8.3), we see the tension illustrated in his emotive appeal for more resources for life-saving transplant surgery and dialysis machines, while he also admits the need for expenditure on prevention. In a sense he wants to have it both ways. He wants unlimited resources to back up his strong sense of the duty to care for those whose lives are at risk, and further resources (if available) for prevention (in justice to the whole population who might become at risk but of whom those affected are only a tiny proportion). Dr Draper's case is based on epidemiological arguments, concerning changes in the pattern of mortality and morbidity in society. Here the control of infectious diseases and effective medical treatment of many life-threatening conditions have left the vast majority of people affected by disorders which are the result of their lifestyle.

These include respiratory disorders and lung cancer caused by smoking, diseases of the circulatory system caused by poor diet, lack of exercise, smoking and alcohol abuse, etc. The argument, based on considerations of justice and the common good, suggests that priority in the allocation of resources should be given to health education and prevention. The policy dilemma of how to deal with coronary heart disease and kidney disease could be resolved on the basis that since most cases of both diseases are preventable, priority should therefore be given to allocating resources to prevention rather than treatment. However, this still leaves the problem of adequate resources for the treatment of patients with renal failure and heart disease unanswered.

Similar difficult decisions have to be faced in dealing with fetal abnormalities. It is possible by antenatal diagnosis to determine that a fetus is defective, but what kind of 'therapeutic' choice is abortion as an alternative to bearing a child with Down's syndrome or spina bifida? There are, nevertheless, still many cases where antenatal tests have not been done or the test refused. Here, faced with the delivery of a spina bifida baby, even one with only a limited hope of survival, nursing staff have to take a position on whether to give the child the necessary care and treatment, or cooperate in withholding treatment. What does the nurse make of the specific demands and rights of the child to treatment, owed a duty of care by the doctor and nursing staff, as compared with the abstract considerations of justice in the management of resources and the common good?

The 'right' of infertile couples to medical assistance to conceive a child would seem to many people to be a fundamental entitlement. However, a helpless defective newborn baby may be denied life-saving treatment because it is thought to be unjust to burden a family or to make great demands on social resources. In contrast to the infant who is unable to defend its rights, forcefully articulate and determined couples may be able to exert great pressure on health services to meet their demands for IVF and assisted reproduction services.

In both cases, difficult decisions may have to be made by health service managers and policy makers, relating to setting limits to what it is reasonable and just for the public to demand from the health services, in view of other demands on time, manpower and financial resources. The objective assessments of the malformed baby's prospects for survival and quality of life have to be balanced against what burden of responsibility it is reasonable and practicable to expect the medical and nursing staff, the child's parents and society to carry. Justice demands that these other interests should be considered in deciding whether expensive life-saving measures should be taken.

In the case of the childless couple, there may well have to be limits set concerning what it is fair to expect public health services to provide. Given the low level of risk involved in remaining childless, it might be argued that, in spite of the emotional cost to the young couple and the 'risk' to their marriage, their 'right' to have a child should not be given priority over other more pressing needs of patients with life-threatening conditions or premature babies requiring life support.

Treatment for infertility may even be regarded as a luxury when the aim is to limit fertility in the interests of population control and the conservation of diminishing global resources; in developing countries, the attempt to set up such services would hardly even be considered. It could also be argued that since the knowledge and technology exist to assist many childless couples to have children (whether by IVF or other means such as surrogate parenthood), in a prosperous society such as that in the UK, this help should be available through the NHS. Alternatively, it could be claimed that people should be able to get the help privately if they can afford it or can raise the money from charity. Even then, would it be reasonable to expect medical and nursing staff to give up time and resources to meet these further demands, which they may not consider to be as important as dealing with life-threatening disease and injury?

Critical to this debate is the following question – who decides what qualifies as a condition 'requiring medical treatment'? For example, who decides that heroic efforts should be made to save the lives of infants with congenital defects or to treat a middle-aged couple requesting IVF? Is this a case where 'money talks' – i.e. those who have the financial resources to pay may claim the 'right' to 'treatment' and those who do not have the resources cannot? This clearly raises the following questions: what is meant by the 'right to health care'; what is the scope of this so-called natural right; and who decides whether or not you can exercise this right? These critical ethical questions will clearly be viewed differently in countries with problems of massive overpopulation and very limited health resources, compared with those with negative population growth, declining fertility and generous state funding for health.

Current speculation about the possibilities opened up by genetic engineering and the cloning of the sheep 'Dolly' at Roslin in Scotland raise questions about the scope and limits of our entitlements to demand assistance from medical science and health services. Cloning may make possible human tissue regeneration and the development of organs for transplantation, but should one have the right to invest in a spare heart or kidney just in case one needs it 'further down the track'? Should anyone be entitled to request that a clone (or multiple copies) of himself be made? The Human Genome Project has set out to map all human genetic types on the planet. This may mean that in the future parents will be able not only to choose the sex of their child but also to order 'off the shelf' (or by mail order!) a child with particular attributes, e.g. beauty, intelligence and scientific ability, rather than plainness, athletic ability and sociability. Discussion of these examples illustrates how, in the interests of the survival of the species and of moral communities in which we tolerate diversity, it may be necessary to strike a different balance between the demands of justice, respect for persons and beneficence.

FRAMEWORKS FOR POLICY-MAKING ON MANAGEMENT OF RESOURCES

The Edinburgh Medical Group Working Party on the Ethics of Resource Allocation (Boyd 1979) put forward five kinds of models or frameworks from which decision-making in health care has tended to proceed. These were identified as the clinical, epidemiological, ecological, administrative and egalitarian approaches. These remain useful ways of conceptualising approaches both to determining priorities and policy planning, and to the actual decision-making about the allocation of scarce health resources. However, the recent introduction of the new economic model of the 'internal market' suggests another framework, namely the business management model. In what follows, we have grouped the ecological and egalitarian models together and introduced the commercial business management model as a fifth. In discussing the nurse as an agent of health and social policy, it will be useful to bear these categories in mind. Nurses have a duty to contribute in a responsible way to public debate on the question of how the health service is to be funded. This includes the issue of private medicine, either within or as an alternative to the NHS, and the relative priority to be given to health education, high-technology medicine, advanced research in exotic areas of medicine, and the need for better primary medical care and community services (cf. Campbell 1978).

Clinical approach (e.g. Murley 1995)

In the previous section, it was argued that because doctors and nurses are trained to care for people in crisis, and not as administrators, they tend to understand their responsibilities mainly in terms of the rights of individuals and their duty of protective beneficence to 'their' patients. They are less concerned with justice to all patients, equitable outcomes for vulnerable or dependency groups and ensuring adequate access to health care for the whole society. The clinical approach tends to give priority to the special knowledge and expertise of health professionals and their presumed right to special authority in decision-making about matters related to health care. The limitations of such an approach are that it tends to be individualistic in dealing with problems which may have complex social origins and consequences; it tends to be crisis-oriented and focused on the short term rather

than on long-term strategic planning. It tends to emphasise the importance of curative and interventionist medicine and rigorous clinical research rather than health promotion, prevention and rehabilitation. Further, it tends to be clinically and morally authoritarian, underplaying the expertise of other professionals and presuming that health professionals and clinicians have special moral insight denied to others (McKeown 1976).

Epidemiological approach (e.g. WHO 1999a)

The epidemiological approach emphasises the need for objective health data on which to base consideration of health priorities. What is required is the scientific study and statistical analysis of the changing patterns of mortality and morbidity in society, including demonstrable trends in the occurrence and recurrence of epidemics and the relative incidence and prevalence of different types of medical disorder. Typically the epidemiological approach is that favoured by community medicine specialists, for planning public health measures and policy directions involves more than individual clinical judgement and requires more objective and universal indicators of both morbidity and health on which to base health care systems for the common good. The main ethical focus of the epidemiological approach is on rational social justice in health care, rather than on individual rights or protective beneficence – for its object is to achieve equality of opportunity in access to services and equitable outcomes for different groups within the population. The public health movement of the mid-19th and early 20th centuries, with the support of the World Health Organization after World War II, campaigned to improve the health of the community of nations and to coordinate international efforts to eliminate the worst killer diseases. *The Ottawa Charter* (WHO 1986) set out to achieve the following objectives together, by a process of enabling, mediation and advocacy with other countries:[6]

● to reorient public health services to better meet actual local needs

- to create supportive environments in which healthy communities can flourish
- to strengthen local community action for health promotion
- to develop the personal skills of people to manage their own health.

The latest initiative by the World Health Organization, namely its proposed programme for *Health for All in the 21st Century* (WHO 1999b), purports to provide a framework and epidemiological data useful to member states in developing domestic health planning and cooperation with neighbouring countries.

The strength of the epidemiological approach is that it aims to achieve objective and universally valid criteria for planning health services and resource allocation. The limitation of the approach is that it tends to be too abstract and impersonal, too far removed from the emotive reality of individual suffering and the demands of individuals to have their rights respected. In pursuit of rational criteria for decision-making, it underestimates the power of medical vested interests and their ability to mobilise media interest in 'miraculous' cures to influence public opinion in their favour, while successes in prevention are largely 'invisible' because well people are not noticed. It also tends to be too far removed from such social realities as poverty, deprivation and ignorance which provide the background to ill-health in contemporary society. It also tends to underestimate the countervailing irrational forces which strengthen patterns of unhealthy living, including stress, anxiety, economic insecurity and the influence of advertisements.

Egalitarian and ecological approach
(Illsley & Svensson 1984, UNO 1993, World Bank 1993)

The egalitarian approach can be identified with the kind of concern for social justice in health care and the rights of all citizens to adequate and appropriate health services which motivated the setting up of the UK NHS and of modern welfare states. In line with the sociopolitical concerns with justice and equity in the egalitarian approach, the focus is not merely on the physical or psychological needs or health of people, but especially on the connection between their health and the socioeconomic and environmental conditions in which they live. For example, Beveridge (1942) saw the welfare state as a means of organising society to combat the 'five giants: want, disease, ignorance, squalor, and idleness'. This approach was classically illustrated in the Black report, *Inequalities in Health* (DHSS 1980). Its two main findings were, first, that nationalisation of the health service in the UK had brought great benefits to British society in the dramatic improvement of the average level of health of the population and in the more equal distribution of health care and resources; and, secondly, that the gap in health status had widened at the extremes between rich and poor in terms of a whole range of health indicators, from infant mortality to causes of mortality that are lifestyle-related. The apparent contradiction between these two theses was explained by the fact that the bulk of the population had moved into social classes III or IV and fewer people were now in social class V than was the case in 1947. The general tenor of the report was that the NHS had been a good thing, but that it needed to be improved and greater resources put into areas of social deprivation if real reductions in the disparities in health between social classes I and V were to be achieved.

In 1984, the World Health Organization commissioned a survey entitled *The Health Burden of Social Inequalities* (Illsley & Svensson 1984). In 1993, two important surveys of world health, economic and social trends were launched at the Second World Conference on Medical Education in Edinburgh, namely:

- The World Bank's *Investing in Health – 1993 World Development Report*
- The United Nations Development Programme *Human Development Report 1993*.

Following in this tradition, Richard Wilkinson's (1996) study, *Unhealthy Societies: the Affliction of Inequalities*, provides an international survey of trends, but challenges the assumption that there is an inevitable connection between health inequalities. His argument is that if you consider the most dramatic contrasts in terms of inequalities in health, e.g. the United States, Hong Kong and eastern European countries, there is no simple correlation between high mortality rates. In Hong Kong in the decade before 1996, there was a marked decline in infant mortality rates, as compared with the United States where levels remained static. In eastern Europe there was a marked increase in infant mortality and suicides among men in heavy industry associated with rapid social and economic change. He puts this down to the presence or absence of hope. In Hong Kong, people saw that there were opportunities and hope and were motivated to value their health, whereas in the other countries this was not the case for the poor and marginalised.

The strength of the egalitarian approach is that it encourages us to look at health within a total social, economic and political context. However, it can become so broad and unfocused in its attempt to address all the problems of society that it loses its cutting edge to deal surgically and effectively with trauma, physical and mental illness and the more specific problems of health service provision.

Administrative approach (e.g. DHSS 1983, Harrison et al 1990)

The administrative approach could be described as being based on the traditional model of the welfare state where health care and welfare are provided by a largely state-controlled and funded service industry, which has to be managed by rational and accountable processes in the public interest. Those employed in the state public sector are charged with the responsibility to provide cost-efficient health services to the community on behalf of the state and are accountable to the public only indirectly through government ministers. Health service planners and managers have an implied social contract with the patient public or 'consumers' of health services, to provide the whole range of medical treatment, rehabilitation and preventive services in return for the payment of tax and/or health insurance. The ethic of public sector administration is one of public service for the common good. While ostensibly governed by

consideration of universal fairness and respect for the rights of patients as consumers, the lack of direct accountability to consumers or the public means that the pattern of management and planning tends to be paternalistic and non-consultative – despite the establishment of bodies such as health councils or consumer rights groups to represent the concerns, complaints and needs of consumers 'to the authorities'. The administrative model gives particular emphasis to organisational and scientific rationality and to the contractual rights of patients and the duties of health professionals to maintain standards and quality assurance, based on models of public accountability.

The strength of this approach is that it encourages centralisation of management, rational planning, data collection and record-keeping to ensure public and financial accountability to parliament or local health authorities through health service bureaucracy. Supported by the medical model of applied scientific method, management is set up to monitor services using largely medical indicators of mortality and morbidity as measures of progress. The effectiveness of medical procedures will, according to this model, be based on proper scientific tests, randomised trials and controlled experimentation. While this model has worked fairly well for hospital medicine and the treatment of disease, it is not adaptable enough for the demands of primary care and health promotion services. While it has provided for systematic collection of statistics to aid strategic planning, rational target-setting, management by objective, sound evaluation and transparent administration, it has been largely insensitive to the desires and needs of consumers, and tends to become overly bureaucratic and impersonal.

Commercial business management approach (e.g. Enthoven 1986, Saltman & von Otter 1995)

The introduction to the UK NHS of the new model of the 'internal market' has also created a new framework within which health service planning, decision-making and delivery are conducted. The two features of this new economy that are relevant to resource management and resource allocation are business paradigms for the 'purchaser/provider' relationship and 'customer focus'. The assumptions of this approach are that in the deregulated market for health service provision, there are 'providers' and 'purchasers' of services.[7] While health authorities or hospital trusts may be providers (possibly in competition with commercial competitors tendering for business), the purchasers are not individual patients, but may be other hospitals, health authorities or general practitioners on behalf of their patients. Individual clients can negotiate their treatment requirements with their doctor or other health professionals, who either provide the service directly or act as brokers in obtaining services from other providers on behalf of their patients. There is a further assumption that health service provision will be determined not on the basis of *a priori* medical assumptions or vested interests, but by market forces and the laws of supply and demand.

The scope of services offered will theoretically be determined by their economic viability on the principle of 'user pays' wherever possible, and in the competition for 'customers' the best units will survive and the worst will 'go to the wall'. The tests of efficiency, from the health authority or state government point-of-view, will be the relative costs and benefits of alternative procedures. These are likely to be measured, like levels of productivity in manufacturing industry, by predetermined 'performance indicators', e.g. numbers of operations or treatment procedures given and bed turnover or discharge rates.

In many respects this approach is a refreshing change from the beneficent paternalism of the clinical model and the directive paternalism of the epidemiological model. It emphasises the autonomy of the patient and the objectivity of her rights, but tends to ignore the fact that the provision of medical and nursing care is not just a commercial transaction like that in any other service industry. The relationship between the contracting parties is inherently unequal and asymmetrical in power terms. The vulnerability and dependence of the patient demand a quality of trustworthy responsibility on the part of the health professional which is unique, because people's lives and health are at stake. Furthermore, the nature of the relationship between 'purchaser' and 'provider' institutions are not like those between manufacturers and suppliers, and there are emerging concerns that 'cosy deals' are being done between institutions to avoid the inconvenience of having to go through tendering processes.

Nurses following a narrow clinical model may favour private medicine because the quality of care for the few patients in such units may appear to be much better than in the NHS. But nurses cannot, as responsible health professionals, be solely concerned about 'their' patients and their income. They must surely, in justice and respect for the rights of all patients, be concerned about the ones who cannot afford private medicine and suffer discrimination because the better off can afford to jump the queue. However, if they sincerely believe that the interests of justice and respect for the rights of all patients are better served by private medicine then they have an obligation to produce the evidence and reasons in support of this view.

How individual countries and health districts cooperate with the World Health Organization in implementing the global and regional strategic objectives of *Health for All in the 21st Century* (WHO 1999b) will be a matter of intense debate, political disagreement, weighing up of alternatives and disputes about competing values. This WHO publication, together with health policies developed locally, sets new ethical and political challenges for nurses, as it does for other health professionals. In discussing each of the questions posed – regarding funding of the NHS, preventive or curative medicine, the relative importance of advanced technology, acute medicine and advanced medical research versus the provision of better primary and community care – perhaps none of the four models taken by itself is adequate. Discussed against the background of three complementary moral principles, each model has to be qualified. This is the very stuff of ethical and political debate.

Politics, as Aristotle observed, is the art of the possible; or, as he suggested in another context, it is the attempt to find the best means to achieve good ends in the light of both practical constraints and our principles and practical experience. The pleasure of politics lies in the challenge to human creativity of finding new and better solutions to old problems. However, the burden of politics is that of knowing that no solution will be ideal and that our principles may have to be compromised to some degree because of the unpredictability and often tragic nature of reality and the intractability of human nature.

In the next section we examine five kinds of issues to illustrate how ethical and political considerations come into management decisions and policy-making at a number of levels:

● Global and local population trends and their ethico-political implications
● Health for all in the 21st century – priorities for health, globally, nationally and locally
● Changing perceptions of the HIV/AIDS pandemic in different regions of the world
● Costs of health services – can they be controlled?
● The impact on microeconomic health issues of macroeconomic and demographic trends.

VITAL STATISTICS: THEIR ETHICAL AND POLITICAL IMPLICATIONS

In exploring some 'political' responsibilities of nurses, it may be helpful to examine some salient economic, demographic and epidemiological facts and to consider the ethical implications of these for nursing services generally and for individual nurses in particular. We might start by

comparing global population trends from the World Bank (1993) report *Investing in Health* (Table 8.1) with local trends in Scotland and the UK (OPCS 1991, HMSO 1992a,b, ISD 1997) (see Table 8.2).

While the rate of increase of the world population may seem (and is) alarming, it is encouraging to note that (for a variety of reasons) this rate is slowing down, even in low-income countries. We cannot be certain why this is happening. Better education and improved social and economic conditions seem to contribute at least as much to people controlling their fertility as any medical or public health measures. However, better understanding of reproduction and sexual health (where nurses and other health workers have made a major contribution), as well as the wider commercial availability of contraceptives and state-provided family planning services, have contributed together to more effective population control.

On the surface, the local figures for Scotland and the UK in Table 8.2 might not appear very interesting, but a closer look will reveal all sorts of hidden implications for future services and training, and these in turn raise interesting moral dilemmas for health service staff and planners.

The overall population of Scotland, which had been steadily declining over the period 1975–1990, has begun to increase in line with the overall trend in the UK. However, there is still a decline in the proportion of the population under the age of 5 years in Scotland, while it is increasing in England and Wales. There is a more dramatic associated decline in the proportion of

Table 8.1 Summary of population trends from the World Bank (1993) report *Investing in Health* (Table A.1, p. 199, simplified)

Country group	Population in millions (including projections from 1993 to 2030)						
	1965	1973	1980	1990	1991	2000	2030
Low-income economies	1776	2169	2507	3066	3127	3686	5459
Average % annual growth	2.5	2.1	2.1	2.0	1.8	1.3	1.3
Middle-income economies	826	997	1155	1379	1401	1608	2273
Average % annual growth	2.3	2.2	2.2	1.8	1.5	1.2	1.2
High-income economies	671	725	766	817	822	864	920
Average % annual growth	1.0	0.8	0.8	0.6	0.6	0.2	0.2
World totals	3281	3895	4428	5262	5351	6157	8664
Average % annual growth	2.2	1.8	1.8	1.7	1.6	1.2	1.2

Table 8.2   Selected vital statistics for Scotland and the United Kingdom 1975–1990. (Extracted from ISD 1997, OPCS 1991, HMSO 1992a,b)

Details	Scotland				United Kingdom			
	1975	1985	1990	1996	1975	1985	1990	1996
Total population	5.2 M	5.102 M	5.1 M	5.128 M	56.2 M	56.6 M	57.4 M	
Males	2.5 M	2.475 M	2.467 M	2.486 M	27.4 M	27.6 M	27.9 M	
Females	2.7 M	2.625 M	2.636 M	2.642	28.9 M	29.0 M	29.3 M	
Under 5 years	7.2%	6.3%	6.3%	6.1%	6.6%	6.5%	6.7%	
0–15 years	26.3%	21.1%	18.75%	12.6%	24.9%	20.8%	19.0%	
16–64 years	60.5%	64.6%	66.33%	66%	61.1%	64.1%	65.3%	
65–74 years	8.7%	8.4%	8.5%	8.7%	9.0%	8.7%	8.7%	
75 years and over	4.6%	6.4%	6.43%	6.5%	5.0%	6.4%	6.93%	
Live births per 1000	13.1	13.0	12.9	11.6	12.4	13.3	13.9	
Fertility rate	1.9	1.7	1.8	1.67	1.8	1.8	1.84	
Deaths per 1000 males	12.8	12.6	12.01	12.0	12.2	12.0	11.2	
Deaths per 1000 females	11.5	12.4	12.11	11.7	11.3	11.7	11.1	
Percentages of all deaths								
Heart disease	33.7%	34.4%	31.8%	29.9%	33.7%	33.0%	46.1%	
Cancers of all kinds	20.9%	22.9%	24.6%	25%	2.1%	23.8%	25.4%	
Motor vehicle accidents	1.3%	1.0%	0.89%	0.6%	1.0%	0.8%	0.88%	
Legal abortions (UK residents, 1000s)	8.381	9.917	10.976	12.307	115.700	150.200	188.300	
Life expectancy at birth (years)								
Males	67.8	70.0	70.7	72.1	69.9	71.8	72.4	(74.1)
Females	74.3	75.8	76.6	77.6	76.0	77.7	78.0	(79.4)

the population under 15 years of age, and while the proportion of people of working age (16 – 64) is increasing, that is projected to decline as the present diminished number of teenagers enter the workforce. The most significant trend is the continuing increase in the proportion of people over retirement age. While death rates have declined slowly, what is significant is that while coronary heart disease has begun to decline, there has been a steady increase in deaths from cancers of all kinds. Although not shown here, there has been a reduction by nearly 3000 in deaths from strokes in Scotland (from 15.7% of all deaths in 1975 to 11.7% in 1996). However, in the same period there has been a steady increase in deaths from respiratory disease, from 6215 in 1975 to 7859 in 1996, or from 9.8 to 12.9% of all deaths. There has been an encouraging but slow decline in deaths from motor accidents, but a steady increase in the number of abortions (rising in Scotland by 12% between 1990 and 1996).

These illustrative statistics taken from official Scottish morbidity records are not meant to give a comprehensive picture of the country's health, but have been selected for their direct implications for planning future nursing services and priorities in patient education and health promotion. The areas where nurses will be in demand will increasingly be in the care of people hospitalised with chronic mental or physical conditions, or dependent elderly people, rather than in the more 'glamorous' areas of maternal and child care, intensive care, and accident and emergency medicine. The significance of changing patterns of morbidity for nurses is both direct and indirect. It is indirect in that planning health services for the future to meet these changes in demographic and health trends will impact on how, when and where nurses are employed. There will also be a direct impact on both nurses in hospitals and (especially) those nursing in the community (health visitors, midwives, mental and occupational health nurses). The changes will impact not only on the focus of their training and work, but also on the different kinds of ethical challenges involved in moving from a largely reactive role, caring for those who present with known morbidity, to being proactive in searching out undisclosed pathology, in screening, prevention and patient education.

The growing proportion of people in the UK aged 75 years and over – the people who suffer the multiple pathologies of old age and who make heavy demands on the health and social services – will demand (and is demanding) a reorientation of approach to the delivery of care. The facts are that, in the industrialised countries, the largest proportion of hospital beds is occupied by patients over the age of 65 years, there is an alarming increase in the number of elderly people needing psychiatric care, and a general increase in the proportion of the elderly in the community. Because infant mortality rates were dramatically reduced in the 20th century and relatively few deaths occur in middle age, today, for the first time in history, most dying is done by the elderly, and in particular by the very old. This trend towards a greater proportion of elderly people in the population is not peculiar to the high-income developed economies, but in terms of sheer numbers is even more dramatically evident in the developing world. Because average life expectancy at birth has been so low, with high population growth in developing countries, even marginal improvements in health are resulting in a massive increase of elderly people. This increase is putting great pressure on health and welfare services budgets of most countries. While we will discuss some of the ethical issues related to resource allocation that arise because of the global HIV/AIDS pandemic, ironically it is the general improvement of health and increased life expectancy that is creating the major headaches and ethical dilemmas for planners at present and into the foreseeable future. Under the joint auspices of the United Nations and the World Health Organization, 1999 was declared 'international year of older persons'. Throughout 1999, major national and international initiatives were launched to research the needs of the ageing population. The object of this research was to improve their quality of life and to take advantage of the potential of retired people to continue to contribute to society and not merely to be seen as a burden on services and national health and welfare budgets. This campaign is, of course, part of an ongoing concern with healthy ageing and the 'health of the elderly' campaign launched in 1990 with the slogan 'Add years to life and life to years!'. It is instructive to visit the WHO website (http://www.who.org/ageing/global_movement/global.htm) to study developments.

As an example, consider the impact of these trends on issues of chronic care and terminal care of aged people, and the disturbing growth of public interest in euthanasia. Because general life expectancy has increased, with an average life expectancy in the UK approaching 75 years, this means that when older people die, their children are likely to be 50–60 years old (or older). These relatives consequently have a diminished capacity to care for their dependent elderly relatives at home, and elderly people are increasingly likely to die in hospital. As more dying is done by the elderly, death and dying become increasingly institutionalised and death becomes increasingly unfamiliar (does not occur in the home or family context). People are older and less able to cope with heavy nursing, and less well prepared for it because of a lack of direct experience of death earlier in life.

Further, these trends impact on nursing. It may be an exaggeration to say that nurses and social workers enter their professions to work with children and end up working with elderly people. However, studies of student attitudes and the general bias of training confirm this, as well as the continuing high status accorded to high-technology and intensive care nursing of all kinds, above psychiatric and chronic care nursing (except for a growing interest in terminal care nursing).

The trend towards separating hospitals and hospices, acute treatment and 'hotel' services for chronically dependent patients, will increasingly affect the pattern of nurse selection, training and employment. This includes an increasing trend, on the one hand, to employ more nurse aids (or nursing auxiliaries) and, on the other, for nurses to become more technically and medically specialised so as to be better able to compete for employment in a contracting labour market. These trends are not only of economic and social importance to nurses, but raise fundamental questions about the nature and *raison d'être* of nursing itself.

Ultimately these are questions about the values for which nursing stands as a profession. They are ethical questions too in so far as decisions have to be made about priorities in education and training, in service delivery and in the relative weight given to working proactively with people who are well, but who may be at risk, as compared with concentrating on nursing the sick.

The altered scene has already been recognised and reflected in health services planning in many countries (as reflected in WHO reports and recommendations). Project 2000 was intended to address some of these challenges for nurses and has to some degree changed the emphasis in training, but a great deal more needs to be done. Here the World Bank report interestingly presents a picture of what concerns should influence health services planning and staff training for the 21st century (World Bank 1993, p. 134):

World-wide, the number of hospital beds rose between 1960 and 1980 from 5 million to almost 17 million, which more than doubled the per capita supply. The number of physicians increased more than fivefold between 1955 and 1990, from 1.2 million to 6.2 million. Such investments have created new opportunities, but they have also led to problems. Once built, hospitals are extremely difficult to close. Once trained, physicians create pressure to be employed. In virtually every developing country, facilities, equipment, human resources, and drugs are skewed towards the top of the health system pyramid [see Fig. 8.1]. Yet the most cost-effective public health and clinical interventions (as shown in this Report) are best delivered at the level of the district hospital or below.

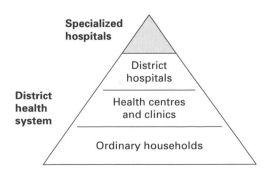

Fig. 8.1   The health system pyramid: where care should be provided.

To the high-income economies, the initial attractiveness of this model, of shifting the burden of care from the state-funded and private hospitals to the local community and family households, was that it appeared to support policies directed to the reduction of state public expenditure. However, in the UK, the Conservative Government's attempt to implement community care policies in the health and social services was not very successful because the cost of making it work properly proved to increase and not reduce public expenditure. The lack of adequate funding for primary care has resulted in many cases in the deterioration of services, particularly for those with chronic health care needs. However, it is true not only in the more technologically advanced countries, but also in developing countries, that governments have been slow to shift resources from hospital-based medicine to primary care. It is not as politically attractive to governments to devolve control and shift resources from the centres of political and medical power to the community, or to invest sufficient funding in skills training to empower families to care for their sick more effectively at home. The achievements of successful primary care and prevention initiatives are less politically 'marketable' and present less 'photo opportunities' than being associated with 'big projects' such as the building of more 'hi-tech disease palaces'.[8]

These mortality and morbidity figures are some of the important facts that need to be taken into account in making well-informed and responsible moral and political policy decisions in the health care arena. However, these are not the only facts that need to be considered. Ethnic minorities and indigenous peoples may suffer specific kinds of social and economic deprivation which impact on their health status. Properly funded and well-conducted research into the social and economic needs of special populations of 'dependency groups' may not be politically popular (nor popular with clinically minded doctors). Nevertheless, these things should be of concern to community nurses, in particular, and they have a professional duty to ensure that policy-makers face their ethical and political responsibility for these issues at local, national and international levels. Here, well-designed and executed local research and familiarity with local area health statistics and trends are moral duties of any responsible nurse, especially those involved in management and policy-making.

HEALTH FOR ALL IN THE 21ST CENTURY AND PRIORITIES FOR HEALTH

The historic 1978 World Health Assembly which met at Alma Ata in Russia reflected on global health needs and epidemiological trends (i.e. changes in the patterns of morbidity and mortality). In response to these needs and trends, the Assembly formulated the *Health for All by the Year 2000* (HFA2000) policy declaration. The World Health Organization then charged its six global regions and all member states of the United Nations to develop relevant local strategies to achieve HFA2000 policy objectives.

Reorienting health services

The key strategy document for Europe, *Primary Health Care in Europe* (WHO 1979), signalled the need for a major shift in resources from high-technology, hospital-based medicine to primary care, and from treatment services to a greater emphasis on health education and health promotion. Health departments of member states were charged with the responsibility to research local needs and to set local priorities and targets for HFA2000. In Scotland, for example, the Scottish Health Services Planning Council, set up under a Labour Government, developed policy and strategic plans to implement HFA2000 objectives. Their first report, *Scottish Health Authorities' Priorities for the Eighties* (known as SHAPE; SHHD 1980), charged Scottish health boards with the responsibility to implement changes and reallocate resources in the light of these policies. Scottish health boards were also required to monitor their success in implementing these policies and strategic objectives, and were obliged to report annually on the results to the SHHD. The Conservative Government which came to power in 1980 was generally hostile to epidemiologically based health planning and placed the emphasis on busi-

ness efficiency and effectiveness, with the introduction of the 'internal market' to regulate the demand and supply of health services in accordance with 'consumer choice and interests'. Despite opposition, the Scottish Health Services Planning Council, before being replaced, collated findings and published the SHARPEN report (SHHD 1990) in which it reviewed health priorities for the 1980s and made recommendations for the 1990s. Paradoxically, under the new Labour Government, the planning approach has been reinstated, along with broad measures to ensure quality improvement and scientific monitoring of health trends. The pro-European Labour Government is cooperating more directly with both the European office of WHO and the WHO headquarters in Geneva to implement the new strategic objectives set out in WHOs (1999b) *Health for All in the 21st Century*.

Changes in patterns of morbidity and mortality will obviously vary from one country to another, even from one region to another, and from urban to rural areas. Thus responsibility for sensible allocation of staff and resources comes right down to the local level. This is why, in discussing the ethical responsibilities of nurses in research, management, public health, patient education and health promotion, the statistical facts of both epidemiology and financial accounting are important in decision-making. In a general textbook like this, we can only examine general information and discuss illustrative examples. Nurses will, however, need to familiarise themselves with the relevant data for their own regions and situations. The World Bank's *Investing in Health – 1993 World Development Report* and the United Nations Organisation Development Programme *Human Development Report 1993* are both very useful resources here.

These reports give detailed facts and statistics on health and economic indicators for all the member states of the United Nations Organisation, and also in-depth analyses of their implications for health services planning for the future. These two non-health-related UN agencies, by amassing the remarkable volume of evidence produced in these reports, have demonstrated for the first time the inescapable connection between poverty and the prevalence of most disease, and the positive correlation between improved health status and economic development. Nurses, as a profession, play a frontline role in most countries not only in nursing the sick but also in disease prevention, public health, health education and positive health promotion. To inform their thinking about policy for the development of services, and in making well-founded administrative decisions about the rational allocation of health and nursing resources in their spheres of influence, they would do well to familiarise themselves with these volumes and the data they contain.

Lifestyles and health

What has become apparent since World War II is that many of today's killer diseases are not the infectious diseases of the past, but are those such as heart disease, many respiratory diseases, and new forms of cancer that are related to people's habits and lifestyles and to environmental factors. While the current AIDS epidemic has raised the spectre of past pandemics, the very nature of the disease and the circumstances of its transmission (mainly by sexual intercourse and intravenous drug abuse) indicate that its prevention is also crucially related to changing people's lifestyles. Nurses trained in general nursing increasingly have to take on new roles as health educators, both in hospital and in the community, to deal with these changes. They are also acquiring more responsibility in helping to decide health policy and in shaping strategic plans for the allocation of staff and resources to deal with future developments. Therefore, the political economy of health can no longer be a matter of indifference to nurses, as it may have been in the past when they thought of it as someone else's problem.

When inappropriate diet, alcohol abuse, smoking and lack of exercise are implicated as major causes of coronary heart disease and other diseases of the circulatory system, the pressure exerted on governments by the multinational food and agriculture industries cannot be ignored by health professionals. Nor can nurses distance themselves from the debate about funding policy in relation to health services, and the role of the private sector in the provision of health services. The very debate about resources for the UK NHS, for example, is a debate about values, not just monetary values, but personal and political priorities. For example, the tenor of conservative political propaganda in the UK for the past decade has been that the cost of the NHS has become more than the nation can afford. The new Labour government has come into power with a promise to increase funding to the NHS, but on what terms? What is the truth about the nation's health, and what bases of comparison should be used when determining the principles on which to base the allocation of economic resources?

For example, in 1990–91, £28.2 billion was spent on the NHS in the UK.[9] That may seem a staggering sum, but that covers the lot – hospital and primary care services, dental, ophthalmic and pharmaceutical services, training and research, and a lot more besides. By comparison, in 1990, UK consumers spent £20.7 billion on clothes and footwear, £19.5 billion on motor cars, and, what is perhaps more significant, £21.7 billion on alcohol and £8.8 billion on tobacco. As a nation we spent more on alcohol and tobacco combined than on the entire cost of the NHS! Similarly, the amount spent by the UK government on social security to assist dependent families and the unemployed, may seem enormous (viz. £55.8 billion), but the amount spent on new company cars as a fringe benefit for senior managers amounted to about a third of that amount.

Now, undoubtedly the government benefits from the excise on alcohol and tax on tobacco (to the tune of £8.1 billion in 1993), which can help to fund some of the services that help to repair the damage they cause. However, the treatment of alcohol abuse and alcohol-related illness alone is calculated to cost the taxpayer about £2.2 billion per year. The combined number of deaths in the UK from heart disease, lung cancer and diseases of the respiratory system (largely attributable to smoking and alcohol abuse) amounts to 406 093, representing some two-thirds of all deaths in 1993.

The good news is that, for England and Wales, Scotland and Northern Ireland, there has been an overall decline in deaths from these diseases taken together – of 7.0% in England and Wales, 7.3% in

Table 8.3   Selected mortality data 1985–1990 (HMSO 1992b)

Disease	England/Wales			Scotland			N Ireland		
	1985	1990	% change	1985	1990	% change	1985	1990	% change
Diseases of circulation	287 054	259 247	−10.7	32 319	29 437	−9.8	8031	7110	−13.0
Respiratory diseases	56 828	61 018	+7.4	7156	7231	+1.0	2511	2781	+10.8
Cancers lung/bronchus	35 792	34 375	−4.1	4307	4123	−4.5	761	771	+1.3
Totals	379 674	354 640	−7.0	43 782	40 791	−7.3	11 303	10 662	−6.0

Scotland, and 6.0% in Northern Ireland – between 1985 and 1990. The bad news is that there have been increases by 7.4% in England and Wales, 1.0% in Scotland and 10.8% in Northern Ireland in deaths from respiratory diseases, and an increase in lung cancer of 1.3% in Northern Ireland as well (Table 8.3). How much the decline in heart disease has been due to health education and health promotion is a matter of dispute, but it would seem to have had some measurable effect.

Preventable morbidity

The bulk of this morbidity is preventable. In the face of these disturbing statistics, the question of the proportion of the health budget devoted to health education and prevention becomes a serious moral and political issue. What are the facts? In the UK, the total allocation for health education for the national bodies in 1991/92 was just under £40 million: Health Education Authority (England), £29.9 million; Health Education Board for Scotland, £5.3 million; Health Promotion Authority for Wales, £3.1 million; and Health Promotion Unit for Northern Ireland, £0.9 million).[10] Again, by comparison, the amount spent by British firms on advertising alcoholic beverages and tobacco products is estimated at between £750 million and £1 billion. The annual budget allocated by the Scottish Office for health education compares with a similar amount (£5.3 million) spent daily by Scots on beer and whisky. These are not just matters of 'political' interest, but ones that impact directly on the work of nurses in hospital, in the home and in the community.[11] Although the proportion of the National Health (sic!) Service budget spent on health promotion has been increased above the level of inflation, it

still remains a tiny percentage of total health service expenditure (e.g. in Scotland in 1997, the HEBS budget of £7.42 million amounted to 0.17% of the total NHS budget of £4.48 billion).

The increase in smoking, especially among women, would appear to have contributed to the increase in respiratory diseases. However, there is increasing evidence of 'passive smoking' and environmental atmospheric pollution being major factors contributing to the increase in respiratory diseases as well. Our uncertainty about direct causal connections makes it important that more research is done on the factors that are contributing to these changes. This is essential if government, both local and national, is to be persuaded to do something effective about controlling smoking in the workplace and places of entertainment and about environmental pollution. While Canada has been willing to 'grasp the nettle' and impose effective sanctions on industries contributing to atmospheric pollution, in the UK there has not been the political will to address the corporate business and industrial sector, for fear of disinvestment. While nurses have a direct responsibility to research and develop more effective methods of patient education and general health promotion for improving the health of their patients, it can also be argued that they should be in the forefront of the campaign for a healthier environment.

Should nurses confine themselves to their clinical roles and responsibilities, or should they become involved in the wider issues? Should the professional associations and nursing unions confine themselves to issues of direct patient care and the 'pay and rations' of nurses, or, like the British Medical Association, for example, become more active in lobbying and campaigning to stop the advertising of tobacco and alcohol in the mass media? Should they follow the example of 'activist' health professionals in the Australian state of Victoria, who successfully campaigned for a hypothecated 'health education tax' of 5% on wholesale price of all tobacco products? This tax has resulted in A\$27 million being made available specifically for health promotion (personal communication, State of Victoria Health Department, 1993). In Canada and Australia, health professionals working in accident and emergency medicine, together with police, have pressed for a change in the law to make hosts and hostesses who allow their guests to drive home under the influence of alcohol liable for prosecution in the same way that hoteliers and bartenders can already be prosecuted for serving people alcohol when they are drunk.

What other strategies ought nurses to be thinking about and what issues should they be campaigning about, as nurses? Which kind of intervention achieves the greatest benefits: attempts to achieve individual behaviour change by direct patient education, or working for changes in the social, economic and physical environment? What kinds of action will reduce the adverse impacts on us of products damaging to our health? Political pressure on local and state government? Marketing health more effectively to change peer group attitudes? Offering financial incentives or sanctions to reduce the impact of tobacco and alcohol marketing strategies? Imposing limits on the general availability of these products by restricting the number of sale outlets and also limiting the places where they can be used? Alternatively, do nurses go along with the general cynicism that dismisses such initiatives as 'politically correct' healthist propaganda?

It is a fact that the majority of nurses do not feel able to contribute individually to health promotion policy-planning or administration, but rather see themselves as engaged in direct patient education on the ward, or in screening and health education in primary care and community settings. Nurses as a group (comprising 78% of the UK health care workforce) can have some real power and influence health policy, directly and indirectly, by collective action. Similarly, influential and respected nurses may also have the power, through representation on health authority committees, to influence health service policy and resource allocation at local and national level. To be effective, both in their 'hands-on' patient education and in local area planning, it is imperative that nurses have access to good evidence, based on reliable local area health statistics (or do the necessary research themselves). Nurses need to know the specific health needs of their own communities, which may be significantly different from those in other areas, despite general trends that are similar.

Scotland has set a very high standard for the collection of excellent local area health statistics, and these provide a good foundation on which to base discussion of the political ethics of health service provision and priorities for health care and health promotion. To illustrate some of the issues which arise in the ethics of planning and administering health services, we will use *Scottish Health Statistics* (ISD 1997), because they provide a good evidential base on which to debate the issues, not only for Scottish nurses, but also for nurses everywhere (see Box 8.4). However, let us first reflect on main trends in Scotland.

The decline in fertility

In Scotland, fertility has been declining and this raises some interesting policy problems. From one point of view, the decline could be seen as contributing beneficially to the health of women and children, and health service staff might be inclined to see this as a triumph of education in matters of sexual health, contraception and family planning. From another point of view, the decline in the general level of fertility signals the possibility of other kinds of problems in the next generation. The ratio of people of working age to the population of dependent and elderly people will be such that we may have difficulty providing adequate health services to meet the needs of the sick, the elderly and handicapped people. Furthermore, it can be disputed whether this change in the pattern of fertility is due to any form of direct medical intervention. The evidence from the World Bank's (1993) report *Investing in*

Box 8.4 'Balance sheet' of main health trends (ISD 1997, p. xv)

Indicators of improvements in health
- There were 59 308 live births in 1996, the lowest number since civil registration began in 1855
- Perinatal mortality rates (9.2 per 1000 live births) have remained stable since 1985
- The number of children with measles reported in 1996 was 764, the lowest since records began
- Life expectancy continues to improve in all age groups (but lags behind England and Wales)
- The incidence of lung cancer in men declined by 15.6% between 1986 and 1995
- Cigarette smoking among adults over 16 declined from 34% in 1992 to 30% in 1994 (a continuing trend)
- The percentage of the adult population with no teeth fell from 45% in 1972 to 25% in 1995

Indicators of actual or potential health problems
- The percentage of births to women aged 35 and over has doubled since 1988 (i.e. 6.4% to > 12%)
- There were 1629 hospital admissions in 1996/97 because of poisoning accidents of children under 15 years
- Notifications of food poisoning have almost doubled in the past 10 years
- Lung cancer was the most frequently diagnosed cancer in males in 1995, at 23.2%
- The incidence of lung cancer in women increased by 18.1% between 1986 and 1995
- In 1997, a third of residents aged 65 and over in private nursing homes suffered from dementia
- A total of 12 307 abortions were performed in Scotland in 1996, an increase of over 12% over the previous decade

---

Health, based on comparative studies of trends worldwide, suggests that this has much more to do with improved general levels of education, better housing, increased prosperity, the commercial availability of the means of contraception, and changing patterns of employment (with more women entering the workforce). With an increasing proportion of women in full-time employment, the trend in the industrialised economies is for women to have children later in life. This brings attendant obstetric problems and potential complications, as well as the increased demand for IVF and other forms of assisted reproduction to deal with declining fertility and problems of infection-related infertility more common in older sexually active women.

Leaving aside the debates about the general ethics of artificial contraception, there remain serious ethical questions about the right of intervention of health professionals in the area of sexual health. First, nurses need to remind themselves that disapproval of artificial contraception is the preoccupation not only of Roman Catholics, but also of some Jewish and many Islamic communities, and in traditional African society, where artificial contraception, if not taboo, is strongly censured. Thus there may be real intercultural conflicts about the appropriateness of these issues being raised, and how they are raised, in antenatal education of mothers-to-be. However, to return to the issue of policy and priorities in sexual health and contraceptive education, questions may be raised about the legitimacy of state intervention in this area. Is it justifiable to implement coercive measures to ensure a one child family policy (as in China); compulsory sterilisation (as was attempted in India); or the less coercive but interventionist policies euphemistically called 'health promotion'? This question should be of vital ethical concern to nurses, for they are the frontline workers responsible not only for caring for people with problems related to their sexual health or reproductive capacity, but also for acting as agents of social control with responsibility for implementing state and local contraceptive or family planning policies.

Increasing use of abortion

In Scotland there were 12 307 legal abortions in 1996. These are not recorded with other mortality statistics, but if they were, they would account for 16.8% of (or 1 in 6) deaths in Scotland. The figure for the UK as a whole was a total of 188 300 legal abortions to UK residents in 1991, representing an increase of 39% over the figure for 1975, and a 21% increase since 1985 (ISD 1997).

Whatever a person's moral convictions may be about the ethics of abortion, these figures should be a cause for concern. Because midwives and health visitors are frontline health educators, they should be concerned that so many unwanted pregnancies occur, that so many women have reason to terminate their pregnancies, and that there are so many failures of contraception or just failure to use any form of contraception. Individual nurses may have to make choices about assisting or not assisting at terminations, and hence should be clear about their own views on these matters. They also need to be aware that there are many economic and political factors – relating to the status of women, the working conditions and terms of employment of women, and environmental and social factors – which complicate the whole problem. Do they become politically involved? As nurse managers, do they adopt a systematic, strategic and long-term approach to dealing with these issues, or just resort to 'first aid' and 'crisis management'?

Other issues arising out of the information in Box 8.4 that bear reflection for nurses are, for example, the dramatic increase in smoking among women and perinatal mortality. The role of nurses in health education here may be crucial (as the evidence is that direct one-to-one counselling by health professionals is 10 times more effective than mass media health education). However, it raises the critical question of whether nurses can be credible role models. The evidence is that nurses as a group tend to smoke heavily, and as the saying goes, our actions speak louder than our words! A different kind of challenge is the question of whether anything can be done by nurses specifically to improve the static level of perinatal mortality in Scotland, while other countries have achieved better rates. To answer this question responsibly is not to debate opinions, but rather it carries with it the ethical responsibility for sound evidence-based research on nursing practice, to see if, for example, the quality of antenatal care or services can be improved. But what other issues of political ethics in planning and administration of nursing services are raised by the summary statistics in Box 8.4?

Improving health services

Many of the questions cannot be settled without considering the relationship between questions of quality improvement in direct patient care or patient education and the social and institutional context in which this is provided. To measure improvement in the quality of services requires not only faithful record-keeping and collection of scientific data, but also careful planning, and the framework and infrastructure to implement quality controls. The setting up in 1990 of the Scottish Quality Assessment and Accreditation Team involved, first of all, work on defining appropriate health and service performance indicators by which progress could be measured. Next it required the setting up of the Scottish Morbidity Record, in order to record, analyse and interpret the data collected. For example, the information in Box 8.5 needs to be factored into our policy planning calculations.

Government bureaucrats and policy planners, concerned with reducing public expenditure and the escalating costs within a country's health services, have been concerned to improve 'cost efficiency' (i.e. the efficiency of services relative to the financial cost) and have used 'discharge rates' (or what used to be called 'bed turnover') as a measure of efficiency. Nurses may question whether this has really brought benefits to their patients. The period of hospitalisation of women in childbirth has been dramatically reduced over the past 40 years, from weeks to days, and now in some cases from days to hours, and this improved 'efficiency' has both provided benefits and incurred

---

Box 8.5 Some indicators of development and improvement in services in Scotland, 1996 (ISD 1997)

- Numbers of in-patient and day-case discharges from hospital continue to increase: almost 1.4 million were treated in 1996/97, up 1.9% from 1995/96 and up 21.0% from 1990/91
- 78% of eligible women underwent cervical screening during the past 3.5 years and 85% in the past 5.5 years to the end of 1996
- Hospital day cases account for over one-half (55.8%) of all elective in-patient and day-case admissions in acute specialities
- The total number of beds recorded in registered nursing homes has almost doubled since 1990/91, with 22 831 beds recorded in March 1997
- 77.5% of NHS complaints were dealt with within 20 working days: 1.8 % of complaints dealt with resulted in a request for independent review
- Medical and dental staff accounted for 12% (13 223) of all staff in 1996, compared with 10% (10 687) in 1980. Female staff accounted for 78% of all NHS staff

costs. Lengthy periods of hospital stay for mothers (unless there are serious complications of childbirth) have been shown by the evidence (contrary to 'old wives' tales') to be harmful to the health of mothers, who do better being encouraged to get back to normal living as soon as possible. Babies, too, benefit from being in the full-time care of their mothers rather than being kept in a hospital nursery as used to be the case. However, there is a 'law of diminishing returns' that seems to apply here. In the rush to be more efficient and discharge mothers earlier from nursing homes, there is evidence that some of the health problems that arise postnatally have to be dealt with in the community. This may be all very well if there are excellent primary care nursing facilities and adequate staff, but it is another question if these services are inadequate, remote, too expensive to afford, etc. Serious, well-researched evidence is required to support a *cost–benefit analysis*, which factors in the human cost and cost to the community of changes in services, as well as the benefits to the productivity of the health services and its customers. If undertaken by nurses, this may be vitally important in factoring in the human dimension into what might otherwise be the manipulation of anonymous statistics and the determination of priorities by 'faceless bureaucrats'.

Similar considerations should be applied to evaluation of the real costs and benefits to psychiatric patients, their families and the community of the so-called 'open door' policy of earliest possible discharge of patients back into the community to be supported by the supposed 'community care networks'. While the problems of institutionalisation of patients with mental disorders have been real in the past, it is questionable whether the 'open door' policy of 'community psychiatry' has been anything more than a 'revolving door' policy. There is a risk that the mentally ill are just recycled through the criminal justice system, as some research has shown.

Again, as a nurse, you might pause reflect on the ethical responsibilities of nurses that may arise out of interpretation of the other findings in Box 8.5. For example, what is the significance of the considerable increase of registered nursing home

beds in relation to the change in the scope and functions of hospitals and the shift in patterns of nursing employment? What is the significance for nurses of the increase in the proportion of doctors and dentists employed relative to the number of nurses, and the fact that 78% of (lower paid) nurses are women? Does this not simply confirm the long-established tendency for women's work to be attributed a lower value and for women to be subject to ongoing 'sexploitation' in the workforce? And what should nurses do about it? Is the encouragement of 'consumers' to make complaints about the quality of service delivery a blessing or a curse? Will it lead to increased litigation? Does it really lead to improvement of services, or is it just part of 'public relations' and largely ignored? Is it ethical to raise the expectations of 'consumers' and then not to fulfil them?

THE CHALLENGE OF THE GLOBAL HIV/AIDS PANDEMIC

To take a different kind of problem, of rather different proportions, let us consider the implications for nursing practice and the delivery of nursing services of the HIV and AIDS epidemic. First, let us consider some salient facts: as of 31 December 1997, the World Health Organization's HIV/AIDS Surveillance Division reported an estimated total of 30.6 million people worldwide living with HIV/AIDS, of whom 1.1 million were children under 15 years of age. By the end of 1997, the cumulative total of deaths from AIDS notified to WHO since the beginning of the epidemic was 11.7 million, including 2.7 million child deaths. The estimated total of new infections in 1997 was 5.8 million, with the overwhelming majority in sub-Saharan Africa (4.0 million) and south and South-East Asia (1.3 million).

WHO's response to the global HIV/AIDS pandemic has been to apply the concept of 'mainstreaming' to its activities. They have encouraged a similar approach in member countries, namely, to bring to bear on the problem scientific knowledge, medical expertise, technology, sound epidemiological data and the energy of various programmes within WHO. The success of such an

Table 8.4 WHO global HIV/AIDS surveillance data – as of end of 1997 (WHO 1999a)

Estimates to end of 1997	Adults and children with HIV/AIDS	Children <15 with HIV/AIDS	Cumulative adult and child AIDS deaths	Cumulative child deaths from AIDS	1997 Adult and child new infections	1997 new < 15 child infections	Cumulative total of orphans
N. America	860 000	8600	420 000	5000	44 000	< 500	70 000
Caribbean	1 300 000	9200	110 000	14 000	47 000	3100	48 000
Latin America	310 000	16 000	470 000	23 000	180 000	5200	51 000
W. Europe	530 000	5200	190 000	2800	30 000	< 500	8700
N. Africa and Middle East	210 000	7000	42 000	4400	19 000	2000	14 000
Sub-Saharan Africa	20 800 000	970 000	9 700 000	2 500 000	4 000 000	530 000	7 800 000
E. Europe and Central Asia	150 000	4600	4500	4200	100 000	700	< 50
East Asia and Pacific	440 000	3200	12 000	1700	180 000	2000	1900
S. and S.E. Asia	6 000 000	89 000	740 000	100 000	1 300 000	47 000	220 000
Australia and N. Zealand	12 000	< 50	7100	< 100	600	< 10	< 500

approach, it is stressed, depends critically on international cooperation in joint planning of technical contributions, systematic data collection, continuous information flow, networking between the various agencies working in the field and a coordinated approach to preventive and treatment services wherever possible. This is not only a medical and administrative imperative, but also a moral one for all who are seriously concerned with this pandemic and other diseases which are becoming the scourge of our overpopulated planet (see Table 8.4).

WHO has established the International Office of HIV/AIDS and Sexually Transmitted Diseases (ASD), with four main objectives:

● to coordinate global, regional and country-level responses to sexually transmitted diseases (STDs) and HIV/AIDS
● to facilitate integration of activities dealing with STDs and HIV/AIDS through provision of technical and normative support, through WHO regional and local offices
● to ensure liaison between WHO and other non-governmental international and national agencies
● to coordinate within WHO and associated organisations the mobilisation of resources to deal with STDs and HIV/AIDS.

At the most basic level, by assisting with the direct care of patients with STDs and HIV/AIDS, and also with conscientious record-keeping and collection of data, nurses contribute significantly

to the overall strategy for controlling this devastating global pandemic.

WHO has cautioned that the reported global number of HIV/AIDS cases in the various health regions is a relatively crude indicator of trends, for the following reasons (DHH&CS 1993):

● less than complete diagnosis in many cases
● less than complete reporting to public health authorities
● delays in reporting inherent in the passive case surveillance approach
● use of different case surveillance criteria around the world
● limited resources in some developing countries for epidemiological research
● the reluctance of some governments to acknowledge the problem or publish data.

The worldwide epidemic of HIV/AIDS has attracted a great deal of attention and concern from both the worried public and health professionals faced with the fact that there is as yet no cure for the disease (antiretroviral drugs AZT, dd^I and dd^C, and other drugs appear to have had some success in delaying the onset of AIDS in those with HIV infection).[12] However, the cost of treatment with these drugs is astronomical and completely out of reach to all but a few of those suffering from HIV/AIDS in impoverished developing countries (e.g. the cost of one course of treatment with AZT is more than the per capita funding available for all medical treatment in Uganda). The absence of effective means of immunisation or treatment of HIV/AIDS has left health professionals feeling relatively impotent to do anything effective in the clinical situation, other than to offer TLC (tender loving care) or palliative care. So the challenge is to address the need for effective primary, secondary and tertiary prevention, and good infection control measures in hospitals and clinics.

Because the primary modes of transmission of HIV/AIDS are sexual intercourse and injecting drug use, effective health education and prevention are the most basic measures required to contain the pandemic. However, these behaviours, which can put people at risk of HIV disease, relate to people's intimate sexual behaviour, drug use and personal lifestyles. What kinds of public health measures are taken, or what style of personal health education or wider health promotion is required, and what forms are socially acceptable, raise the question of the limits of personal rights to privacy and autonomy when the health of children and the general public is put at risk. Primary prevention is no 'quick fix' but aims to change people's attitudes and behaviour over time in relation to various forms of high-risk sexual behaviour and substance abuse. While some spectacular success has been achieved in the USA and Australia, particularly among highly motivated and better educated homosexual men, the main thrust of preventive services has been in encouraging the practice of 'safe sex'. This has been mainly through encouraging the use of condoms or other protectives, and through the establishment of needle exchanges to prevent the transmission of HIV infection through sharing of injection equipment. Caring by carers for people living with HIV/AIDS, in both the pre-terminal and terminal stages of the disease, has been a model in many countries of how support for the dying and the bereaved can be improved generally. Many nurses have been in the forefront of efforts to humanise the services dealing with people suffering from AIDS.

Few diseases have challenged health professionals more radically in recent times. On the one hand, they have had to come to terms with their own risk of infection in their day-to-day work (and the panic in the early days of the epidemic verged on the hysterical). On the other hand, they have been challenged by HIV/AIDS, perhaps more than any other disease, to confront the taboo issues of sexuality, death and drug dependency. Nurses have had to examine their own attitudes to these issues and their own sexual behaviour, recreational use of drugs and how they deal with the death of people of their own age. They have also had to choose between their responsibility to care for and protect vulnerable HIV/AIDS patients in their immediate care, and their wider responsibilities to the family and the sexual partner(s) of the patient and to the patient's employers and workmates. Health professionals, in their anxious attempts to change people's sexual behaviour or use of drugs, for their own good and to protect society, risk becoming intrusive, officious or authoritarian in their methods and approaches to the delivery of services. Many classical ethical problems in nursing and caring relationships have reappeared in painful form in the face of the HIV/AIDS pandemic. These include issues around contact tracing, screening for HIV, pre- and post-test counselling, antenatal and postnatal care of mothers and children with HIV/AIDS, segregation of AIDS patients from other patients, treatment of AIDS patients in prisons, and issues of voluntary or compulsory reporting and treatment of people with HIV infection.

These moral quandaries and ethical dilemmas related to working with HIV/AIDS can arise for nurses at two rather different levels – at the more intimate personal level and at an institutional level in the context of their professional work. At a personal level, the challenge is that before nurses can work effectively with people with HIV/AIDS, either in clinical nursing or in health education roles, they have to confront their own fears and fantasies (including homophobic prejudices) and questions about their own sexuality and lifestyle that have a bearing on how they relate to these patients. Evidence from work done in Britain, training health professionals for AIDS and drugs-related counselling, brought to light considerable resistance among nurses and other health professionals to working with patients with HIV/AIDS and problems in confronting these issues themselves.[13]

Even before the HIV/AIDS epidemic, working with heroin addicts and other intravenous drug users was an unpopular 'no hope' area for both medical and nursing staff, partly because of scant evidence of successful treatment or rather depressing evidence of regular relapse. Staff would complain of the difficulty of working with patients who appear unreliable, who are often dishonest and willing to steal, who would threaten health care staff to get money or drugs, and whose lifestyles are often very chaotic and usually very different from those of the health care staff. The limited success of detoxification programmes, with or without counselling or psychotherapy, and the risks of overdose in patients being treated on the new 'wonder drug' naltrexone have made most health authorities reluctant to invest large sums of money and staff time in dealing with these 'very demanding', 'manipulative' and 'unrewarding' patients. Few nurses are prepared to make the extensive investment of their time and energy required in working with these people, who often resent being treated as 'patients', and they have not surprisingly been inclined to favour policies of risk minimisation, rather than hope for cures.

At an institutional level, other kinds of issues arise in the 'management' of people with HIV/AIDS. In the early stages, in the clinical situation (in the clinic, patient's home or hospital), the issues of confidentiality and invasion of privacy are the most important. Later on, the questions for nurses are what kind of care, staff training and practical support for the carers are the nurse's responsibility. Nurse managers should be contributing to overall HIV/AIDS policy, but would also be expected to help determine how these policies are implemented at ward and overall hospital level, e.g. policies on general infection control, on record-keeping and confidentiality, on segregation of patients and access by relatives and significant others. They also have to decide on relevant in-service and AIDS awareness training for staff. Health authority managers have had to develop AIDS policies on a number of issues: employing affected health professionals and service staff; workers' compensation for nurses infected through needlestick injuries or contact

with patients' blood or body fluids; training policies; and issues of prioritising the allocation of staff and resources to deal with the often neglected areas of sexual health and sexually transmitted diseases.

HIV/AIDS is a good example of an issue where knowledge of the local culture, religious background and health data is critical for the development of appropriate services, training relevant to working with affected and at-risk individuals, and development of sound ethical policies for local HIV/AIDS prevention and patient education. Let us consider some comparisons between Australia, Scotland and Botswana, as countries with different general health status, socioeconomic and cultural traditions (see Table 8.5):

- Australia, with the largest population (18.25 million), has the highest income level (GNP per capita of US$18 720), about 35% of its population is of reproductive age, and has a birth rate of 14 per 1000 and an average life expectancy at birth of 78 years. The ratio of people living with HIV/AIDS in Australia is 0.06%.
- Scotland, with a population of 5.13 million, has a similar income level (GNP per capita of US$18 500), about 28% of its population is of reproductive age, a birth rate of 12 per 1000, and an average life expectancy at birth of 78 years. The ratio of people living with HIV/AIDS in Scotland is 0.05%.
- Botswana, with the smallest population (1.52 million), has the lowest income level (GNP per capita of US$3020), more than 40% of its population is of reproductive age, a birth rate of 36 per 1000, and an average life expectancy at birth of 52 years. The ratio of people living with HIV/AIDS in Botswana is 12.5%.

Many inferences could be drawn from these comparisons, but perhaps some of the most significant are that, in the high-income economies, people are motivated to control their fertility and, presumably because of the ready availability of condoms and other contraceptives, this is possible. With comparable proportions

Table 8.5 People living with HIV/AIDS (WHO 1999c)

Country (population)	Category of persons	People with HIV/AIDS	Cumulative AIDS cases	Cumulative AIDS deaths	Deaths in 1997	No. of orphans	Transmission
Australia (18 250 000)	All adults Women Children	11 000 550 < 100	8300	6000	610	–	MSM IDU Hetero
Scotland (5 128 000)	All adults Women Children	2676 644 28	890	684	26	–	IDU MSM Hetero
Botswana (1 518 000)	All adults Women Children	190 000 9300 7300	50 000	43 000	15 000	28 000	Hetero

MSM, men having sex with men; IDU, injection drug use; Hetero, heterosexual.

of their populations of reproductive age, the contrast between Australia and Botswana is most dramatic. It is also significant that injection drug use (IDU) is a major contributor to the incidence of HIV/AIDS infection in the developed economies, but not in Botswana (where the drugs are neither available nor affordable) and heterosexual transmission is the primary route of infection. The most striking differences between Australia and Scotland are that, in Australia, men having sex with men (MSM) accounts for the greatest proportion of all cases of HIV/AIDS, followed by IDU and heterosexual sex. However, in Scotland, IDU has overtaken the incidence of HIV/AIDS associated with MSM, and MSM is now almost level with heterosexual sex as the second most important route of infection. While it would appear that the peak of the epidemic was reached in Scotland in 1986, and that in Australia in 1994, and it is now in decline in both countries, in Botswana the epidemic (of tragic proportions) is still on the increase, with no immediate end in sight. Evidence that, with massive support from WHO and international aid agencies, the epidemic is beginning to recede in Uganda is encouraging, but the implications for the future health and prosperity of sub-Saharan African countries are dire.

Here you might reflect on how differently the incidence and prevalence of HIV/AIDS in each of these countries might affect your approach to dealing with the disease if you were a nurse working in these countries, e.g. in relation to (a) nurse training, (b) hospital services, (c) preventive services, and (d) planning for the future.

The HIV/AIDS pandemic can be useful to illustrate the themes in nursing ethics that we have attempted to illustrate in this chapter, namely:

● Ethical decisions have to be made in health care at a number of different levels, and at each of these levels nurses may be involved and have to accept responsibility for decisions:
  – micro: at the 'bed face' in decisions affecting the direct nursing care of AIDS patients
  – macho: in multidisciplinary team decisions about the clinical management of people who are HIV-positive or with end-stage AIDS, and who on the team takes responsibility
  – meso: in hospital or clinic level decisions about policy and procedure for dealing with infection control or prevention, treatment or after-care
  – macro: in decision-making and policy-setting at local authority, regional and national levels affecting the deployment of nursing services to deal with HIV/AIDS relative to other needs.
● The second theme concerns the competing values in the workplace which shape our priorities and determine choices relative to: the care of individuals; working in teams; management of resources; and shaping health care policy. Where we place the emphasis will determine the priority we give to nursing

people with HIV / AIDS, relative to other services or to groups of patients with different needs.

● Nurses at a more senior level, managers and those in positions of power and authority have a responsibility to be informed about the basics of public administration, the alternative possible frameworks and principles which underlie approaches to policy development.

Here, public panic about the incidence and prevalence of HIV / AIDS may result in poorly informed judgements about the allocation of resources.

● Finally, nurses have a fundamental professional responsibility to ensure that their practice is based on sound behavioural and scientific research, and that it conforms to the highest standards of probity and ethics.

 ## further reading

Different contemporary models and values for the caring professions
Bowden P 1997 Caring: gender-sensitive ethics. Routledge, London – *a readable analysis by a feminist philosopher of nursing, mothering, friendship and political involvement of women*

Campbell A V 1985 Paid to care. SPCK, London – *an ethical and theological critique of the function, institutionalisation and professionalisation of care in modern society*

Freidson E 1994 Professionalism reborn: theory, prophecy and policy. Polity Press, Cambridge – *a revamped analysis of the social and political role of the professions in modern society*

Phillips S S, Benner P 1996 The crisis of care: affirming and restoring caring practices in the helping professions. Georgetown University Press, Washington, DC – *a critical look at the caring professions and the pressures they are under from increasing commercialisation of care services*

Windt P Y, Appleby P C, Battin M P, Francis L P, Landesman B M 1989, Ethical issues in the professions. Prentice Hall, Englewood Cliffs, NJ – *a useful collection of articles on different types and levels of professional ethics*

The political ethics of resource allocation in health care
Enthoven A 1986 Reflections on the management of the National Health Service. Nuffield Provincial Hospitals Trust, London – *a critical analysis of the delivery of health services the model of microeconomic reform and the creation of an 'internal market' in health*

Mishra R 1984 The welfare state in crisis. St Martin's Press, New York – *a readable defence of the concept of a welfare state, challenging some of the prevailing theories*

Murley R (ed) 1995 Patients or customers: are the NHS reforms working? Institute of Economic Affairs Health and Welfare Unit, London – *a useful collection of articles presenting a number of views and critical perspectives on the application of business management models in health care*

White R 1985 Political issues in nursing. Wiley, Chichester, vols 1 and 2 – *a readable and helpful introduction to some of the key political issues facing nurses in the health industry*

Frameworks for policy making and resource allocation
Downie R, Tannahill C, Tannahill A 1996 Health promotion: models and value. Oxford University Press, Oxford – *an overview of different approaches to public health and planning based on various social and medical models*

Harrison S, Hunter D J, Pollitt C 1990 The dynamics of British health policy. Unwin Hayman, London – *an informed and critical administrative perspective on the problems of resource allocation*

Kitson A, Campbell R 1996 The ethical organisation: ethical theory and corporate behaviour. Macmillan Business, Basingstoke – *a readable introduction to the ethical issues in business management and commercial activity, from a corporate rather than personal perspective*

Taylor-Gooby P 1985 Public opinion, ideology and state welfare. Routledge & Kegan Paul, London – *a critique of the political economy of health and welfare from a social justice perspective*

end notes

1 Summary of government expenditure on social services and housing, 1990/91: education, £22.15 billion; National Health Service, £28.19 billion; personal social services (social work), £5.6 billion; social security, £55.8 billion; housing, £4.6 billion (see World Bank 1993).

2 Reproduced with permission from Thompson & Harries (1997).

3 Gilby T, 1964, *St Thomas Aquinas – Philosophical Texts*, Oxford University Press, London, paras 332, 958, 961

4 Dr Fiona Stanley, Director of the West Australian Research Institute for Child Health, speaking in Canberra, was quoted in *The West Australian* of 22 July 1992 as saying: 'Australia cannot afford to waste its scarce health dollars on inappropriate technology such as IVF. Money could be better spent researching the causes of infertility or the effectiveness of surgery in treatment of infertility in women. The evidence of the Canadian Royal Commission on in vitro fertilisation is that women who drop out of IVF programmes have the same chance of becoming pregnant as women who stay in the programmes. My major concern is that there has been no randomised control trial, comparing IVF with either doing nothing or doing other things, for example surgery for tubal problems. Without adequate trials we do not know either whether these techniques are really effective, nor do we know what the risks and complications are likely to be.'

5 Reviewing the research on IVF and its use in assisted reproduction and the 'treatment' of infertility in Western Australia, Grayson remarks on the fact that Australia as a nation with a heavy reliance on stock breeding in farming not only led the world in the application of IVF to stock breeding , but also 'led in the commercialisation of IVF [for humans] with the establishment of the first company to market reproductive technology'.

'The direct transference of IVF from animal to human application is illustrated by the fact that veterinarians can be found working in prominent positions in IVF clinics,' she said.

She points out that IVF is commercially very profitable for the private operators (who in WA charge A$1500 per treatment cycle, and an average IVF confinement costs A$57 000), but about half of these costs are borne by the state and the taxpayer. In addition to the cost/benefit issues, there are in her view deeper problems relating to the role and identity of women in this medical commercialisation and aggressive marketing of services for assisted reproduction: 'Motherhood is thus portrayed as at once a biological imperative and a right, but one which is acknowledged only in women in certain approved circumstances. Women who are married, heterosexual and affluent are portrayed as requiring children, regardless of the cost to society or to their own finances and health. A danger of new reproductive technologies may be that such contradictory rhetoric may serve to reduce women's reproductive choices to a function of their social situation.' (cf. O'Brien M 1981 *The Politics of Reproduction*. Routledge & Kegan Paul, Boston; and Singer P, Wells D 1984 *The Reproductive Revolution: New Ways of Making Babies*. Oxford University Press, Oxford.)

6 The *Ottawa Charter for Health Promotion* was published in Ottawa at the 1st International Conference on Health Promotion, jointly sponsored by the World Health Organization, the Canadian Health and Welfare Department, and the International Public Health Alliance.

7 The system is open to wide abuse in the public service because of the wide flexibility possible in defining who is 'purchaser' and who is 'provider'. In the Australian Capital Territory, for example, the State Justice Minister required the Director of Public Prosecutions to sign an agreement with him as 'purchaser' to provide prosecution legal services to the state on the terms required by the Minister, in return for an appropriate budget!

8 A phrase coined by Dr Ralph Hendrikse, a Paediatric Health Consultant to the World Health Organization.

9 The figures quoted here and in the following two paragraphs are taken mainly from *Annual Abstract of Statistics* (HMSO 1992b) and from *Social Trends* (HMSO 1992a).

10 Taken from annual reports of the respective national bodies.

11 From available evidence in 1991, the UK tobacco companies spent a total of £67 million on promoting their product – £42 million on advertising and £25 million on sports sponsorship. The alcohol industry spent a total of £680 million on advertising and sponsorship.

12 Antiretroviral drugs: AZT = Azidothymidine (zidovudine); dd^I = didanosine; and dd^c = dideoxycytidine (Zalcitabine).

13 Unpublished reports of the Health Education Authority and Health Education Board for Scotland, relating to the national in-service training programme, brought these problems to light and led to much greater emphasis being given in AIDS awareness training to exploring personal feelings and fears relating to sexuality, death and drugs, and less emphasis on purely information-based courses. Similarly, in skills training the focus was on personal exploration and growth in self-insight, before moving on to more specific skills training.

some suggestions on method

Different levels of ethical decision-making
As an initial assignment, students could be asked to work in small groups to 'map' the structure of decision-making in their local district, from the level of direct patient contact to health authority policy-making. They should produce examples of different types of ethical problems and dilemmas that arise at each of these levels. When they report back to the class on their findings, these could be grouped and analysed under the headings of micro – personal, macho – team, meso – organisational, and macro – inter-agency issues. (This is particularly relevant to decision-making in the new 'internal market'.)

Competing values in the workplace
To start with, the class could be asked to brainstorm examples of applications in nursing of 'a caring ethic', 'a service ethic', 'the ethic of public office' and 'the business ethic'. The class could be divided into four groups (or more if they identify other types of ethic operating in their environment). They should be asked to think about what position they would adopt if asked to argue the case for proposed cuts in staff or resources, or the relocation of funds from treatment services to screening or health promotion. When they are prepared, they could be asked to simulate a committee discussion around a specific case, with the requirement that they defend their position as cogently as they can, discuss the merits of the case of their 'opponents', but seek to arrive at a group action plan by negotiation.

Frameworks for policy decision-making
Given the theoretical frameworks that have been identified, groups of nurses could be assigned the task of interviewing representatives of each of the following types of approach:

- clinical – senior doctor/ICU staff nurse
- epidemiological – a public health doctor
- egalitarian and ecological – union branch executive
- administrative – a senior nurse manager
- commercial business management – business manager of the hospital or hospital trust.

The aim would be to identify the assumptions and methods which they apply in their decision-making. When completed, the class could report on and discuss their findings, identifying similarities and differences between the different approaches.

Researching health and demographic data
The class could be assigned the task to visit their nearest library or health records officer, in order to investigate the facts about any of a number of issues: deaths from smoking, alcohol abuse and drugs, facts on abortion, euthanasia and terminal care, facts on local health budgets and expenditure on nursing.

Alternatively, the class could be set the task of collecting data on HIV/AIDS in their country or region, to establish what local policy is on HIV prevention, and what nurses are doing about it locally. Specifically the class should be asked to investigate the role of nurses in the community, in health education, in hospital nursing to apply infection control precautions, in nursing/treating patients with AIDS, and in the terminal care of people with AIDS.

9

Nurses and society: agents of health and social policy

AIMS

This chapter has the following aims:
1. To introduce nurses to some of the key issues in the political ethics of health care which impact on nursing, namely:
    – how policy decisions are made
    – how to set sound ethical policy
    – when nurses are justified to go on strike
    – whether the welfare state is in terminal crisis
    – whether NHS reforms have worked or not.
2. To encourage nurses to be better informed about the ethics of management, policy-making and the administration of health care and nursing.
3. To encourage nurses to recognise their ethical duty as professionals to contribute to public debate about the political economy of health.

LEARNING OUTCOMES

When you have read and worked through this chapter, you should be able to:
■ Give a good account of key current issues in the political ethics of health

care that impact on nursing and explain how they do so

■ Give an informed account of local health policy and funding of services, and demonstrate knowledge and practical understanding of how both raise vital ethical questions for nurses

■ Use the POLICY model in reference to some matter of direct concern to yourself, and demonstrate that you know how to apply it to other nursing issues

■ Demonstrate ability to debate the pros and cons of nurses going on strike in such a way as to show that you understand the ethical issues involved and can make informed judgements about different kinds of proposed strikes

■ Show evidence of having researched some of the issues related to the funding of services in your hospital, clinic or local authority, and should understand the issues at stake in the political debate about the future of welfare states.

SHOULD THE STATE BE RESPONSIBLE FOR HEALTH CARE?

During the 20th century, there was a growing public belief and expectation that everyone is entitled to good health. This faith was based on some of the spectacular developments in medicine, in pain control, microsurgery, chemotherapy and biomedical technology. However, it was perhaps more solidly grounded on observed reduction of mortality and morbidity, and improved general health and life expectancy of people – at least in the developed countries.

Both within more technologically advanced societies and in developing countries people have come to demand access to health care services as a political right. After World War II, several welfare states were established more or less contemporaneously with the founding of the United Nations

and the launch of the UNO Declaration of Human Rights. In Article 25 (UNO 1947) it states that every human being has a right to adequate health care, and, by implication, all governments have a duty to provide it. Health was seen increasingly not only as a quality of life, but as a necessary means to achieving one's life goals as a human being, and therefore as a fundamental human right. Likewise, the UK National Health Service Act (1947) was based on two assumptions: citizens have a right to basic health care, and the state has a duty to provide health care for all, on a sound and equitable basis (HMSO 1976).

The 'political ethics of health care' has been characterised by public debate about the scope of the state's responsibility for health care. With changes in the pattern of morbidity and mortality in developed countries, politicians have also had to address the practical changes in services required by these trends along with broadening public expectations of the responsibilities of governments in this area. Both the health and personal social services have become the arena in which debate about personal rights and public policy, and the best means to achieve health for all, has been

---

Box 9.1 Issues in the 'political ethics' of health

● What forms of 'treatment' or 'therapy' should be covered, and what range of services should state-funded health services provide? (For example, should these include transplants? In vitro fertilisation? Cosmetic surgery?)

● To what extent should the state attempt to define 'quality of life' for any group in the population? (For parents in relation to child care? For people with mental or physical handicaps? For elderly people?)

● How actively should the state be involved in health-related social engineering and social control to promote health? (For example, by active economic development? By reverse discrimination to overcome inequalities in health? By community development? By fiscal/legal inducements or controls?)

● What scope should state-provided preventive services have? What definition should be given to 'health promotion'? (For example, initiate proactive screening and preventive programmes? Compulsory immunisation? Health education in schools? By programmes of lifestyle and behaviour change?)

focused. There are perhaps four levels at which the political debate has been conducted (see Box 9.1).

Policy decisions taken by governments or local health authorities about each of these issues will impact on the work of nurses, whether they like it or not. In that sense, nurses cannot escape from the practical implications of health policy. For this reason they should be actively involved in contributing to informed debate about the political ethics of health care – within their spheres of influence. To become involved in politics, by active participation through their unions and professional bodies and as policy-makers (where this applies), is something nurses can hardly avoid, for not only is it in their own interests as nurses, but it is also a moral duty flowing from their responsibility for the well-being of their patients. In each of the areas mentioned in Box 9.1, the political debate will be partly about theoretical and ideological issues, and partly about practical means. For example, in relation to 'quality of life' issues, from one point of view, it is arguably the duty of the state to provide sheltered housing to protect frail elderly people from harm or self-neglect; from another point of view, the state should not interfere in the lives of older people and patronise them. From this latter perspective, the state should seek to promote the ability of frail elderly people to live independent lives, perhaps providing them with money from national insurance, as is the case in Germany, to buy in the services for social care they want or need, rather than institutionalising them.

The National Health Service (NHS) is a major institution and service industry in the UK. It is the largest employer not only in the UK, but also in the whole of Europe. Health policy and the political economy of the NHS are, or should be, matters of great importance to nurses, both as health professionals and as citizens and taxpayers. In a sense, as taxpayers, we are shareholders in this vast enterprise, whether privatised or not, and have a right to demand a say in what priority is given to health in public expenditure and what proportion of our gross domestic product (GDP) is 'invested' in health. For example, the UK Department of Health is one of the biggest spending departments in government, the proportion of total government expenditure on the NHS being about 6.1% of GDP, or a sum of £28.2 billion in 1990–91 (compared with £20.8 billion spent on defence). The comparative amounts spent on other social services in 1990–91 are set out in Table 9.1.

From another perspective, when politicians claim the cost of health services in the UK is excessive, the proportion of GDP spent on health in the UK, compared with other countries (Table 9.2), becomes a matter of ethical and political interest. So does the proportion of health services funded by private health insurance as compared with state funding. These matters may seem remote from the practical concerns of nurses, either in their professional roles or as voters, but policy decisions about these matters have profound implications for how health services will be provided and determine the context and availability of employment for nurses (DoH 1991a).

There are several reasons, from an ethical point of view, why it is helpful to think of the NHS as an industry, or even as a vast business corporation. By this we do not simply refer to the advent of the

Table 9.1   Summary of government expenditure (£ billions) on social services and housing (HMSO 1992a)

Department	1980–81[*]	1985–86[*]	1990–91[*]
Education	13.04	16.68	22.15
National Health Service	11.94	16.31	28.19
Personal social services	2.23	3.47	5.59
Welfare foods	0.035	0.113	0.115
Social security	24.43	43.246	55.8
Housing	6.30	4.64	4.6
Total government expenditure	57.975	84.459	116.445
Central government share	41.72	65.44	
Local government share	16.27	20.52	

[*] Years ended 31 March.

Table 9.2 Health spending (as a percentage of GDP in selected OECD countries) (OECD 1987)

Country	Public	Private	Total
United Kingdom	5.3	0.8	6.1
Canada	6.3	2.0	8.3
Germany	6.4	1.7	8.1
Italy	6.1	1.1	7.2
Sweden	8.6	0.7	9.3
United States	4.3	6.3	10.6

general manager and introduction of the internal market and business systems into the administration of hospital and primary care services. These innovations will ultimately be judged by whether they deliver the boons and blessings promised (or even the cost savings required). The imposition of new government financial discipline and quality assurance requirements on health authorities and health boards all have the potential to improve efficiency and financial accountability, but whether they will result in a better and more effective service has yet to be proved.

Many people feel that the idealism that attracts people into the caring professions and the ethic of service to others are put at risk by the values of 'economic rationalism' currently driving the reorganisation of health and social services. However, it is precisely these issues and challenges that demand we eschew a narrow personalist view of morality and develop a more adequate approach to professional and corporate ethics and ethical policy development.

'RATIONALISING' THE COST OF HEALTH SERVICES IN THE UK AND SCOTLAND

To readers of the previous edition it will be apparent that we have retained this section virtually unchanged. Why, it may be asked, have we not updated this material, given the major changes in the UK NHS during the period 1991–1999? And to this question two different kinds of answer can be made. On the one hand, the general ethical issues of rationalising scarce health resources and responsible management of the health budget are questions that apply equally validly to any other period one might choose to examine, whether it be before 1975, or from 1975 to 1991, or

from 1991 to 1999, and so it can be argued that the period 1975–1991 is as good as any other to illustrate the points to be made.

It can also be argued that the period from 1975 to 1991 in the UK is particularly interesting because it illustrates the end-stage of the application of what we referred to earlier as the administrative and epidemiological approaches to the political ethics of resource allocation and health services planning. After 1991, not only did the Conservative Government move rapidly to implement the new business-based mode of the 'internal market', based on a deregulated and competitive market in the provision of health services, but the method of collecting data also changed. This has made it much more difficult to make the kinds of comparison we developed in the third edition between spending and service priorities in Scotland and the rest of the UK.

We have decided to retain the analysis that follows for its illustrative purposes, recognising that it is now mainly of historical interest. The type of administrative rational planning model which it exemplifies rather well was popular during the 1970s and 1980s in many other countries, e.g. Sweden, Canada, New Zealand and Australia. This has been replaced in the 1990s in most of these countries by the fashionable new 'purchaser–provider' type of economic management. And, because the latter operates on the liberal model of the free market, public spending in the health and social services is supposed to be regulated and controlled by 'market forces'. These forces are mainly consumer demand and free competition between suppliers or 'providers' of health and social services – many of which already were, or were to be, privatised. What the new system did not provide for was an adequate method of collecting comparative data to monitor the quality of services or to ensure responsible reporting of results of this vast social experiment.

Before discussing the success or otherwise of the 'internal market' in achieving its objective to cut public expenditure while improving the quality of services and increasing the range of consumer choice, let us review the issues within the previously applicable system and model. Consider the distribution of the health budget in both Scotland and the UK, shown in Table 9.3.

Table 9.3 Costs of health services, 1975 to 1990–91 (HPSS 1990/91/92, ISD 1991, HMSO 1992a)

Details	Scotland (£ million)			United Kingdom (£ million)	
	1975	1985	1990–91	1985	1990–91
Total cost of health services	591	1963	2973	19 750	28 190
National insurance contributions	45.5	176.9	390.5		
Exchequer contribution	545.9	1775.9	2582.9		
Health board administration	23.5	55.5	104.5	11 730	18 150
Hospital and community services					
Revenue	389.3	1297	1912.5		
Capital	38.9	117.8	162.0		
Hospital running costs	358.0	1297	1912.5		
Salaries					
Medical and dental	37.0	127.5	193.0		2043
Nursing	128.8	436.0	639.9		6509
Community nursing	35.9	49.5			
Family practitioners	101.3	365.8		4227	
Central health services					
Revenue	15.3	53.3	92.0		
Capital	3.6	11.6	20.1		
Ambulance service	7.8	24.9	Privatised		
Blood transfusion	3.4	13.4	Privatised		
Health education	0.5	3.0	5.2	15	40
Administration	0.3	2.1		142	271
Training	4.2	15.3	30.0		
Research	2.6	5.3	5.56		

These statistics, illustrating government health service policy and priorities on allocation of resources, impact directly on nursing services, hospital management and standards of patient care, and therefore should be of vital concern to nurses. Senior nurses have a responsibility to be informed about these matters, in order to contribute intelligently to debate about health service priorities.

Notable changes in the distribution of costs over the period 1975–1991 are, first, the fact that 7.06% of the cost of the NHS in Scotland was paid for from National Insurance contributions in 1975, compared with 9.6% in 1985 and 13.13% in 1990, with proportional reduction in the contribution of the Exchequer. Secondly, between 1975 and 1985 costs of administration of the health boards in Scotland were reduced from 4 to 2.8% of the total costs, but rose again in 1990 to 3.5%. Thirdly, the proportion of total NHS expenditure on nurses' salaries in Scotland increased from 21.8 to 22.2% from 1975 to 1985, but dropped back to 21.5% in 1990 (the proportion for the UK in 1990 being 23.1%). Fourthly, the proportion spent on health education has steadily increased – from

0.08 to 0.15 to 0.17% in Scotland, i.e. from £0.10 to £0.59 to £1.02 per head per annum (the percentage spent on health promotion in the UK has increased from 0.07% in 1985 to 0.14% in 1990–91, i.e. from £0.27 to £0.70 per head per annum) (ISD 1991, HMSO 1992a).

These facts and figures alone do not enable us to decide on priorities in resource allocation. We have to clarify and prioritise our values as nurses in order to make responsible ethical decisions about economic priorities in nursing. The duty of care and considerations of justice and the rights of patients are all relevant to the debate, and the different weightings given to these principles will influence policy about resource allocation in profound and subtle ways. Clearly, in making decisions about policy and in attempting to influence policy at local and national level, different nurses will have different priorities, based on their political leanings and how they rank their ethical principles. As responsible professionals, they cannot avoid contributing to debate about these issues or attempting with their colleagues to achieve a consensus within their unions or professional body which contributes to the debate about the political ethics of nursing within the health care system.

Doctors and nurses, trained to deal with the patients who present to them for care and treatment, and experienced in crisis management, naturally tend to see their first priority as saving life. Their conditioned reflexes are to give priority to the duty to care (in a response which emphasises their sense of commitment to individual patients). This represents a clinical rather than an epidemiological view of the problem, and a personalist rather than an organisational set of values. Where the health of the public is at risk from an epidemic (e.g. HIV/AIDS), or where medical research has to be undertaken in the interests of all patients, or where demographic change or changes in the pattern of morbidity necessitate it, the duty of care for individuals must be qualified by considerations of justice and the rights of others, to ensure equity in the allocation of resources.

SHAPE: regional health priorities for Scotland: a case in point

The need for an overall approach to planning that is both rational and grounded in epidemiological research, rather than driven by short-term political agendas, is perhaps well illustrated in the policies developed by the Scottish Health Services Planning Council's SHAPE and SHARPEN reports – respectively, the *Scottish Health Authorities Priorities for the Eighties* (SHHD 1980) and the *Scottish Health Authorities Revised Priorities for the Eighties and Nineties* (SHHD 1990). Senior nurses represented the interests of nursing and nursing services on both councils.

Implementing such policies inevitably encounters resistance from vested interests, and in the case of the SHAPE and SHARPEN reports there was considerable resistance from established medical and conservative nursing interests to effecting the redistribution of manpower and resources required in the light of the Council's priorities for the 1980s (Box 9.2).

In the SHAPE report, existing services were divided into three categories, A, B and C, according to their priority, and indications given of what

---

Box 9.2 SHAPE categories

Category A
- Prevention
- Services for the multiply deprived
- Care of the elderly and elderly with mental disability
- Care of the mentally ill, mental and physical handicap

Category B
- Maternity services
- Primary dental care

Category C
- Child health
- Acute hospital services

---

the likely cost and staffing implications would be of the changes proposed in shifting resources from other sectors. Essentially this meant shifting resources from high-technology hospital-based medicine to primary care, and from treatment services to a greater emphasis on health education and health promotion in line with WHO's 'health for all' strategy. A strenuous rearguard action was fought by medical and nursing staff, particularly in obstetrics and gynaecology, and in the acute sectors of general medical and surgical services. In the areas of psychiatry and mental handicap nursing, there has also been considerable resistance to moves to de-institutionalise patients, and to move towards maintaining more patients in the community, in pursuit of policies of 'normalisation' and 'community care'. Some nurses have argued against these developments on the basis that these dependent patients 'need institutional care' and would be 'put at risk if discharged' into the community, and that the staff and facilities in the community are inadequate.

The first problem is that the term 'community care' signifies rather different things to those working in health and social services, and also to health service planners, on the one hand, and health care staff on the other. Development of high-quality non-residential services is an understandable priority for social service planners and for professionals in this field. Community care has tended to mean, therefore, the development of good community services as a prelude to reduction in the number of institutional places. From a medical and health service point of view, on the other hand, community care has been primarily a means to releasing 'blocked' beds. This refers to the problems created for hospitals by elderly or mentally handicapped people who are admitted as patients for medical reasons, and who then cannot be released back into the community for largely social reasons, because, for example, the facilities to which they will be released are not regarded as satisfactory. The pressure from the health service has therefore simply been to off-load these dependent people into community support schemes, thereby releasing the beds which doctors want for other purposes. Furthermore, the White Paper *Care in the Community* (DoH 1988) envisaged local authority social work services taking on more of the role of managers than direct providers of care in the case of such groups as elderly and mentally handicapped people. The local authority's role would be that of a purchaser and coordinator of services provided by a range of other suppliers, including private and voluntary health and accommodation services, and primary care and hospital-based health services, for these clients.

These opposing perceptions of the same phenomenon have, not surprisingly, led to very different priorities in and approaches to planning. One group is less concerned with the kind of service, and accordingly presses for the release of patients back into the community. The other side has tended to be more cautious and to resist attempts to discharge large groups of people into the community without the development of services of the appropriate type. In this regard Baker & Urquhart (1987), in surveying the needs of adults with mental handicap in Scotland, brought to light considerable disparities between the perceptions of need of relatives, medical and nursing staff, social workers and the mentally handicapped themselves.

Professional self-interest may induce certain groups to argue, for example, for the retention of patients in hospital, when this is not strictly necessary. Research undertaken by the Scottish Health Service Information Services Division indicated that staff assessments of patients' ability to live in the community with minimal support ranged from 83 to 3% (with the mean being 40%). The sample population was 1000 mentally handicapped persons in 19 psychiatric hospitals and five mental handicap units. Certain medical and nursing staff, in units facing closure or reduction in capacity, were opposed to the discharge of patients into the community. This appeared to have more to do with fear of job losses than concern to protect patients. Local authorities, with limited resources at their disposal to cope with the problem, have also been reluctant to press for their release. Joint planning has failed to create an appropriate service for a group of patients who might be expected to be the prime beneficiaries of collaborative arrangements (Baker & Urquhart 1987).

To the extent that these practical and policy decisions relating to the management and re-allocation of staff and resources have been argued by nurses on ethical grounds, it has been primarily by an appeal to the primacy of their 'duty to care' for these vulnerable patients. Alternatively they have argued on the grounds of 'respect for the rights of dependent people' to better standards of care. Some of the support from nurses for the policy of 'giving patients more choice' and for the move towards more private health care provision has to do with defending their territory in these 'threatened' areas. Part of this is, quite understandably, defending their personal 'investment' in continuing to work in the more glamorous areas of nursing. It is perhaps also true that some nurses have been reluctant to change with the times, to undergo retraining and to change their methods and working practices to accommodate the realities of changing health care needs and different expectations of people as patients/clients/consumers of health services.

From Table 9.4, it can be seen that despite resistance, the SHAPE programme priorities have been implemented with some degree of success. There has been increased hospital-based provision for elderly people, particularly those with mental disability, and also for people with severe physical handicaps. There has been a marked acceleration of discharge rates for elderly people (66.8%) and elderly people with mental disability (183%), but much lower rates in child health (12%) and general and acute medicine (15.4%). Whether the reductions achieved in hospital provision for people with mental illness and mental handicap (10.5 and 17.9%, respectively) have been matched by adequate alternative 'community care' is questionable and is of continuing concern to nurses, carers and the public. During this same period the numbers of medical staff have risen by 6% and that of nurses by 8.3%. To the extent that this was also intended to contain health service costs (of which medical and nursing salaries form one of the largest components) the exercise has been of doubtful success. However, this may have had a lot to do with the effectiveness of the political activity of unions representing medical and nursing interests. Attempts have been made in recent surveys by the Scottish Office to establish whether the SHAPE recommendations were being implemented.

It is difficult to evaluate the success of the earlier reforms associated with the Conservative Government's introduction of the 'internal market'– including the establishment of hospital trusts, fundholding GP services and the 'contracting out' of ancillary services. This is because the model was designed to free up health services from the constraints of both 'bureaucratic planning or administration' and the 'conservative medical or public health planning approach' that insists on scientific or epidemiological justification for determining health priorities.

There was growing concern during the decade of these 'reforms' that the determination of health priorities or the regulation of public expenditure could simply be left to 'market forces'. It was argued that unless we have a naive faith in Adam Smith's 'hidden hand' guiding the free market, it might seem reasonable to ensure that scientific, epidemiological and administrative rationality play a more significant role in determining priorities in health care. Without research-based planning, the implementation and monitoring of the political economy of resource allocation in health care tend to be blind and unprincipled. In response to public concern about abuses in the system, the Nolan Committee was set up to investigate complaints and allegations of impropriety and fraud. Their investigations brought to light some serious problems in the way things were being operated within these supposedly 'reformed' public services. The Commission recommended in its three reports on standards in public life action by the authorities to ensure greater respect for standards of probity and accountability in public life, and more rigorous forms of corporate governance to be put in place if corrupt

Table 9.4 Comparison of SHAPE categories 1980 and 1989 (ISD 1991)

SHAPE category	Hospital beds			Nursing staff		
	1980	1989	% change	1980	1989	% change
A. Care of elderly	9764	11 213	+14.8			
A. Psychogeriatric	2742	5574	+103.3			
A. Mental illness	17 040	15 275	−10.4	9752	11 429	+17.2
A. Mental handicap	6617	5435	−17.9	3428	3882	+13.2
A. Physical handicap	470	532	+13.2			
B. Maternity	2689	2327	−13.5	4593	4457	−3.0
B. Maternal/neonatal	3315	2873	−13.3	4593	4457	−3.0
C. Child health	1257	1051	−16.4			
C. General/acute	19 745	17 672	−10.5	35 479	37 902	+6.8
Total	58 208	54 051	−7.1	53 251	57 669	+8.3
A. Community nursing	4907	5648	+15.1			
B. Family practitioners	3256	3694	+13.5			
B. Dentists	1280	1572	+23.1			
B. Ophthalmic services	583	831	+42.5			
C. Pharmacists	1107	1125	+1.6			

abuse of the system is to be prevented in large public institutions.[1]

There has been considerable change in the pattern of health service funding and management of services in the UK since 1991, and again since New Labour came into power with an overwhelming majority in 1997. The very fact that the public signalled considerable discontent with the way the previous Conservative Government had handled the health and social services was taken by the new administration as giving them a mandate to institute yet another round of reforms. What this meant was that the 'reforms' associated with the introduction of the 'internal market' had hardly had time to bed in before being subject to further 'reform' by the policy-makers of the New Labour administration. The new administration has attempted to retain many 'good features' of the previous government's reforms while attempting to address some of the deepest-felt public grievances about how they were working (HMSO 1997a,b).

Some appraisal will be made of the effectiveness of the 'internal market' at the end of this chapter, but suffice it to say that a major area of public concern about the introduction of the internal market was the lack of public accountability of the new 'autonomous' hospital trusts and privatised services. What New Labour has attempted to introduce is an element of 'policy directed management' into the supposedly 'free' economy of their predecessors. This is to be achieved by replacing the free 'internal market' with direction of the political economy of health by NHS Management Executive Groups to be set up in Scotland and in England, Wales and Northern Ireland. Health service providers (e.g. hospital trusts and group practices providing primary care services) are to be financially accountable to these Management Executive Groups through a programme which requires them to publish and benchmark their costs on a consistent basis. Regardless of the political rhetoric of the new administration's policy documents, they are interesting because they attempt to factor ethical considerations of care, equity and respect for people's rights into their statement of objectives.

In *Designed to Care [Scotland]* (HMSO 1997b), for example, the value priorities asserted to be essential to achieving their objectives are (para 13):

- improving reliability and co-ordination of care through use of new technology;
- improving clinical effectiveness by ensuring that performance meets agreed standards and that these standards are driven upwards;
- promoting the adoption of more effective care based on evidence;
- involving patients to a greater extent in decisions about their own care and treatment;
- providing patients with more information about their health and about the options for treatment when they are ill.

Significantly, in *The New NHS: Modern, Dependable* (HMSO 1997a, Ch. 7), the move towards a 'one-nation NHS' involves a 'national drive to improve quality and performance' by providing 'national leadership to support local development', the establishment of a new 'National Institute for Clinical Excellence' and a new 'Commission for Health Improvement'. The internal economy of health care is to be managed by continuing to apply the principles of quality improvement and total quality management introduced by the previous administration, but with more rigorous accountability to the NHS Management Executive Groups on the basis of sound 'benchmarking' and 'performance management'. The requirements are stated in HMSO (1997b) as follows:

115. Health services should be provided efficiently and effectively. Benchmarking and performance measures have a key role to play in achieving this goal and will help:

- inform the process of setting priorities, objectives and targets
- enable monitoring of progress against objectives and targets
- promote the use of best practice; and
- improve the public accountability of the service to patients and the wider public.

In clarifying the rationale for introducing these procedures into the administration of health care, the policy-makers have sought to emphasise the ethical justification for the requirements, rather than simply legislate that they are to be followed (HMSO 1997b):

116. The Government believes the main areas in which performance measures are relevant are:

- *the clinical effectiveness of services:* for instance, the extent to which services achieve reductions in mortality, morbidity and disability;
- *the quality of services:* for example, waiting times for outpatient appointments and for diagnosis and treatment;
- *the efficiency of services:* the costs incurred in delivering services, and the use made of staffing, beds and other resources;
- *access to services:* the availability of services in different areas of the country;
- *inequalities in health:* differences in morbidity and mortality between socio-economic groups;
- *the appropriateness of services:* the type of services provided for patients – for example, the use made of day cases.

This is all very fine on paper, but the question is how well this will be implemented in practice. It is too early to assess whether these more ethically and community medicine-based criteria are being implemented and effectively applied to management of the political economy of the UK as it enters the 21st century. However, it provides us with an interesting model for discussion of the question of how we develop sound ethical policy.

DEVELOPING ETHICAL POLICY FOR ONESELF AND SOCIETY

Review and reorganisation have been features of life in major public sector organisations during the past decade, as governments have sought to reform and corporatise (or privatise) the management and financing of major institutions of the welfare state. Formulation of 'mission statements', 'values statements' and 'strategic plans' has been the order of the day with the introduction of business models of 'total quality management'.[2] In the major business corporations on which these forms of organisational development have been modelled, ethical policy and standards development have been found to play an important role in giving direction to change (Fig. 9.1).

Ethics is not an optional extra in business or health services management, but should be a routine and integral part of sound strategic planning and management. Corporate statements of an organisation's mission, vision and values mean little if they cannot be 'cashed out' in workable corporate and operational ethical policies, and if these are not applied in a hospital's or clinic's ordinary everyday business. This is because an organisation's choice of values plays a crucial role in defining both its short- and long-term goals and the practical meaning of 'quality' in its service delivery and the products it supplies. Clarifying values also serves to determine what kinds of processes and systems are most appropriate to achieve its objectives, and to monitor its performance.

Sound strategic ethical management is based on the application to a whole organisation of the methods of continuous quality improvement where strategic planning and management are directed by the values that are fundamental to the organisation. In such an organisation, its values play a central role in defining its leadership style, employee development, the way it does business and the quality of its products or the services it delivers. In order to accomplish this, it is necessary to get away from a narrow individualistic model of ethics and to recognise the various levels where ethical problems arise:

- External stakeholder level – ethics in strategic planning and inter-agency relations
- Internal stakeholder level – ethics in corporate management of human and financial resources
- Team leadership level – ethics in interdisciplinary cooperation and teamwork
- Individual level – ethics in personal decision-making and employee development.

In addition, those who are to exercise leadership, administrative and management roles in corporate life require skills in a number of practical areas of moral competency, namely:

- skills in clarifying and applying values to everyday operations
- skills in making sound and well justified ethical decisions
- skills in setting organisational standards, ethical policy and rules of conduct.

Developing competence in practical ethics also requires understanding of fundamental ethical

(A) Process improvement/Ethical policy development cycle

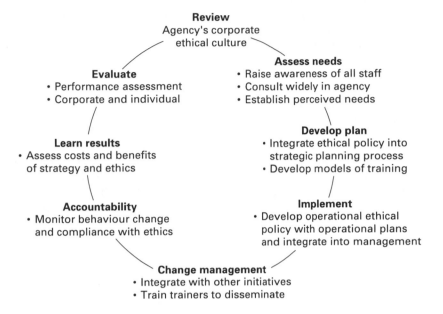

Review
Agency's corporate
ethical culture

Evaluate
• Performance assessment
• Corporate and individual

Assess needs
• Raise awareness of all staff
• Consult widely in agency
• Establish perceived needs

Learn results
• Assess costs and benefits
of strategy and ethics

Develop plan
• Integrate ethical policy into
strategic planning process
• Develop models of training

Accountability
• Monitor behaviour change
and compliance with ethics

Implement
• Develop operational ethical
policy with operational plans
and integrate into management

Change management
• Integrate with other initiatives
• Train trainers to disseminate

(B) Integrating ethics in corporate planning progress

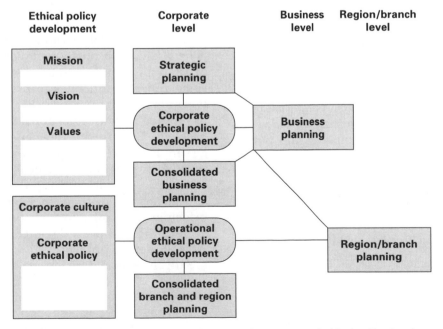

Fig. 9.1   RADICALE model for continuous improvement. **A**: Process improvement/ethical policy development cycle. **B**: Integrating ethics in the corporate planning process.

principles (e.g. the principles of justice, respect for personal rights and beneficence or responsible care). Sound management practice presupposes that these principles are applied competently with discrimination and judgement at individual, team and corporate levels.

Skills in clarifying and applying values to everyday operations

In previous chapters, we have discussed the importance of values for ethics and of critical self-assessment of the goals to which one is committed as an individual and as a nurse. Because our choice of values determines the means we adopt to achieve our short- and long-term goals, it is also crucial that in any business or organisation there is clarity about the values which operate within it – at the corporate management, professional and individual levels. It is also important that employers and employees not only have insight into the competing (and sometimes conflicting) values which operate in any moral community, but also have the necessary skills to deal with and resolve serious conflicts of values. One way this can be effected is by engaging the key stakeholders (or their representatives) directly in the process of ethical policy development. Codes of ethics or codes of conduct are of little avail if there is not real ownership of them by all the staff in an organisation. This process also enables people to understand how the fundamental principles and values should influence decision-making and policy-setting in the organisation.

Skills in making ethical decisions

In the first chapter we pointed out that ethical decision-making is not some kind of mysterious or occult process, but a type of problem-solving process which requires practice and skill to apply well. We stated that whether you are a detective, lawyer, scientist, doctor, counsellor, nurse, accountant or public servant, you follow broadly the same steps in problem-solving:

- collect and assess the evidence and define the problem

- consider what principles and values apply to the case
- review the options and choices available in the situation
- devise an action plan, with clear objectives
- act effectively to implement the plan and observe the process
- analyse and learn from the results.

We will be discussing ethical decision-making in greater depth in the next chapter and will be examining a number of models that can assist us in understanding and applying problem-solving methods to ethical problems more effectively. The main point which needs to be emphasised here, however, is that making ethical decisions must be carefully distinguished from making ethical policy, or setting standards and laying down rules. Ethical decisions are always directed to solve particular problems, involving oneself or other specific individuals, at a particular time and place. Decisions, like incisions, cut into the texture of life and change things, often irrevocably. Choosing one course of action also cuts out the possibility of pursuing some other course of action, for the time-being and maybe for ever. Policies and rules, however, are general and apply not to single acts, but to classes of acts or problems. They are designed to give us some general guidelines to prevent identified types of problem from recurring; or, if they recur, to provide us with rules for dealing with such problems. Because rules are general, they cannot be simply or directly applied to particular situations. To do so requires practical wisdom and life experience, so that we can choose the best available means and methods by which to apply our principles and rules to each problem so as to achieve the best possible outcome (this is how Aristotle defines prudence).

Skills in ethical decision-making are not confined to skilled application of problem-solving methods in making *personal* ethical decisions. In any organisation, business or government department, most decision-making *is an activity of committees or teams* and requires complex skills in analysis and negotiation to explore the interests of concerned stakeholders. At a corporate level, chief executive officers and senior managers are involved in the complex diplomacy and politics of negotiations with government and in inter-agency consultation and collaboration. Devising means to consult with and involve relevant external stakeholders in the process, and suitable methods for taking account of different agencies' policies and procedures, makes ethical decision-making at these levels even more complex, and we need training and skills to do it properly.

Skills in setting standards and ethical policy

Skills in setting sound ethical policy or determining standards or 'performance indicators' also have to be learned. Policy development requires that an organisation has clarified its values, where there are people with experience of making responsible ethical decisions, and where staff have sufficient relevant experience to develop sound policies, i.e. policies that will work and will be 'owned' by all affected by them. 'Management by memorandum' or 'making policy on the hoof' is a case not of assertive management, but of incompetence, for in such cases, managers mistake government by edict as fulfilling the responsibilities of policy-setting. This is actually the least effective way to manage people and is frequently unethical in both its demands and methods of implementation. Because 'policy' is often 'handed down from on high', people often think the term 'policy' refers either to aspirational statements of organisational ideals or simply to the autocratic demands of the boss. The former are thought to be vague and applying to everything in general and nothing in particular, the latter to be unreasonable and arbitrary. Policies are often thought to be impractical because such vague general statements cannot be directly translated into operational rules and procedures and that can have measurable impact. It is often said of policy, and the policies of governments in particular, that 'the way to hell is paved with good intentions' (or 'carpeted with copies of unfulfilled election promises').

This could not be further from what is intended by the term 'policy' in a sound business or public administration environment. Policies are useless unless they are workable, i.e. they can be operationalised in everyday practice. If they are practical in this sense, they can result in real benefits to all stakeholders, employees and customers (e.g. better working conditions, increased income and productivity, reduced costs and less inefficiency). Policies are useless unless the effects of their implementation can be measured. The new jargon of management – 'benchmarking', 'strategic planning', 'target setting', 'effective implementation' and 'performance management' – is part of the process of applying sound policy to the systems and procedures of any operation. Sound policy-making can be applied at a personal level to one's own work or family finances or to one's professional performance; or it may relate to the operation of one's team and the operation of a whole corporation. Policies would not be worth the paper they are printed on if they did not 'cash out' in assessable and ethical procedures, improved systems and methods of dealing with conflict, change and the proper monitoring or audit of performance.

An ethical policy is an official statement, on behalf of stakeholders or recognised authority within a moral community, which outlines a general ethical approach to dealing with recurrent types of problems or difficult situations. An adequate ethical policy must fulfil a number of conditions, namely:

- specify the class of problems it is meant to address
- set out the overall ethical approach and objectives adopted
- list standard procedures and the ethical justification for them
- provide a framework for decision-making and conflict resolution
- set criteria for monitoring performance and implementation of the policy
- indicate a clear strategy to achieve endorsement of policy by stakeholders.

What we suggest is that application to personal or organisational practice of these general requirements of sound policy can be helped by adopting a standard procedure or protocol for conducting

---

Box 9.3 POLICY model for setting standards and ethical policy

P – Problem type that requires standard policy/procedure
- What type of problem do you face and what is its scope?
- What are the main causes of this type of problem?
- What do you propose to do about it?

O – Outline ethical approach and objectives to be recommended
- What ethical principles are directly relevant?
- How will you consult about the overall approach to be taken?
- What are the objectives of your proposed policy?

L – List the standard procedures to follow and their ethical rationale
- What practical steps or procedures must be followed?
- What is your ethical justification for each step/procedure required?
- What incentives/sanctions will apply for compliance/non-compliance?

I – Identify methods to resolve conflict over policy's implementation
- What channels are there for identifying problems or discontent with policy?
- What measures are to be used for negotiation, or to resolve disagreements?
- What procedures are there for dealing with grievances or appeals?

C – Check out the effectiveness of policy to achieve its objectives
- By what measures will you test the effectiveness of your policy?
- How will you assess personal or team performance in relation to policy?
- How will you measure or audit performance of the whole organisation?

Y – Yes to policy! Strategy to ensure 'ownership' by stakeholders
- By what means will all stakeholders be informed of the policy objectives?
- How do you propose to get endorsement of the policy by stakeholders?
- When and how frequently should the policy and procedures be reviewed?

Box 9.4 Charter: promote responsive public services

- *Paradigm* – guaranteeing service standards; quality assurance; inform clients
- *Client* – empowered to claim their rights by proactive professional help
- *Professional* – responsible and accountable; acts as custodian of public rights
- *Principle* – equity: equality of outcome for groups

---

policy or standards development. In Box 9.3 we set out a checklist that helps to give a practical focus to the steps that need to be taken in setting ethical policy.

CORPORATE ETHICS IN HEALTH CARE

In earlier editions of this book, we developed an analysis of different models or approaches to professional ethics, based on *code, contract* and *covenant*. With the advent of the 'contract culture' in the welfare state and public services, there has been a new emphasis on the commercial imperatives of income generation, quality assurance, customer focus and respect for the patient or customer's 'right to choose'. There has also been a greater emphasis on the responsibility of health service providers to demonstrate competence in management of the resources funded from the public purse and to guarantee the quality of professional services provided to consumers. In order to do justice to the ethical demands of public accountability, it has been necessary to introduce a fourth model–that of *charter* – as we saw in Chapter 4. In corporate ethics, the charter model (p. 76) has tended to be expressed as in Box 9.4.

For better or worse, then, we have entered the era of 'citizen's charters'! We have charters for all kinds of 'consumers' – for parents of schoolchildren, for taxpayers, for business clients, even for prisoners and patients! *A Patient's Bill of Rights*, originally developed in the United States by the American Hospital Association (1973), can be seen as an ancestor of the *Patient's Charter*, and it has spawned a variety of new charters of patients' rights (see, for instance, DoH 1991b). While cynics might see these as merely an extension of public relations and marketing, the more serious ethical purpose behind this model is to emphasise the duty of public accountability in large business corporations and public sector services. If charters are to mean anything, then clear standards have to be set for the delivery of services, and commitments made not only to maintaining those standards, but also improving them in the light of consumer criticism and market research. While the duty to provide the highest quality service possible for the benefit of clients/patients has always been implicit in the very concept of professionalism, what this new emphasis on quality assurance and quality improvement does is to make this duty explicit and open to public scrutiny.

There has been a movement in the management of business and public sector organisations which has been referred to as the 'new corporatism' (French 1995, Kitson & Campbell 1996, Beauchamp & Bowie 1997). There are risks in the new corporatist approach to the ethics of organisations, in so far as it may lead simply to reinforcement of corporate self-interest or may be expressed in closed and authoritarian institutions. On the other hand, there is a real potential to rediscover an holistic approach to ethics as an enterprise of the whole organisation, based on equal opportunities policies and fair and equitable power-sharing between people, in a working community that sees itself as a moral community (see Box 9.5). What this approach means in terms of management of health services is adopting ethical policy and standards development as an integral part of organisational and staff

---

> **Box 9.5** Adopting a holistic approach to corporate ethics
>
> - Instead of corporate ethics being seen as merely necessary for dealing with discipline, corruption or fraud, it becomes an integral part of the agency's ethos, strategic and operational planning.
> - Operational systems, procedures and training programmes are set up in such a way that ethics is introduced into the bloodstream and contributes to the ongoing life of the body corporate, its planning for growth, organisational change and employee development.
> - Sound ethical policy is seen to contribute to both corporate and individual well-being, and thus collective commitment to the new ethos of ethical management and practice is seen to be advantageous to all, to be secured by negotiation rather than edict from above.
> - Quality assurance, standards setting and peer review are seen to be a normal part of ethical management – encouraging development of skills and confidence in self-audit or monitoring, thus reducing dependency on legalistic, authoritarian, `disciplinary' approaches.

---

development. This can have as many benefits for health service structures as it has for business and industry, and it need not be motivated by anti-liberal policies. However, there are rather different ideologies that inform Anglo-American and European models of management of public services within a developed capitalist economy and industrial society.

The political ethics of corporate responsibility has been marked by a heated debate centred on the concept of 'stakeholders' – there being an inherent tension between the traditional liberal model of unrestricted competition in a 'free' market economy and the emerging sense of moral accountability of providers of public services to 'clients' and 'consumers'. These 'stakeholders' in public services –whether as tax payers, contributors to health insurance, or purchasers of services – have rights that have to be respected. Defenders of a more traditional capitalist ethic argue simply *'caveat emptor* – buyer beware!', making it the responsibility of the purchaser to check out the quality of the product and to know better next time.

Capitalist business ethics, following the classic Anglo-American economic analysis of Milton Friedman, has contended that a business exists solely to maximise profits for its 'stockholders', namely those who invest venture capital in a business, carry the financial risks and therefore deserve to profit from its success. Managers who contribute to 'good social causes', unless it can be justified as 'promotional advertising', are, to put it bluntly, guilty of theft. From this point of view the corporation is simply a nexus of contracts with various parties. Other 'stakeholders' do not count and do not have any special rights. As long as employees are treated fairly, consumers are happy and contracts to suppliers and the state are met, then the firm has no other financial responsibilities to the community at large, other than to generate profits and pay the required taxes to the state.

There are those who argue that for a corporation to be a responsible corporate citizen it must recognise that it not only has rights (as a corporate 'person'), but also duties to other stakeholders besides the stockholders with investments in the company. From this point of view, a corporation is a responsible member of the wider moral community and not only owes a duty of care to its employees, suppliers, customers, the local economy, local and state government, but also has a duty not to pollute the environment and to contribute to the common good of the wider community which it both serves and on which it depends for its labour, markets and goodwill. These obligations on a corporation correspond to a range of rights claims of varying weight for different 'stakeholders.[3] Along the same lines, Michael Albert, in his book *Capitalism against Capitalism* (1993), distinguishes between what he calls the 'Anglo-American' and 'Rhine' models of capitalism; he sees the former as aimed at the achievement of 'individual success and short-term financial gain', the sole function of a business being 'to generate profits', whereas the latter in continental Europe 'tends to look beyond the bottom line and see the company as fulfilling a variety of needs which range from job creation to the enhancement of national competitiveness' (p. 13). While the Anglo-American 'stockholder' model is individualistic and profit-orientated, the Rhine 'stakeholder' model of capitalism sees its organising principle in a community of interests between a company and its employees, and a company and its consumers. Alex Robertson (1997) argues that this approach has its roots in the European Catholic tradition of social solidarity, compared with the more individualistic culture of Anglo-American Protestant variety.

Clearly, applying each of these different models to the management and financing of health care has a different ethical rationale, and each would have different consequences. It is the task of critical and professionally applied ethical policy development to weigh up such ideological alternatives and choose between them in the light of evidence and sound argument. Those implementing policy, procedures and practices, whether as administrators or ministers of state, owe it to the public to give both a clear rationale and intelligible ethical justification for the position they adopt, and to assure consumers that their practice will be transparent and their financial management open to critical scrutiny.

Firstly, ethical policy development can play a crucial part in the life of small or large corporations in the context of their organisational review and development. Developing a 'mission statement' and 'values statement', if developed as a whole corporation community enterprise, with effective consultation and participation at all levels, can be a powerful and invaluable means of building corporate solidarity. Staff commitment to and 'ownership' of the ethical policy can give a new sense of purpose and direction to their work and help create a new sense of corporate identity and integrity. However, if this is merely a cosmetic and public relations exercise, it is bound to fail, to deepen divisions and to reinforce workforce cynicism. Properly integrated into organisational development, corporate ethical policy can embrace not only agency–customer relations (including quality assurance and charters of client rights), but also internal policy on human resources management, the ethical accountability of management, staff discipline and fraud control.

Effective ethical review and policy development require staff with the necessary skills and authority to implement the policies and monitor compliance. The skills required are 'people management skills', competence in the core skills in applied ethics mentioned above, skills in working out with staff appropriate performance targets and methods of performance assessment (including matters of financial and ethical probity). Applying the now familiar stages of the problem-solving process to corporate ethical review and ethical policy development is necessary – from collective needs assessment, joint planning, teamwork in implementation to meaningful corporate ethical audit and performance assessment. In this way the conditions for the well-being of the whole corporation can be identified, means found for promoting those ends, and energy and resources committed to achieving them. Ethical policy development is about corporate and individual behaviour modification. To work, it requires sincere commitment of management and staff to collaborate in the process, and a major commitment to developing skills in applied ethics, the management of change, conflict resolution and dealing with resistance to change.

Secondly, corporate change can only be effected through fostering a sense of collective or corporate responsibility for that change. Ethical policy development is a key means of building a sense of moral community among those working in an organisation. What is required is training to develop skills in group work and in facilitating meaningful power-sharing in groups. Without these, there will not be credible ethical direction of the organisation or constructive resolution of conflict. A genuinely ethical culture is necessary for the development of trust and commitment to joint action for the common benefit of the corporation, for its members and the client population it serves. If real teamwork and collective commitment to common values and standards are achieved, policing of staff performance and behaviour becomes virtually unnecessary. It can be regulated in most instances by peer review and constructive support and skills training for staff in personal profiling and individual performance review. Disciplinary and grievance procedures will always be necessary. However, these are relegated to much lesser importance if the emphasis in ethical policy development is on meaningful participation. This brings positive benefits to all staff and to the business, which flow from working by ethical standards, rather than working to rule.

This may sound overoptimistic, for in medicine and nursing there has been a great reluctance to make peer review really work. Too often there has been a 'closing of ranks', out of a misguided sense of loyalty, to defend colleagues from criticism or charges of incompetence (e.g. where the person concerned has a serious alcohol or drug problem, or a psychiatric disorder). If peer review is to work, there has to be more than token commitment to the policy. It is a prime example of a situation in which involvement of all stakeholders in developing the policy and in endorsing its implementation is necessary if all parties are to 'own' it and apply it in their everyday practice. Recent scandalous cases in Britain – of unacceptable mortality rates among newborns in Bristol, due to incompetent surgery on infants with heart

defects, and misdiagnosis or late diagnosis of breast cancer in Kirkcaldy in Scotland due to poor record-keeping – are cases brought to light by independent critical peer review of local practice. However, if operating on a regular basis and in a constructive and non-threatening environment, these problems can be prevented and those whose skills need to be improved can be identified and given the necessary help.

Thirdly, the well-being of corporations depends critically in practice, as well as ethically, on the corporation's commitment to the personal and professional development of its whole workforce. Justice and equity in access to training and opportunities for self-improvement not only foster a sense of being valued by all staff, but also mean that they give value for money in terms of service in return. The 'great discovery' of General Motors (as a giant multinational), in making its comeback from near economic ruin, was summed up by one of its chief executives as 'Train, train, and again I say train your staff'. Ethics is fundamentally about human beings, about valuing human beings, and if human resources management is not a priority in any firm, it would be questionable whether this was ethical, however much stress is placed on 'quality assurance' and 'quality improvement'. The time invested in training personnel in interpersonal skills, in group work and communication skills, in effective support and supervision of others, in skills in developing their potential, pays off not only in better understanding, trust and cooperation, but in effective teamwork and higher productivity.[4]

The process is more concerned with the definition of the positive values of the corporation (the commonly held beliefs about what will promote the well-being of the organisation, its staff, its clients and the wider community), rather than policing misconduct. In a health care setting, the ethical goal could be summarised in terms of health care institutions themselves becoming health-promoting for all involved. There are perhaps obvious contradictions in hospitals or health centres being stressful and unhappy places to work. Where little consideration is shown for the physical, mental, and social well-being of staff, where working conditions are poor, canteen food unhealthy, smoking is permitted and staff relations conflictful, these institutions are likely to be illness-inducing rather than health-promoting.

If ethics is about securing the conditions for human flourishing, promoting human well-being, then the 'health-promoting hospital' (health centre or health authority) is not only a requirement for congruence between health policy and practice, but is also a necessary ethical ideal as well. However, where the fabric has been neglected, working conditions and pay are poor, where morale is low and absenteeism is high, the malaise may have more to do with the institution's management than with the performance of staff. It may be that the hospital organisation is 'sick' rather than that the staff are 'malingering'. Concern about the health of the institution and the environment in which they have to work is a quite proper ethical concern of nurses. It is just as important as concern for their patients' health and well-being. In fact the health and well-being of patients, and the quality of service they receive, may have more to do with the 'health' of the institution and 'healthy' management/staff relations than with strict hygiene and efficient routines. Given serious concern by nurses about the poor state of health of an institution, and if, additionally, management or local government will not negotiate or cooperate in making improvements, nurses may have to contemplate collective action, including strike action if necessary, to ensure that attention is given to the problems.

Ethics ought to be an integral part of industrial relations in the management of hospitals and the running of health services. Sound ethical policy should be developed to cover both responsible and publicly accountable service delivery, management of staff and the allocation of resources. Ethics applies both to the management side and the staff side. It is not only about regulating behaviour, disciplining substandard practice or malpractice, eliminating fraud or resolving industrial disputes; it is also about building an ethical culture in an organisation, promoting cooperation based on real consultation and mutual accountability, encouraging delegation of responsibility to self-directed teams, and building a real sense of community and commitment among staff. Ethics is thus not just about the imposition of management values, corporate ethical policies and standards development on an organisation; it is also about the rights of workers to participation in decision-making, recognition of good service, justice and fair dealing with staff, equal employment opportunities, and good mechanisms for conflict resolution and management (see Box 9.6).

Box 9.6   'The house that ethics built'

Focus on 'how?' rather than on 'what?' (in quality improvement and ethical policy development)

Corporate ideals
- Corporate values statement
- Statement of ethical principles
- Human resources development
- Communication systems

Ethical review procedures
- Review corporate culture
- Management styles (managers)
- Accounting and accountability
- Specific work procedures
- Individual responsibility
- Performance review

Opportunities
- Professional development
- Quality of life at work
- Relevance to promotion
- Working time and toil

Scope for participation
- Goals and targets setting
- Skills training
- Planning and audit
- Enhanced responsibility
- Debriefing and feedback
- Rewards and recognition

Monitoring measures
- Ethics discussion document
- Staff involvement – aiming for
- Self-regulation/peer review
- Structures of support

Statement of ethics
- Ethics in the workplace
- Business/organisational ethics
- Ethical review procedures
- Revisable code of practice
- Disciplinary processes
- 'Fraud management'

INDUSTRIAL ACTION, OR THE 'RIGHT' OF NURSES TO STRIKE

In the course of the last half-century, strikes and various forms of so-called 'industrial action' have become commonplace among health care workers, whereas previously their interpretation of the 'caring ethic' meant that strikes were virtually unheard of before World War II. In the past 20 years, forms of industrial action have been taken by a variety of health care workers ranging from medical consultants to junior hospital doctors, nurses and a variety of professions allied to medicine, ambulance drivers and paramedicals, hospital porters and catering staff.

Historically, nurses have been reluctant to take strike action, although from the earliest times they have staged demonstrations. Until 1987 the traditionally conservative Royal College of Nursing (RCN) was opposed to nurses taking industrial action, particularly in pursuit of wage claims. The RCN has favoured 'no strike' wage deals with nurses, based on guarantees from the government that it would underwrite nurses wages and working conditions by having them index-linked to the rate of inflation or comparability with other professions such as civil servants. During the 1987 National Conference of the RCN, however, this policy was changed in favour of qualified support for nurses taking industrial action in circumstances where standards of patient care and staff morale are so badly affected by poor pay and working conditions that the health and well-being of both are put at risk.

The earlier 1977 RCN *Code of Professional Conduct* unequivocally rejected strike action as a legitimate weapon to be used by nurses, particularly if such action put at risk the safety of patients (RCN 1977, Clause 4). On the subject of industrial action, most students surveyed in 1977 by the RCN believed that they had a primary duty to ensure the safety of patients when nursing colleagues or other health care workers withdrew their labour. Some student nurses thought they might be justified to take industrial action, but only in extreme situations when necessary improvements in standards of care were not being

made by their local health authority. This action would only be contemplated where patient care was compromised, and even then they thought action should only be taken in units where patients' lives would not be at risk, e.g. in day hospitals. The problem that remained for nurses who objected to strikes 'on principle' concerned the attitude they should adopt towards health workers who did – whether in pursuit of wage claims or objecting to unacceptable working conditions.

Attitudes in the nursing profession in the UK have changed under pressure from a number of quarters, mainly caused by changes in the political economy and management of health care introduced by the Conservative Government of Mrs Thatcher. However, attitudes have also been influenced by the critical reports of public commissions of enquiry into (mainly long-stay) hospitals, by the example of successful industrial action taken by other health care and ancillary workers and by break-away nursing unions with more radical policies than the RCN.

In the wake of the enquiry into the appalling conditions at the Normansfield Mental Hospital (HMSO 1978a), nurses were publicly criticised, both in the report and in the national media, for not doing more to draw the attention of the authorities (or the public) to the fact that standards there had deteriorated to levels that were unacceptable. It was argued that nurses as public officers charged with the care of patients have a duty to protect the interests and welfare of patients and, if necessary, to take industrial action when the standards of available patient care fall below acceptable levels and endanger the health and safety of patients. The Normansfield enquiry found that the appalling standards of patient care were partly attributable to the intolerance and high-handedness of the responsible consultant, but also to the poor state of buildings and equipment, poor staffing levels and poor morale. Whether demoralised nurses in such a hospital could have organised effective industrial action may be doubtful. However, considerations of justice and the interests of the long-term safety and well-being of the patients demanded that some drastic action should have been taken by nurses. The risk of short-term inconvenience to patients would have been justified in the context of the longer-term interests of psychiatric services in the district.

A series of 'work-to-rule' campaigns by nurses at a major psychiatric and several general hospitals in Scotland during the 1980s, by way of protest at 'unacceptable cuts in staff, which put both patients and staff at risk', were clearly motivated by concern about standards of patient care and the nurses' own working conditions. But the rhetorical question asked by politicians through the media was: Are nurses, as a profession committed to caring for the most vulnerable people, ever justified in taking industrial action, working to rule or going on strike? The various trade unions representing nurses in the UK adopted different policies on this issue over this period.

Strikes by hospital porters and ambulance staff, with sympathetic support from nurses, helped to radicalise nurse opinion on the matter, and the example of the strike in 1991 by UK junior hospital doctors had a direct impact on nurses. Their strike was over the injustice to patients and to medical staff of having to work 108 hour/week contracts without adequate medical back-up. (Similar strike action is being contemplated in Australia as we write in 2000!)

In both cases, junior doctors have argued (with the backing of their national medical associations) that working such long shifts while being on call at night has meant unacceptable fatigue with loss of judgement, putting the health and safety of patients at risk. Despite the fact that they earned extra money for working these unreasonable and antisocial hours, the junior hospital doctors led by those at Edinburgh's Royal Hospital for Sick Children and at other hospitals in the UK took industrial action. Supported by nurses and by skilful use of the media, they succeeded in bringing to public attention the risks to vulnerable patients where the competence of staff could be seriously compromised by sheer exhaustion. It was accepted that they had made a good case for changes to their contracts and improved working conditions. Immediate changes were made and a ministerial review was instituted to re-examine the general terms of employment of trainee doctors.

However, it is mainly the social, political and economic changes in the past 20 years that have forced changes in the attitudes of nurses and their perception of themselves within the workforce. In particular, in the 1980s, the introduction in many countries of a political economy of health based on monetarist policies of economic rationalism raised the temperature and blood pressure of nurses. With staff reductions (or 'down-sizing'), with forced cuts and/or 'contracting out' of many services and the application of 'user pays' policies to health service consumers, the mood has changed and nurses in many countries have become more militant in defence of their patients and in preserving their hard-won standards of pay and working conditions.

With the introduction of the 'internal market', a contract culture and charters of patient's rights, all the parties to the contract, purchaser, provider and client, have acquired new rights and obligations. The fact that these duties and quality assurance standards have in many cases been imposed from above without negotiation, and have been policed by management without the consent of the workforce, has led to industrial action of various kinds to protect the rights of nurses and other health care staff, and to clarify the terms of 'performance appraisal', including the requirement that management themselves should be more accountable, and their performance audited too. The innovations were in many cases shown to be unworkable without meaningful consultation, and therefore unlikely to achieve their intended 'reforms' either in the employer's or in the patients' or consumers' interests. It was increasingly being argued in the political climate of the 1990s that the question of the right to strike was becoming an obligation to strike by nurses – on clinical, moral and commercial grounds – if they felt that clients were not getting a fair deal, or they were unable to fulfil their obligations as 'providers' of health services under the charter of patients' rights.

It can be argued that nurses have been caught in a double bind – partly because the majority are women, but also because there is an inherent contradiction between the attitudes to industrial democracy and the right to strike in the occupational ideologies applicable to being a 'health worker' and being an independent 'professional' (Friedson 1994). From the standpoint of other occupational groups and the unions representing them, nurses have been criticised for having weakened their bargaining position by wanting to be treated differently as 'professionals'. These critics point out that nurses do not in fact enjoy the autonomy which self-employed people in the traditional professions have been able to exercise. If other industrial workers have the right to strike, then nurses, as employees of the largest single 'industry' in Europe, should also have the right to withdraw their labour – if negotiations with their employers over pay and working conditions have reached an impasse and there is no other way of achieving a settlement.

It has also been argued that the non-striking posture of 'professional' nurses lays them open to exploitation by the employing authority, and the idealism and dedication of nurses make them vulnerable to moral blackmail in pay negotiations, where their compliance with their duty only delays the necessary improvements (Ashley 1976, Johnstone 1994, Davis 1995).[5] This is a risk which is especially great in a huge nationalised industry like the NHS, where decisions about the allocation of resources are taken by bureaucrats or politicians in Whitehall, far removed from the actual working conditions of nurses. It has to be pointed out to those who argue that nurses are not morally justified in taking strike action on their own behalf, but only if patients are at risk, that it is impossible to separate issues of patient care from the pay and working conditions of health care staff (especially in large institutions).

The claim that low staffing levels and poor working conditions affect staff morale, resulting in deterioration of the standards of patient care, has often been made by nursing unions when negotiating nurses' salaries and employment conditions. But these claims have often been dismissed by management as self-interested and based on anecdotal evidence, while they point rhetorically to the dedication of other nurses working under difficult conditions! However, there have been several reports by independent bodies which have borne out this causal link, e.g.

the already mentioned Normansfield Hospital Enquiry and the critical report by the Scottish Mental Welfare Commission on the state of the mental hospitals at Lennox Castle and Larbert in 1991, where, they observed, patient care had suffered because of the demoralisation of the nursing staff. More objective scientific evidence for this connection is presented in an important study by Robertson et al (1995). In this in-depth observational study of four psychogeriatric hospitals, over a period of 4–5 months, in which quality of care was studied through standardised recording of staff's feeding, toileting and bathing of a stratified sample of patients, they found:

The findings point to a very strong relationship between job-satisfaction and the quality of patient care. Staff and patients in high-satisfaction (HS) wards proved more likely to initiate a conversation or other interaction. HS staff also offered patients more choice, independence, personal attention, supervision, information and privacy, and were more likely to converse with patients during feeding, toileting and bathing. Toileting and bathing appeared especially sensitive to these effects. Despite these differences, HS staff took no longer to feed, toilet or bathe their patients. These relationships are suggested to be mainly attributable to management practices, particularly at ward level, which influence both job satisfaction and quality of patient care.

How do we sort out the moral imperatives? The RCN code gives ultimate priority to the principle of beneficence, or the duty to care, when discussing the nurse's obligations. In a sense, this is the easy, more respectable and least controversial line to take. It is in accord with the model of the nurse unselfishly sacrificing herself in the service of humanity. However, beneficence alone does not define moral duty, as it does not take account of the rights of others or the requirements of justice either to nurses or to their patients.

The principle of respect for persons requires that the nurse recognises the patient's rights, including the right to adequate treatment. Where treatment is below standard to the point of endangering the health or even the life of the patient, the nurse has a duty to do something about it. This overrides her duty merely to continue to perform her prescribed institutional duties. The patient's right to privacy and respect for his dignity is compromised in overcrowded, poorly staffed hospitals, and the right to know is violated if patients are kept in ignorance of the fact that they could expect a better standard of care. The principle of respect for persons also applies to nurses themselves. Nurses are entitled to decent working conditions and a fair wage, within the limits of available resources, and they are entitled to protect themselves against being unjustly exploited. What this means in specific situations would have to be examined. The form of protest or strike action taken would have to be proportionate to the degree of risk to patients if action were not taken and to the degree of exploitation or intimidation suffered by nurses.

The principle of justice might also take precedence over the principle of beneficence in specific circumstances where patients suffer gross injustice owing to inadequate staff or medical resources which puts them at risk, or where health care staff suffer gross injustice which threatens their well-being and standards of patient care. Again the action taken, if it were to be morally justifiable, would have to be proportional to the risk suffered by patients or the injustice suffered by staff. However, in the real world the issue cannot be decided just by appeal to abstract principle, but questions of proper representation of stakeholder and power interests must be decided in advance, as well as a suitable framework for negotiation. These are matters of the political ethics of membership of a profession, which cannot be divorced from more personal aspects of responsibility.

Here it is easy to exaggerate, and the rhetoric of pay negotiations, for example (especially when they are conducted in front of the media), invariably exaggerates the risks and injustice involved. It is relatively easy to envisage the kind of extreme situations where strike action would not only be justified but become a moral duty. If nurses were terrorised and threatened with loss of their jobs and banishment if they did not do their duty, even though paid only starvation wages, then they would be justified in staging a revolt. However, in less dramatic circumstances, it is often more difficult to determine whether the nurse's duty to care

should take priority or whether nurses should withdraw their labour in pursuance of justice and proper respect for their rights and those of their patients.

On the matter of strikes, the law in the UK is rather confused. Discussing strikes and the NHS, Gerald Dworkin (1977) observed that in terms of Section 5 of the Conspiracy and Protection of Property Act of 1875, 'it is a criminal offence for any health service employee wilfully and maliciously to break a contract where there is a risk to a patient's life or limb'. However, he went on to point out that industrial action within the NHS has in some instances attempted to remain technically within the law by adopting two strategies: (1) work-to-rule or work-to-contract, so that the letter if not the spirit of the contract is honoured, and (2) undertaking to deal with 'emergencies' so that those who are at risk are not affected by action taken.

The risk in such strategies is that they become hypocritical. The work-to-contract is in reality a strike with serious implications for many patients – in terms of unfair delays, deterioration in standards of care, or worse. The 'emergencies only' policy is a farce, when porters or ambulancemen decide which cases are emergencies. Even doctors cannot in good faith justify a policy of selective action that is designed to affect administration rather than clinical care. As Lord Amulree said in a House of Lords debate: 'The decision to treat emergencies is…humbug, because one cannot tell what is an emergency' (RCN 1977).

It is part of the rhetoric of industrial disputes to talk glibly about 'the right to strike'. There is no such right in law where there is risk to the health and safety of other people, and a strike is even less acceptable in moral terms if it puts others at risk. The fact is that the talk is loudly about 'rights' when we wish to draw attention to injustice or felt justice of our cause, but rights cannot be rights if they are exercised at the price of harm to others. Here the considerations of formal justice have to be tempered by respect for persons and the duty to care for others. The alleged 'right to strike' is not enforceable in law; on the contrary, it often means using extralegal means to bring pressure on employers or the state to yield to demands.

Writing in the 1970s, Professor Kahn Freund argued that instead of trade unions being the victims of a repressive system of legislation which discriminates against them 'the danger has shifted. It seems that there is a spreading belief that the law cannot put any limits on any action taken in the course of an industrial dispute' (Freund 1977). His argument was that if any kind of industrial action for whatever cause, however trivial, justifies extralegal action, then there is a serious risk that the law and legal institutions will be brought into disrepute and society will be thrown into anarchy. On the other hand, there were those at the time who argued that such revolutionary action was necessary, because the structure of a capitalist society and economics was inimical to the health of people and was leading health services to a state of collapse.

However, the majority of people did not agree and certainly did not consider that such extreme measures were justified to achieve the necessary reform and improvements in society. A majority of the electorate endorsed measures taken by Mrs Thatcher's government in the 1980s to prohibit secondary picketing (i.e. support by workers of one union for industrial action taken by another) and to restrict the rights of trade unions under law. Public support was based on successful exploitation of views like Freund's in party propaganda, rather than on any considered moral position. Government trade union reforms aimed at restricting the power of trade unions were justified by appeal to such views and by the successful appeal to the fear of voters that trade unions were in the business of either pursuing selfish ends or promoting anarchic political action, possibly even by intimidation.

The rise in unemployment in the 1980s (in labour-intensive industries) and the corresponding fall in union membership, and the fragmentation of unions by the device of introducing local 'enterprise bargains', undermined organised labour's political power. This was rationalised in terms of 'increased productivity' and the need to reduce 'overmanning' (particularly in the service industries). The risk is that if such action is taken too far and the power of organised labour is undermined to the degree that workers have no real power or legitimate mechanisms to negotiate over pay or working conditions, then the situation becomes ripe for riot and anarchy. To be both fair and equitable, on the one hand, and politically realistic and effective on the other, a nice balance has to be maintained between the power of governments, employers and workers if the demands of justice and the common good are to be properly safeguarded. For service industries such as hospital and health care services, or education and social services (where women make up the vast majority of workers), there are particular risks that the hard-won legal and political rights of workers and trade unions are lost, to the particular detriment of women.

If, from a moral point of view, nurses are only justified in taking strike action if, and only if, there is serious deterioration of services and risk to the lives of patients, then it is more difficult to establish a credible case based on arguments that poor wages for nurses threaten the health of patients. The danger is that the use of the rhetoric of 'campaigning for better standards of patient care' tends to be heard by politicians and the general public as special pleading and is often regarded with scepticism by those commanding the control of resources. It might well be more effective, and appear more honest to the public, for nurses to separate the issues of standards of patient care from disputes about their own wage claims. Each issue can be the basis of responsible protest (or even strike action) in appropriate circumstances.

THE 'CRISIS' OF THE WELFARE STATE AND THE NHS

The welfare state in the UK emerged out of a process which began with the Liberal reforms of the Victorian period and in reaction to the Bismarckian reforms in Germany in the late 19th and early 20th centuries. These had resulted in piecemeal improvements to welfare rights and services before World War I. While the Beveridge report (1942) is often taken to mark the establishment of the British welfare state, a good argument can be made for the fact that Beveridge simply consolidated and rationalised existing welfare provisions begun by the Liberal reformers. These included, for example, labour reforms affecting working hours and old age pensions (1909) and family allowances (1930). The Beveridge report was not so much a revolutionary as an evolutionary development of ideas that were emerging in Europe. Beveridge's vision was of a society organised to tackle what he imaginatively called 'the five giants': want, disease, ignorance, squalor and idleness. He also held out the promise that these could be conquered by the development of appropriate public services, such as social security, health and education, and the application of government policies to ensure full employment. The British welfare state evolved into five public service divisions: health, education, social security, housing and social work (or the personal social services), which could be seen to address Beveridge's 'five giants'.

Beveridge's proposals proved extremely popular, probably because they were in tune with the universalist spirit of the postwar years and also because the scheme's social insurance basis enabled people to regard their benefits as entitlements, thus removing the stigma of the hated 19th century Poor Laws. What he contributed was a good administrative base on which to establish an integrated and universal system of health, education and welfare provision to be funded by a single form of national insurance. The development of the British welfare state continued post-Beveridge, too, e.g. with the provisions of the 1948 Child Protection Act.

While the various forms of welfare state that came into being after World War II remained relatively unchanged for the succeeding 40 years, during the past decade these systems have been put under considerable strain, as governments have wrestled with the 'blow-out' of welfare costs and the impact of alternating periods of inflation and recession. It has become almost a cliché to say that welfare states all over the world are in a state of 'crisis' and that health services in particular are in a state of crisis. We have to ask ourselves if this really is the case, and if so, what the ethical implications are of the various policy options which are being offered as 'solutions'.

Robertson et al (1992) offer three broad hypotheses for the 'crisis' in welfare, namely:

● the financial crisis of welfare
● the crisis brought about by major social and demographic changes
● the crisis of confidence in the ideological rationale for the welfare state.

The *financial crisis* of welfare is usually explained as resulting from the gap which it is alleged has developed between people's unlimited expectations and demands for state-provided welfare services – in health care, social security and education – and the limited resources available to governments to service these 'needs'. The major *social and demographic changes* which are putting health care systems under stress are, paradoxically, the results of their very success. People are living longer to survive in increasing numbers into extreme old age, and more people born with physical or mental handicaps or who have suffered handicap as a result of trauma or disease are also surviving. The cost to health and welfare services of this vastly increased number of elderly people and growth in other 'dependency groups' was not planned for in projections of costs of the welfare state. The *crisis of confidence in the ideological rationale for the welfare state* is perhaps marked by a shift in political and moral priorities from the postwar universalist concern with social justice and equity to a privatised morality which is more concerned with the fulfilment of personal rights and material success – where the demographic changes have been reflected in changes in socio-economic outlook and expectations. The broad internationalist and socialist vision which inspired the postwar founding of welfare states has yielded, in part, to 'new right' economic rationalism, combined with uncritical belief in the self-regulating nature of the free market. This has come to be expressed in a new hard-line managerial conservatism ('let the mangers manage'), a defence of personal autonomy (for those that can afford it) and the unfettered right to pursue one's own financial advantage in the speculative generation of wealth.

Concerted efforts have been made by 'new right' politicians to persuade us that their diagnoses of the malaise of the welfare state and their prescriptions for its treatment represent the only possible and correct interpretation of the facts. However, evidence from social attitude surveys shows continuing public support for the welfare state, and it is important to recognise that other interpretations of the facts are possible, that alternatives to 'new right' policy options are available, and that we are not driven by necessity to accept their conclusions. Vic George and Peter Taylor-Gooby (1996), in their book *European Welfare Policy: Squaring the Circle*, argue that other alternatives are possible to those offered by economic rationalism. We can always reshape history and society by our choices. Some of these choices will be ethical choices, or choices with important ethical and social implications. Consider the various assumptions that are listed in Box 9.7.

The claim that the welfare state is in a 'state of crisis' is as much a matter of persuasive definition and tendentious political rhetoric, as it is a matter of 'fact'. The claim is put forward as if it were an unquestionable scientific truth, but it is based on a number of questionable assumptions which need to be challenged and justified before they are accepted. These assumptions are not only matters of economics, but involve value judgements which relate to our fundamental beliefs about ourselves and human society. For economics itself is not a value-neutral science, nor is economic policy ever independent of political and ideological considerations. The economic debate about the future of the welfare state is also a debate about the future of human society, about the terms and conditions for human coexistence and cooperation, and the future of human life on this planet. Ethics is at the heart of this debate (Robertson 1996).

Driven by doctrinaire 'new right' economic and political assumptions, governments have instituted major reforms and repeated reorganisations, which have left people working within these systems feeling 'punch drunk' with change, insecure and depressed at their seeming powerlessness to bring about constructive change. People working in the human services have

---

Box 9.7 Questioning assumptions about the welfare state

That human beings are necessarily selfish and, given half a chance, they will exploit the welfare state to their own advantage
The myth that society is crawling with people who are parasitic on the health services, who are social security scroungers and tax dodgers, is a creation of political propaganda and is not borne out by the evidence (Cartwright & Anderson 1981, Cartwright & Smith 1988).

That we pay too much tax already, and that we cannot afford the welfare state or the National Health Service
The question here is a matter of perception of priorities. On the one hand, Bacon & Eltis (1976) have argued that the growth of welfare has resulted in resources being diverted to social development rather than investment in industry. On the other hand, when the UK spent £18 billion per annum on alcohol in the 1980s, the total cost of the NHS at £23 billion might seen relatively modest given the services provided. Besides, the UK spends less on health relative to GNP than do Italy, Germany, Sweden, Australia and Canada (OECD 1987). The issue is a matter of contention between those who favour a change to a greater proportion of private provision of health care, and those who want to retain the health service as a national welfare service (Klein 1989).

That the Beveridge plan and Keynesian economic principles on which the welfare state was based either no longer apply or are discredited
The debate between 'monetarist' and 'Keynesian' economists is not dead, but rather it is the case that the latter is experiencing a revival after the dominance of the former during the Thatcher years. This is not the place to enter into discussion of economic theory, but suffice it to say that the debate is not merely technical, but ideologically and value-based, with real personal and political choices to be made here (Robertson et al 1992).

That the crisis of the welfare state was inevitable once the economic going got tough and economic growth gave way to recession
Ian Gough has argued that the apparent success and stability of welfare states from 1944 to 1974 was made possible by 'the long boom' – a period of unprecedented worldwide economic growth. From this perspective the commitment of governments and people to the concept of the welfare state remained good only so long as welfare provision seemed to help lubricate the machinery of industrial development and mitigate its worst social effects. The collapse of popular support for Communism in the USSR and 'Eastern Bloc' countries could be interpreted as a delayed expression of the same process. Gough takes a critical and sceptical view of capitalist 'democracies' and their ability to deliver a

just and equitable society. Once again, the pros and cons of alternative forms of social and economic organisation are matters of legitimate ethical and political debate by professionals and people generally (Gough 1979).

That the concept of welfare is workable in small communities where face-to-face accountability is possible, but in large, impersonal and bureaucratic states people do not have the same investment in preserving the common(wealth)
The large-scale pooling of resources and sharing of risk which is the mark of collective welfare is based on assumptions of fair give and take, by individuals and between generations. The postwar welfare states were set up by a generation who believed overwhelmingly in their duty to provide, first and foremost, for the needs of young people by substantial family allowances, free education and health services, low-rental housing and subsidised interests rates. What has happened in the past 25 years, however, is that 'the welfare states for youth have been abandoned, and replaced by welfare states for the ageing'. This 'ageing' of the welfare state has been explained by some social historians (e.g. Thomson 1992) as a cohort phenomenon, where those who have grown up with the welfare state have come to take the security it provides for granted, without recognising a corresponding duty to contribute to the well-being of generations who come after them.

That the huge sums of money raised by states through taxation, to finance welfare, could be more usefully put at the disposal of the private sector
The question of who benefits (*cui bono?*) from the privatisation of welfare, and how, is an important issue of political ethics in the contemporary debate. There are, as the moguls of industry say, 'big bucks to be made from privatising welfare'. The increasing power of mega-multinational business conglomerates, especially in the pharmaceutical, medical technology, medical insurance and private health care areas, to dictate policy to governments is a matter of concern to various analysts (Gough 1979, Taylor-Gooby 1986).

That the private sector is always more efficient and cheaper than public sector services can be, and that the application of business management to the delivery of health care, education and social welfare will be better
The myth that costs of administration in the NHS are disproportionately high was exposed in the 1979 Royal Commission Report on the NHS, where it was shown that, in the NHS, a smaller proportion of the total budget was spent on administration than in most businesses. Furthermore, comparisons that tend to be made between public and private sector hospitals do not usually involve comparison of like with like, for the private sector tends to have concentrated its services on the high-profit, high-turnover sectors of health care rather than on the

perennial burden of chronic medicine, mental illness and care for highly dependent groups – where care is labour-intensive and bed turnover inevitably slow. What measures are used of 'costs' and 'benefits' or 'efficiency' are of crucial moral and social importance here (Wicks 1987).

increasingly seen themselves (as much as their clients) as victims of actions taken by distant politicians or faceless bureaucrats. We must ask whether people in the caring professions are not becoming victims of the same type of 'learned helplessness' (Seligman 1975) that they see in their institutionalised patients and multiply deprived clients. The question is what to do about this depression and professional malaise? It may well be that the problem is not a personal problem, but a structural one requiring new forms of health and welfare provision (George & Taylor-Gooby 1996).

'Reorganisation', 'restructuring' and 'rationalisation' have been the order of the day, not only in the UK but in most of the capitalist democracies which had previously adopted forms of welfare services. Attempts to reorganise and restructure health, education and welfare services have occurred in the UK, New Zealand, Canada, Australia, the United States and other democratic countries. While these are described as being 'revolutionary' and as marking 'fundamental change', they have also been described as instituting a new type of managerialism which operates a system of 'management by insecurity'. Do these changes represent real change and progress, or just a shift in ideology and political rhetoric with little real benefit to the public or improvement in the provision of services? Concerned about the impact of so-called reforms on mental health services, Annie Altschul (1989) encapsulated the challenge in her Mental Health Guest Lecture: 'Let's not be afraid of change, but let's have some REAL change for a change!'

What we have had for the past two decades has not been real change, but rather 'Stop!–Go!' responses to what has been a fundamentally stagnant economic and political situation. 'Inflation–deflation–reflation' has been a repeated pattern of attempts to 'manage the economy' and to 'manage social policy'. The reality has been little real change in the sense of real improvement in social services. Rather, what has changed is that the moral and political consensus which has sustained and supported health, education and welfare services for a generation has been undermined, and the new breed of politicians have politicised health, education and welfare. From being rather marginal to the political process, these issues have been brought back to the centre of politics in a way that has not been the case since World War II. If this change results in politicising professionals in the health, education and welfare services, so much the better – maybe then we will get some real change for a change! However, while political activity without passion is empty, political activity without principles is blind. What fundamental principles are involved in the work of the caring professions and in politics? What policy options do we have? What approaches are possible to solving the 'crisis' of the welfare state and the NHS? What moral and ideological beliefs do we think should inform the process of reorganisation, reforming or restructuring of the NHS?

RESPONSES TO THE 'CRISIS' OF THE WELFARE STATE AND THE NHS

Broadly speaking, there have been two different kinds of political approach to the crisis of welfare, namely social corporatism and market pluralism (Mishra 1984).

Under *social corporatism*, workers' and employers' organisations work within a framework of shared collective responsibility for all decisions concerning both social and economic policy. Representatives of employees and employers, as the major economic interests, work in partnership with the government, seeking to arrive at an agreed course of action in respect of the principal objectives of welfare capitalism. These are to maintain full employment and social programmes, as well as ensuring profitability, low inflation and economic growth. Among the primary advantages claimed for such a system are that it avoids government overload and it enables social and economic policies and objectives to be chosen together.

The evidence suggests that a social corporatist strategy enabled Austria and Sweden to maintain near full employment during the recession of the 1970s and 1980s, while also pursuing policies that entail high social spending and taxation. This has not been without strain on their economies, but their overall economic performance and level of growth did appear better than those of other countries during this period. More recently, Sweden has had to make adjustments to its system under the impact of economic recession and 'new right' political thinking. In general, the social corporatist approach requires a wide social consensus on which to base a 'social contract'. This 'social contract' seeks to guarantee profits for employers in exchange for jobs and state welfare provision for their workers. It would thus seem to have offered an effective basis for securing the future of the welfare state (Robertson et al 1992).

Advocates of *market pluralism* seek to strengthen the 'capitalist' element in the present system of welfare capitalism. They believe in a return to the disciplines of the marketplace and rely on market forces to rectify the economy. They see economic and social policies as largely independent of each other and regard the first priority of government as that of 'getting the economy right'. Under market pluralism, the industrial area is marked by free collective bargaining. Organised groupings are seen to pursue their sectional interests with a view to affecting policy decisions in ways that will maximise advantages for themselves. Market pluralism has clearly gained prominence in the debate over the future of welfare states.

British Conservative governments from 1979 to 1991 worked under these assumptions, and would seem to have been striving to achieve the following general objectives:

- to reduce public expenditure
- to create an environment and attitudes conducive to individual enterprise
- to reduce the public sector in both industry and social services.

Robertson et al (1992) pointed out that there has been a determined attempt to increase the role and the size of the private sector in the fields of education, housing and health. As far as housing policy was concerned, tenants in local authority housing were encouraged to buy their houses at prices some way below the market rate: a measure which proved popular but which has also created a shortage of housing for those persons who cannot afford to buy their own home. With regard to education, the government set up the 'assisted places' scheme which gave assistance to families on low(er) incomes, if they so choose, to send their children to private schools (this has since changed). So far as health is concerned, the privatisation programme has hitherto taken two forms: (1) privatising some hospital ancillary services, e.g. laundry, catering and cleaning services; and (2) measures to encourage extension of private health insurance.

The White Paper *Working for Patients* (DoH 1989a) introduced a number of major changes, under the principles of the 'internal market' which the Conservative Government sought to promote, following the Enthoven report (1986). For example:

● Health authorities (or health boards), instead of planning hospital services for the geographical region for which they were previously responsible, were to buy services from the hospitals they judged to be offering the most attractive terms, wherever those were located.
● The health authorities/boards were required to make an annual surplus on the budget allocated to them by the government, by various forms of income generation.
● In an experimental trial, a number of volunteer general practices were allocated a budget to provide drugs, hospital care, etc. to the patients for whom they were responsible. They then had to buy these services on behalf of their patients at the rates they found most favourable.
● A proportion of hospitals were encouraged to opt out of the local health service management system as 'hospital trusts'. By this means, for example, they were given greater powers to manage their own budgets and special powers over the hiring and firing of their medical staff.

The 1983 Griffiths report, *Community Care: Agenda for Action*, sought to extend the principles of the internal market to personal social services, in particular for elderly and handicapped people. Griffiths suggested that instead of a diversity of people having responsibility for their care, one single official should be responsible for the coordination of their care in the community, comparable to the role of GPs in primary care. In order to streamline community care, the following changes were proposed (DHSS 1983):

● Central government should play a clearer strategic role through the appointment of a Minister for Community Care.
● Local authority social services departments should become the lead agencies in coordinating social care, facilitating and enabling the planning and delivery of care by relevant agencies. Their responsibility would be to assess the needs of particular clients and devise 'packages' of services appropriate to their needs, and to monitor how appropriate and effective these proved to be.
● In the delivery of these customised packages of care, the social services would have authority to buy in appropriate services, as well as provide these, where indicated. Instead of being a monopoly provider, the social services were to acquire the role of consultants and brokers of services, using statutory, commercial and voluntary providers.
● Local social services were to be encouraged to make maximum use of this range of services provided by the private, voluntary and statutory sectors to 'encourage competition', 'broaden scope for choice' and supposedly 'reduce costs'.

The 1983 Griffiths approach to social care planning sought to focus on the needs of the individual, rather than on the organisation of services available. It represented a development that has some parallels with the shift from task-oriented nursing care to patient-centred nursing care, with its emphasis on the responsibility to develop individual care plans for specific patients.

The White Papers *Care in the Community* (DoH 1988) and *Caring for People* (DoH 1989b) accepted the general thrust of the Griffiths proposals. Of considerable importance to nurses is the underlying distinction which these official policy documents make between 'health' and 'social' care, and the implied redefinition of which professional groups have responsibility for care of various groups of disabled people in their homes and non-institutional settings in the community. Social care is defined as the responsibility of the social services, including home-help services, occupational therapy and the provision of aids and adaptations for disabled people, adult training centres, day care, respite care and residential nursing home care. Health care is defined in this context as including long-term residential medical care for people with high levels of dependency, hospice care, and assessment of mentally handicapped and mentally ill people for discharge into social care, and these are the responsibility of the health services.

This redefinition challenges nurses to re-examine the scope of their own definitions of nursing, and the relationship between physical nursing, psychological care and counselling, and concern with the social well-being of their patients. The fact that the administrative redefinition has been driven mainly by the attempt to save on salary costs for professional staff and to shift a greater burden of care onto relatives, volunteers and the community should be a matter of concern for both health policy and ethical reasons.

The fiscal policies of the Conservative governments after 1979 attached importance to attempts to increase the efficiency of the various social services and, in particular perhaps, the health service. This has been in line with a traditional stream of Conservative thinking in relation to the welfare state. Thus, we have seen the introduction of general managers at both regional and local levels of the NHS. Their main tasks have been, for example, those of reducing costs by means of using staff resources more effectively, 'rationalising' use of hospitals or beds, etc. Part of general managers' remuneration has been based on performance-related pay, i.e. dependent on savings made.

There has been a regular reduction in the powers and independence of those sectors of civil society – local government and the trade unions – which might behave in ways that contradict the overall thrust of government policies in the service areas we have been considering. For example, in the case of local government this has been achieved through (Robertson et al 1992):

- introduction of limits on financing of local authority services
- councillors being subject to financial penalties if they exceed funding targets
- reduction in the planning and management functions of local government through measures which give management powers to 'users'.

Robertson et al (1992) ask whether the state acceptance of responsibility for the health and welfare of its citizenry will prove to have been just a passing phase in the evolution of the capitalist democracies, or whether the problems which the welfare state was intended to solve are not permanent aspects of our social life and political organisation in post-industrial society. They suggest that the ethical and political debate about the common good and the ends and means for achieving it will continue. As for the relative merits of the popular alternatives currently being offered, much could be said for and against these options, and detailed comparison and analysis of their relative effectiveness may have to be left for some time until their outworking in new systems can be properly evaluated (Mishra 1990).

Social corporatism has sought to spread the costs and benefits of adaptation across the population. Rather than pursuing economic and social objectives largely independently of each other, countries such as Austria and Sweden have set up arrangements which permit representatives of identified interests within society to seek solutions that harmonise economic and welfare aims. The pressures of economic recession and public reaction to high rates of taxation to pay for health and social welfare (drummed up by new right politicians) have necessitated changes to the systems of both countries which mirror developments in the UK and/or Germany. Kersbergen Kees' (1995) study of *Social Capitalism* and Michael Albert's (1993) *Capitalism against Capitalism* explore the possibilities for adaptation of social corporatism to the needs of Europe in the 21st century (cf. Robertson 1997).

Market pluralism, on the other hand, has tended to favour the upper classes, and imposes considerable costs on the poor and the lower strata generally. In the view of not a few critics of the actions of the Thatcher governments, developments since the late 1970s have seen a move back towards the principle of 'less eligibility' and the harsh assumptions of the Victorian Poor Law. In support of this contention one can point, for example, to the considerable burden that has been placed upon the poorest and most disadvantaged members of British society by policies that have been pursued during that time. The cuts that have occurred have consistently been concentrated in services for needy minorities, e.g. in housing and unemployment benefit, discretionary grants within the social security system, local authority residential accommodation and the home-help service. Demands imposed on clients by the social fund are a striking example of this tendency.

EVALUATION OF THE 'INTERNAL MARKET' REFORMS OF THE UK NHS

The practical achievements of the Thatcher experiment seem rather modest when set against the claims originally made for it. During the years of Thatcher governments and attempted savings in public expenditure on the major social services (social security, health, housing, social work and education), the only area in which real cuts in spending were achieved was that of housing. [Here over half a million council houses were sold off between 1979 and 1985, these sales being effected with an average direct subsidy of more than £10 000 per house (Taylor-Gooby 1986).] Scrutiny of the take-up of such forms of private welfare cover as private health insurance, occupational pensions and sick pay schemes, schooling and commercially rented (as opposed to local authority) housing suggests that the long-term expansion of private welfare has been relatively little influenced by the policies of the Thatcher era. In the health field, for example, take-up of private insurance has been largely linked to occupational schemes. The take-up has tended to be corporate

rather than individual. The evidence is that people tend to use private medicine for the treatment of more minor ailments, to avoid the sometimes lengthy waiting times in the public sector. When more serious or life-threatening conditions are involved, the public system is overwhelmingly preferred (Klein 1989).

Robertson (1996), in an important paper, sets out to evaluate the apparent benefits and problems involved in implementing the 'internal market' reforms of the UK NHS, initiated by the Conservative administration between 1989 and 1997.

Benefits of internal market reforms Robertson (1996) summarises the evidence and lists the apparent benefits under a number of headings:

Responsiveness to patients. On improved responsiveness to patients' needs, he quotes Smee (1995) who claims there is:

...much evidence that individual Trusts are taking advantage of their freedoms to innovate and improve services. These changes cover a very wide range of activities, from patient hotels, through new forms of care for people with learning difficulties, to fuller utilisation of hospital theatres.

He notes that Kennedy & Nichols (1995), a fundholding GP and hospital consultant respectively, argue on the basis of their experience that GP fundholding has brought benefits to patients – in particular reduction in the numbers of 'long-waiters' and expansion of 'in-house services' to patients; and Glennerster et al (1994) claim that GP fundholders have a greater financial incentive than do non-fundholding GPs to engage in health promotion and ensure that their patients are healthy.

Improved links between different service sectors. Kennedy & Nichols (1995) claim that due to regular meetings between key clinicians, hospital managers and community care teams, there has been an improvement in inter-agency liaison.

Increased awareness of quality issues. Appleby et al (1992) claimed early on that 81% of district general managers reported that the new contract culture had led to improvements in the quality of services. However, this evidence was challenged in a BBC Radio Scotland programme on 21 November 1996. Joss & Kogan (1995) remark that the introduction of quality assurance regimes and techniques, driven by market pressures, have put managers on notice that consumers expect more information on quality and performance in the NHS and that these developments have strengthened the hands of managers; whereas Kennedy & Nichols (1995) claim that the reforms have led to wider acceptance of medical audit and patient satisfaction surveys.

Accountability. Against the background of some favourable comment on improved standards of accountability, Robertson observes that democratic accountability in the NHS has always been rather weak, and therefore marginal improvements may appear more significant than they really are. Measures that are cited by various authorities as contributing to improved accountability are the obligation of 'providers' to report to district general managers (Appleby et al 1992); the contestability of contracts (Robinson & Le Grande 1995); and the fact that the work of consultants is open to scrutiny in a completely new way (Kennedy & Nichols 1995).

Improved use of resources. In this area, Glazer (1995) reports that 'in some aspects of care the NHS is better run, wastage is less and patients and GPs are getting a better deal'. Smee (1995) claimed that in the first 2 years of operation, hospital trusts outperformed other hospitals, with increasing numbers of patients receiving treatment. Glennerster et al (1994) review evidence that fundholding GPs were using their purchasing power to pressurise providers into improving services if their custom was not to be withdrawn in favour of others.

Problems of internal market reforms On the negative side of the 'balance sheet', Robertson (1996) draws attention to he following problem areas:

Adverse selection. Johnson (1990), Hudson (1994) and Saltman & von Otter (1995) are cited as providing evidence of 'cream-skimming', i.e. that 'providers' and 'purchasers' would be reluctant to take on the type of patients who would require substantial resources for their treatment and ongoing care. Kennedy & Nichols (1995) found that patients were nervous of the implications for themselves if they required expensive treatment or care. Smee (1995) expresses concern about the 'potential perversity' of some of the incentives facing fundholders, and that hospitals might be tempted to concentrate on 'profitable patients'.

Administration and transaction costs. Glazer (1995), Kennedy & Nichols (1995), Robinson & Le Grande (1995) and Smith (1996), each produces evidence of increases in administrative and transaction costs of various kinds accruing to purchasers and providers as a result of having to operate under the new internal market requirements: increased management, support and transaction costs; time and resources spent on bidding for and negotiating new contracts each time round; costs of installing appropriate information technology for data processing and communications to operate the system; the inability of purchasers or providers to rely on long-term contracts to provide stability of service of the kinds that are possible in the commercial sphere. Here Glennerster et al (1994) conclude that 'GP contracting seems to be better, but to cost more'.

'Commercialisation' of NHS values. Appleby et al (1992) and Glazer (1995) question whether the ethos of public service and a caring ethic can be sustained and defended in an environment of increasingly cut-throat competition for contracts, cost-cutting and general economic rationalism.

Lack of public accountability. In contrast to the optimistic first reports on accountability in the new contract market system, Glennerster et al (1994) and Collison (1995) observe that so far as accountability to the public is concerned, financial transparency and accountability are sadly lacking, with appeal to 'commercial confidentiality' being used as an excuse not to divulge information of political interest to the public, and Collinson points to the fact that because the CEOs and trustees of the hospital trusts are not elected or democratically accountable, but appointed by the trusts (with the approval of the Secretary of State), there is a risk of cronyism and misuse of public resources, as evidenced by the findings of the Nolan Committee (1995).

Problems with contracting. Most serious problems of the internal market relate to the fact that it is not (and probably never can be) a truly free market. Munro (1996) conducted a review on behalf of the Scottish Office Health Department, which provided evidence of the fact that purchasers and providers were not really contracting, there was limited 'competition' for contracts, a tendency to use 'block contracts' and for health boards to award contracts to their own provider units.

'Fragmentation' of the NHS. The 'fragmentation' resulting from privatisation of services, contracting out and the establishment of a mixed economy of NHS hospital trusts and other hospitals under district health authority control etc. is criticised on two grounds: first, that it has complicated access for patients; and second, that it has made overall strategic control, management and public accountability more difficult (Glennerster & Matsaganis 1992, Munro 1996, Durham 1997).

While, on the one hand, there is evidence that the 'internal market' model has limited application and relevance to the actual relations between hospitals and their 'clients' (whether individuals or fundholding GP practices), on the other hand there is no substantial evidence that GPs have either the skills or the desire to take on the role of purchasing, or consultants the role of entrepreneurs (Durham 1997).

Furthermore, available evidence also points to a continuing high level of public support for the welfare state (Golding & Middleton 1981, Taylor-Gooby 1986, Ranade 1994, Jowell et al 1995). However, these selfsame surveys also indicate that such endorsements of public provision often coexist with a degree of acceptance of the private sector.

Taylor-Gooby's (1986) discussion of the results emerging from his extensive investigation of British attitudes towards the welfare state confirms a picture of ambivalence by highlighting the frustration people feel with the regulations and restrictions of the 'nanny state'. However, he also stresses the importance they attach to what they see as an 'adequate' level of welfare state provision, and their resulting opposition to real cuts in a system of services which they value. His conclusions remain valid and may be summarised as follows:

● The public would thus by and large appear to wish to retain the welfare state.

● Government attempts to dismantle the welfare state have been largely ineffective and regarded with deep ambivalence by the electorate.
● Current attempts at health service reform provide a good case in point. The internal market the current government is attempting to promote falls some way short of 'new right' ideals of a private market in health care.
● Widespread opposition to the reforms themselves reflects both a popular commitment to the ideal of public health service and the electoral peril awaiting parties which attempt substantially to modify that ideal (Robertson et al 1992).

It should be obvious that nurses cannot remain indifferent to these issues, nor avoid taking sides in the political debate about the political ethics of health care. To remain indifferent would be an abrogation of their duty to care (for their patients or for their own future as a profession) and it would represent a failure to exercise the proper civic responsibility which goes with the public office of a nurse, given his or her unique knowledge of health care at the sharp end. Fundamental ethical principles must be applied to the public and political domain as much as to the private and clinical domains. The only problem is that we feel less competent to deal with the former, and tend to rely on instinct and intuition to deal with the latter. To become more skilled and competent in deciding on matters of ethical policy and practice is an issue to which we turn in the next chapter. In it we examine some of the practical skills in ethical problem-solving and decision-making which all responsible professionals require, if they are to move beyond instinct and intuition and to apply the same degree of informed and practised competence to moral decision-making that they do to clinical judgements. We also look at what is involved in the process of ethical policy and standards development, as part of the responsibility of managers and staff in the new corporate cultures of the late 20th and early 21st century.

further reading

Role of the state in providing health care
Ashford D E 1986 The emergence of the welfare states. Blackwells, Oxford – *useful historical background to state involvement in health care*

Illsley R, Svensson P G 1984 The health burden of social inequalities. World Health Organization (European Office), Copenhagen – *classic WHO study with recommendations to UNO member states*

Olsson S E 1990 Social policy and welfare state in Sweden. Arkiv förlag, Lund, Sweden – *a useful reminder to British readers that Sweden has a proud record of state health provision*

Robertson A, Thompson I E, Porter M 1992 Social policy and administration. Health Education Open Learning Project, Keele University, Keele, Staffordshire – *a self-learning resource for nurses*

The nature of sound ethical policy
Allsopp J 1996 Health policy and the National Health Service: towards 2000. Longmans, London – *a challenging look at possible future directions for health policy in Britain*

Harrison S, Hunter D J, Pollitt C 1990 The dynamics of British health policy. Unwin Hyman, London – *a useful classic analysis of the policy development process in Britain*

Joss R, Kogan M 1995 Advancing quality: total quality management in the National Health Service. Open University Press, Buckingham – *a valuable introduction to TQM principles*

Kitson A 1993 Nursing art and science. Chapman and Hall, London – *raises some more general issues about the nature of nursing that should impact on policy formation*

When can or should nurses go on strike?
Jackson M P 1987 Strikes. St Martin's Press, New York – *a historical overview of strikes and lockouts and the various kinds of rationale that can be given for workers taking industrial action*

Johnstone M-J 1994 Bioethics: a nursing perspective. WB Saunders/Baillière Tindall, London, ch 13 – *a critical analysis of ethically sound and bogus reasons for going on strike*

Kerridge I, Lowe M, Mc Phee J 1998 Ethics and law for the health professions. Social Science Press, Katoomba, NSW – *a review some of the ethicolegal issues for health workers taking strike action*

Deciding priorities for health spending: counting the cost of health
Campbell A V 1978 Medicine, health and justice: the problem of priorities. Churchill Livingstone, Edinburgh – *an early but still useful introduction to the ethics of resource allocation*

Caplan A H, Callahan D 1981 Ethics in hard times. Hastings Centre Series on Ethics. Hastings on Hudson, USA – *a collection of philosophical essays providing good background for this chapter*

Mooney G 1992 Economics, medicine and health, 2nd edn. Harvester Wheatsheaf, Hampshire – *a classic analysis of the political economy of health by a respected health economist*

Wilkinson R 1996 Unhealthy societies: the affliction of inequalities. Routledge, London – *an encouragingly hopeful analysis of the world situation which also deals with 'nitty gritty' examples*

World Bank 1993 Investing in health – 1993 World Development Report. Oxford University Press, Oxford – *much quoted in this chapter, but introductory chapters are essential reading*

The future of health services – socialised or privatised health care?
Baggott R 1994 Health and health care in Britain. Macmillan, London – *a useful general overview*

Hudson B 1994 Making sense of markets in health and social care. Business Education Publishers, Sunderland – *a critical analysis of the effectiveness of market economics in health care*

Mishra R 1984 The welfare state in crisis: social thought and social change. St Martin's Press, New York – *a provocative, now classical, analysis of the crisis facing welfare states*

Saltman R B, von Otter C V (eds) 1995 Implementing planned markets in health care: balancing social and economic responsibility. Open University Press, Buckingham – *an excellent student's guide to the concepts behind the reforms*

end notes

1   See the reports of the (Nolan) Committee on Standards in Public Life, Vols 1–3, *On Standards* (1995 CM2850-I), *Local Government* (1996 CM3702-I0) and *Local Public Spending Bodies* (1997 CM3270-I), HMSO, London.

2   James P 1996 *Total Quality Management – Introductory Text*. Prentice Hall, New York.

3   See Beauchamp T L, Bowie N 1993 *Ethical Theory and Business*. Prentice Hall, New York – see the debate between Milton Friedman and R. Edward Freeman on stockholder versus stakeholder rights in Chapter 2.

4   This is the boast of both multinational companies such as BP and 'caring companies' such as Body Shop, based on their commitment to ethical policy and practice, and consumer audit.

5   Ashley's early work, *Hospitals, Paternalism and the Role of the Nurse* (1976), analyses some of the structural reasons for the political weakness and reluctance of nurses to take industrial action, in the American context, namely subjection to an ideology of duty, obedience and submission to administrative and medical authority. Johnstone's chapter, 'Taking a stand', in *Bioethics: a Nursing Perspective* (1994) is particularly good in the analysis it gives of the dilemmas as seen from within the profession in Australia. Davis's 1995 book, *Gender and the Professional Predicament in Nursing*, extends and continues the debate, examining it from the perspective of nursing in Britain.

some suggestions on method

Role of the state in providing health care
Students might find it illuminating to research the historical origins of health care provision in their country, or even the history of their hospital and the funding of its services. Given access to suitable library services, or archival resources at a local newspaper headquarters, students could be assigned the task to investigate the history of policy and funding for their institution or health services, and to report back to the class. Students could work individually or in groups, on local or national issues, dividing up the task with the tutor.

The nature of sound ethical policy
Here the tutor could come prepared with a number of current problems facing the nursing college, hospital or local health authority, and get the group to role-play a committee formulating policy about the type of problem indicated, using the POLICY model as a prompt and pro forma to ensure they cover all the key requirements of a good policy. This could be practised more than once to gain confidence in using this and similar policy-setting models.

When can or should nurses go on strike?
Class exercises around this question should deal with several levels of ethical exploration of the issue. They could first of all be asked to brainstorm as a group what ethical principles they think should be taken into account by nurses in deciding to strike or not to strike; secondly, to work in pairs and share with one another (in confidence) what kind of issues would be important enough to make them take industrial action, or

whether they never would. On being invited to share with the whole group, they might be encouraged to indicate whether they agreed or disagreed about nurses going on strike, and what principles and criteria they used to reach their shared or differing positions.

Deciding priorities for health spending
Examine a hypothetical proposal from the district health authority to shift resources from cosmetic surgery and IVF treatment to improve services to elderly people with dementia. The class could be asked to debate the merits and difficulties of this proposal for a range of interested 'stakeholders':

● local health authority
● local health consumers council
● individuals or pressure groups concerned with the needs of infertile couples, and carers of people with Alzheimer's disease
● local midwives and consultant obstetrician
● local long-term nurses and geriatrician.

Socialised or privatised health care?
Students could be asked to form a line in which they stand where they feel most comfortable on the continuum between total privatisation and total management by the state, and then be asked in turn to give a brief reason for the position they adopt. Next they might be asked in small groups to discuss the pros and cons of the 'welfare state' versus the 'internal market' as models for the funding and delivery of health care services, and then to report these back to the whole group for discussion.

Moral decisions and moral theory

10

Making moral decisions and being able to justify them

AIMS

This chapter has the following aims:
1. To clarify what is involved in making a specific decision, as distinct from seeking agreement about general ethical policies
2. To explore the variety of approaches necessary for the effective teaching and learning of competence in practical ethics
3. To explore methods of problem-solving in ethical decision-making and parallels with problem-solving elsewhere
4. To examine the necessary and sufficient conditions for free, purposeful and responsible action as moral agents.

LEARNING OUTCOMES

When you have read and worked through this chapter, you should be able to:
■ Describe and analyse typical situations demanding real decisions, rather than notional agreement about rules and policy

- ■ Discuss critically the role of 'conscience' and 'intuition' in our moral experience
- ■ Demonstrate understanding of different approaches to teaching ethics and skills in ethical decision-making, and ability to apply these in conducting tutorials
- ■ Demonstrate ability to apply the given models of problem-solving to specific cases taken from nursing experience
- ■ Demonstrate ability to make critical appraisals of the extent of a person's responsibility for his or her actions, by considering specific cases
- ■ Demonstrate understanding of what it means to give a systematic and comprehensive account of the reasons and grounds for a moral decision.

HAVING TO TAKE A MORAL DECISION

It was remarked in Chapter 5 that we tend, when discussing ethics, to focus on the 'big dilemmas', the urgent and dramatic situations where we have to take big and risky decisions. While it is perhaps understandable that we should focus attention on particularly painful problems and the difficulty experienced in taking decisions relating to them, this does tend to skew our perception of decision-making. For, in everyday life and in routine work, we take decisions as a matter of course, with little awareness of doing so, and without stopping to reflect particularly deeply on *what* we are doing, *why* we chose a particular course of action, and *how* we arrived at our decision or how we would justify it to someone else.

It is interesting that in Greek the word 'crisis' originally just meant 'decision time', not a time of drama, but a time *when we have to make a judgement about what to do next*. Obviously, when we are faced with life-threatening and urgent problems and have to do something, we are faced with a crisis in both senses, but the critical need is to take a decision. We commonly use the word 'crisis' to refer to major life events, turning points in our lives

or turning points in the course of an illness. Commonly, these events are associated also with making difficult or painful decisions. However, most decisions we take in life are neither dramatic nor dangerous. In performing routine work, numerous minor decisions are taken every day, including routine moral decisions.

It is important to stress that not all moral decision-making is associated with drama and crisis. On the contrary, most of us develop remarkable skill at making rapid moral assessments of the problems facing us in the practical situations in our lives and in taking the appropriate decisions. Some decision times will be crises for us, but like the insurance company's advertising slogan, it is important generally 'not to make a drama out of a crisis'!

In general, our family upbringing and experience of school, work and the wider community equip us with knowledge of the moral values and rules in our society, and we develop by trial and error practical skills in applying them in our daily lives. Some of these values and rules we will adopt as our own, to others we may simply show the respect that is necessary to get on with people, but others again we may actively criticise or reject. Whatever we do and whichever lifestyle we choose, our decisions and actions, our moral judgements, will embody and express our value judgements. Like learning to walk or run, where we employ the principles of physiology, mechanics and kinaesthetics without being aware of these, in routine decision-making we are applying scientific knowledge, practical experience, and organisational and moral principles in a highly complex process which we would find just as difficult to explain as the man challenged to explain how he manages to walk.

We do not normally reflect critically on what we are doing when we make decisions, particularly those decisions which involve application of our own or society's established moral values, unless we are faced with a crisis. In this sense, a 'crisis' may be interpreted as a situation which demands a decision, where we are challenged or forced to reflect on what we are doing, and where we are challenged to give a clear explanation of our reasons for deciding and acting as we do or have done.

Several factors may cause us to experience decision time as a crisis:

- *The first kind of crisis is where we are entering unfamiliar territory*, e.g. when the trainee nurse first encounters the practical and moral problems of nursing a dying patient, or when the experienced nurse acquires new responsibility as a ward sister or manager. Here, lack of appropriate knowledge or skills, unfamiliarity with established rules of practice or ignorance of likely outcomes may undermine the confidence of nurses and force them to examine carefully how and what they are doing and why they choose, or chose, to act in a particular way.

- Related to this is a *second kind of crisis*, namely *where an individual suddenly finds himself faced with greater-than-usual responsibility*, or is obliged to act on his own, without the usual opportunities to check things out with colleagues or friends. Here the urgency of the problem that has to be dealt with and the need to accept personal responsibility may challenge us to seek a clearer justification for what we have done so as to be able to answer criticism if things go wrong, or to give reasons for our actions.

- *The third type of crisis concerns the nature of decisions themselves* – namely, that choosing one thing or one course of action forecloses other options (the word 'decision', coming from the same root as 'incision', has the connotation of 'cutting off' other possibilities). Deciding to accept one job rather than another or to marry one person rather than another has long-term implications for one's life and limits one's other decisions (although it may open up new possibilities as well). Choosing a particular treatment option for a patient may mean excluding other options, and following one course of action may often mean that one cannot go back later to try another course of action. Confronted with situations where decisions are irreversible or where the consequences will be far-reaching, we are faced with awesome responsibility, and these circumstances may also cause us to pause and reflect.

- *A fourth type of crisis is where we are faced with a genuine moral dilemma* – an irresolvable conflict of duties or a painful choice between two equally unacceptable moral outcomes. Here we are forced to reflect critically, not on the circumstances in which the decision is demanded, nor on the degree of responsibility demanded of us, nor on the likely consequences, but on the relative priority to be given to our moral principles, on how they are related to one another and how we are to act if we cannot resolve the conflict. Such cases of real dilemmas certainly do arise, and if we are faced with a crisis, namely a situation where a decision *has* to be taken, then we can be in a terrible quandary. We have to face up to the challenge to make a decision and to act as wisely and professionally as we can, without the comfort or security of familiar rules or established procedures to guide us. We also have to be prepared to accept responsibility for the outcomes, particularly if we have misjudged the kind of response required to deal with the crisis. Fortunately, such situations are fairly rare. Most moral choices relate to situations that recur in various forms in our routine work. If we deal with moral problems routinely in a responsible, systematic and disciplined way, we should be able to give a good account of ourselves and the evidence and reasons why we acted as we did when we are faced with real dilemmas as well. These decisions may in turn serve as a guide or basis for future action. Even though there may not be solutions to moral dilemmas, there are still methodical ways we can examine our options, marshal evidence and reasons, clarify the underlying moral principles and act with forethought rather than impulsively or just following blind prejudice.

- *A fifth type of moral crisis arises when we are forced to re-examine and justify our whole moral position*, as when someone demands that we justify our fundamental moral principles and values, or when some event in our lives causes us to call into question and to doubt the whole basis of our established moral beliefs. We are forced back to a more basic level where we are obliged to examine the presuppositions on which our moral beliefs are based and the reasons and evidence we could produce to justify them. While confrontation by another person, or a personal moral crisis, may represent a painful challenge to our moral beliefs, the discipline of philosophy is a systematic way in which we can study these questions and test solutions against those worked out by others over the centuries. This particular aspect of decision-making – namely, that concerned with moral theory and the justification of our fundamental moral principles – is the subject of Chapter 11. At this stage, however, we return to the analysis and description of the more basic characteristics of routine decision-making, and the justification of moral decisions and actions.

CONSCIENCE, FEELING, INTUITION AND MORAL JUDGEMENT

Since we do, in fact, make moral judgements all the time – about what we consider right and wrong in general, what we consider the best course of action in a specific situation – or make judgements about our own or other people's actions and characters, we tend to resist attempts to analyse the process involved (because we do this semi-automatically). We tend to appeal to 'the voice of conscience' or 'intuition', or say that 'it just felt right'. While these expressions have an important and proper place in our moral discourse, they can also represent a 'cop-out', a refusal to look at the underlying reasons why we act or have acted in a certain way.

However, our use of these phrases expresses our sense that moral judgement, decision and action are as natural a part of living and doing as breathing. We all grow up in some sort of moral community. We adopt some of its values, making them our own, while perhaps rejecting others. We form dispositions and learn routine patterns of effective action, by habit and practice, so that they become, as Aristotle said, 'second nature to us' – these are what we have traditionally called 'virtues' and 'vices', or 'competencies' in modern parlance. We have routine ways of justifying what we do to others and ourselves and/or making excuses for ourselves if things go wrong. Because our moral experience is coextensive with the rest of our human experience and permeates all we are and do, it seems perhaps rather artificial to try to

analyse it and separate out the moral decision-making bit from the rest of our daily living. We thus often appeal to the 'voice of conscience', 'gut feelings' or 'intuition' in justifying our actions, just because these terms express how much of all this has become second nature to us.

However, appeal to conscience or intuition to justify a moral decision can also be a form of mystification (as we suggested in Ch. 4), suggesting that decision-making is a kind of impalpable and private, even occult, process. The discussion at this point often echoes the school of thought which claims that 'nurses are born not made', that the attributes required of 'good' nurses – empathy and sympathy, sensitivity to the patient's real needs, gentleness, competence, efficiency – cannot be taught. Of course, some people have natural predispositions to care for people, and others do not. But if we can rationally understand and describe the nature of the skills required, then in principle we should be able to teach them. Likewise, some people may start with certain advantages of stable family life and moral upbringing, relevant experience and practical wisdom and may therefore appear more competent and confident in making decisions and exercising moral responsibility. However, even the most confident person can be shaken in a crisis, but it is equally true that most people can be trained to exercise or carry responsibility. They can be trained to cope better with routine decisions and crises. They can learn to give an account of what they have done, how and when they did it, and why they did it. However, this all presupposes the need for some awareness of training approaches, methods and management procedures, and it is this need that this chapter addresses.

In ethics, it is important to demystify moral decision-making, both for the sake of clarity and truth and to encourage people to address those forms of knowledge and skill that can be learned and taught. Ethical decision-making may be difficult to do well and methodically, but there is nothing occult about the process. Moral decision-making is but one particular form of problem-solving activity among other forms. We can learn a lot in ethics from studying other methods of problem-solving and then apply them to moral problems specifically. But there are also dangers that follow from failure to pay attention to the particular nature of moral decision-making, or from trying to force ethics to fit the demands of inappropriate methods.

The mathematician and philosopher Spinoza hoped to achieve the same degree of certainty in moral judgement that we can achieve in mathematics by reasoning about ethics *'more geometrico'*, i.e. by attempting to make moral arguments fit the 'procrustean bed' of geometrical reasoning and deduction. The result was either a gross oversimplification of the complexity of moral arguments, or just simply a caricature of them. Other philosophers have tried to apply the methods of the empirical sciences to ethics, to attempt to develop a 'scientific' ethics, based on 'facts' (usually of psychology or sociology), and which they supposed could be proved by scientific experiments. Neither of these approaches has been very successful or very helpful. We have to recognise the distinctive nature of ethics and the kinds of problem-solving methods that would be appropriate to dealing with moral decision-making. Aristotle, in the middle of the 4th century BC, suggested that 'it is the mark of a civilised man to demand only that degree of certainty in ethics that the subject matter allows'. We could hardly do better than to heed his advice. His own methods and approaches have stood the test of time remarkably well, and there is currently a considerable revival of interest in what he taught.[1]

There are many different approaches to problem-solving, which we use in different domains of our lives, some, if not all, being relevant to moral decision-making by nurses as well:

- experimental methods in the sciences
- logical analysis in mathematics
- probabilistic methods in statistics
- historical analysis in archaeology, social and personal history
- cultural analysis in anthropology and political science
- the methods of jurisprudence in law
- what Sherlock Holmes called 'deduction' in detective work.

In medicine, the doctor takes a medical history, examines the patient, seeks to elicit signs and symptoms, consults his theoretical and practical knowledge of medicine and allied sciences, and then proceeds to make a diagnosis, determine a course of treatment, monitor and evaluate the effectiveness of his interventions, and perhaps venture a prognosis. The 'good' doctor, from the standpoint of his colleagues, will make a general assessment of the success of his treatment of a patient in the light of his original assessment of the evidence and prediction of outcomes, taking into account actual outcomes. He should then incorporate what he has learned into his ongoing practice. However, whether the doctor is a 'good' doctor from the standpoint of his patients will depend on his possession of other skills and attributes as well.

The *Nursing Process*, for example, besides being a method of planning nursing care in an intelligent and rational way, also represents a way of demystifying nursing care. This is important to get away from the idea that nursing cannot be taught. However, rigid and unimaginative application of the Nursing Process will not guarantee either the quality of care or the competence with which it is given. Here feminist critics of rational models of decision-making which ignore feelings and relationships have some point, but caring for individuals alone is not a sufficient basis for making sound nursing decisions (Bowden 1997). The Nursing Process presupposes the nurse will apply knowledge and intelligence, as well as skill and sensitivity to the needs of individual patients in their particular situation. The knowledge and skills components can perhaps be directly taught, but the common sense and sensitivity are not so much taught as caught – learned by imitation of others with more experience of life and practical wisdom. Just as Aristotle suggests that we require both the intellectual and moral virtues to be complete and balanced people, the same could apply to nursing. The use of the Nursing Process as a problem-solving method in practical nursing is meant to improve practice.[2]

Whether one is talking about methods in medicine or nursing, religiously following the method does not in itself guarantee that you will be a 'good' doctor or a 'good' nurse. At the very least, however, it should help to ensure that you are a 'competent' or 'efficient' doctor or nurse. Similarly, the application of problem-solving models or moral theory to decision-making does not guarantee that the decision taken will be either wise or morally sound. Following a method, analysing a decision or planning a course of action in a systematic way only ensures that it is done in a more rational manner and enables clearer reasons and coherent justification to be given for what has been done. Acting responsibly means being able to give an account of what has been done and accepting that you are accountable (i.e. liable to have to give sound reasons for your actions). Following an appropriate problem-solving method for making moral decisions will help considerably in demonstrating intelligent and practical accountability. We would suggest that many of the arguments introduced by Roper et al (1981), in their book *Learning to Use the Nursing Process*, to justify the adoption of systematic care planning also apply to ethical decision-making.

Before continuing with the exploration of methods and requirements for effective moral decision-making and responsible moral action, it is perhaps worth pausing to consider the origin of expressions like 'conscience', 'intuition' and 'feeling'.

While the 'voice of conscience' may mean anything from the echo of parental authority to Freud's superego or the voice of God, the 'inner voice of conscience' seems, on the one hand, to refer to the sense of conviction we have about our moral beliefs and the internal authority they have for us in deciding what is right and wrong, and, on the other, to stand for collected and collective moral wisdom or practical experience, which lends weight to our feeling that a course of action is right. However, it is noteworthy that the original meaning of the word 'conscience' (from Latin *cum* = 'with', and *scientia* = 'knowledge') means 'having comprehensive theoretical and practical knowledge'. Conscience in the classical sense is that faculty which integrates awareness of moral values with theoretical knowledge and practical experience, enabling a circumspect view of things before taking action.

The most influential thinker on the subject of conscience in the English-speaking world is the philosopher and theologian Bishop Joseph Butler,[3] who in the 18th century defended the rationality of moral judgements as based on appeal to conscience as a faculty of the mind or 'principle of reflection' instilled by God in us all. Let us consider a classic passage from his *Sermons*:

... man cannot be considered as a creature left by his Maker to act at random, and live at large up to the extent of his natural power, as passion, humour, wilfuness, happen to carry him; which is the condition brute creatures are in; but that, *from his make, constitution, or nature he is, in the strictest and most proper sense, a law unto himself.* He hath the rule of right within: what is wanting is only that he honestly attend to it ....

But allowing that mankind hath the rule of right within himself, yet it may be asked, 'What obligations are we under to attend and follow it?' ... Your obligation to obey this law, is its being the law of your nature. That your conscience approves of and attests to such a course of action, is itself alone an obligation. Conscience does not only offer itself to show us the way we should walk in, but it likewise carries its own authority with it, that it is our natural guide, the guide assigned us by the Author of our nature.' ...

Conscience and self-love, if we understand our true happiness, always lead the same way. Duty and self-interest are perfectly co-incident; for the most part in this world, but entirely and in every instance if we take in the future, and the whole; this being implied in the notion of the good and perfect administration of all things.

Fundamental to this concept of conscience is that it is not some mysterious 'voice' in our heads, but rather the rational capacity to reflect on our nature and constitution as rational beings, and to intuit what is our duty in a particular situation if we are to act in harmony or accord with our true nature. For Butler, the fact that conscience is instilled in us by God is important because it gives conscience an authority that transcends mere subjective feeling or intuition. However, his account of conscience could be defended even if we did not believe in God, but merely affirmed that we share a common and given human nature, and have the capacity to intuit what that is and to judge accordingly.

The same could be said of 'intuitionism'. 'Intuition' literally means 'to look inward' (from the Latin verb *intueri* = 'to look at intently'). In moral philosophy (and the poetry of Coleridge) it has been interpreted as an integrative ability of the imagination to take the confusing variety of data and phenomena in a situation and make some kind of sense out of them. The faculty of intuition not only helps us to locate our experience in space and time, in relation to preceding and subsequent events and other similar or different situations, and enables us to imagine the possible outcomes of alternative courses of action, but it also assists us in 'making sense' of our experience.

'Feeling things are right' is not necessarily or exclusively a statement about private feelings (like 'I just had a gut feeling that it was the wrong/ the right thing to do'). It can also be taken to refer to the sense of having one's bearings, of being oriented, having a sense of direction about where one is going – a settled conviction that in relation to what you know and your past experience this is the most appropriate thing to do (Campbell 1984b). However, feelings are as important in ethics as they are in life. We ignore the feelings of others at our peril, and ignoring our own feelings can lead to our acting in bad faith or hypocritically, as both feminist and existentialist philosophers have emphasised. Much of what existentialist philosophers have sought to correct in the rationalist tradition, which grew up with modern science, concerns the importance of people's feelings as well as their cognitions in the life choices they make. Augustine (354–430 AD) said, 'If you wish to know what a man is, ask what he loves.' Our interests define who we are, what kind of people we are, what we consider worth living for and what we would be willing to die for. Because feelings are so personal and ephemeral, taken by themselves they are not a sufficient basis on which to base our judgements or our moral lives. Clearly, we need other evidence, reasons and principles on which to base our moral beliefs and decision-making. However, the logic of our feelings should also be taken into account. As French philosopher Pascal (1623–1662) said: 'The heart has its reasons, of which reason knows not.' For St Augustine there is a given order (ordo) in nature and a corresponding hierarchy in our loves, and it is the 'primary task of the moral life to determine our lives

in accord with the proper order of priority amongst our loves'.[4]

Exploring what is meant by decision-making in terms of 'conscience', 'intuition' and 'feeling' can only lead so far. Each term, as we have seen, is a metaphor for the possession of some kind of insight – whether self-insight into one's own motives and intentions, or the values one has made one's own, or insight into the demands of the overall moral situation and one's own feelings about how things are. Obviously all these kinds of insight are important and necessary, but unless we can 'give a reason for the faith that is in us' or give reasons for acting as we do, then we act blindly and we cannot really expect people to take us seriously – especially if we have to defend ourselves before a disciplinary enquiry or in court. What we need to consider next are the kinds of training or formation that will help us to become more competent and responsible moral agents, and better able to give an account of our decisions and actions.

DOES A GOOD MORAL AGENT NEED SOUND METHODS OR SOUND CHARACTER?

Opinions tend to be divided on which is more important – to teach people decision-making skills or to teach them virtue (if the latter can be taught!). The debate about this issue is as old as philosophy.

Socrates (469–399 BC) challenges us with a number of conundrums of the kind posed in the heading above. On the one hand, he suggests that we cannot be responsible moral agents without self-insight ('know thyself'), and on the other hand, he questions 'Can virtue be taught?'. Alternatively he suggests that 'virtue is knowledge', but also suggests that 'wisdom begins in the admission of your own ignorance'. These puzzles take us to the heart of ethics (Rouse 1984). Moral educators through the ages have tended to go for one or other of the two alternatives below, often to the exclusion of the other:

- emphasising knowledge of moral principles and methods of problem-solving as essential to the competent moral agent as decision-maker

● emphasising the need for self-insight and the cultivation of the personal habits and dispositions, which ensure integrity of character, consistency, dependability and responsibility in actions of the moral agent.

Aristotle (384–322 BC), in his *Nicomachean Ethics*, develops a system requiring two kinds of complementary skill or competency necessary for the balanced moral agent, namely what he calls the 'intellectual and moral virtues'. The intellectual virtues involve the acquisition of competence in a variety of methods and approaches to decision-making or problem-solving, while the moral virtues relate to the habits of character required for reliability, effectiveness and efficiency in action. The relationship between the intellectual and moral virtues in the character of a moral agent, and the need for a balance between them, is symbolised in an arch with two legs, joined by a

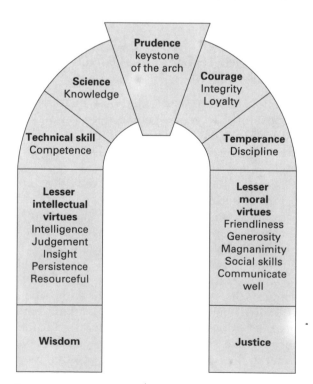

Fig. 10.1 Symbolic representation of Aristotle's view of the relationship between prudence and the intellectual and moral virtues.

keystone which is the faculty of prudence (Fig. 10.1). In what follows, we shall use this model to develop an approach to decision-making which takes account of methods necessary to develop both types of competency.

APPROACHES TO TEACHING ETHICS

Approaches to teaching ethics in the professions of nursing, medicine, law and accounting (as well as other professions) could be classified as falling under one of the following four models:

● The moral instruction school
● The ventilatory school
● The critical thinking school
● The situation ethics school.

Each of these approaches is often presented as if it were the only way to approach the pedagogy of ethics, and the others either dismissed as irrelevant or ridiculed. On the basis of our experience we believe each model has something to offer, but we also believe that none of them is adequate taken on its own. Each emphasises a different but valid part of our moral experience, but not one of these can be normative for the rest. Taken together they are capable of illuminating different aspects of our moral experience and helping us learn the different kinds of insight and skills that are relevant to responsible ethical decision-making. They tend in reality to complement each other.

The moral instruction school

This traditional approach focuses on instruction based on codes of ethics and rules. It reminds us that ethics is not just a private matter, for we are all born into a morally structured environment and a world of rules and regulations. Families have their rules, schools are rule factories, clubs and professions have their rules and partnerships, and corporate institutions have their codes of ethics, rules, regulations and well-tried procedures. Ethics education has to be, among other things, an initiation or induction into the 'rules of the ball game' – whether these are unwritten rules of etiquette, or codes of conduct, formal rules or legal requirements. The 'moral instruction school' focuses on these deontological elements in any profession or institution, which serve to define the principles on which we are supposed to act and on our rights and duties. Induction into the values and 'culture' of a profession may also serve to make us more aware of our own moral beliefs and values and the moral baggage we bring with us into adult professional life. We also need to understand the structure of power and authority within the profession or institution in which we work, to understand the etiquette and 'pecking order' as well as the assumptions on which the ethical culture of the organisation is based. We need instruction in the etiquette and both the implicit and explicit values and rules which underlie the ethical culture of institutions. It is just as important as learning the formal rules or disciplinary code of conduct that apply to our profession. These issues are basic to the process of being socialised into a profession and accommodating oneself to the 'culture' of the hospital, firm, public sector institution or corporation in which one practises.

Encouraging familiarity with our own moral beliefs, the ethical culture of the institutions in which we work, and the code of conduct of our profession are all individually important and help us to develop insight and confidence that we can 'work the system'. However, this approach, far from exhausting the meaning of ethics, also does not help us very much with learning practical skills in moral decision-making in nursing practice, nor does it prepare us to carry the responsibility involved in doing so.[5]

The ventilatory school

This approach focuses on how people feel about the ethical dilemmas they face or the decisions they have made, and not just on rational considerations alone. It recognises the need, for those who will have to make painful decisions in stressful situations, to be able to debrief with colleagues and, if necessary, receive professional counselling. It also recognises that sharing experiences of successes and failures with more experienced professional colleagues can help us to improve our skills and develop insight into our strengths and limitations, and those of our prejudices, values and

moral beliefs which influence our conduct and performance. It may bring to light for managers what support or further training and supervision staff need. Structured case conferences and case-based teaching from real-life examples certainly have an important part in training in applied ethics, whether based on simulation, role-play of hypothetical situations or actual and current cases. This approach gives rightful importance to the exploration of the practical relations between feelings, attitudes and moral values in practice, and between the psychological and skills-based aspects of our work.

By providing scope for regular debriefing, training in counselling skills and group work, this approach can use 'ventilation' of feelings about one's performance (and perhaps the stress involved), not only to promote catharsis and deepen rational insight, but also as a method of processing experience so that we learn from it in the most successful way. Most importantly, it acknowledges that we are not disembodied minds, but have feelings and experience, anxiety and stress, satisfaction and frustration in our work. Finally, it creates opportunities for people to explore the nature and scope of their moral commitments and the extent and limits of their responsibility in practice, in a supportive and non-threatening environment.

The critical thinking school

The critical thinking school has emphasised the importance of teaching moral theory and knowledge of moral principles. It has rightly emphasised the cognitive and rational aspects of ethical decision-making. While this approach can be overcerebral, its importance lies in offering a different approach to one that simply appeals to authority, or to the rules enacted by authority. It also counteracts an oversubjective approach, which the first and second approaches can each encourage. The critical thinking school strives for objectivity in making moral judgements and decisions, based on universal standards and rational problem-solving methods. The critical thinking school emphasises that ethical decision-making is a set of skills that can be learned. It represents a type of problem-solving with direct resemblance to other problem-solving activities, and it is only realistically grounded if it takes serious account of the demands of the specific situation and circumstances surrounding the action in question, as well as having clear and assessable objectives. Kohlberg and Gilligan see such a model of 'rational justice' as representing a typically male perspective on ethics – in opposition to an 'ethics of care' with its focus on the impact of decisions on interpersonal relationships, which they identify with the 'different voice' of women in dealing with ethics (Bowden 1997).

At its best, the critical thinking school equips students and practitioners with a repertoire of practical skills and insight arising out of supervised practice. Ideally it assists them to integrate moral theory and knowledge of principles, through rehearsed practical experience of choosing and applying different means and methods, action planning and evaluation of their actions. If practised regularly, this can lead to the development of competence and reliability in application of standard procedures.

The situation ethics school

In summary, the situation ethics school, at its simplest, suggests that all we need to do is pay attention to the demands of the specific situation and attempt to address it in the most relevant and appropriate way. It's *raison d'être* is to criticise the myth of impartial objectivity and the pretensions and implicit reductionism of universalist grand theories which tend to treat each case as a specimen of a type, instead of recognising that each situation demands to be addressed on its own terms. The rational justice or duty- and rule-based ethical approaches are seen as trying to force situations to fit preconceived ideal templates.

The situationist approach has its roots in the tradition of Christian agapeistic (love) ethics and in confessional and legal casuistry, in the antinomian ethics of existentialism and modern 'situation ethics'. It has recently been appropriated by the advocates of an 'ethics of caring', which can be described as having the following features (Bowden 1997):

- emphasis on the irreducible specificity of real-life situations in which we have to make moral choices
- willingness to identify the specific character and needs of individual 'stakeholders', their personal background and history, and the way they interrelate with one another within the fabric of their society
- aiming to achieve insight and understanding of the unique features of the situation for participants
- flexibility in the face of the constantly changing and developing nature of human situations, of action and reaction and mutual adjustment, being willing to live with ambiguity and ambivalence
- sensitivity to gender stereotyping in the rational justice model (seen as predominantly masculine) and encouraging respect for others, avoiding the merely instrumental use of care
- requiring a willingness to look at situations on their own terms (phenomenologically) so as to be open to the unique ethical possibilities of each situation and the type of care each demands
- openness to recognise that one's own self-understanding or sense of identity can change and develop.

The type of pedagogy best adapted to this is perhaps illustrated by the use of traditional casuistry in case-based individual or group training for pastors, counsellors or nurses, and in practical jurisprudence for legal practitioners. Its object would be to broaden the capacity of trainees to empathise with other people in their situations, develop personal insight and skills in caring for the needs of people. This care should be on the clients' terms, rather than seeking to define their problems for them, and should help them find their own solutions to their problems rather than prescribing our own. It would correspond to some models of non-directive client-centred counselling, based on 'unconditional regard' for the other person and a 'non-judgemental' approach, facilitating the client's own self-discovery and problem-solving, resisting the temptation to rush in and give people 'advice' (Campbell & Higgs 1982).

Box 10.1 Kohlberg's stages of moral development

Pre-conventional level
Stage 1 Punishment and obedience orientation
Stage 2 Instrumental relativist orientation

Conventional level
Stage 3 Interpersonal concordance ('good boy'/'good girl') orientation
Stage 4 'Law and order' orientation

Post-conventional, autonomous or principled level
Stage 5 Negotiated social contract, legalistic orientation
Stage 6 Universal ethical principle or rational justice orientation

---

Moral development – can virtue be taught?

There is a growing literature on moral education and moral development, both in general educational literature and specifically related to the teaching of ethics in business, medicine, nursing, social work, accounting and law. The now classic work of Kohlberg (1973, 1976) on moral development caused a stir at the time it was published, mainly because he advanced a theory that moral development in individuals follows a series of developmental stages from the most immature and unsophisticated to the most mature and sophisticated, and because of his conclusion that women rarely reach the highest stage in his hierarchy of universal rational justice thinking (!) (see Box 10.1).

The usefulness of Kohlberg's theory may be seen not in terms of its merits or limitations (for it has been heavily criticised from the point of view of the scientific validity of his research methods and results), but more particularly because of the almost naïve philosophical assumptions he makes, from within the deontological German tradition, that a universalist and rational justice view of ethics must be superior to say a utilitarian or hedonist one. Gillon (1981, 1986) and other philosophers have pointed out that Kohlberg's 'scientific' theory begs the question, by making unjustified value judgements, about which values we ought to aspire to as human beings. His conclusions conveniently reflect and reinforce his own uncriticised value assumptions based on a (Kantian) view that critical thinking in terms of universal principles is the highest stage of moral development. [His approach incidentally also affirms a North American view of personal autonomy as the highest good for the individual (Beauchamp & Childress 1994, Beauchamp & Bowie 1997).]

Educationists have criticised both his theoretical presuppositions and his practical methodology, for lack of proper controls in selection of his subjects, hasty generalisation from inadequate empirical evidence and for following Piaget too slavishly – Piaget's work again being heavily dependent on Kantian rationalism. Feminists have attacked Kohlberg's model for canonising a male stereotype of dominative, competitive and critical intelligence as the highest and best model for ethics, namely a type of critical thinking concerned with 'proof' or 'winning arguments'.

Gilligan (1977) attempted to repeat his research using a sampling method that was controlled for social class and gender bias, and was unable to confirm his findings. Instead she found that there were significant differences between the way women and men respond to moral experience and the responsibilities of moral decision-making. She found that there is empirical evidence that women are more concerned with conflict resolution, acceptance of responsibility to one another and caring for others. She argued that Kohlberg's model fails to do justice to these important social values.

It is not our purpose to enter here into the debate about Kohlberg's alleged stages in the moral development of individuals, for some of the reasons already given by his critics, but mainly because we believe that moral character is much more complex and that the balance achieved in different individuals gives wonderful diversity to the different ways in which human beings express moral maturity. We believe that Aristotle's model of the complex possible interrelationships between, and combinations of the intellectual and moral virtues in different individuals has greater potential to account for the complexity of moral character and the various forms of moral competence in human beings of both genders, including the behaviour of moral recidivists!

Our purpose here is to suggest the relevance of educational and training methods which are appropriate to the development of the moral and intellectual virtues in people, and which have particular relevance to the debate about the form in which the ethics education and development of competence in ethical decision-making may be taught. Whatever specific methods may be used, it is necessary that they provide scope for learning about and being able to handle the following:

- relations between personal and public, professional and corporate ethics
- application to clients, professional colleagues, management of hospitals and inter-agency business
- ethical theory, in practical moral decision-making, setting policy or standards and in ethical audit.

Methods of moral instruction: relations between personal, public and professional ethics

The proper concerns of the 'moral instruction school' require implementation of pedagogical approaches that focus in particular on power and authority, roles and rules in social settings. The aim of such an approach would be to provide learning opportunities for critical examination of:

- the content of our background personal moral formation – family, school, religion, etc.
- the process of formal socialisation into an institution or community
- the process of professionalisation and role of codes of conduct
- personal commitment to a set of values – applying codes of practice to actual cases
- learning to resolve conflicts between personal, professional and institutional values.

The objectives of moral education in this mode would be to help develop knowledge, insight and skills in individual nurses, to help them deal with the complex and competing demands of personal, professional and institutional values. The kinds of method for which relevant exercises would need to be developed are (Preston 1994, Kiersky &

Caste 1995, Thompson & Harries 1997, Grace & Cohen 1997, MacAdam & Pyke 1997):

- personal, professional and institutional values clarification
- social role analysis and definition of responsibilities
- force-field analysis of institutional authority and power structures
- functional analysis of the role of 'codes', 'contracts', 'charters of rights' and 'covenants' – between professionals and their clients
- skills in negotiating procedures and boundaries of responsibility at work
- individual and team decision-making and conflict resolution.

Methods of psychological debriefing: ethics in everyday nursing practice and corporate life

With the focus of the ventilatory school being on the interrelations of feelings, attitudes and values, in the exercise of personal moral responsibility in practice, training in this area would be aimed at enabling people to explore the feelings and conflicts which arise in their management of particular cases, and to develop skills relevant to dealing with them and enabling others to cope with similar difficulties. The aim here would be to achieve:

- development of insight into personal feelings and attitudes
- understanding of differences between moral problems and dilemmas
- development of models for case analysis and case conferencing
- understanding of the dynamics of teams and groups
- recognition of the value of experiential and participative learning.

Development of competence in these areas would require the use of a range of methods, which would give nurses practice in the following:

- skills in case analysis and conducting case conferences

- skills in teaching ethical decision-making, using various models
- application of problem identification and problem-solving skills
- skills in counselling, group work, support and supervision of colleagues
- skills in conducting experiential workshops exploring moral concerns.

Logical and critical thinking approach: ethics in theory and in practical moral decision-making

Generally speaking, academic teaching of ethics has tended to be overly theoretical and focused on the study of moral philosophy, rather than on the development of practical skills in applied ethics. When we are challenged to justify a moral decision, the proper response is not to appeal to moral theory, but to explain the practical steps we have taken. These would normally involve:

- assessment of the facts and values relevant to the case
- recounting what options we have considered or examples from past experience
- setting out our reasons for our decision or action
- explaining how we would evaluate whether our action was successful or failed.

Moral theory becomes relevant only when we are challenged to provide backing or justification for our underlying moral beliefs and for the very values or principles we employ in everyday moral decision-making. In practice, people tend not to perceive the relevance of moral theory until they are fairly confident about their basic values and principles and have had practical experience of applying them. To address at the outset of training moral theory and the higher-level or meta-ethical questions, which are the concern of moral philosophy, is educationally unsound and generally unproductive; whereas dealing with them when people know the rules and are reasonably confident players of the ethical 'ball game' can be useful in broadening their tolerance of different points of view and deepening their understanding of the roots of ethics.

Developing critical insight and analytical skills in the area of moral decision-making would require a number of different kinds of training. In developing competence in this area, the training objective would be to develop understanding of:

- the methods of logical and critical thinking
- the logic of decision-making in general, and in ethics in particular
- the types of decision procedure appropriate in different contexts
- the value of role-play, simulation and regular practice of skills in problem-solving methods and their application to values clarification, ethical decision-making and policy-setting
- the range of moral theories and what aspects of moral experience these theories address (e.g. intuition, a sense of duty, rule-governed behaviour, consequences, the role of love, etc.).

To facilitate the acquisition of skills and competence in these areas, the kinds of method for which relevant exercises would need to be developed are as follows:

- exercises in the use of different models of problem-solving
- exercises in context or situation analysis to determine the most appropriate decision procedures
- exercises in constructing a sound justification for a decision or action
- simulation exercises to ensure that people can discriminate how boundaries of responsibility/accountability shift with context
- exercises to demonstrate the relevance of different moral theories to understanding different aspects of the decision process.

Situation-based ethics – paying attention to the demands of the specific situation

The critical importance of situation ethics is twofold. First, it seeks to counteract the tendency of deontological ethics, whether in the form of authority-based codes of conduct or the rational justice model, to be too abstract and general. Its protagonists argue that the other approaches lose the particular in the universal and ignore the role of personal feelings and motives in their attempt to avoid relativism and to achieve universal moral rules. Second, it attacks the 'manipulative', 'managerial' and 'controlling' elements in a teleological or utilitarian ethics that is only concerned with calculating costs and benefits, effectiveness and efficiency. Economic rationalism, with its supposedly value-neutral approach, would be the object of particular criticism. In contrast, a situationist approach (like virtue ethics, to which it is related) focuses attention on the moral agents, and their competence and ability to handle responsibility. It examines the specific conditions and limitations under which they have to operate, and what means and methods are available to them as decision-makers.

The aim of teaching based on the situationist model would be to create a suitable learning environment in which students can gain experientially based knowledge and critical insight into:

- their own strengths and limitations in handling ethical decisions in real-life situations
- what skills training they require to overcome their weaknesses or strengthen their repertoire
- the nature of their own moral prejudices, ethnic and gender biases
- the way institutional structures and practices can be shaped by people's values and prejudices
- the hidden complexity of situations in which there may be a variety of stakeholders.

The kinds of method which could be used to facilitate experientially based learning in these areas might include some or all of the following:

- Self-assessment, as well as peer-group and departmental assessment, using, for example, SWOT exercises (assessment of strengths, weaknesses, opportunities and threats) as a tool
- Groupwork to explore issues of prejudice and gender bias in their immediate experience, e.g. how they perceive the way the nursing college itself is structured and how it operates
- Observation reports in which individual students, or paired groups, are briefed,

charged to observe and then report back to the class on their observation of various routine situations, e.g.
  - admission and history-taking from a patient
  - informing a patient of a bad prognosis
  - dealing with bereaved relatives or a mother who has had a stillbirth
  - a domiciliary visit to a patient in a community setting
  - interviewing student applicants for nurse training
- Training through role-play and structured debriefing, with or without the use of CCTV, to practise interviewing and listening skills, followed by supervised practice in interviewing clients
- To practise as a group the task of setting practical and workable performance indicators – for their academic performance, and ethical conduct as individuals and as a college.

These are only a selection of a potentially unlimited range of methods which can be employed. We cannot attempt here to be comprehensive, but wish to emphasise that if ethics teaching is to be more than 'chalk and talk' or 'grandstanding of opinions' then it does require some imagination and creativity in designing methods and approaches that will be effective in achieving successful education and formation of nurses. A summary of approaches and methods is given in Box 10.2.

In conclusion, ethics is no 'quick fix' and there are no shortcuts to effective training to ensure the development in people generally, or in nurses in particular, of the necessary skills and competence in ethics or ability to function as responsible moral agents. The knowledge and theory which can be taught is, in the case of ethics, perhaps far less important than learning skills which allow people to develop their own character, competencies and critical intelligence in the light of experience of applying moral principles in their professional work.

The model suggested above for the possible construction of teaching programmes is very complex and would require a great deal of time if

---

Box 10.2   Four approaches to teaching applied ethics

Approaches to teaching ethics have tended to be based on one of four different models:

- Moral instruction school – ideological formation
- Ventilatory school – therapeutic approach
- Critical insight school – rationalist model
- Situation ethics school – existentialist/feminist model.

Each approach has something to offer, but equally none of them is adequate taken on its own. They complement one another, each drawing attention to different aspects of moral experience.

The moral instruction school
Personal/professional values clarification
Developing an integrated curriculum
Promoting a whole-school approach
Developing community links/involvement
(Corporate ethical policy development)

Skills required
Values clarification skills
Curriculum development in ethics
Awareness of systems theory
Community building skills
Policy negotiation and development

The ventilatory school
Exploring personal feelings and attitudes
Building competence in applied ethics
Training in ethical decision-making skills
Practice in teaching applied ethics
(Professional development for teachers)

Skills required
Counselling and helping skills
Skills in personal problem-solving
Case-work and practical experience
Groupwork and interpersonal skills
Training for trainers and teachers

The critical insight school
Ethics integrated across the curriculum
Comprehensive life-skills approach
Familiarisation with values and principles
Practice in ethical problem-solving
(Developing pupil competencies)

Skills required
Cross-curriculum needs assessment
Training in life-skills transfer
Critical thinking skills
Practical experience of work with peers
Support and supervision skills

The situation ethics school
Assessment of personal strengths and limitations
Skills training and personal development
Insight into moral prejudices and gender bias
Analysis of corporate ethical 'culture'
Observation of nurse practitioners at work
Improvement of interviewing and listening skills
Developing performance indicators

Skills required
Practice in self- and peer-group assessment (SWOT)
Interactive group work and formal debriefing
Role-play and functional analysis of actual practice
Examine dissonance between professed values/practice
Practice in applying systematic methods of appraisal
Role-play then supervised practice with feedback
Group project for self-assessment and audit of institution

---

offered as a separate ethics 'module', but that need not be the case. Many of these methods and approaches are already used in our training programmes. What is required is not so much the adding on of a new subject to the overcrowded curriculum, but raising of the awareness of ethics in every dimension of ordinary basic training and in ongoing staff development. The effective use of the kinds of methods and approaches outlined above to address the moral content of everyday nursing practice, and not merely 'hard cases', can be powerfully effective in developing the necessary skills and competencies 'on the job'. The need for formal instruction in ethics remains, but the

place for attention to relevant moral theory will emerge as people wrestle with the actual complexities of life.

Competence, skills and discrimination in applied ethics can only be learned through a combination of knowledge, practice and experience. The development in us all of a combination of theoretical and practical moral wisdom, and an ability to integrate it and apply in our lives what Aristotle called 'prudence' is probably the crucial kind of competence to be emphasised. In Aristotle's arch of the virtues, prudence is the keystone linking the moral and intellectual virtues, and is the special type of virtue or competence most relevant to being a wise and responsible moral agent. He defines prudence as the knowledge and ability to apply universal principles to the demands of specific situations, in such a way that we choose the best means to achieve a good outcome. Prudence cannot exist, however, without achieving a balance between the scientific or intellectual virtues and the practical or moral virtues. The former include critical analytical and logical skills as well as relevant theoretical knowledge and practical life experience. The moral virtues include self-discipline, courage, temperance, honesty and integrity, justice and fairness, and a range of social and interpersonal skills (see Fig. 10.1 and fuller discussion in Ch. 11).

In developing personal insight and the moral virtues, we need all that can be learned from the methods of the 'moral instruction school', the 'ventilatory school' and the 'situation ethics school'. However, if we are to develop the intellectual virtues or methods of logical and critical thinking then we need training in the methods of the 'critical thinking' school as well. All this needs to be subject to critical research and empirical testing of the relative efficacy of the various methods suggested if we are to be sure in the future about what is most effective in facilitating the learning of skills in applied ethics, and the acquisition of the intellectual and moral virtues. Here the research of Fry (1989a,b) and McAlpine (1998) is both pioneering and exemplary.

PROBLEM-SOLVING APPROACHES TO ETHICAL DECISION-MAKING

As we indicated earlier, there are many kinds of problem-solving method which we employ in different domains of human activity and knowledge. When we come to consider what models to apply to ethical decision-making we have to recognise that there has been a long history of effort to develop and refine appropriate methods to deal with the complexity of moral arguments and judgements. These range from the classical analyses of Plato and Aristotle, through rabbinical and early Christian moral theology, to the sophisticated moral casuistry of the mediaeval confessors and moral philosophers (Gill 1985). They take

in the attempts of rationalists and empiricists to bring moral discourse within the 'logics' of either mathematics or empirical science (Macintyre 1981). They include the attempts of modern philosophers to understand the nature of moral argument by analysing the 'language of morals' (Hare 1964, 1981), to consider 'the place of reason in ethics' (Toulmin 1958), or recent attempts to revive interest in casuistry (Jonsen & Toulmin 1988).

What is specially interesting about the earliest efforts of Plato and Aristotle is that they are concerned to give a three-dimensional account of moral argument and decision-making, as concerned with both living ideals and the practice of living. Plato writes about philosophy in dramatic dialogue form, which enables him to illustrate the point of intersection between theory and practice, between moral theory and life. His great teacher Socrates is shown to be not only a subtle thinker, but also a courageous man who was prepared to put his life on the line for what he believed. Plato's *Republic* begins with Socrates asking the question: 'What is justice?'

On the surface this looks a relatively innocent question, but in this dialogue and in several others, Plato demonstrates that by merely asking the question, Socrates put his life at risk. Socrates' persistent challenging of people, politicians and self-styled experts, his asking the question with ultimate seriousness was felt to be subversive. Found guilty by the popular court of undermining popular confidence in Athenian justice, because he challenged its institutions in the name of a more ultimate justice, Socrates was condemned to death.

Plato is concerned not only with logical consistency in argument, but also with moral consistency or congruence between what people profess and how they act. Thus, in the dialogue, *The Gorgias*, Socrates and Callicles (a disciple of Gorgias) are shown locked in argument about the nature of rhetoric and truthful communication. The bystanders become frustrated that the argument is not leading to agreement between the two men. Socrates is challenged to agree with Callicles, but retorts that the problem is not to get Callicles to agree with Socrates, but to get Callicles to agree with himself, both in the sense of avoiding contradicting himself and, more importantly, in the sense of practising what he preaches. Plato is concerned to emphasise that what a man says should square with what he is, and what he does with the fact that he is saying it (Hamilton 1950).

Similarly, Aristotle's analysis of what he called the 'practical moral syllogism' should be considered alongside what he says about the practical nature of ethics – as being concerned with the conditions for human well-being and flourishing, and the responsible exercise of power for the good of individuals and the community. The 'practical syllogism' is both a form of argument and a statement about the need for congruence between thought and action, between the intellectual and moral virtues. As a form of argument it represents a scheme in which the minor premise is a statement of the case, the major premise a statement of the relevant moral principle under which the case could be said to fall, and the conclusion the judgement of what ought to be done. It is not so much a means of calculating what to do, as a summary of a complex process in which we have to deliberate carefully, weighing up the pros and cons like a judge in a law court, and ultimately have to make a prudent choice, based on the evidence, relevant principles, our past experience and what we believe will be the best means to a good end (Thomson 1976).

Moral decision-making can be compared with clinical judgements in both medicine and nursing, in both the stages and complexity of their problem-solving methods. Clinical decisions in medicine involve taking a medical history, examination of the patient, diagnosis and prognosis, treatment, ongoing observation, further tests and investigations, and evaluation and learning from outcomes. In making clinical decisions in nursing, the four stages of the Nursing Process have been taught as one means to clarify what is required to plan patient care in a systematic way. These four stages are:

- *assessment* of the problem situation
- *planning* what to do about it
- *implementation* of the planned decision
- *evaluation* of the success of your action.

Adopting such a systematic approach enables nurses to act in a responsible way and to have clear treatment aims in terms of which outcomes can be assessed and as a result of which they can learn from the process (Roper et al 1981).

In just the same way, moral decisions have to make provision for careful rational deliberation on the available evidence, consideration of relevant moral principles, appraisal of options and possibilities, monitoring of effects and consequences of our actions, and identification of what we can learn for the future from our successes or failures in the past to achieve our goals. This requires models which not only do justice to the complex logic of moral decision-making, take account of the complexity of the situation and the roles of various players in the drama, and make provision for learning and improving our performance in the future. An obvious difficulty with the naïve view that decisions are just either 'right' or 'wrong' is that they fail on all three counts to do justice to the process of moral assessment, deliberation, decision, action and reflection on outcomes.

The four-stage Nursing Process problem-solving model has the virtue of being simple and easy to remember. However, it tends to abstract 'the problem' from the context of the existential encounter between individual nurse and patient, and relationships with significant others. If the problem is primarily seen as a clinical one, it can also result in significant socio-economic and cultural variables being overlooked. While the nursing process has these limitations, it also has features in common with many other models, so it makes for useful comparisons. In what follows we will elaborate a number of models which can be useful in moral decision-making, using the Nursing Process as our starting point, because of its assumed familiarity to nurses (see Johnstone 1991).

Because of the complex nature of the nurse's interaction with the patient (and perhaps the patient's family and community), moral decision-making in nursing has to do justice to several things at once:

1. the need to address a particular patient's problem, explore treatment options, give

treatment and ongoing care, monitor progress and evaluate outcomes

2. the need to be sensitive to the interpersonal encounter and the nurse's ongoing relationship with the patient, based on trust and confidentiality, and the patient's need for support

3. the need to attend to the wider social context of the patient's life, family relationships and work situation, and to the various 'players' in both the patient's management and ongoing life.

In dealing with (1), scientific and legal parallels suggest themselves as useful. In dealing with (2), however, models taken from psychotherapy and counselling may be more appropriate, and in dealing with (3) social context and force-field analysis may be required to deal with the complex variety of variables. A comparison of various models may bring out the strengths and limitations, similarities and differences between various problem-solving models (see Table 10.1).

From an ethical point of view, what is revealing about the Nursing Process is what it leaves out. Obviously, nurses meet patients and have to interact with them at a personal level. They often form significant relationships with patients and have to face the termination of those relationships, whether the patient recovers or dies. The fact that these features are not 'up front' in the Nursing Process model is revealing. First, it suggests that nurses see their relationship with patients as derived from or secondary to the patient's relationship with the doctors. Second, it suggests a possible concern with the clinical aspects of the contract-to-care, and neglects the interpersonal aspects of the interaction. The beginnings and endings of such relationships may be crucial from an ethical point of view. The psychologist, Eric Berne (1966, 1973) (father of transactional analysis), has said that learning to say 'hello' and 'goodbye', and to do it properly, are two of the most fundamental skills in life. The way we greet new life and the way we say our farewells in the face of death are two of the most important rituals in every human society. Similarly, calling each other names can be part of intimate love play or verbal abuse. John Bowlby's classical studies of separation anxiety in hospitalised children cut off from contact with their mothers has helped to change policies on admission of mothers in children's hospitals, but he has also taught us to recognise more generally that the pathology of our emotional life and relationships relates to how we cope with 'making and breaking of affectional bonds' (Bowlby 1979). The challenge of beginning and ending relationships, as well as sustaining them, demands not only understanding and self-insight, but many kinds of skills and coping strategies.

Table 10.1 Comparison of stages in different problem-solving models

Legal	Scientific	Medical	Counselling	Nursing
Crime alleged to be committed by accused	Definition of the problem for investigation	Patient presents with problem or symptoms	Meet client who comes for help with crisis	
Indictment and specific charges	Formulating alternative hypotheses	Take medical history	Elicit nature of 'problem'	ASSESSMENT
Prosecution case and defence case	Design of experiment(s)	Examine patient – initial diagnosis	Clarify nature of problem(s)	
Cross-examine witnesses, other forensic evidence	Experimental investigations (repeated)	Tests, investigations, treatment, prognosis	Explore options available, transforming problem	PLANNING
Argument on points of law	Analysis of results/outcome	Monitor patient's progress	Assist client in choosing solution	IMPLEMENTING
Deliberation and judgement	Considering new implications	Evaluate final result/recall	Support client in coping with results	EVALUATION
Sentence: convict or discharge		Discharge patient	Leave client to get on with life	

Ordinary problem-solving methods have at least to take account of this interpersonal context, if they are to be adapted to help us with ethical problem-solving. Furthermore, they must do justice to the ongoing history of such relationships.

THE NURSING PROCESS AS A MODEL FOR ETHICAL DECISION-MAKING

Box 10.3   Ethics and the Nursing Process

Initial steps – clarify and define the nature of the problem

What is the crisis (or dilemma) requiring a decision?

(note – *crisis* means 'decision time' in Greek)

Assessment – identify key facts and values applicable

What are the crucial facts of the case?

What *moral principles* are at issue here?

What decision procedure is appropriate?

Planning – what are the right means to reach our goal?

What is the primary aim or *good* for which we are acting?

What objectives, *benefits*, moral goals are achievable?

What previous cases or contingencies should we take into account?

Implementation – decision: commitment to action

How do we begin, continue and finish the process of intervention?

How do we assess *costs/benefits* of the intervention?

How do we monitor *success/failure* in the overall process?

Evaluation (with reference to aims and objectives)

What means have we set up for debriefing and feedback?

Have we used the 'right' means to a 'good' end?

How do we review the pros/cons for the action taken?

Final steps – retrospect (apply the following tests)

Could I/we provide a reasonable ethical justification for the course of action taken?

Can I/we identify what we have learned from applying this model to decision-making?

How do we integrate this learning into the next decision-making cycle?

In the context of nursing care, the application of the Nursing Process is not simply a technical method of directing clinical practice in terms of rational care plans, as if moral considerations did not come into it. In any care plan, or application of the Nursing Process, all sorts of moral considerations are taken for granted and are often explicit. The purpose of pursuing this analogy with the Nursing Process in analysing moral decision-making is not only practical, in seeking to clarify the processes involved, but also to stress that the nurse's moral experience and nursing experience are one and the same. But what, then, are the practical implications of using this model for the analysis of the moral aspects of decision-making in nursing? (Box 10.3 illustrates the model.)

Assessment

Just as nurses are expected to take a detailed history from individual patients and carefully note their general circumstances as well as the specific problems they are experiencing, and to apply a general knowledge of the principles and practice of nursing to the interpretation and assessment of the situation, so a similar process is involved in making moral decisions.

First, we have to clarify the facts of the case: what are the background conditions affecting the life of the patient in question; what are the immediate causes of the specific crisis demanding a decision; what alternative options and means are available; and what are the likely outcomes?

Consider, for example, a community nurse visiting a bed-bound elderly patient at home, or a casualty nurse in an ambulance team attending victims of a railway accident in a remote place, or a nursing officer dealing with acutely ill patients in an understaffed ward. In the first case, it may be as important for the district nurse to have good knowledge of the housing conditions, financial state and family supports (or lack of them) of the bed-bound patient as it would be to know what resources could be called upon to assist in providing good nursing care. In the second case, it is essential to know what effective care can be given, and even what it would be right or wrong to do. Giving emergency first aid to accident victims in a remote place, where only minimal resources are available, will be quite different from doing so in a well-equipped hospital. What can be done and what ought to be done will be determined and limited by the circumstances. In the third case, where a charge nurse is faced with staffing shortages, his moral obligations would be different from those where there was normal cover. The charge nurse would have the same duty to care for his acutely ill patients, regardless of the circumstances, but what he can or cannot be do will be determined by what resources are available. The nurse cannot be held responsible for what he cannot do (for 'ought' implies 'can'). He may feel guilty later that more was not done for patients in a particular crisis, but his only obligation might be to try to ensure the problem does not arise again.

Secondly, we have to clarify what kinds of knowledge and skill are relevant in deciding what to do. This will include consideration of the relevant rules and moral principles relating to one's personal and professional duties. Merely to provide nursing care for the bed-bound patient (e.g. to administer a routine bed-bath or pain relief, or to recommend hospitalisation) would be irresponsible if no attempt were made to ensure that family members were provided with what support they needed to enable them to manage better on their own. The community nurse might have an obligation to liaise with social services to ensure that the patient's entitlements, e.g. to a home-help, disability allowance and provision of physical aids, are respected. The nurse's duty of care to the patient, interpreted narrowly as simply providing nursing care, would not be sufficient to clarify what should be done. Similarly, in the case of a nurse working at the scene of a railway accident, some painful decisions might have to be taken about who to treat, who can be left to cope and who to leave to die. Here the most responsible and caring thing to do would be to recognise first what can and cannot be done, given limited resources, and then to give assistance by applying a policy of triage. This would not involve treating all patients equally. Instead it would mean giving what comfort is possible to those who are too far gone for help; reassuring those who are likely to recover without help; and

concentrating efforts on those who have a chance of recovery but who are unlikely to do so without help. Here the demands of the duty to care may have to take precedence over considerations of justice or respect for the rights of individuals. A nursing officer without sufficient staff to operate an acute ward, by contrast, might have to take political action – e.g. threatening to walk out unless help is urgently forthcoming. Here a nurse's action might be guided by considerations of justice and respect for the right of all committed into his care.

Planning

Once the problem has been clearly defined (by a careful assessment of the general circumstances, the needs of the specific individuals, available means, and the general nursing and moral principles relevant to the situation), then it may be possible to plan a course of action. This will involve several stages:

- consideration of the specific knowledge and practical procedures known to be relevant to the defined problem
- retrospective examination of past experience of the success or failure of alternative courses of action for dealing with similar problems
- prospective anticipation of the likely consequences of alternative courses of action in this specific situation
- choice of the best and most appropriate means to achieve the desired goal, including ensuring that adequate resources are available
- formulating a definite plan of action with clear objectives, including possible contingency plans if things go wrong and circumstances demand a change of plan.

The ability to make sound action plans requires the particular combination of knowledge, skill and practical experience that we call practical wisdom (or what Aristotle and the classical philosophers called the 'virtue of prudence'). Prudence is defined as the knowledgeable and skilled ability to apply general principles to particular situations, so as to choose the best and most appropriate means to achieve a good end (outcome or goal)

(Thomson 1976). However, having a good plan and all the experience of a lifetime cannot protect us against the unexpected or chance developments that may throw everything awry. Prudence requires flexibility, resourcefulness and adaptability too, and good planning will allow for contingencies as well (Pieper 1959).

Implementation

How effectively and efficiently decisions are implemented and plans worked out in practice will have a great deal to do with their success or failure. Aristotle identified a specific virtue or skill (solertia) which is associated with being confident, decisive and courageous in carrying through a decision or action plan. This virtue is something people can learn with experience, enabling them to avoid timorousness and indecisiveness, while nevertheless remaining sensitively responsive to changing situations without being over-rigid in keeping to their plans at all costs (Pieper 1959).

Implementation is the key part of 'action', but it cannot be considered in isolation. From a moral point of view, we are concerned with observing and monitoring the soundness of the whole process against set objectives or targets. Implementation includes ongoing responsible assessment of the prevailing circumstances throughout the process and the changing moral demands of the specific situation. Several factors are involved in effective and efficient implementation of practical decisions. These include responsible monitoring of progress or failure of the action taken to achieve defined objectives; honest evaluation of the actual consequences or outcomes of the action, and its general costs and benefits. At each stage, moral deliberation and judgement will require application of relevant knowledge and skills to management of the implementation process.

Evaluation

The term 'evaluation' can be applied to the attempt to judge each stage in the process of decision-making, but it is more commonly used in a restricted sense to apply to assessment of the consequences or outcomes of an action. Competent evaluation of a decision and its implementation will always involve consideration of whether the actual consequences of an action are the same as the intended consequences. Judging whether the consequences are better or worse than hoped for, and whether the long-term effects of a course of action will be successful, is necessary in order to clarify whether the action taken would justify its becoming standard practice. Evaluation in this sense is part of a learning process. Feedback from experience, if consciously integrated into understanding of what we are doing, should equip us to act more effectively when faced with similar situations in the future.

In this way, the feedback in the learning process helps to build in habits (virtues) which make decision-making potentially easier as we gain in experience and confidence. However, there is a broader aspect of evaluation of importance to moral judgement. This relates to the cost–benefit analysis of alternative courses of action, not merely whether they are efficient in achieving our desired ends. Evaluation of costs and benefits, like 'quality of life' assessments, is not simply a requirement of sound economics and practical management of professional tasks; it is also a demand of sound moral judgement. This brings us back full circle to the re-examination of the fundamental principles and values we espouse in the belief that they promote human flourishing. In nursing, clinical nursing and promotion of complete physical, mental and social well-being are one and the same activity. Moral considerations are inseparable from proper application of the Nursing Process, and thus by building in the moral dimension we can not only use it to deal with moral problems when they arise, but it will also ensure that nursing work can be undertaken in a way that is both morally responsible and accountable.

Finally, there is the inclusive sense of evaluation. This covers the whole process of decision-making (including assessment, planning, implementation and evaluation). Evaluation is concerned with judgements both about how well individual steps in the process have been completed and about how successfully the whole process has been in practical and moral terms. Ethical disagreements can arise at each of these stages in the process. There can be disputes about facts and values in relation to assessment of what ought to be done, how it should be done, whether the right means have been chosen, how well it is actually done, and whether the specific outcomes or general consequences are good. The words 'ought', 'should', 'well' and 'good' belong to the vocabulary of moral judgement and relate to rules, duties and values for the assessment of performance and general costs and benefits, respectively. [As will be seen in the next chapter, disputes at the level of moral theory relate to the different ways in which we justify our moral judgements in each of these contexts (Nowell Smith 1957, Hare 1964)].

SOCIAL CONTEXT ANALYSIS IN ETHICAL DECISION-MAKING

In the early work of Dorothy Emmet, philosophers and those interested in practical ethics were reminded that we cannot treat human situations abstractly, divorced from the social context in which they occur (Emmet 1966). She suggested that if we are to do justice to the demands of each case, we must examine four interrelated factors or variables that are involved in practical decision-making: the demands of the specific situation; the roles of the different participants; the variety of rules applicable to the exercise of these roles; and the arbiters to whom we are accountable for our actions – or, simply, *situation, roles* and *rules* and *arbiters*. In sound ethical decision-making, each and all of these factors must be taken into account (see Downie 1971).

Situation. The details of a specific moral situation are important. It will involve some general factors common to most human situations and some that are unique to this particular situation. In institutions such as hospitals, there are general factors common to most patients: their vulnerability and dependency; their need for nursing care and medical treatment; their relative lack of privacy; and in a particular ward perhaps the same kinds of medical problem. In a patient's home,

the nurse and patient stand in a different kind of relationship. The district nurse or health visitor is a kind of guest, and the patient, however ill, is more in control. In a health clinic where people come voluntarily for help or screening and can 'vote with their feet' and leave if they are unhappy with their treatment, the situation is once again different. Further, each individual has a unique medical history, specific identity and social status, a particular set of family or social obligations. Both general and specific factors in the situation, including those relating to the stay and available resources, need to be taken into account. Situational analysis attempts to focus on the specific case and to avoid the tendency to treat every case as simply a specimen of a species or an example of cases of a particular type, and encourages us to address it on its own terms.

Roles and rules. These tend to be interconnected. The roles of patient, doctor, nurse, porter, administrator and relative all tend to be governed by different implicit and explicit rules and conventions relating to permissible and non-permissible behaviour. We also need to consider the general rules governing the institutions in which we work, the more general rules and laws governing society, and the universal moral principles in terms of which we attempt to order and make sense of all these other rules. People in a given situation may play more than one role at a time. A patient, besides being a patient, may be a father, a lawyer, a champion bridge player and a Protestant. The nurse may be a man, a qualified SNO, a union member and a Roman Catholic. The doctor may be a young woman, feminist, keen golfer and atheist. In the developing action of a particular case, the rules governing these various roles may appear as more or less important. The value conflicts implied in these different roles may not only complicate the process of decision-making and interaction between the various 'players' in the 'drama', but also set up conflicts within the individuals themselves. Here objective values clarification may be necessary before the various parties can collaborate effectively in dealing with the problem in hand.

Furthermore, the roles of doctor, nurse, social worker, other health professionals, the patient, friends and relatives may all change as the drama unfolds. For example, an unconscious and seriously injured victim of a road traffic accident may first be admitted by ambulance to the accident and emergency department for immediate life support or first aid, then sent to the X-ray department or elsewhere for tests, transferred to the operating theatre for emergency surgery, be returned to the ward for postoperative care and treatment, sent to a specialist unit for rehabilitation, and discharged home into the care of his family, the local doctor and community nursing services. At each of these stages, the value priorities governing interactions between health professionals and the patient may be different. (The television programme *Casualty* makes compelling viewing not only because life-and-death crises are being portrayed, but also because the situations are inherently dramatic and constantly changing. Also, different players occupy central stage at different times, and the roles of nurses change from being part of the crash team to bedside care, from stage management to playing the role of the chorus. Just as acting out a specific role on the stage is governed by the script and the rules of the production, so the varying roles and rules of action in health care are dramatically varied and complex.) Downie (1971) points out that all these factors relating to roles and rules are relevant to moral decision-making, but to different degrees, depending on what is at issue. Eric Berne has developed a whole school of psychology, namely transactional analysis, based on the various 'transactions' between people interacting with one another while 'acting out' different roles. His analysis of the rich diversity of human interactions in both conflictual and cooperative relationships can be illuminating for ethical interpretation of complex situations.

Arbiters.   When we make moral decisions we also have to consider to whom we are responsible and accountable – in other words, those persons to whom we relate as arbiters of our actions. While nurses are *responsible for* their patient(s) (although not in quite the same way as the doctor), they would not normally be *responsible to* the patient(s) (although they may feel they are). Nurses are directly *accountable to* their line managers, but also indirectly to their peers and to the doctor responsible for giving instructions relative to the patients in their care. Nurses can also be held accountable to, or responsible to, the patient's relatives and ultimately to society through the courts. The most immediate arbiter of the nurse's professional work and general behaviour would be the charge nurse or the line manager. In life, we invariably 'look over our shoulder' to consider who is watching our actions and to whom we are expected to be able to give a proper account or justification for them.

Because we generally operate in professional life under authority, we have to consider whether our actions are appropriate or authorised, given our status, role and responsibilities. Thus, in making moral decisions we are obliged to consider those to whom we are responsible and accountable, those who are arbiters of our actions. Generally nurses must 'obey orders' where these are appropriate and ethical, and will feel that they should bear in mind what their line manager or the doctor may think of their actions. However, it would not be appropriate for them to act simply to please their line manager or the doctor if they believed the situation demanded a different response. Whether or not nurses are acting directly under orders, they would most likely take the arbiter of their actions into account in deciding what it is appropriate for them to do, or they might wish to consult the person concerned before acting on their own responsibility.

Because each situation is different, all these factors are variable. People play different roles, numerous different rules apply, and we are accountable to a variety of people in different ways. Moral decision-making is complex – especially in an institutional setting. Having the ability and confidence to make responsible decisions is a matter of knowledge and growth in experience and sophistication, sensitivity and wisdom (Emmet 1966, Thompson 1979a). The model illustrated in Figure 10.2 is suggested as a framework for such decision-making. It can be useful in making a careful assessment of one's own decisions and actions, and is also a useful aid to collective moral decision-making in the team management of complex cases or in deciding moral policy on a committee.

Ethical decision-making. A model for group decision-making

Application of this model depends on identifying the inter-relations between four factors in the social action context:

Situation	- the unique factors in this case, here and now
Roles	- the key players in this piece of action
Rules	- the specific rules of this 'ball-game'
Arbiters	- who is accountable to whom or who 'calls the shots'

Further, it involves applying to the specific ethical situation the four operations of this problem-solving process:

Assessment	- identifying main facts and values involved
Planning	- rehearsing options, and goal setting
Implementation	- accepting responsibility for decision or action
Evaluation	- accessing outcomes, costs and benefits

Using both sets of indicators it is possible to build up a more three-dimensional model for the decision-making process.

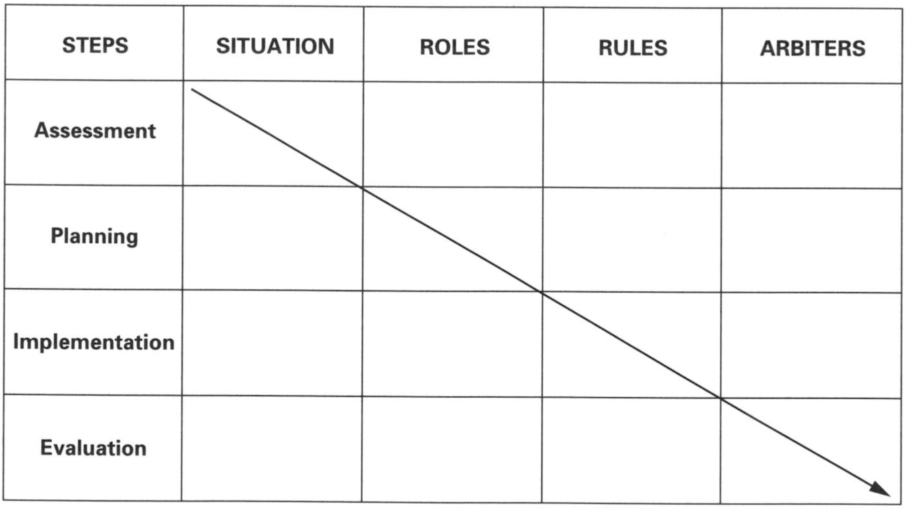

STEPS	SITUATION	ROLES	RULES	ARBITERS
Assessment				
Planning				
Implementation				
Evaluation				

Fig. 10.2 Combined social context and problem-solving analysis.

STAKEHOLDER ANALYSIS

The process of stakeholder analysis is a useful method for clarifying the nature of the ethical problem(s) which need to be tackled, by clarifying what rights and duties apply to the various 'players' in a given situation. Ethical problems frequently arise because the rights of one party or another have been infringed or they have not received their proper entitlements. (In most situations it is sufficient to identify the rights of the patient/client and the duties of the decision-maker (nurse or doctor), but in more complex situations it may be helpful to consider both the rights and responsibilities of the patient/client and the duties and rights of the health professional who has to make the decision about the delivery of the service.)

In working through the process, it is important to recognise that there will be duties that the decision-maker will have to the wider public and to his or her employing authority, as well as the spe-

Stakeholders (for example)	Stakeholder's rights	Charge nurse's duties	Charge nurse's rights	Stakeholder's duties
1. Patient				
2. Family				
3. Ward patients				
4. Ward staff				

Fig. 10.3   Matrix of rights and duties of stakeholders.

cific duties owed to the patient or client. The grid in Figure 10.3 can be a helpful aid to setting out the matrix of rights and duties of the stakeholders, so that a more informed judgement can be made about the real nature of the ethical problem(s) involved.

If the decision is being taken by a team of people, and particularly if the team is made up of people with a variety of kinds of professional expertise, it may be necessary to disaggregate their different conceptions of what 'the problem' is, what different kinds of action or 'interventions' are necessary, and what 'outcomes' or 'solutions' they each anticipate (see Fig. 10.4).

In a complex situation, it is possible that there may be little initial agreement about what the

problem is or how it is to be dealt with. If there are serious disagreements at this level, then it would be necessary to explore how serious the differences are and what scope there is for a negotiated agreement about definition of the problem and the course of action to be followed in dealing with it. For example, in dealing with a staff member with a 'drug problem', the doctor may see it as a problem of addiction, needing detoxification; the psychologist may see the problem as a dysfunctional way of coping with life problems, and requiring psychotherapy; the nurse manager may see the problem as one of chaotic behaviour and unreliability, requiring discipline; the chaplain may see the issue as one arising out of marital problems and financial difficulties,

Team member (for example)	Value base or expertise	Definition of 'the problem'	Proposed intervention	Expected outcome
1. Head nurse				
2. Medical registrar				
3. Psychologist				
4. Chaplain				

Fig. 10.4   Disaggregation of the different conceptions held by members of a team of decision-makers.

requiring sympathy; while the prosecuting police may see it as a problem of law-breaking and criminal conspiracy, requiring punishment. If all were involved in a 'case conference' about how to deal with the person, it might be important to discover first what common ground there was for cooperation in decision-making and management of the problem. Sometimes the complexities that emerge in the course of stakeholder analysis are due to the conflating of several problems, each of which needs to be tackled separately and in order of importance or urgency. Sometimes the complexities are due to the different ways in which the same problem is conceptualised and represented by different members of the team of people involved in making the decision.

THE DECIDE MODEL FOR ETHICAL DECISION-MAKING

In the literature on biomedical and applied ethics, there is an increasing number of decision-making models, each of which has certain advantages and limitations (cf. Beauchamp & Childress 1994, Johnstone 1994, Grace & Cohen 1998, Kerridge et al 1998). This is not the place to evaluate them, but as we have seen, there are common features to problem-solving methods as these are applied in a variety of fields. The DECIDE model (Box 10.4, Fig. 10.5), which we recommend here, is a refinement of the original SPIRAL model published in previous editions of this book. The usefulness of this model, as will be more fully discussed in the next chapter, is that it provides a practical method of making prudent value judgements and ethical decisions. This is in line with Aristotle's definition of prudence as *the knowledgeable and skilled ability to apply general principles to specific situations, in such a way that we choose the best available means to a good end*. Also, following Aristotle, we recognise the 'causes → means → ends' structure of all intentional acts, and that any sound method of ethical decision-making must take account of all three aspects of purposeful and deliberate acts.

What Aristotle means by 'causes', 'means' and 'ends' needs to be clarified:

> **Box 10.4** The DECIDE model
>
> **D – Define the problem(s)**
> What are the key facts of the case? Who is involved? What are their rights, your duties? What is the main ethical problem to be addressed?
>
> **E – Ethical review**
> What ethical principles have a bearing on the case and which principle or principles should be given priority in making your decision?
>
> **C – Consider the options**
> What options do you have in the situation? What alternative courses of action? What help, means and methods do you need to use?
>
> **I – Investigate outcomes**
> Given each available option, what consequences are likely to follow from each course of action open to you? Which is the most ethical thing to do?
>
> **D – Decide on action**
> Having chosen the best available option, determine a specific action plan, set clear objectives and then act decisively and effectively
>
> **E – Evaluate results**
> Having initiated a course of action, monitor how things progress, and when concluded, assess carefully whether or not you achieved your goals

- 'Causes' refers to the *background conditions* that determine the specific context in which one has to act or make a decision. These include both the external causes and psychological conditions which precipitate the 'crisis' (i.e. a time where we must make a decision). However, the term also refers to the 'rules of the ball game' or principles applicable in the specific situation in which we must act.

- 'Means' refers to both the agent(s) responsible for implementing the decision or action plan and the choice of means and methods required to achieve one's goal. In a sense, the moral agent is the primary means by which principles are applied to specific situations in order to decide what action(s) to take or what changes to effect in the situation by one's intervention. However, in any given situation, one may need the help of other people or additional resources in order to act effectively. They become instrumental means to implement one's intended action. Choice of

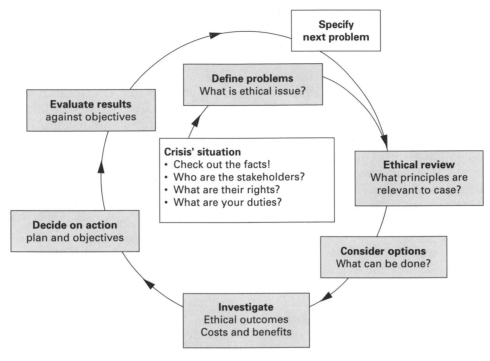

Fig. 10.5   The DECIDE model for ethical decision-making.

appropriate 'means' may also mean careful consideration of the best methods to use, based on one's past experience of what works and what does not.

- 'Ends' refers to both the purpose or goal of the action taken and the intended consequences or outcomes of the action. Responsible action is not only purposeful, but is based on realistic and achievable objectives. It is no good having a grand goal or end in view if it is impractical or not achievable, either because one lacks the knowledge, skill or power to act effectively or because one does not have available the necessary resources to achieve one's goal. Sound decisions and intended actions must have not only a purpose, but also realistic objectives. If intelligently planned, then the success or failure of the action can be measured against the set objectives. Without clear objectives, there can be no proper evaluation and we cannot learn from our experience.

The six steps of the DECIDE model relate to the various aspects of the 'causes → means →

ends' structure of intentional acts, in the following way:

- the first two (D, E) review the background causes and principles applicable in the situation
- the second two (C, I) involve an appraisal of available options, means and methods for action
- the third two (D, E) involve purposeful action and evaluation of results in the light of objectives.

MORAL AGENCY – WHEN ARE WE RESPONSIBLE FOR OUR ACTIONS?

Having discussed systematic methods by which we can make considered and well-justified moral decisions, and having considered the virtues needed in the moral agent, it remains to examine another question: under what conditions can we hold a person responsible for her actions, and what factors would serve to excuse someone from blame? Aristotle pointed out that we do not apportion praise or blame for actions unless a person is sane and has acted purposely, knowingly and voluntarily. We also assume people must have some sense of the boundaries of permissible action set by the moral community in which they live, and understand what their rights and duties to other people are. People cannot be held responsible for their involuntary behaviour, or when they do not know what they are doing, or when they act in complete ignorance of the likely consequences of their actions, or do not know what the 'rules of the ball game' are. Although we might want to refine Aristotle's criteria, his commonsense rules are still useful for most practical purposes.

However, when we speak of people as responsible moral agents, we are making a number of assumptions which may be challenged. Perhaps our most fundamental assumption is that human beings are not robots, that they can make independent choices and decisions, that they possess 'free will'. Another assumption we make concerns the nature of moral rules, namely that they are not simply personal, but apply to all human beings, that they are universal. In fact, many people would want to assert that moral principles are absolute, not relative to each person or culture, and that our moral duties are unconditionally binding, not dependent on time, place or circumstances.

To discuss and reflect upon these issues of moral responsibility and the binding nature of moral obligations is to engage in meta-ethics or moral philosophy, i.e. the higher-level activity of critical reflection on the presuppositions of everyday practical ethics and moral action. In moral philosophy, we explore what kinds of reason or evidence can be offered for believing or not believing in moral freedom, or in moral obligation, the universal applicability of moral rules and fundamental human rights. Some of these theories derive from religious or metaphysical beliefs about the nature of human beings and their relation to God and the universe; others from analysis of what is implied in the concept of human reason or the nature of love and the obligations these impose on us. Other philosophers are more concerned with the logic of the process of moral decision-making and focus on methodological questions. (We will say more about these matters in the next chapter where we explore the nature of moral theory.)

The enlightenment philosopher Kant (1724–1804) insisted that ethics could not get started without three fundamental beliefs or postulates: God, freedom and immortality.[6] He argued that the existence of God, as a transcendent source and point of reference for ethics, is necessary to guarantee that ethics is universal and above individual and cultural differences. He argued that personal immortality is necessary if human life is to have any ultimate meaning, if truth and virtue are to have abiding value and if there is to be any final justice and reward for a life of virtue rather than vice. Finally he argued that the concept of freedom is logically necessary both as a foundation for ethics as such, and as the only basis on which we can argue that people are morally responsible for their actions. Given the importance of this concept of human freedom (or 'free will'), we shall undertake a brief examination of the debate about whether human beings are free or determined, before we get into the discussion of specific moral theories.

The determinist argues that while people may think they are free, they are in reality wholly determined in what they do by forces or causes beyond their control. Determinism can have its roots in religion, in the belief that we are created and controlled by some superior being, an omnipotent God, who wholly predetermines how we will act; or belief that one is bound to the 'wheel of fate' and that one's *karma* is determined by forces outside the control of one's will. Alternatively, we may adopt a secular 'scientific' determinism based on the belief that a universal law of causality operates in nature so that cause and effect are necessarily connected in such a way that effects follow inevitably and without exception from their causes. From this point of view, we are so programmed by our genetic constitution, the accidental circumstances of birth and the social conditioning to which we are subject within our culture, that everything we do is causally determined, predictable and unavoidable.

The language of law and morality, as well as everyday speech, assumes the distinctions between active and passive moods, assumes that human beings can be both active agents initiating actions or passive 'patients' at the receiving end of the actions of others. For most ordinary purposes we describe our actions from the standpoint of actors or agents who do things for reasons, and with definite aims or objectives in mind. When we explain our actions, stand back and reflect on how and why we acted as we did, we analyse the rules and evidence on which we operate. We may indicate external forces that caused us to act in a particular way, or we may seek to justify or excuse ourselves by pointing to particular features of our inherited constitution, experience (or ignorance) or limiting factors in our environment that restricted our freedom of choice.

In attempting a retrospective analysis of past actions, we adopt the standpoint of spectators towards our own actions. As spectators of our own actions we see them as determined (or caused) by our wills, as resulting from the decisions we make – based on the complex reasons, facts and evidence we take into account before we act, and which we can offer by way of explanation or justification for what we have done. When we attempt the same kind of analysis of the actions of other people, we are easily persuaded that the explanations of how and why they acted as they did are compelling; that, given foreknowledge of the persons, their background and acquired knowledge and attitudes, and the prevailing circumstances, we could actually predict how they would behave. Husbands and wives, lovers and enemies often believe they know one another so well that they can predict exactly what the other will say or do. Strangely, if we really could predict how another person would behave, we would have good reason to doubt that the person was really alive and not just a robot. Someone who is alive is always capable of surprising us.

It does not follow from the fact that people can give explanations for their actions that the reasons they give are the direct causes of things happening the way they do. Reasons are not to be confused with causes. Anticipatory and subsequent explanations of actions tend to have a different logic.

The person who offers reasons for acting in a particular way sees the events in terms of his or her self-determining action as a free agent. Retrospective analysis of the reasons or causes of an action, or analysis of the necessary and sufficient conditions for an action to occur, tends to define the events as determined, the outcome predictable and the scope of choice limited. It is rather like looking at the world with Alice 'through the looking glass', for determinist arguments see everything retrospectively, in reverse, through the frame of the spectator's mirror. With the 'wisdom of hindsight', things can have a dreadful inevitability.

The type of theology which argues from the existence of an omnipotent, omniscient God to the conclusion that people cannot in any sense be free or responsible for their actions follows a similar 'logic'. To argue that because all our actions must be foreknown and therefore predestined by God, the predestinarian adopts the radical spectator point of view. Theological determinists assume that they can personally adopt a God's-eye-view of things, the privileged position from which they can view the universe as a whole, understand what is going on, and declare that moral effort is pointless because everything is predetermined anyway. The argument assumes that: (1) if you have complete knowledge of someone (omniscience); (2) if you can be constantly present to her (omnipresent); (3) and if you can comprehend and control all the variables in her life (omnipotence); then you could determine in advance everything she would do.

The argument rests on a number of big 'ifs', but it also makes a dubious logical assumption, namely that foreknowledge is coercive or compelling of future outcomes, and it is for this reason that other theologians, and most notably Augustine (354–430 AD), have argued that God's omnipotence and other divine powers do not necessarily entail that human beings cannot have free will or that we are predestined to act in a way that we cannot resist.[7]

Arguments for determinism which rest on appeal to the 'law of universal causation' are particularly attractive to those who attempt to offer comprehensive scientific or historical explanations of world events, natural processes and the behaviour of human beings. These arguments rest on the faith that a law of unexceptional causality applies throughout the universe. By its very nature, this is an unverifiable metaphysical belief. It is tempting to extrapolate from causal processes in contained and finite systems to the universe as a whole, but this is not logically justified. Causal inference is a method we apply to the analysis of processes in nature that we can control or observe under repeatable conditions, and which display predictable regularity. It is a conceptual tool which we freely apply to the ordering of our experience in an attempt to make sense of the finite and observable world, or systems we can control. We cannot argue that our choice, or a scientist's choice, to employ cause and effect explanations is itself determined by the law of cause and effect, without getting into a circular argument or infinite regress.[8]

The types of argument developed in some forms of determinist psychology (e.g. Freudian or behaviourist) or some forms of sociology (e.g. Marxist/Leninist) appear to offer very powerful explanations of why people behave in certain ways. For the Freudian, neurotic behaviour in adult life is seen to be caused by traumatic emotional disturbances in childhood, or, more generally, human beings are inevitably determined by their particular heredity and environment. For the strict behaviourist, such as Pavlov, all human and social action is the result of 'conditioning'. It is argued that repeated experience of trial and error, success or failure (or rewards and punishments) builds into our behaviour conditioned reflexes or learned responses. These are not free or spontaneous, but determined by the particular conditioning to which we are subjected by life and experience. Alternatively, Marxist 'social scientists' would explain all human and social processes as the result of external historical and economic forces acting upon individuals, over which they have no control. However, the Marxist claims that dialectical materialism gives us privileged insight into these processes and thus ability to direct and control the social and economic forces operating in history, liberating us to some extent from the forces of historical determinism.

The fact is that the terms 'free' and 'compelled', 'active' and 'passive' are correlative terms. We cannot make sense of one term without presupposing the others. For this reason, to speak of 'absolute freedom' or 'absolute determinism' leads us into nonsense. Similarly, to assert that there is evidence of some logical or empirical connection between factors or events which we label 'cause' and 'effect' does not mean, as Hume (1711–1776) pointed out, that the connection is either logically necessary or that some compulsion operates between 'cause' and 'effect', or that being able to predict (with a high degree of probability) what the result of some action may be forces the outcome (Lindsay 1951). The freedom required for moral action is the power of self-determination in a world where, in order to act, we have to (Downie 1971):

- choose between the various causal factors operative in a situation
- understand our own limitations and the constraints placed on us by circumstances
- reflect on the present situation confronting us, in the light of past experience
- deliberate on what resources or means we need to achieve our goal
- calculate the likely outcomes of various alternative courses of action
- choose ourselves to become causes or determinants of other effects (Fig. 10.6).

The questions we need to ask of the 'free-willer' or 'determinist' are perhaps those raised by Nietzsche (Cowan 1955), who comments on the irrelevance of the free will/determinism controversy to ethics (even though it might have entertainment value in metaphysics and theology):

Why should anyone want to delude themselves that they enjoy absolute freedom? Such a view is literally 'out of this world' and has more to do with individual will-to-power and delusions of grandeur than a responsible view of man's moral and political duty! Why should anyone want to maintain that all men are slaves to economic or material necessity? Unless their ulterior motive is to control people by encouraging them to abrogate their moral responsibility or to persuade

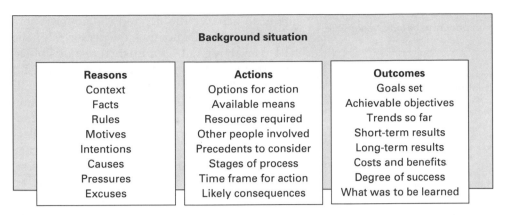

Fig. 10.6   Constraints and possibilities in moral choice.

oppressed people that they really are slaves and can do nothing to improve the world or their lot! So, we have to choose [sic] whether we are going to believe in our freedom to make decisions, and accept responsibility for the results or outcomes of our actions; or we must pretend that we are victims of circumstance or forces beyond our control and excuse ourselves from moral responsibility! [paraphrasing Nietzsche]

Aristotle distinguished between voluntary, involuntary and non-voluntary actions. Voluntary acts are those knowingly and purposefully undertaken to achieve a particular goal, e.g. forming and executing a plan to go to town to buy some clothes. Involuntary, or reflex, 'actions' are those such as jumping up with a shout of pain when you sit on a sharp tack, or knocking a cup off the table because you withdrew your hand suddenly on contact with a hot kettle; both are mechanical reactions, or forms of behaviour, resulting from internal or external causes which are neither purposeful nor subject to conscious control. Non-voluntary actions are actions which are done either through ignorance or in a state of intoxication, when you are not fully aware of what you are doing. Alternatively, you act non-voluntarily when you are compelled to do something against your will, e.g. at gunpoint or when subjected to forces you cannot control. [Aristotle's own example is of the captain forced to jettison his cargo in a storm to avoid his ship being swamped (Thomson 1976).]

In general terms, we cannot be held fully responsible for actions which we were caused to do by external factors or forces beyond our control. Determining the degree to which someone can be held responsible for her actions in a particular case will therefore involve careful assessment of the full circumstances in order to establish whether or not the person acted knowingly or in ignorance; voluntarily or involuntarily; or while subject to external (or internal) compulsion.

When a person actively causes things to happen which would not have happened without her intervention, we normally regard the person as the responsible agent. When a person is the passive object of external forces acting upon her, or simply reacts in a mechanical or reflexive way to external causes, then we do not regard that person as responsible. Obviously there may be difficulty in determining for certain the degree to which a given person acted freely or under duress in a particular situation, or to what extent her ignorance, state of intoxication or inner sense of compulsion could serve as excusing conditions if she were being tried for a serious crime. Making these assessments is part of the day-to-day business of juries and law courts, and also of the assessments of staff performance for disciplinary or promotion purposes. (Aristotle showed some interesting reservations in the treating of ignorance, drunkenness or inner

---

Box 10.5   Conditions for people to be held responsible for their actions

Knowledge of:
- Background circumstances
- The nature of the situation requiring action
- What alternative courses of action are available
- What resources or means are necessary (and available)
- The likely consequences of one's actions

Ability or power to:
- Act purposefully and in a goal-directed way
- Control oneself or one's own actions
- Achieve the type of action required
- Mobilise the necessary resources to achieve one's goal
- Control the process and determine the outcome

Freedom from:
- Physical compulsion or duress exerted by someone else
- External restraints on one's ability to act
- Internal psychological compulsion
- Intoxication or drug-induced confusion or stupor
- Delusion or ignorance of what one is doing

Freedom to:
- Choose one's own course of action
- Determine one's own goals and act on them
- Exercise decision-making responsibility in the situation
- Appropriate the necessary means to implement the action
- Own one's actions and accept responsibility for what one has done

---

power to achieve the desired outcome. Where these conditions are not met, the person might be said to be acting with diminished responsibility. For Aristotle, one's competence as a moral agent increases with one's general growth in intelligence and realisation of one's powers as a human being, but also more specifically as one gains control over oneself through mastery of the intellectual and moral virtues. Because people may vary in their degree of moral maturity (as with physical and psychological development) they may be more or less responsible, depending on the stage of their development. However, he also recognises that a person may suffer from 'weakness of will' due to a failure to develop the intellectual and moral virtues. Such people could be indirectly responsible, and therefore to blame, for not having cultivated themselves or made the effort to develop their potentialities. Box 10.5 summarises the conditions for purposeful and rational action to be praiseworthy or blameworthy.

The difficulty in assessing the degree to which 'voluntary' acts are actually 'free' acts – given the many factors which limit freedom and predetermine scope for action – may lead us to question more radically whether human beings are free at all. Do human beings have free will or are they wholly determined? It is important to note that both law and social morality rest on the assumption that people are normally responsible for their actions. Those wishing to plead diminished responsibility have to produce strong evidence that they were temporarily insane, incapacitated, acting under duress, or the like. Excusing conditions in law or morality are often offered by way of extenuating circumstances to lessen the degree of guilt or blame for an act, or to reduce the penalties exacted. Moral and legal discourse take for granted that it is possible to discriminate between voluntary, non-voluntary and reflex behaviour.

compulsions as excusing conditions – regarding human beings as at least partially responsible for their own ignorance, excessive drinking or tendency to give way to irrational compulsion.) (Downie 1971).

To act responsibly, and therefore to be in a position where one can be held responsible for one's actions, and praised or blamed for the outcomes, one would normally be held to have acted purposefully with knowledge, freedom and the

further reading

Considering moral decisions or moral policy
DeBono E 1990 I am right – you are wrong. Penguin Books, Harmondsworth – *a popular discussion of practical problems in moral argument and how to address them*

Hare R M 1981 Moral thinking, its levels, methods and point. Oxford University Press, Oxford – *a more advanced discussion of the issues from a philosopher bent on being practical*

Jonsen A R, Toulmin S 1988 The abuse of casuistry: a history of moral reasoning. University of California Press, Berkeley, CA – *a fascinating survey of the history of casuistry, but with most helpful practical applications*

Toulmin S 1981 The tyranny of principles. Hastings Center Report 11(6): 31–39 – *critical discussion of a naïve approach to moral judgement based on appeal to principles*

Toulmin S 1986 The place of reason in ethics (reprint). University of Chicago Press, Chicago – *a classic discussion of the logic of moral reasoning with real value in its practical application*

Are good nurses born, bred or educated?
Benner P 1984 From novice to expert: excellence and power in clinical nursing practice. Addison-Wesley, Menlo Park, CA – *critical examination of the 'breeding' of nurses, effects of gender stereotyping and power issues*

Crittenden P 1993 Learning to be moral: philosophical thoughts about moral development. Humanities Press, London – *a more advanced philosophical examination of the issues in moral development*

Johnstone M-J 1994 Bioethics: a nursing perspective. WB Saunders/Baillière Tindall, London, chs 1–6 – *a useful summary and overview of the issues involved in nurses acquiring skill and expertise in ethics*

Melia K M 1988 Learning and working: the occupational socialisation of nurses. Tavistock, London – *an empirical study of the process by which nurses are socialised into a professional role and set of values*

Methods of teaching applied ethics
Ketefian S, Ormond L 1988 Moral reasoning and ethical practice in nursing: an integrative review. National League for Nursing, New York – *review from a nursing perspective of ethics education in nursing*

Lamb M 1987 Nursing ethics and nursing education: past perspectives and recent developments. Perspectives in nursing 1985–1987. National League for Nursing, New York, p 3–21 – *a practical assessment by nurses of approaches to ethics in nurse training and practice*

Macintyre A 1990 Three rival versions of moral enquiry. University of Notre Dame Press, Indiana – *a critical appraisal of approaches to teaching ethics by a great contemporary moral philosopher*

Thompson I E, Harries M 1997 Putting ethics to work: a training resource pack. Public Sector Standards Commission, Perth, WA – *a practical guide to teaching applied ethics, values clarification, ethical decision-making and setting standards and ethical policy, especially applicable to the public services*

What is conscience?
Beauchamp T L, Childress J F 1994 Principles of biomedical ethics, 4th edn. Oxford University Press, Oxford, ch 8 (esp. p 475–483) – *a brief and readable account of conscience and conscientious objection*

Butler, Bishop Joseph 1970 Sermons, 'On conscience', iii. In: Roberts T A (ed) Fifteen sermons preached at the Rolls Chapel. SPCK, London – *a classic analysis of conscience*

D'Arcy E 1961 Conscience and its right to freedom. Sheed and Ward, London – *a classic and accessible discussion of the concept of conscience by a Catholic moral philosopher*

Johnstone M-J 1994 Bioethics: a nursing perspective. WB Saunders/Baillière Tindall, London, ch 13, p 449ff – *a very useful explanation of different theories of conscience and their application in nursing ethics*

How do we make sound ethical decisions?
Jonsen A, Siegler M, Winslade W 1992 Clinical ethics: a practical approach to ethical decisions in clinical medicine. Macmillan, New York – *a very practical guide which, while directed at doctors, is useful for nurses too*

Kerridge I, Lowe M, Mc Phee J 1998 Ethics and law for the health professions. Social Science Press, Katoomba, NSW, chs 4 and 5 – *gives some useful models for reviewing clinical ethical decisions and principles*

Steele S M, Harmon V M 1983 Values clarification in nursing, 2nd edn. Appleton-Century-Crofts, Norwalk, CT – *a most illuminating discussion of values clarification; also provides a rich variety of suggested types of exercise*

Thompson J, Thompson H 1985 Bioethical decision-making for nurses. Appleton-Century-Crofts, Norwalk, CT – *intended to be a practical guide to learning what decision-making means and how to do it*

Assessing moral competence
Kohlberg L 1984 Essays on moral development: the psychology of moral development: nature and validity of moral stages, vol 2. Harper & Row, New York – *a classic modern work on the process and stages of moral development*

Kurtines W, Gewirtz J (eds) 1984 Morality, moral behaviour and moral development. John Wiley, New York – *a collection of essays by a variety of authors reflecting on Kohlberg's theory, its usefulness and limitations*

Macintyre A 1981 After virtue, 2nd edn. Notre Dame University Press, Indiana – *a view from the perspective of virtue ethics, critical of the Kantian assumptions underlying Kohlberg's thesis*

end notes

1 Baruch de Spinoza (1632–1677), in his *Ethics* (Gregory 1955), developed a deductive system in which he sought to reduce ethics to a kind of mathematics. Utilitarians like John Stuart Mill (1806–1873), in his *Utilitarianism* (Lindsay 1957), sought to develop a kind of science or calculus by which 'the greatest good for the greatest number'could be determined empirically. Aristotle (384–322), however, in his *Nicomachean Ethics*, develops a system based on developing two kinds of skill or competency required by the moral agent – the intellectual and moral virtues. The intellectual virtues involve the acquisition of competence in a variety of methods and approaches to decision-making or problem-solving, while the moral virtues relate to the habits of character required for reliability, effectiveness and efficiency in action.

2 See previous note and Book 3 of the *Nichomachean Ethics*.

3 Bishop Butler (1692–1752), a critic of 18th century deism and psychological hedonism, believes conscience is both a God-given guide for action instilled in us by the Creator and the basis for the assurance that God is concerned for us and our ultimate well-being, giving us a more reliable compass to find our way to happiness than the assumption of the hedonists that we blindly follow the promptings of pleasure and pain and some vague general feeling of benevolence towards others. Conscience is not some irrational impulse, but the capacity to intuit the rational basis for acting in conformity with our God-given nature.

4 See Blaise Pascal's *Pensées,* iv, p 277 (Stuart 1950) and St Augustine's *City of God* (Healey 1968).

5 Freidson E 1994 *Professionalism Reborn: Theory, Prophecy and Policy*. Polity Press, Cambridge

6 Kant I (tr. Abbott T K), 1889, *Critique of Practical Reason*, Longmans Green, London

7 Augustine St (tr. Pontifex M) 1955 *The Problem of Free Choice (de libero arbitrio)*. Newman Press, Westminster, MD

8 Stebbing L S 1950 *Modern Introduction to Logic*. Methuen, London (chapter on causality); Toulmin S 1957 *Metaphysical Beliefs*. SCM, London, pt 1 (contemporary scientific mythology)

some suggestions on method

Considering moral decisions or moral policy
Students could be divided into small groups and assigned cases on a range of topics, requiring decisions about particular patients. These could cover cases of conflict over breaching patients' confidences in their interest, requested termination of pregnancy, a request for euthanasia or a patient needing to be given involuntary treatment. The exercise would be to first establish what decision needs to be taken and on what grounds it could be justified in the particular case. The second task would be to discuss what policy or legislation the students consider should be put in place to deal with the issue, and the justification for such legislation.

Are good nurses born, bred or educated?
The class could be engaged first in a general discussion of whether moral character is innate, the product of (unconscious) social conditioning or the product of deliberate education and training. Following this discussion, the class could be organised into three groups to prepare talks and to debate the question given as the title for this section.

Methods of teaching applied ethics
Having explained to the class the advantages and limitations of each of the given four approaches to teaching ethics, the class could be divided into four groups and assigned the task of preparing a lesson using one or other approach. The purpose would be to give students experiential understanding of each approach, followed by a critical debriefing on the advantages and disadvantages of each approach.

What is conscience?
The class could be introduced to the topic by contrasting the views of conscience as 'superego', 'intuitive awareness of moral principles', 'the voice of God in one's head', 'the virtue of prudence', 'the cognitive ability to integrate knowledge, experience and principles applying these to specific situations'. Alternatively, the class could be asked to debate the question by presenting a case to illustrate what they mean by conscience in practice.

How do we make sound ethical decisions?
Understanding of the value of using problem-solving models to assist us in making moral decisions can only be gained by repeated practice in applying them to real-life cases. Clearly the model would need to be explained and the tutor should assist by working through an example with the whole class. Thereafter, students should first be encouraged to practise use of the models in small groups, and then set examples to work through on their own.

Assessing moral competence
In order to bring home the issues involved in determining the degree of responsibility attributable to a person (or excusing conditions for the person's incompetence), it may be helpful to start with cases of patients with learning difficulties or mental disorder, and to progress to examining the issues in relation to more 'normal' patients, using case studies (preferably suggested by the students).

11

The relevance of moral theory: justifying our ethical policies

AIMS

This chapter has the following aims:
1. To assist students to understand the nature of philosophical disputes about ethical policy and the justification of ethical policies and rules
2. To develop in students a sympathetic understanding of the variety of ethical theories, what they seek to emphasise about our moral experience, and their strengths and weaknesses
3. To clarify the nature of deontological ethical theories and their attempt to provide a ground for universal principles, rights and duties
4. To clarify the nature of pragmatic theories and their function in drawing attention to the moral agent, personal responsibility for our actions and the choices we make of means and methods
5. To clarify the nature of teleological ethical theories and the importance they give to the values and goals which determine our actions, as well as the consequences of our actions
6. Finally, to emphasise the role of ethical policy and skills in developing rules and standards in professional life, business and society at large.

THE RELEVANCE OF MORAL THEORY

The reputation of ethics for being a subject where everything is contestable is perhaps well deserved, partly because of the nature of the subject, and partly because of confusion about the role of moral theory in ethics.

On the first point, Wittgenstein observed, 'Philosophy is not a theory but an activity.'[1] What he was concerned to emphasise was that philosophy (or ethics) is *not* a body of doctrine or truths that give ready-made answers to the questions of life. Rather, he was concerned to stress that philosophy is concerned with skills in analysis and with rational methods of addressing the various kinds of problem with which life presents us. In ethics, as we have observed before, people often look for moral certainty and simple 'right/wrong' answers to everything. Because life is full of uncertainty and complexity, people do not want to wait to work out rational solutions to problems – hence the appeal of fanatical religious and moral fundamentalisms with their simple certainties. Here we should perhaps remind ourselves of Nietzsche's advice: 'Beware of the dreadful simpli-

fiers!' However, it is also true that there is a lot of confusion about the nature of ethics: first, because 'problems' are tackled which are not single problems but complexes of problems, and second, because people misunderstand the role of moral theory.

In the previous chapter, we were concerned to clarify both what is involved in making ethical decisions and under what conditions people can be held responsible for their actions. We also considered a number of different approaches to teaching ethics and introduced a number of practical problem-solving methods to assist us in making sound ethical decisions.

In relation to making moral decisions in everyday life, we argued that if our decisions are to be well-founded and ethically justifiable, then we normally would be expected to be able to give an informed and intelligent account of the following:

- the background facts of the case and the nature of the problem faced
- the principles and rules which were applicable in the specific situation
- the means and methods we considered and used in making the decision
- what possible consequences of the action taken we took into account beforehand
- what specific objectives we set as the basis for our action plan
- what provision we made to monitor and evaluate the success of our action.

We pointed out that *moral theory plays relatively little or no part in justifying particular actions or decisions in specific situations*, but when we come to consider how we justify our general ethical principles and the policies we develop to deal with general types (or classes) of recurrent problems, moral theory does become important. In this chapter we proceed to consider the relevance of moral theory and both how we set general ethical standards and policies and how we justify them.

JUSTIFYING OUR MORAL PRINCIPLES AND BELIEFS

In the previous chapters, we discussed practical moral dilemmas in nursing in terms of the rights of patients and the duties of professionals, and discussed also the broader social responsibilities of nurses in terms of the Principles of Respect for Persons, of Beneficence and Justice. In doing so, we have not questioned the concepts of rights and duties, and have taken for granted that what was said about respect for persons, beneficence and justice would be commonly understood. In other words we have taken for granted that there is a broad consensus in our society about the meaning of these fundamental moral concepts and principles. We have argued against a superficial relativism that the principles of beneficence, justice and respect for persons are essential to all human societies – because they relate to the fundamental relationships of power and responsibility that people share in all moral communities. We maintain this is true despite the different weighting these principles may each be given in different cultures and the different conventional forms in which protective care, justice and respect for the rights and dignity of people are expressed.

However, it must also be obvious that people may not only challenge the way these principles (of beneficence, justice and respect for persons) are applied in practice, but also demand adequate theoretical justification for our believing in these principles at all. Some moral disagreements in society, as between conservatives, liberals and socialists, are about the relative weight given to various competing claims, e.g. of personal rights and liberty versus the state's duty to protect its citizens and maintain law and order, or between personal autonomy and the demand that everyone 'should have a fair go'. Some groups will challenge the established moral consensus about sexual mores or the use of drugs, as when people campaign for gay rights, the legalisation of abortion or the liberalisation of drug laws. Alternatively, we may question the very basis of morality and the moral beliefs we have come to accept as the basis for living. This may occur because of some major personal crisis, social dislocation, experience of war and revolution, exile or imprisonment, or the impact of a different religion or culture on ourselves.

To engage in critical reflection, discussion and analysis of these issues is to engage in the activity that we call moral philosophy. Ethics, as we have said, is the activity of systematic reflection on the principles, moral rules and values on which we act; thoughtful examination and practice of decision-making skills; and learned discrimination in choosing appropriate decision procedures for different action contexts. The systematic study of the means we use to justify moral actions and decisions is what we call ethics. However, the critical study of the theoretical underpinnings of our moral systems, beliefs and principles is what we call meta-ethics, or moral philosophy.

The aim of this book is practical and therefore, as we indicated in the Preface, we have attempted to keep the amount of moral theory or moral philosophy in it to a minimum. In this chapter, however, we will now turn to consider some of the more important and commonly used moral theories, and to discuss both their strengths and weaknesses, to what aspects of moral action they draw our attention, and what they tend to overlook.

Most stable societies have a long tradition of law and custom which embodies the established moral consensus of that society. Obviously, laws and customs do change and develop with the times and may change dramatically in times of war or revolution or rapid social change. Moral rules are not unchanging, nor do we start from scratch and have to invent them anew with each generation. From the time we are born we find ourselves in a morally structured environment, in our family, school, community. Some features of that moral environment we accept or tolerate, others we rebel against and may try to change. Negotiating and renegotiating the boundaries and limits of the moral community is a sign of life in a moral community, as people do not simply accept the imposed social order (say communist or capitalist, democratic or authoritarian) but seek to reinterpret or change society's moral priorities, by appeal to 'higher' moral ideals. Moral communities, even the most traditional and conservative, are not static, but do change and evolve with time – some more dramatically and radically than others – and some, after periods of apparent liberalisation, revert to fanatical and conservative fundamentalism. With the dramatic changes in the geopolitical order in the past decade, the revival of religious and political conservatism may well be an understandable defensive reaction to insecurity and too much change. However, moral and religious bigotry are essentially dysfunctional ways of dealing with moral disagreements and cultural differences in society.

Whether societies can change and adapt to major shifts in moral attitudes will depend on the adaptability of their underlying assumptions about human nature and society. Social institutions cannot function without some stability in laws and customs. Some kind of moral consensus is necessary for the ordered functioning of society. In a relatively stable society we do not constantly question the moral beliefs of our community. For all practical purposes we take these for granted in our day-to-day decision-making, unless and until we are faced with a crisis of some sort. This may be a major social crisis or a personal moral dilemma where our moral convictions are at odds with what we are required to do, or where the majority viewpoint differs from our own. Here we are forced to consider the kinds of reasons and evidence we would advance to defend our moral beliefs.

SUBJECTIVE, CONVENTIONAL AND OBJECTIVIST ACCOUNTS OF ETHICS

Birth, copulation and death affect our private lives most intimately, and these have traditionally been the areas most carefully hedged about with taboos to protect the rights and vulnerability of individuals. These are also the areas where modern society has challenged the traditional taboos most fundamentally and where modern technology has opened up whole new areas of ambiguity in the traditional moral consensus. Fertility control, assisted reproduction by artificial insemination, ovum donation, in vitro fertilisation and embryo transfer, genetic engineering, organ transplants, artificial life support and the possibility of cryopreservation of human beings comprise some of the current issues debated in medical ethics. If we are challenged to say why, as a matter of policy, we think any of these things are wrong and should be

prevented, or why we think they are morally justifiable, we may adopt one of a number of different strategies:

- We may say that we just 'feel' it is right or wrong, but do not really know why and would prefer not to discuss it. In so doing we may give expression to the view that moral beliefs are private and subjective, based on our feelings or intuition, and that they cannot be settled by argument or appeal to evidence.
- We may argue that moral beliefs are decided by convention and that these differ from one society to the next. Different societies arrive at a consensus, or some sort of social contract, by reasoning together and agreeing to certain rules for their mutual protection and benefit. Other societies may have different kinds of convention based on similar or different reasons and may or may not recognise the validity of one another's conventions.
- We may claim that moral beliefs are grounded in the objective nature of things or the inherent structure of human reason, and must be universally valid. From this point of view, the first approach (subjectivist) leads to arbitrariness and irrationality, the second (conventionalist) to relativism. The 'objectivist' argues that morality is based on the objective 'laws' which govern our given physical and psychological nature as human beings. If morality can be grounded in nature in this way, then it can be argued that ethical principles have interpersonal validity and a kind of objectivity that the other two approaches do not allow.

Moral principles, however we seek to justify them, are important for our day-to-day living and decision-making. They help in the ordering of moral experience and provide some sort of systematic basis for decision-making. They are both psychologically necessary to help make sense of our lives and moral experience, and practically useful in enabling us to make value judgements in a non-arbitrary manner. In both senses, they assist us in our communication with others and in the rationalisation of cooperative action. It is because they perform this primitive ordering function of knowledge and action that we call them principles. They also serve as starting points for reasoning about action and the methods and rules we should adopt to make responsible decisions. It is doubtful whether anyone can do without principles and continue to function in society or as a member of a moral community.

Agreement about moral principles is obviously highly desirable and makes social life a lot easier and tidier. But how do we arrive at agreement, and what is meant by 'agreement'? The view that moral principles are entirely private and subjective, although commonly held, is an inadequate basis for any kind of social or professional ethics, for ethical decisions would be arbitrary and capricious. Such a view would lead to inconsistency in individual practice, make social cooperation very difficult and ultimately lead to anarchy in society. The fact is that while we may agree to disagree about matters of taste, we do continue to argue about moral principles and try to persuade others to our point of view. That is because we recognise implicitly that for moral rules to have any validity, to be binding on us and on other people, then they must apply equally and universally to everyone. The legal system and other social institutions could not function without universal rules. In practice we cannot claim our rights as members of any moral community without making a personal commitment to the values and ground rules which operate in that moral community, and without accepting responsibility to uphold and defend the principles we hold in common.

Underlying our moral disagreements and continuing arguments about moral issues is a conviction that moral principles must in some sense be universal and objective. We continue to seek reasons and evidence to establish moral agreement. We could take refuge in irrationality, but that does not help either to justify the moral position we adopt or to defend us against the attempts of others to impose their moral beliefs on us. We have to continue to reason together, in the attempt to find rational grounds for interpersonal agreement and social cooperation. We try to establish some kind of intersubjective validity for moral principles, and by appealing to common

sense and universal features of human experience seek to justify and give objectivity to our moral judgements.

In whatever way we attempt to defend our moral principles, we are bound to adopt one or other of these three strategies, or a combination of them. The reason is that each strategy emphasises an aspect of moral experience that is important in itself. Ethics does relate in a special way to what it means to be a subject, to be an autonomous moral agent, to have ownership of a set of values and principles for living. However, it is also concerned with the social conventions which govern the way we relate to one another and which serve to define our social duties and rights. And, finally, we act out our purposes in the real world, where our actions impact on other people and bring about objective changes in reality, with both desirable and undesirable consequences.

The *subjectivist* is perhaps less concerned to emphasise the private and non-rational nature of moral judgements than to stress that moral principles are something we must choose ourselves and make our own. No-one can decide for you what values you must adopt, or on what principles you must base your life. You have to make your own commitment to them and try to live your life in accordance with them. In this sense the subjectivist points to the necessary moral autonomy of the mature person. Moral principles and values are always very personal in this sense – in so far as they are believed in and acted upon by persons who may feel very strongly about them and may stake their very lives on them. Because of this very personal identification with a moral point of view, we may not like our feelings about moral matters or our commitments to be challenged. However, this personal aspect of moral commitment does open us to accusations of subjective bias or moral prejudice. Part of what the other approaches emphasise is the necessity for external checks.

To the *conventionalist*, the most important fact to emphasise is the public and social character of our moral beliefs and their function as necessary conditions for social intercourse and cooperation. Conventionalists do tend to point out the variations in moral conventions between different societies, not primarily to stress the relativity of all values, but rather to emphasise the need for tolerance of other people's values. The universality of moral principles, in this view, is achieved by negotiated rational agreement between people of different cultures and traditions and learning to be tolerant of diversity.

Objectivists are concerned to avoid the dangers of irrational subjectivism and a relativism which they see as threatening to undermine the sense of public moral accountability and the imperative and unconditional character of moral principles. Objectivists seek to anchor the concepts of value and obligation in the real world and not in personal feeling or mere social convention. For them, moral principles must in some sense correspond to the demands of reality, as they believe the universality of moral principles and their objectivity can only be guaranteed in this way. They tend to argue that moral laws are fundamentally laws of our nature, given with the very structure and dynamics of human life in the world. Alternatively, the objectivist argues that the principles of morality are derivable from the given structure and nature of reason, as imperatives which we logically must obey if we are not to contradict our nature as intelligent beings, or which we must follow if we are to achieve fulfilment of our nature as rational beings.

Plato suggested in his dialogue, *The Gorgias*, that there are five kinds of 'agreement' that are necessary in honest and rational moral discourse and which can serve as a foundation for moral consensus in society. (Hamilton 1950). These kinds of agreement might be called the five C's:

- Our individual actions should agree with one another, i.e. be *consistent*
- Our lives should have unity and integrity, agree with what is good, i.e. be *coherent*
- Our actions should agree with the demands of the situation, i.e. *correspond* to reality
- Our thoughts and actions, profession and practice should be *congruent* with one another
- Our ethics should be capable of agreement with the general human *consensus*.

The demand that our moral life and acts should display these forms of agreement, namely self-consistency, coherence and correspondence with the demands of reality, relate to some of the objective tests we might apply to someone's ethics. Congruence and consensus relate more to subjective and conventional forms of 'agreement'. The test of congruence is a test of sincerity and agreement between subjective intention and action. Consensus, or agreement in principle with others, is the necessary foundation for social contracts and conventions. We need to consider all five aspects of moral experience when we speak of justification in ethics. These different senses of agreement each emphasise an important aspect of moral experience, but none is adequate by itself to cover the whole complex subject of what it means to lead a moral life in company with other people.

VARIETIES OF MORAL THEORY

Many different kinds of ethical theory have been put forward in the course of history to justify an existing moral consensus or to justify particular moral principles, and, as we have argued, these can be classified under the headings of 'subjective', 'conventional' and 'objective' theories. Introducing the DECIDE model for ethical problem-solving in the previous chapter, we suggested an alternative way of classifying types of ethical theory, based on analysis of the 'causes → means → ends' structure of intentional acts (see Box 11.1):

- *Causes* – ethical theories that focus on the antecedent conditions or principles which serve as the foundation for our moral duties and rights, and which we must take into account before we act. These theories are called 'deontological' from the Greek *deon* (= 'duty'). Typical of these theories would be divine command theory, natural law theory and rational intuitionism.
- *Means* – the second class of theories which focus on action and the moral agent as the primary means by which ethical principles are applied to the world of moral experience can be called pragmatic theories. They include

theories which focus on the practical means and methods required for our actions to succeed. Typical of the first type would be virtue ethics, which focuses on the integrity and competence of the moral agent; and of the second type, prudential ethics, pragmatism and situation ethics (including a love ethic such as Christian agapeistic ethics), which focus on the specific demands of the situation.

● *Ends* – this final class of ethical theories focuses on the intended goals and outcomes of our actions, and is called 'teleological' from the Greek *telos* (='goal' or 'end'). Typical of these theories would be Aristotle's theory that all human action aims at happiness (teleological eudaemonism); utilitarianism, which recommends the practical criterion of 'the greatest happiness for the greatest number'; and consequentialism, which determines whether moral actions are good or bad by assessing their consequences, costs and benefits.

DEONTOLOGICAL ETHICAL THEORIES – FOCUS ON PRINCIPLES, RIGHTS AND DUTIES

Divine command theories

In virtually every known society, ethical codes have had their origin in religious traditions and

---

Box 11.1   Classification of types of moral theory

'Causes' – prior conditions and principles

Deontological ethics
Divine command theories
Natural law theories
Duty- or rights-based theories

'Means' – agency, means and methods

Pragmatic ethics
Virtue ethics (integrity of agent)
Prudential or casuistic ethics
Agapeistic and situation ethics

'Ends' – goals and consequences

Teleological ethics
Teleological eudaemonism
Utilitarianism and hedonism
Consequentialism

---

practice. This is not just a matter of anthropological interest, but also of philosophical significance, which tells us something important about the nature of ethics. If moral principles and rules are to command our respect and to be equally binding on all members of society, then their authority must be based on something more than personal caprice or the arbitrary edicts of kings or tyrants. The authority of moral principles and rules depends on them being understood to have an authority that transcends the self-interest of individuals, however important or powerful. A divine or suprapersonal basis for the authority of moral rules would seem to guarantee their universally binding character, ensuring that they can serve as the foundation for unconditional rights and obligations.

Further, if morality is not to be dictated simply by the edict of the king, high priest or clan leader, and enforced by that person's authority (as has often been the case), then these powerful figures themselves must be subject to some higher authority and not allowed to be 'a law unto themselves'. Only submission of king and citizens alike to the same ultimate source of moral authority will ensure that moral rules are respected and obeyed by all. Divine command theories appear to provide such an ultimate and transcendent basis and sanctions for the authority for law and morality.

In Judaism, it is claimed that the Torah – the Law of Moses and the Prophets – ultimately came from Jahweh (the God of Abraham, Isaac and Jacob). The Jewish leader Moses, who led his people from oppression and slavery under the Egyptians into the Promised Land, claimed that the Ten Commandments were given to him by God on Mount Sinai. The Ten Commandments were to form part of a covenant between God and His people. According to Moses, God agrees to care for and to protect His people as long as they obey His commandments. The Jewish law developed over the centuries as a complex body of religious, dietary and social rules as well as basic moral principles. While this Law was particularly binding on the people of Israel, the Jews believed these laws were universally applicable to all human beings and that it was their mission to teach all people to obey the laws of God.

For both the Christian religion and for Islam, the Ten Commandments remain the foundation of their ethics. However, each of these world religions developed an ambivalent attitude to the rest of the Jewish tradition of the Law and the Prophets, including the Commentaries by rabbis and legal scholars over the ages. Rejected by orthodox Judaism, both these movements developed in time into independent religions.

Jesus of Nazareth, believed by Christians to be the Son of God, was not only a reforming prophet, proposing a more radical obedience to the spirit rather than the letter of the law, but he also set out in his teaching, and particularly the Sermon on the Mount, a new ethic of love and forgiveness, which was to serve as the foundation for the movement that he started. While Christian ethics is founded on the teaching of Jesus and the two Great Commandments – to love God and to love one's neighbour as oneself – it is also an example of a divine command theory, in so far as Christians believe Jesus spoke with the authority of God Himself. It is on the basis of this claim that Christians maintain that their ethic of love has universal application, and believe that they are called to preach the gospel of love to all people everywhere.

The followers of Mohammed, and his teachings as recorded in the Koran, make similar claims for the ethical teachings of Islam, namely that they are directly revealed by God to his Prophet, have universal applicability and are binding on all humankind. While Muslims do not believe Mohammed to be divine, they do believe that in a special sense he was the primary channel through which Allah revealed the ultimate principles of human conduct and the truth about human destiny. 'Islam', which means obedience to the will of God, Allah, reasserts a radical monotheism (belief in one God) in opposition to what they see as tritheism in the Christian belief in Father, Son and Holy Ghost.

All three world religions emphasise the fundamental importance of ethical living and obedience to the moral law as necessary conditions for salvation and eternal life. However, divine command theories are not exemplified only by these three religious traditions; in many other religious traditions, appeal is made to some supernatural source of authority for the moral law. In Aboriginal Dream-time, the ethical and religious traditions of the people are supposedly communicated by the Spirits of the Earth to the ancestors, and by the ancestral spirits to the elders and then to the people, in dreams and re-enactments of the timeless rituals of the people. The authority of ancestral spirits is invoked in African animism and ancestor worship, as the basis for ethical and religious practice, and to reinforce the authority of the moral law and tradition.

Natural law theory

The second form of deontological theory is the type that claims that the moral law is in some sense written into the constitution of things. It is claimed that just as the laws of physics govern the operation of the natural world and serve as the foundation of order in the universe, the moral order is founded on the laws given with and inherent in human nature.

In its classical form, natural law theory is difficult to disentangle from traditional religious beliefs, in both the Graeco-Roman and Judaeo-Christian traditions. In the 5th century BC, the Greek tragedian Sophocles portrayed his heroine Antigone as standing up to the injustice and arbitrary rule of King Creon in the name of natural justice (Fagles & Knox 1982). Antigone defies Creon and gives her brother the proper burial rites, despite the King's edict forbidding the burial of her brother because he had raised a rebellion against Creon's tyrannical rule of Thebes. To justify her apparent impiety in opposing the will of the King, Antigone appeals to the Justice which governs the universe, and which not only the King and all people, but even the Gods, must obey.

Plato, commonly regarded as the father of Western philosophy, drew a clear distinction between 'nomos' or conventional law, based on social custom and popular agreement, and 'phusis' or the inherent laws of our own nature as human beings. He argues that 'phusis' or natural justice is more fundamental than 'nomos' or conventional law and morality. He advances two different kinds of reason for this claim. The first is that unless there is a more fundamental basis for justice than the arbitrary edicts of tyrants and the fickleness of public opinion, there can be no rational basis for objecting on moral grounds to unjust laws or unjust acts. He concludes that because we can conceive of the possibility of rational justice there must be some kind of transcendent standard or form of justice against which unjust actions and laws can be judged and found wanting. Secondly, he argues that what makes order and harmony in the cosmos, society and personal life possible is that they are all governed by natural laws inherent in the structures and dynamics of being itself. 'Dikaiosune', the ideal form or standard of justice, is, he believes, the principle of order and harmony in things. His belief in this more fundamental natural justice was inspired by the practical example of the life and death of his master Socrates (469–399 BC). Socrates not only made himself unpopular by interrogating politicians and lawyers, by demanding to know the true nature of justice, but was also accused of 'corrupting the youth', because he challenged traditional religion for its lack of moral standards. He voluntarily drank the hemlock, acting as his own executioner, because he said he did not wish the city of Athens to commit an even greater injustice by killing him as an innocent man. By accepting his fate and voluntarily drinking the executioner's cup of poison, Socrates bore witness to his belief in an eternal and incorruptible Justice which ruled the Universe, transcending the corrupt justice of men (see Rouse 1984).

Within the Biblical tradition, we have the figure of Job, in the biblical allegory of that name (Ch. 19, vv. 25–29), who is portrayed as an ideally righteous and innocent man who suffers what Shakespeare called 'the slings and arrows of outrageous fortune'. Despite the injustice and humiliation he suffers at the hands of men, the abuse of his friends, the challenging and questioning of his integrity, and the injustice of the fate which God allows to befall him, Job believes that God, who is ultimate justice, must be consistent with his own nature and will therefore come to his aid and vindicate him. His words have become an expression of hope to many people in despair: 'I know that my redeemer lives, and that he shall stand at the latter day upon the earth... that you may know that there is justice.' In a different vein, the Old Testament prophets rail against the corruption, abuse of power, immorality and injustice of kings and people in the name of the God of Righteousness and Justice. The clear implication of the Judaeo-Christian tradition is that human laws must be subjected to the test of congruence with this more universal divine justice, by which the 'justice' of men and their laws are often found wanting.

This belief in a universal cosmic justice, more fundamental than the arbitrary justice of men, is common to many religious and cultural traditions. It has much in common with divine command theories, except that it does not attribute the moral law directly to some kind of divine edict, but rather sees the natural moral law as built into the very structure of things in the way an intelligent Creator, in designing things to serve a specific purpose, constructs things so as to reflect intelligent and therefore intelligible purposes. What distinguishes natural law thinking from divine command theories is that while the latter requires simple obedience to the will of God, the natural law tradition requires us to use our intelligence or reason to analyse the laws which govern the Universe and our own nature. It is claimed that by the exercise of human reason, and without supernatural revelation, we can discern from our experience and study of human nature what requirements we have to meet if we are to fulfil our species being and achieve the purposes for which we were made the way we are.

The Greek and Roman Stoics argued that the universe is rationally intelligible because it is a cosmos, i.e. an ordered whole governed by rational laws. Human reason is just a part of the Divine Reason, the basis of this rational order in the universe. That is why human reason can understand this order. It is claimed that rational beings must live in accordance with this given rational order in nature if they wish to achieve fulfilment, happiness and a state of harmony with others and the world. Here again, the appeal to a moral law written into nature is made, first, to resist the arbitrariness of personal edicts and the relativism of social conventions and, second, to explain the universality and interpersonal validity of moral principles (Cowen 1961).

When the Roman Empire expanded to include numerous other societies and cultures, Roman jurists found it necessary to develop a distinction between the conventional law of the societies they ruled (e.g. the Mosaic Law of the Jewish people) and the universal principles of law which they believed were applicable to all societies and by which the justice of conventional laws might be judged. The former was called the *jus gentium* (law of the people), the latter the *jus naturale* (the natural law). This *jus naturale* became the basis of what in the tradition of Roman–Dutch Law was called 'natural law'. Two traditions developed in Roman–Dutch Law: the first emphasised the Stoics' view that the rationality of justice derives from it being grounded in the rationality of the order of nature; the second, later tradition sought to ground the rationality of justice in the rationality of human beings and in the social contracts they develop to express that rationality.

The Roman Catholic tradition of law and morality has traditionally been based on a doctrine of natural law which tends to be reinforced by arguments taken from revelation. In its classical form, the doctrine is similar to the Stoic one. The argument rests on a number of connected premises:

- God created the world an ordered harmonious whole, governed by natural laws
- human beings have the intelligence to deduce these laws of nature from their experience
- they can infer what it is necessary for them to do if they are to fulfil their species nature
- they can choose to live a fully human life following these natural laws, or live a life of frustration and ultimate self-destruction by acting against the laws of their nature.

Thus natural law theory presupposes that people can arrive at knowledge of the natural law

from observation of Nature and their own make-up, and hence deduce what is necessary for them to flourish as human beings, and what to avoid if human life is not to be inhuman or subhuman, or if life in society is not to be dehumanising and people treated in an inhumane way (see d'Entrevres 1951, Finnis 1999).

The strength and appeal of the natural law tradition exists partly in the fact that it represents an attempt to ground ethics in something objective and more stable and enduring than individual caprice or changing and culturally determined social conventions. Of course, the various interpretations of natural law principles and precepts will have culturally determined features or emphasis, but this 3000-year-old tradition has endured and a lot of its precepts have found their way into the common law, public and international law, declarations of human rights and the constitutions of various states.

However, natural law theory is not without its problems. Perhaps the most hotly debated issue is what do we mean by 'nature' or 'natural' in the context of ethics and law? Is surgical intervention to prevent a maternal death in the case of ectopic pregnancy a natural, unnatural or non-natural intervention? Further, even if we can agree general and broad guidelines or statements of fundamental rights, based on natural law, how these are 'cashed out' in terms of operational rules, laws and moral decisions in particular cases may still leave much room for argument and disagreement. The mere fact that moral debate has to be related to the features of the world which we share in common, and is not based on arbitrary subjective opinion, personal or mob feelings, or fickle conventions, is some guarantee that as we negotiate democratically with others the mutually acceptable boundaries of the moral community, what we will arrive at has some objectivity.

In Christian ethics definition of the natural law is often supplemented in practice by appeal to revelation – to the laws given by Moses and the teachings of Christ. When Catholics condemn abortion or contraception as evil, because they claim it is 'unnatural', it is not always clear whether they do so on the basis of natural law or biblical teaching, or a combination of both (Gill 1985, Gilson 1994).

Historically, natural law theory in ethics and jurisprudence has had an enormous influence on the development of both our social and legal institutions. Against the view that statutory law enacted by a sovereign parliament has ultimate authority, people have appealed to the concept of natural law and natural justice to challenge unjust laws or what they see to be the tyranny of the majority. When Americans seek to test the validity of laws by their consistency with the Constitution (which embodies a declaration of human rights), or when appeal is made to English common law, appeal is being made to principles of natural justice which are considered more universal than statutory law. The United Nations Declaration of Human Rights and other modern attempts to formulate universal human rights make implicit or explicit appeal to the idea of rights as grounded in the nature of humans as such, to natural law.

Belief in the absolute sovereignty of parliament (on the basis that it represents 'the will of the people') can be dangerous if it means that enacted laws or statutes can be thought to override any other considerations of justice or morality. Talmon (1966), in *The Origins of Totalitarian Democracy*, traces historically how this doctrine has led to totalitarianism and tyranny. He also predicts that unless constitutional safeguards are built in, such as the principles of natural law, many modern democracies based on the claimed ultimate sovereignty of parliament can be led down the same road – attempting to define by legislation the scope of social morality, without the possibility of a higher court of appeal against unjust laws (cf. Arendt 1967).

Duty- or rights-based theories

The German Enlightenment philosopher, Kant, the most famous proponent of this type of theory, argued that it is not the end result or consequences of an act which make it right or wrong but the goodwill or intention of the agent. It is the intention to do one's moral duty which determines whether an action is morally praiseworthy. To get

to this view, Kant developed an argument about the rational nature of moral principles and moral obligation, which has been of the greatest importance for ethics.

He maintained that for a moral principle to be binding as a duty, in other words for a principle to be *moral*, it must be (a) universal, (b) unconditional and (c) imperative. Kant said we can never arrive at the notion of obligation from an empirical study of the tendencies built into nature, or from the psychological study of man's feelings about pleasure and pain. The concept of duty, he argues, follows as a logical consequence from our notion of rational practice. Human actions cannot be consistently rational unless they obey rules which are universal, unconditional and imperative. In his determination to combat moral scepticism and relativism, Kant set about demonstrating, in his *Groundwork to the Metaphysic of Morals*, that there are universal principles presupposed in, and necessary to, the formulation of any coherent system of ethics (Paton 1969). He argued that any system of ethics based purely on empirical observation of human psychology, of human nature, or study of the practical consequences of actions cannot lead to certainty. At best, such reasoning can lead only to probabilistic conclusions. Similarly, an ethics based on feeling risks being as arbitrary or fickle as capricious emotion. Unless moral duties are certain and absolute, there is no way to avoid the apparent relativity of all moral values. The way seems open to moral scepticism.

Kant's confidence in human reason and rational order in the universe was grounded partly on religious and metaphysical beliefs, partly on the logical proofs provided in his *Critique of Pure Reason*. Here he had demonstrated to his satisfaction that without the *a priori* categories of pure reason, we cannot make sense of the jumble of impressions we receive from our senses (Kemp Smith 1973). Furthermore, he adduced from this given rationality in the world of our experience that this order must have its origin in a suprapersonal cosmic reason. In the *Critique of Practical Reason*, Kant argued that there are three essential and necessary presuppositions of all morality, namely God, freedom and immortality (Beck

1949). God, he infers, is a necessary postulate for morality, for without a god it would not be possible to ground the moral law or the absolute duties of the moral life, or to ensure the universal, categorical and imperative nature of moral obligations. Without freedom or the power of self-determination and choice, we cannot speak intelligibly of moral action or moral responsibility, for all our behaviour would be automatic, reflex or socially conditioned. Kant considered immortality of the rational soul necessary to guarantee the enduring and universal validity of moral values and rules, and the ultimate significance of the moral life for individuals.

In addition to these metaphysical arguments for the existence of God, human freedom of will and the immortality of the soul, Kant developed some powerful formal arguments about the essential logical requirements for an ethical system to be consistent and coherent. What he did was to explore what he called the *constitutive and regulative principles* of ethics as such. In more modern terms he set out to clarify the logical basis of ethics as a universe of discourse in its own right. If ethics is a way of speaking about the world and human actions in it, what are the rules of this 'language game'? Kant adduced several concepts which are in his terms 'constitutive' of ethics as such:

- the concept of a moral law
- the concept of a universal and coherent system of such laws
- the concept of a person
- the concept of a kingdom of ends.

Kant was struck by the fact that moral duties are not conditional in form (If...then...) but categorical (Thou shalt.../I must do...). The moral 'ought', he argued, is categorical and imperative, but it is also, and must be, universal. Moral duties cannot be accepted as binding unless they are understood to apply universally, to be equally binding on everyone. The concept of duty and universally binding moral laws follows logically, Kant believed, from the concept of a rational agent as such. Rational beings are those who know by introspection that they must act rationally in conformity with their own rational nature and the rational structure of the universe, if they are to live a life that is rationally self-consistent, moral and thus satisfying to a rational being.

The concepts of 'personhood' and a 'universal kingdom of ends' are more substantive and less purely logical principles of an ethical system. As explained in Chapter 4 , Kant argued that ethics cannot get off the ground without the concept of a person, not merely as a rational agent, but as a bearer of rights and responsibilities. In the *Groundwork to the Metaphysic of Morals*, the definition of personhood he gives is abstract and formal. In order to apply respect for persons as a regulative principle of ethics, this formal definition of 'person' has to be filled out with named human attributes and the details of specific situations, before it can be 'cashed' in concrete 'moral transactions'. Thus, for example, we will arrive at somewhat different definitions of fundamental human rights, depending on whether we define human beings as 'rational animals' (Aristotle), 'having a capacity to love' (Augustine), or as 'capable of creative work' (Marx). There are, however, obvious links and interconnections between these attributes, and differences are mainly about which should be given priority in the definition of human rights or duties.

Similarly, behind his very abstract discussion of the *principle of the universal kingdom of ends* there is something like the ideal of an all-embracing rational good or common goal for which all rational beings are striving. Behind the principle of universalisability as well is the demand that the laws which apply to one should apply to all for the sake of the common good. Implicit in these two concepts is the principle of justice, or universal fairness. Finally, in his concept of doing our duty, based on the principle of reciprocity ('do as you would be done by'), Kant offers a social justification for the principle of beneficence, namely the demand that we should care for other rational beings in order to assist one another to achieve fulfilment as moral and rational beings.

Deontological theories of ethics are often linked to religious beliefs and tend to be absolutist in form. The absolutist character of moral principles or duties can derive, as in Kant's case, from metaphysical and formal arguments about their logically necessary character, or they may be claimed to be absolute because commanded by God or based on sacred scriptures or pronounced by figures representing divine authority. Some kinds of Christian ethics are based on such absolutist deontological principles – exemplified by advocates of total pacifism, or 'pro-life' opponents of abortion or euthanasia under any circumstances – but Marxists and proponents of other secular ideologies may adopt similarly absolutist positions on people's categorical duties to the state or to other citizens. Such deontological theories can take two forms: act deontology and rule deontology.

Act deontology is based on the claim that one can intuit directly one's moral duty, what one ought to do in a particular situation, by rational introspection. It represents a personal and subjective view of duty that attempts to determine whether particular actions are right or wrong on the basis of whether one's motives are pure or one's intentions good and conform to what one believes is one's duty. The appeal by Quakers to the Divine Light, and the appeal of others to the 'light of conscience', as well as some forms of rationalist belief in the illumination of rational intuition, are all variants of act deontology. As such, they are virtually indistinguishable from intuitionism and do not necessarily make claims about the universal validity or applicability of moral rules to all rational beings.

By contrast, *rule deontology* is the position outlined earlier which tries to emphasise the universal, unconditional and imperative character of moral laws or rules and moral duties. In this sense, rule deontology attempts to establish that ethics has an objective, suprapersonal character, based on the universal rational structure of the universe and represented in microcosm in human reason. In terms of rule deontology, actions are right or wrong in so far as they conform to the universal, categorical and imperative character of moral rules within a coherent and consistent system of ethics. Alternatively, they must satisfy what Kant called the 'principle of universalisability', namely that any general rule by which I act in a given situation can only be said to be moral if it can be universalised. That is, I have to ask myself: 'Could the rule on which I am acting now become the basis of a universal law, and therefore applicable to everyone?'

The value of both forms of deontological ethics is that they draw attention to the fundamental role of the concept of obligation in ethics. Other systems of ethics (e.g. teleological and utilitarian, hedonist and subjectivist theories) focus on personal life goals, striving for personal fulfilment, concern with the well-being of the majority and pursuit of personal happiness or pleasure. These theories do not do justice to the reality of duty or obligation to others, as fundamental to our experience of membership of a rational moral community. They also fail to explain the sense in which duty transcends personal interest or possible pleasure or gain. It is exemplified by selfless service to others or personal sacrifice for a transcendent ideal. Ethical absolutism has a prophetic quality in offering uncompromising opposition to what is seen as evil. While other more pragmatic approaches may appear to compromise or to be vacillating and indecisive, an absolutist acts confidently and often courageously in the conviction that he is right. However, absolutism may lead to rigidity, intolerance and self-righteousness. In this sense, 'absolutism without prudence is empty and formal, and worldly-wise prudence without principle is blind' (with apologies to Kant).

Deontological theories, and Kant's in particular, are often criticised for empty formalism. This is both the strength and the weakness of this type of theory. The strength of formalism lies in its universality and its emphasis on the suprapersonal, supranational character of moral laws. It is thus no accident that there is a direct line of connection between Kant, the later Idealists, and the principles which underlay the first attempts at world government in the League of Nations and the United Nations Declaration of Human Rights (UNO 1948). The weakness of the theory lies in the fact that the gap between the theoretical principles and their practical application is so wide that other lower-level concepts and principles are required to enable us to work with such a formal system of ethics in practice. A related difficulty is that if we interpret all moral laws as universal and unconditional imperatives, then there is no way we can sensibly decide which rule to obey if we are faced with a conflict of duties (e.g. between telling the truth and lying to protect someone from a person who wishes to kill him). However, the abiding insight of deontological theory is that ultimate (rather than derivative) moral principles must be universal and binding on us all, if they are to serve as a basis for both individual and social life (Maritain 1963).

Kant's deontological ethics has often been described as a form of *rational intuitionism*. As such, it represents a form of subjective theory of ethics which maintains that we arrive at moral principles by rational introspection, by looking into our own minds and grasping what we find there. 'Intuition' means direct perception, insight. In popular terms, we know what is right by consulting our consciences.

Rational intuitionism is the view that by direct inspection of our own minds we can know what to do. Intuitionism comes in both simple and sophisticated forms, and perhaps there are elements of intuitionism in all ethical theories. For example, how in natural law theory one knows which elements of order are relevant to moral experience is a matter of moral insight. Similarly, knowing what is the most loving thing to do in a particular case means considering all the relevant factors and arriving at a judgement by some kind of intuition, rather than crude calculation. At its crudest, intuitionism may represent a refusal to give reasons or evidence for a moral point of view, and can represent a retreat into inarticulate irrationality. But, more seriously, it is an attempt to draw attention to the activity of the moral subject as an essential factor in moral judgement. Computers cannot make moral judgements; it has to be a human subject, or moral agent, that alone can do so.

Intuitionists have traditionally tried to avoid the charge that moral principles are the products of random, arbitrary and capricious judgement by arguing that there are given structures in the mind or moral experience which we can intuit. For Plato, moral principles are in some sense innate. We are born with certain implicit moral ideas which it is the function of reason to make explicit in consciousness. For the early Quakers and certain Reformers, we know moral principles by illumination from the Divine Light or Holy Spirit. In defending the ultimate authority of personal conscience against the moral authority of the Pope or the Church, they appealed to direct intuition of moral principles. For Kant, intuition is the introspective rational activity whereby we grasp the principles which alone make reasoning and a rational moral life possible. This process gives us insight into the form of the moral law. Intuition of what he called the unconditional and categorical *a priori* forms of reason is the ultimate basis on which we justify moral principles. He claimed, as we have seen, that moral principles are ultimately grounded in man's rational nature as such, and further that the categorical, or unconditional, nature of moral obligations is guaranteed because finite reason is rooted in the Infinite Reason which is the source of all things.

Intuitionism emphasises two important features of moral experience: first, that our consciences are pre-formed in some way before we come to make moral judgements for ourselves; and, second, that to be regarded as responsible moral agents we must have internalised a set of moral values and made them our own. We may explain the pre-formed character of conscience as did Plato, the Quakers or Kant, or we may explain conscience in terms of the process by which we are educated and socialised into the acceptance of a set of values. In practice, it is difficult to separate intuitionism from theories which explain the 'origin' of moral principles in social convention and social conditioning. When someone says, 'That is just not cricket', he appeals implicitly to the moral consensus among the English as to what is acceptable behaviour and what is not. The 'intuition' of what is right or good tends to be filled out in practice by content drawn from religious tradition or social convention. However, as has been said, there is an element of personal judgement or intuition in the way moral principles are both understood and applied, and it is important we recognise this.

PRAGMATIC ETHICAL THEORIES – FOCUS ON MEANS AND METHODS

Virtue ethics – an ethics of personal and corporate integrity

Virtue ethics is as old as Aristotle (384–322 BC) and as new as Alastair Macintyre's (1981) defence of virtue ethics in his book *After Virtue*. What it does is to focus attention back onto the moral agent rather than the abstract principles, rights and duties on which we base our judgements or on the practical consequences or outcomes of our actions. Virtue ethics concentrates on the moral agent as the person who is responsible for deciding how to apply general moral principles to specific situations in order to bring about the desired consequences. Among the various means and methods used in effecting change through actions, the moral agent is the primary means or channel through which things get done.

What virtue ethics emphasises is that the quality of the action produced is affected by the integrity and competence of the moral agent. If the agent is corrupt, the action is likely to be corrupt. If the moral agent is incompetent in either a practical or a moral sense then the action is likely to be less than satisfactory. If you lack the skill or competence to perform a particular act (e.g. to insert a catheter or intravenous drip) then it would be morally irresponsible and unjust to patients to subject them to your incompetence. If you lack any or all of the basic intellectual or moral virtues, then the quality of your action is likely to be compromised. Here we have in mind Aristotle's classification of the forms of *intellectual competence* (or virtues), which include relevant scientific knowledge, technical skill and experience, intelligence, discriminating judgement and practical wisdom; and his list of *moral competencies* (or virtues), which include honesty, temperance or self-discipline, courage, justice and fairness, magnanimity and wisdom.

There are close links between virtue ethics and the emphasis on professional competence in modern competency-based training, and the emphasis on striving for excellence in corporate management, business and public administration. The popularity of virtue ethics in contemporary business ethics links with the quality movement in business management (including 'quality assurance', 'performance assessment', 'continuous improvement' and 'total quality management'). Here, the notion of 'quality' is linked directly to striving for excellence at the levels of individual virtue (or competence), corporate virtue (or integrity) and continuous improvement in the quality of services delivered or products manufactured.

In his book *After Virtue*, Alastair Macintyre challenged the dichotomy set up in contemporary moral philosophy, between *deontological* and *teleological* theories, and suggested that virtue ethics represents a bridging third type of ethical theory which has been neglected in the debates between deontology and teleological utilitarianism.

The way debate about ethical theory has been presented as a choice between deontology and teleology as mutually exclusive alternatives has led to unproductive adversarial conflict between these two schools of thought. The polarisation of these two approaches was greatly influenced by Kant, who reformulated the agenda for philosophical ethics by setting an absolutist ethic of principle and duty against anything else that relativises ethics, and against pragmatic or utilitarian arguments in particular.

Kant was concerned, above all, with the clarification of the logical foundations of ethics and the defence of ethics as a rational discipline against the psychologising tendency of the Scottish empiricist David Hume. Hume had argued that there can be no necessary connection between facts and values, and that we cannot deduce moral laws from the laws of nature. His most famous sceptical remark about previous attempts to found ethics on 'natural law' was to say that we cannot logically derive 'ought statements' from descriptive or 'is' statements. Instead, in his *Treatise of Human Nature*,[2] Hume fell back on our subjective feelings as the basis for our value judgements, and human sympathy and rational self-interest as the basis for ethical conventions. 'Custom', he said, 'is the great guide of human life' (Downie 1971).

For Kant, custom or practical utility cannot be an adequate basis for ethical obligation, or a basis for the universality of rational ethical principles. His attempts to provide rigorous logical proofs of the 'constitutive' and 'regulative' principles of ethics, in his *Groundwork to the Metaphysic of Morals*, presuppose that reason and logic are the final arbiters of ethics. He argued that we cannot base moral obligation on conditional principles ('*If* I do … *then* … will result'). Contingent facts – like whether the results of my action will turn out well or badly – he insists are irrelevant. Moral principles have to be universal and *unconditionally binding* on everyone. Thus Kant emphasises the concept of duty, based on rational rules, to the exclusion of anything else. Utilitarian arguments that attempt to justify moral actions by their outcomes, costs or benefits, either beg the question of what goods are to be regarded as 'benefits' and what evils as 'costs', or tend to use the end to justify the means chosen for our actions. Kant maintains that we should act out of a motive of pure duty for duty's sake. He will have no truck with doing your duty for some kind of personal reward or benefit.

Macintyre believes that by reducing ethics to a choice between deontological and utilitarian ethics, modern philosophers have undermined public confidence in ethics. He criticises Kant's ethics for its arid formalism and abstract intellectual approach to our moral experience. He sees Hume's ethic of sympathetic feeling as leading to subjectivism and moral scepticism. The hedonistic utilitarianism of Bentham and Mill he sees as attempting to substitute calculation of the relative importance of various pleasures and pains for oneself and society for the exercise of personal moral responsibility. He argues that contemporary ethics has been reduced to either barren explorations of the logical grammar of the language of morals or to the arbitrary subjectivism of emotivist theories of value. What both schools do is to treat moral judgement abstractly, i.e. both traditions ignore the existing historical subject or person who is a member of a particular society or moral community with a defined role, and who, as a good, bad or incompetent moral agent, makes actual decisions and acts in the world for good or ill.

What Macintyre attempts is to rehabilitate the *concept of virtue*, rescuing it, on the one hand, from sanctimonious and pious religious associations, and on the other, from empty formalism. He encourages us to return to the foundational work of Plato and Aristotle on ethics, where virtue is linked to the striving for excellence and the attain-ment of knowledge of being. Like them he focuses attention on the key *concepts of intellectual and moral competence.* He also points out that virtue can only be defined in a social context, in relation to a person's role and duties or responsibilities in a moral community. In focusing on virtue, or those personal qualities of the moral agent that serve as indispensable *means* for the effective translation of abstract principles into action, bringing about good or bad effects in the world, he is saying in effect: 'a plague on both your houses'! From another point of view, he is describing the moral agent as the bridge between principles and practice, and the virtue of prudence as central to moral judgement and achievement of the good life.

The Greek notion of virtue as an 'athletic' concept, both literally and metaphorically, linked with moral strength and vice with moral weakness. The perfection of bodily development, mastery of skill and balance, and the achievement of outstanding performance all serve as a model for 'virtue' when applied by Plato and Aristotle in the moral domain. Perhaps the main interest of Macintyre's work here lies in its immediate relevance to contemporary attempts to address the issues of quality improvement and the achievement of excellence in business and professional practice. His emphasis on virtue as related to the performance of a role in society gives importance to the determination of standards for performance appraisal. Thus it has considerable relevance to corporate ethics and concern with the qualities of leadership and teamwork in business.

Because most modern business is corporate in nature, often involving large national and multinational corporations, a focus on individualistic ethics is likely to miss the mark in terms of what is needed for our times. Here Aristotle's and Plato's emphasis on moral agents as not being a complete 'law unto themselves', but as needing to cooperate in organisational life, becomes relevant. Besides, such a non-absolutist approach to ethics, which focuses more on discrimination and judgement and less on simply abiding by the rules, is more appropriate to situations where people have to exercise leadership and responsibility.

Prudential or casuistic ethics

Prudential ethics (like jurisprudence in law) has its roots in the tradition that goes back to Aristotle, who argues that we cannot solve ethical problems simply by deductive argument from given principles or by applying universal principles directly to any and every issue. The process of ethical problem-solving is a complex one, both logically and in so far as it requires skill, knowledge and experience. While deontologists want to defend the universal and categorical nature of moral principles, Aristotle and the advocates of a prudential and casuistic approach to ethics are concerned to emphasise that decisions always relate to specific individuals acting in particular situations. Further, because no two situations are precisely identical, it requires discrimination and judgement to make appropriate decisions.

Prudential ethics emphasises that ethical decision-making is a problem-solving activity requiring knowledge, skill and experience to do well, and thus has two parts: the first focuses attention on the nature of problem-solving and the logic of decision-making, and the second focuses on the types of competency required in the decision-maker – what Aristotle calls the virtue of prudence (or practical wisdom). *Casuistic ethics* is related to prudential ethics. It develops within the tradition of prudential ethics and legal practice. What the casuist maintains (as pointed out in Ch. 5) is that ethical issues have to be decided on a case-by-case basis. From this it follows that we cannot simply apply universal rules to each and every case of the same type without considering the specific features of each case. This means, on the one hand, taking account of the specific demands of the situation, the affected parties or players in the drama, and the nature of the crisis requiring a decision; on the other hand, the casuist questions the value of universal principles and is sceptical about whether we can achieve more than well-founded precedents based on repeated experience of dealing with similar cases. This means that moral judgements cannot claim to be certain or indubitably right, but rather that they are probably correct, or that a decision based on serious consideration of similar cases is at least likely to be the best practical solution, given our past experience (Beauchamp & Childress 1994, Ch. 2, p. 92ff).

Aristotle's ethics combines the emphasis of virtue ethics on the integrity and competence of the moral agent with a detailed analysis of the virtues (or competencies) necessary for sound moral judgement and effective moral action. His analysis of the structure of moral problem-solving, which we have already touched on several times, is developed on the foundation of the intellectual and moral virtues. In Figure 10.1 (p. 262) we illustrated how Aristotle conceives prudence as the keystone of an arch made up, on the one hand, of the intellectual or theoretical virtues and, on the other, of the moral or practical virtues. Aristotle makes it clear that he believes that the fully competent moral agent will possess both types of virtue in a proper balance, held together by the virtue of prudence or practical wisdom, and that ability to exercise these intellectual and moral virtues is a necessary condition for competent decision-making. So what are these virtues?

The intellectual virtues (or competencies)

The intellectual virtues required by the moral agent to make competent decisions are listed and discussed by Aristotle as follows:

- *Science* – theoretical and practical knowledge of the world, human psychology, and of oneself
- *Technical skills* – practical expertise and life skills, acquired through experience
- *Discrimination* – a variety of minor intellectual competencies including intelligence, judgement, self-insight, persistence and resourcefulness
- *Wisdom* – the ability to integrate all the above and apply them to one's personal life.

For competent nurses, possession of the intellectual virtues necessary to perform their job well and to make sound ethical decisions would include all these virtues. They would need to have a sound grounding in the medical sciences (e.g. anatomy and physiology, genetics, endo-crinology and pharmacology), in the behavioural sciences (e.g. social science, psychology and ethics), and in self-understanding gained through participation in training which facilitates personal growth. In addition, they would have to have had extensive supervised ward-based and community experience in which they had learned to apply theoretical and practical knowledge in clinical situations and developed an appropriate level of competence to be 'let loose' on patients. Finally, their performance would be subject to regular assessment to establish that they were developing their intelligence, skills and confidence in judgement, self-insight, reliability and resourcefulness. Growth in wisdom would be evident in the extent to which all this had become 'second nature' to them.

Competence in ethical decision-making within this tradition requires knowledge and skill in a number of different areas, and all these require discrimination and judgement. The knowledge required is knowledge of the world, how things work, of human nature, and of the basic values and principles that apply to all human societies, as well as our own specific moral community. More than mere intellectual knowledge is required. We also require understanding of their scope and application. Of the skills required, the following are the most important:

- *Ability to identify the facts of the case, the nature of the problems and their causes.* In reality, what may present as one problem may be several entangled problems. The ability to sort these out and identify which is most important to tackle first is the primary task and skill. This may only come with life experience and practice in decision-making.
- *Ability to identify and prioritise the ethical principles relevant to the problem.* Because real-life problems are often complex, several ethical principles may have a bearing on the resolution of a difficult case. Having the ability to rank the relevant principles aids clarity of thought and responsible decisions.
- *Ability to consider the variety of available means and possible options for action.* Possession of

acquired life and social skills will increase the repertoire of possible and relevant responses we can make to a situation. Life experience will also give us insight into what we can and cannot do ourselves, with or without the help of other people or resources.
- *Ability to appraise the relative value of these options, based on past experience.* In making an assessment of which is the best option, or the least bad option in a difficult situation, requires that we make competent and informed value judgements. Knowing the rules is not enough; the question is how best to apply them, especially if there is no rule that conveniently fits the problem at hand.
- *Ability to act with resolution and clear achievable objectives, to execute an action.* Indecisiveness is not only a sign of weakness and lack of competence, but may actually be dangerous. To be decisive means having the courage to take risks and to accept personal responsibility for the outcome. 'Decision' (like the doctor making an *incision*) means moving out of the comfort zone of 'head-talk' into the real world of real people trying to find real solutions to real problems. Provided one has applied appropriate knowledge and skills, the risks may be reduced, but they are never eliminated. Decisions may be wrong, dreadfully wrong! They may also be the right decisions, which bring rich benefits and rewards to oneself and others.
- *Ability to review actions in the light of one's objectives and to learn from one's mistakes.* Skilled problem-solving, as Aristotle recognised, builds the 'feedback' loop into the process, as part of the learning cycle, ensuring that past experience is put to good use in future decision-making.

The moral virtues (or competencies)

Moral decisions cannot be taken by robots or puppets, but only by persons who act freely, understanding what they are doing, and who are committed to a clear set of values and principles on which they stake their choices and perhaps even their lives. The person who simply does what he is told acts either unthinkingly or under the compulsion of an externally imposed rule. Kant regarded this state of *heteronomy* as the enemy of responsible moral action, which he insisted was based on *autonomy*.[3] The ideal of moral autonomy is not just, as the media would tend to suggest, being able to do what you want. Autonomy does not mean licence or even just liberty 'to do your own thing'. Autonomous moral choice and action means *acting on a basis of values and principles which you have made your own*. Without moral commitment there is no real personal responsibility.

But what are the personal moral qualities that make the difference to whether my performance is outstanding, mediocre or poor? These *competencies* correspond to what have been called the 'moral virtues', in contrast to the 'intellectual virtues' we have just discussed. What, then, are the key moral virtues? These classically were defined as temperance, courage, justice, sociability and prudence.[4]

Temperance.   This traditional virtue points to a kind of inner strength of the individual that is expressed in self-mastery, self-discipline and self-control. Like tempered steel it is not brittle, but flexible and resilient. It does not mean being a 'teetotaller' but does convey the sense of being a balanced person and one of moderation rather than excess.

Courage.   This virtue is of particular importance to the person who has to take responsible decisions. It means being able to strike the right balance between timidity and recklessness, based on sound knowledge and experience of life. Courage is linked to loyalty and integrity – in the sense that the courageous person is someone reliable and consistent at work, and faithful to friends and colleagues. The courageous person is also able to stand up for what he believes is right and good, and stand by his decisions and take responsibility for his actions.

Justice.   As a personal quality or virtue, justice has to do with the perception that one acts fairly towards others, is even-handed, listens well, respects the rights of other people, and shares power equitably with other people. Justice has to do, above all, with ability to act always with the good of others in mind, and not to discriminate against or abuse people. However, it also has to do with the need to exercise authority where it is necessary to ensure that the interests of others and the moral community are protected from harm.

Sociability.   In addition to the *cardinal virtues*, Aristotle taught us that the morally competent person also has a range of social skills and that his understanding of human nature is based on ability to get on with other people and co-operate with them in both work and society. Good communication and social skills are traditionally seen to be essential to the decisive and responsible person. These skills are necessary for one to be able to think clearly and express one's thoughts. They are also essential if one has to seek help from others or persuade them of the merits of one's plans. These skills are also related to the way we best acquire knowledge of other people, how they think and how they are likely to act normally and in a crisis.

Prudence.   As a moral virtue, prudence is the ability to integrate the moral and intellectual aspects of one's life, and to apply one's knowledge and skills with appropriate concern for the good of the moral community and oneself. As a state of excellence, prudence involves possession of a range of particular skills. These are traditionally described as follows:[5]

- Clear-sighted objectivity, decisiveness, ability to learn from real experience, and to be flexible
- Accurate recollection and recording of facts; gives reliable testimony; checks things out
- Humility to learn from others, recognising the need for help and advice from others
- Foresight – a sense of timing and ability to recognise likely outcomes of one's actions
- Cunning or worldly-wise, without being cynical – 'as wily as serpents and harmless as doves'.

The virtue of prudence[6] is closely linked in Aristotle's thought with what we would call an *informed conscience*. Conscience in classical philosophy did not mean some 'voice of God' or 'voice of parental authority' echoing in one's head, but an intellectual faculty. This *faculty* or *ability* to make sound practical judgements includes both theoretical knowledge of moral principles and practical skill or experience in their application. It also includes the idea that sound moral judgement requires an ability to properly assess the particular facts of a situation, and also to be able to *see the big picture* – past, present and likely future possibilities which have a bearing on a decision. To describe prudence as a 'faculty for practical judgement' implies that it is a virtue that has to be developed by habit and practice. It is not an innate ability, nor is it something that has been programmed into us. Prudence is described as the measure of the other virtues, in the sense that its role is to maintain a proper balance in life, or sense of proportion between the other virtues. Prudence is also said to inform the other virtues, i.e. it provides the knowledge base for other virtues. It plays a crucial role in moral judgement because it is based in practical life experience, of trial and error, and is concerned with the choice of the best ways and means to achieve our goals.

We may paraphrase Aristotle's definition of prudence in its practical application in moral decision-making as follows: *prudence is the knowledgeable and skilled ability to apply universal principles to the demands of particular situations, in such a way that we choose the most appropriate means to achieve a good result or outcome.*

For Aristotle, prudence is the key virtue, determining both the general competence of the moral agent and that person's specific competence in making effective moral decisions. Failure to develop this capacity or potential, or allowing it to atrophy through lack of practice, results in *weakness of will* (or *akrasia*) and *indecisiveness.* These, like the other vices, express essentially a lack of developed competence or a negative state of unfulfilled potential. As the keystone of the arch, prudence not only is the bridge between the intellectual and moral virtues, but holds them together, giving strength and resilience to the whole character of the person.

Finally, to return to casuistry, this is really best understood as an adjunct to a prudential ethics, where the existence and importance of universal ethical principles are still recognised, but they have to be adapted and applied in a relevant way to the needs of particular situations. Casuistry without principle has justifiably been the subject of ridicule – for it becomes indistinguishable from an ethic of convenience and compromise. However, it is equally true that an ethic of principle which does not take account of or learn from particular cases can be criticised for being inhumanly rigid, out of touch with reality and abstractly formal.[7]

Agapeistic ethics or an ethics of care

We have encountered the New Testament Greek term *agape*, for caring love of another, in two other contexts in this book already – first in discussing the strengths and limitations of 'caring ethics' in Chapter 5, and then in Chapter 10, in discussing the situationist approach to teaching ethics. In both contexts we emphasised that agapeistic ethics *focuses on the concrete relationships between particular people at a particular time and place*; thus (from Ch. 5):

In the attempt to do justice to the needs of specific people in particular circumstances, the Judaeo-Christian love ethic has emphasised the kinds of obligation that are rooted in caring for others, rather than a more legalistic approach. In fact, St Augustine, in his commentary on 1 John 7: 8, summed up Christian ethics in the challenging phrase 'love, and do as you like' (Clark 1984). An ethics of caring (or agapeistic ethics) which strives to determine what is the most loving thing to do in the circumstances serves three different kinds of purpose:

- First, it offers an alternative to an impersonal rule-based ethics of duty, emphasising that the obligation to care for individuals, as we would want to be cared for ourselves, is more important than obedience to formal rules.
- Secondly, it emphasises that caring love demands that in decision-making we pay attention to the specific individual rather than society in general, to the particular circumstances rather than universal conditions and requirements.
- Thirdly, it underlines the fact that our actions have to be measured by their effects on particular people and situations rather than their conformity to general rules and duties.

Judaeo-Christian ethics has tended to take one of two forms: either to build theistic elements into the doctrine of natural law, making the mind of

God the source of the intelligible order in the universe and human life; or to opt for a love ethic (or a combination of both). The tradition of agapeistic ethics is mainly Jewish and Christian, but is not confined to these world religions. Its foundation in the Jewish tradition is summed up in the Shema Israel – the call to the people:

Listen O Israel: Yahweh our God is the one Yahweh. You shall love Yahweh your God with all your heart, with all your soul, with all your strength.
(Deuteronomy 6: 4)

You must not exact vengeance, nor must you bear a grudge against the children of your people. You must love your neighbour as yourself. I am Yahweh.
(Leviticus 19: 18)

In contrast to the natural law tradition, which emphasises the rationality of human beings above everything else, the Judaeo-Christian tradition seeks to define the essential nature of human beings in terms of their capacity to love. In theological terms, the argument is that God is love, and since people are made in the image of God, the most important thing about people, the most important value in human life, is love. In terms of this theory, love is not only the essence, the very 'power of being' in human life, but it is also the ultimate test and justification for our moral decisions and actions. Love can also be the specific norm we apply to every situation and on which we base our moral judgements, and decide what is the most loving thing to do in particular circumstances.

In the theological tradition, there has been disagreement about the extent to which we can infer, from the essential nature of God as love, that human beings, supposedly made in the image of God, are capable of disinterested and forgiving love of the same kind. Thinkers who reflect on the evil in the world and human society, and the apparently depraved nature of man, are reluctant to conclude that imperfect human beings are capable of agape love without supernatural assistance. Anders Nygren, in his book *Agape and Eros* (1953), distinguishes radically between 'eros' as natural human love and 'agape' as a form of supernatural caring love only made possible through the action of divine grace in our lives. Martin D'Arcy, because he does not accept the total depravity of human nature, argues in the

Heart and Mind of Love (1962) that both 'agape' and 'eros' are natural to human beings, although he would agree that the example of Christ and divine grace makes it easier for us to practise care and forgiveness towards others. The contemporary Jewish philosopher, Emmanuel Levinas, despite his experiences of the Nazi Holocaust, argues passionately in his *Ethics and Infinity* (1985) for the recovery of ethics, not as an intellectual enterprise, but as the actual engagement of person with person, face to face: 'Access to the face is straightaway ethical.' In his book *Responsibility for the Other* (1982), Levinas argues that love is an unconditional commitment to the other for the other's sake, and is made possible by the gift of personhood which the other makes to me *en face* – making me self-consciously aware of myself as a person in relation to another person and therefore directly responsible to that person as the other.[8]

From a more practical and historical perspective, agapeistic ethics has developed in reaction and opposition to legalistic ethics within both Judaism and Christianity. Appeal has been made to an ethic of love when ethics has become a matter of fearful obedience to the law, or a matter of empty or superstitious ritual. Agapeistic ethics is a protest against the conception of God as a remote and merciless judge who demands strict justice and ritual purity from adherents, and has insisted that God must be a loving God who cares for us in our frailty. Against moralism, as the morality of false guilt and taboos, and legalism, as the observance of the letter rather than the spirit of the law, agapeistic ethics has demanded authenticity, truthfulness and openness in religious and moral life. Love-based ethics claims that we cannot force concrete human situations, in their everyday variety and uniqueness, to fit the requirements of abstract general laws. Love demands recognition of the particular character of each unique human person, his situation and the painful complexity of the moral choices he makes in real life. To live by love rather than by the demands of the law is liberating, it is claimed, while living by law is restricting and guilt-inducing (Pontifex 1955).

The second important emphasis in agapeistic love-ethics is on the importance of the affections in our moral life. The emotions are, as the word 'e-motion' suggests, what get us going and motivate us to act in the first place. The master-psychologist St Augustine (354–430 AD) describes human life as being in the state of *inter-esse*, i.e. as 'being-in-between', meaning that we are not self sufficient but contingent beings, or creatures in his terms. All our interests arise from our state of *inter-esse*. It is because we are incomplete and therefore needy creatures that we have feelings of desire. Our desires relate to our fundamental needs, and these desires drive us to act to satisfy our desires. Augustine, like his master Plato, observed that desires are insatiable, they are potentially infinite while realisation is always finite. A particular meal, or experience of sexual delight, may satisfy us temporarily, but sooner or later we seek further satisfaction of our desires. The problem then becomes how we regulate our desires and loves and do not become slaves to impulse.

The critics of an agapeistic love-ethics – which seeks to determine how we should act by simply asking what is the most loving thing to do in the circumstances – argue that one cannot live without rules, that this anti-nomian, anti-law, form of love ethic leads to anarchy. In response to the charge of anti-nomianism, advocates of agapeistic ethics have adopted two different approaches. The first is to say that *there is logic to our loves* which does provide some guidelines as to how we should act. The second, more radical, alternative is to say that we do not need rules at all, that rules prejudge human situations and moral experience, that *we must therefore approach each situation as far as possible without preconceptions* and allow love alone to dictate to us what to do.

There are several examples of the first kind of love ethics. The moral philosophy of St Augustine is perhaps the most famous and has been the most historically influential, while the writings of the American Methodist philosopher Paul Ramsey (1980) have perhaps been the most important of recent theories. Augustine argued that since God is love and people are made in the image of God, then it is their capacity to love which characterises their essential nature. 'If you wish to know what a man is, ask what he loves.' From this

it follows that in one's concrete historical existence, the problem is to work out and achieve the right ordering of one's loves, as he says: 'the primary task of the moral life is to achieve the right order of priority amongst one's loves'.

But how do we know what is the right order of human loves? Augustine argues that God has created nature as an ordered hierarchy of beings: from the lowest physical elements to plants, insects, animals and humans, and, he would add, angels at the top of the hierarchy! Corresponding to this order in nature is an order in human life, of the physical, emotional, intellectual and spiritual. Human loves can be ordered in their moral importance accordingly. All lower loves must be subordinated to *agape* – love of God and love of neighbour. Friendship, the desire for personal fulfilment, erotic love and the basic physical appetites are each important in their own place, but unless each is subordinated to the other, in the proper order, then chaos is likely to result. Basic physical appetite must be subordinated to, and controlled by, the others, or it leads to selfish exploitation of others and to one's own harm. The desire for self-fulfilment has to be subordinated to the demands of friendship and the higher duty to care for the well-being of others under God, and so on. Evil for Augustine is but deranged love, giving undue importance to lower loves at the expense of higher (Jaspers 1962, Frankena 1964, Healey 1968).

The second type of love ethics, what has been called 'situation ethics', can also be traced back to a saying of Augustine: '*dilige et quodvis fac*' – 'love and do as you please' (Clark 1984). What Augustine suggests is that love alone is a sufficient 'law' by which to live, and that if we are faithful to the nature of agape caring love, then we will always find the most appropriate and loving way to deal with each situation. By emphasising that love is a sufficient criterion by which to judge all other moral rules, St Augustine shows remarkable faith in the ability of human beings to live by the principle of agape love and to discern how to apply it in each and every situation.

In its 20th century form, situation ethics owes a great deal to existentialist philosophy, in particular to Sören Kierkegaard, Friedrich

Nietzsche, Jean-Paul Sartre and Albert Camus. They share a common detestation of hypocritical bourgeois morality, moralism and an ethics of respectability. In their quest for moral authenticity, they each stress in different ways the need to approach each situation on its own terms, without moral prejudices, and to be open to its possibilities and unique ethical demands. Joseph Fletcher (1979a), in his book *Situation Ethics*, served more than anyone else to popularise a situation-based love ethic. He also attempted, in his book *Humanhood: Essays in Biomedical Ethics* (Fletcher 1979b), to apply this kind of love ethic to medicine. Broadly speaking, he argued that all that doctors and nurses need, by way of moral equipment, is their personal knowledge, skill and expertise as health professionals, a commitment to a love ethic and a sensitivity to what each human situation demands. Deciding what is right to do in each case would then mean simply taking account of the unique circumstances of each patient, the nature of the responsibilities of the caring relationship between the health professional and the needs of each individual patient.

While also advocating a love ethic, Paul Ramsey, in his book *Deeds and Rules in Christian Ethics* (1983), and William Frankena, in his various writings on agapeistic ethics, criticise Fletcher's position as simplistic and ultimately untenable. Ramsey argues that a love ethic cannot avoid the need for rules, as any case which serves as a precedent, or any general requirement of love, is itself a rule of a kind. He goes further to demonstrate that just as Augustine suggests that there is an ontological basis for determining a hierarchy of love, so in everyday life when we apply the love principle, we prioritise our love commitments. As a result of this criticism, Fletcher has somewhat qualified his position in his later work. What all three authors wrestle with is the tension between an ethic based on love which attempts to be faithful to the demands of the situation and the needs of the specific individual. Frankena (1964) and Ramsey (1983) both attempted to answer the need for rules in Christian ethics as well as caring love by developing the idea of 'covenantal love' (Ramsey's expression), namely the varying kinds of commitments we make to others in relation to the norm.

David Hume's ethics of sympathy and the logical positivist emotivist theory of value can each be seen as secularised versions of agapeistic ethics.[9] For Hume, 'reason is and ought to be the slave of the (sympathetic) passions', by which he means that sympathy is not only what binds society together, but also the criterion and norm of what is ethical. For the positivist, moral judgements are but covert expressions of our feelings of approval or disapproval of actions. While this 'boo-hurrah theory of value' is easy to satirise, it too emphasises the importance of our feelings as motivating our actions, influencing what we value and thus our value judgements. However, its limitations lie in the fact that it evacuates ethical discourse of any meaning or significance. In *Language, Truth and Logic* (1958), A. J. Ayer puts forward the positivist empirical meaning criterion, namely that 'every meaningful proposition is either analytic or empirically verifiable', and he revels in the fact that according to this criterion the propositions of ethics and theology are literally nonsense.

What all these pragmatic ethical theories have in common is that they pay primary attention to moral agency. Virtue ethics focuses on the moral agent and the competencies the agent requires to act effectively and ethically. Prudential ethics focuses on the nature of practical, effective and prudent decisions, and the practical means required to implement our decisions. Agapeistic and situation ethics concentrate on the demands of love, the feelings and desires that motivate us to act, and the specific requirements for appropriate and authentic action in each given situation.

TELEOLOGICAL ETHICAL THEORIES – FOCUS ON ENDS, GOALS AND CONSEQUENCES

Teleological theories (Greek *telos* = 'end' or 'purpose') seek to justify moral principles *either* in terms of some overall goal or sense of purpose in nature or human society *or* in terms of the consequences of actions, their results or outcomes relative to goals.

These two approaches relate to two different senses of 'goal' or 'end' in our experience. The latter type of justification relates to *purposeful acts*, which have specific goals. The former is less familiar, although it has been very influential, namely that of some kind of *built-in purpose or design in nature.* This is seen as either God-given or inherent in nature, perhaps linked to the evolution and development of species.

Teleological eudaemonism – the end of human life is happiness

Aristotle (384–322 BC) was the son of a doctor, and was perhaps first and foremost a biologist. His ethics is described as a form of teleological eudaemonism –'teleological' because of his belief in a built-in *telos* or purpose in nature and in human beings, and 'eudaemonistic' because he saw human life as fundamentally motivated by the quest for happiness or well-being (from Greek *eudaimonia* = happiness). This system of ethics has been one of the most influential in the history of Western culture and has greatly influenced Christian ethics, particularly that of the Roman Catholic tradition.

As a biologist, Aristotle is struck by the fact that living things grow and develop, and so he built into his ethics and philosophy developmental concepts that he derived from his observations of nature. For example, he observed that all living things have a built-in tendency to fulfil their genetic potential, to develop from embryonic form to the fulfilled mature form of their species. Plants and animals begin as tiny seeds and grow into what may be large trees or gigantic elephants or whales, progressing through various developmental stages towards the fulfilment of the form of their own species. Acorns do not turn into apple trees nor caterpillars into people. Each species seems to strive toward the fulfilment or perfection of its form and reproduction of its kind.

For Aristotle,[10] human beings appear to be goal-directed in two senses; first that they are capable of *purposeful and self-directed action*, and second, that they appear to *strive towards some ultimate end or telos*, namely happiness or the fulfilment and perfection of their essential nature as human beings. This striving or built-in tendency to fulfil all the potentialities of our species being (to achieve physical, emotional and intellectual well-being) is both innate in us and also capable of being recognised and then rationally and voluntarily self-directed by each person. The goal which governs this striving is the pursuit of happiness, both in terms of personal well-being and fulfilment, and in terms of the happiness of the rest of society, since, as 'political animals', we cannot be happy in isolation.

Aristotle distinguished between 'pleasure' and 'happiness'. Whereas pleasure and pain are physical sensations or psychological states, happiness is a state of being. Pleasure and pain may be transitory and may relate to a part of the body or to particular feelings. Happiness, however, relates to the state of the whole person, is more enduring, and may persist even if the person is experiencing pain. Happiness relates to purposeful action and, as a disposition or orientation of a person's whole being, is directed towards some ultimate goal or ultimate good. Ethics as a whole is concerned with goal-directed action and the ordering of life and life's priorities towards the achievement of this ultimate good and personal fulfilment. Virtue and vice are defined in terms of whether they promote or frustrate the flourishing of individuals or society, and promote achievement of personal fulfilment and the general health and well-being of society.

According to Aristotle, *the quest for pleasure and the avoidance of pain are needs-directed, whereas happiness is goal-directed, relates to being and action directed towards our self-fulfilment and self-actualisation as human beings.* Aristotle recognised that our basic human needs drive us to pursue pleasure and that it requires effort to rise above this level to pursue a life of rational reflection. This bears comparison with Maslow's *Hierarchy of Human Needs* (1970). According to Maslow, we can only pursue the higher levels of personal and intellectual self-actualisation when we have successfully met our lower needs. These needs, in descending order of importance relative to the necessities for survival, are:

● the need for intellectual and personal self-actualisation
● the need for self-esteem and social recognition

- the need for social role, identity and employment
- the need for personal security – health, emotional and material security
- basic physical survival needs – food and water, clothing, shelter, etc.

From Maslow's point of view, Aristotle has a somewhat elitist view of happiness. As a relatively wealthy Greek citizen or freeman, he could afford a view of personal happiness based on the leisured pursuit of the intellectual pleasures of philosophy, whereas his slaves would be prevented from experiencing happiness, to the extent that the practice of philosophy is a necessary means to achieve it. However, this criticism does not completely invalidate what Aristotle says about happiness. For him, all people, including slaves, strive for happiness, even if the conditions of their life frustrate the full realisation of their potential. For happiness is not simply a matter of feeling, but *contentment arising out of fulfilment of one's potentialities as a human being.* Happiness is more enduring than pleasure, because it is concerned not with a part but the whole of one's being, and may thus persist even if the person is an oppressed slave or is experiencing pain. Happiness as a disposition consists in the active orientation of one's life towards some ultimate goal or ultimate good. Ethics has as its primary goal the ordering of life and life's priorities towards the achievement of personal and social fulfilment, health, well-being and happiness. Virtues and vices are defined in terms of whether they promote or frustrate the flourishing of individuals or society. Personal growth through the development of the intellectual and moral virtues serves to promote both one's own health and well-being and also that of our whole society, for, according to Aristotle, as 'political animals', we cannot but be concerned about other people, for our fulfilment is involved in theirs, and theirs in ours.

In many respects, this theory has common elements with natural law theories, in emphasising that the tendency to strive for happiness is built into our nature as a law of our very being. It is not just a matter of subjective feeling or personal desire, but a given characteristic of human nature.

Aristotle's theory has been called utilitarian, in so far as his test of the rightness of actions and moral principles is whether they are ultimately conducive to the greater good and happiness of men and society. However, his ethics was more tied to his biology and philosophy of nature, and his view was that the tendency to strive for happiness is inherent in human beings and not a matter of choice by individuals or agreed social policy. He would have agreed that human beings have to understand and strive consciously to achieve fulfilment, but he would have argued that we also have a natural tendency to do so. Whereas the psychological hedonist considers people to be completely determined and un-free, Aristotle believed we are capable of self-determination and thus of moral choice concerning our life and destiny.

Ethical and psychological hedonism

Happiness can and has been interpreted as a desirable psychological state (of pleasure or pain), rather than as a general state of being, and pursuit of a life of pleasure can be seen as a rational goal personally chosen, rather than something built in by nature. This interpretation of happiness was accepted by Epicurus (341–270 BC) and his followers in antiquity, and by Jeremy Bentham and John Stuart Mill in the 19th century. Theories which make the quest for pleasure and the avoidance of pain the basis for making moral choices have been called *hedonist* (from the Greek *hedone* = pleasure). *Utilitarian* theories seek to base moral judgements or policies on their usefulness or practical value in adding to our pleasure, diminishing our pain, and thus adding to the sum total of human happiness.

The pursuit of pleasure as a principle for living can take both selfish and altruistic forms. The kind of hedonism associated with Epicurus and his followers was not self-indulgent, as common proverbial use of the term 'hedonist' would suggest, but Epicurean hedonism was associated with a disciplined form of community life devoted to pursuit of the higher intellectual pleasures and long-term 'happiness' of the community, rather than indulgence in short-term carnal pleasures. Epicurus believed that people ought to pursue a life of pleasurable happiness and avoid pain, and that this could only be achieved by subordinating lower pleasures to higher ones, especially choosing pleasures that contribute to the enrichment of friendship. This kind of hedonism is called moral hedonism to distinguish it from psychological hedonism – the theory that human beings have no choice but are in fact always motivated by the instinct to seek pleasure and avoid pain.

Modern utilitarianism is associated with the reforming movement of 19th century, Liberalism. It is associated in particular with Jeremy Bentham (1748–1832) and John Stuart Mill (1806–1873), who as members of the Philosophical Radicals or Whigs (later the British Liberal Party) were widely influential in parliamentary reform.[11] In 1832, Bentham played a prominent part in the passage of the Reform Bill, which removed control of the House of Commons from the landed aristocracy and gave more effective political power to the new urban bourgeoisie.

Jeremy Bentham states in his *Introduction to the Principles of Morals and Legislation* (1789):

Nature has placed mankind under the governance of two sovereign masters, pain and pleasure. It is for them alone to point out what we ought to do, as well as to determine what we shall do. On the one hand the standard of right and wrong, on the other the chain of cause and effects, are fastened to their throne.

He goes on to define the *Greatest Happiness or Greatest Felicity Principle* as follows:

That principle states that the greatest happiness of all those whose interest is in question, as being the right and proper, and only right and proper and universally desirable, end of human action: of human action in every situation, and in particular that of a functionary or set of functionaries exercising the powers of Government.

As a reformer, his main point was to stress that politicians and administrators should not act out of self-interest, nor to their own advantage, but in the interests of their subjects, aiming always to achieve the greatest happiness for the greatest number.

Bentham takes it as self-evident that pleasure is good and pain is bad, and attempts to ground his ethics on this apparently objective fact of human psychology. His initial claim is that the worth of actions can be determined by the degree to which they promote pleasure and prevent or reduce pain. He further assumes that the greater the quantity of pleasure, the better things will be. While he enthusiastically promoted the idea of a 'felicific calculus', the problem he faced was how to determine or measure the quantity of pleasure produced or pain avoided by an action or policy. He failed to give specific criteria to define 'pleasure' and 'pain', or to enable us to distinguish them from one another. He uncritically assumed that their meanings were self-evident and that they are intrinsically good and bad, respectively, whereas we might want to argue that some forms of pleasure are bad (e.g. associated with cruelty to animals) or that some forms of pain are good (in that they signal warnings to us, or are associated with processes like strenuous exercise or corrective surgery that are meant to do us good).

Thus, his attempt to provide a purely quantitative criterion runs into difficulties as soon as an attempt is made to apply it to actual calculations or discriminations between what are to count as 'pleasures' and what as 'pains'. In the absence of criteria for making sound value judgements about what pleasures are to count as 'normal' or 'pathological', 'good' or 'bad', we cannot get very far. His utilitarianism seductively suggests that these issues can be decided by reference to facts – falling foul of Hume's argument that an 'ought' statement cannot be logically derived from an 'is' statement. Like other self-styled 'scientific' theories of morality, what Bentham does is to covertly import his own values into his supposedly 'objective calculations' and appraisals of pleasure and happiness. Far from being value-neutral, his 'felicific calculus' begs the question of the real nature of happiness and tends to promote the interests of majority public opinion. Without qualitative moral criteria, his hedonistic calculus proves of little practical worth and tends to be based on arbitrary interpretations of the pleasure principle.

Bentham, like modern utilitarians, was more concerned to emphasise the psychological rather than the ontological nature of happiness – identifying it with feelings of pleasure and freedom from pain. He stresses that the pursuit of happiness, whether as an individual goal or a social policy, is a matter of rational choice or social contract. At a simple everyday level, the general utilitarian formula – 'choose the course of action which causes the least pain and maximises happiness for the greatest number' – seems to be a useful guide to decision-making and dealing with moral dilemmas. However, when we look at the formula more critically, it raises a number of questions: What do we mean by 'pleasure' and 'pain'? Are pleasures better if more intense or longer-lasting? How do we calculate the degree or quantity of 'pain' or 'pleasure'? Can we use pleasure alone as a criterion to determine that intellectual interests are preferable to physical pleasures? How do we distinguish between normal and abnormal pleasures? Why should sadomasochistic sex not be better than enjoyment of what we call 'normal' sex? How is pleasure related to happiness? Do we concern ourselves with the 'happiness' of just those around us or with the whole of society? Furthermore, when we attempt to apply the 'general happiness' formula to specific actions, are we talking just about the immediate psychological effects of our actions or the long-term benefits (rather than costs), to us and to society, of utilitarianism as a policy for action?

John Stuart Mill recognised the obvious defects of Bentham's formulation of the Greatest Happiness Theory, but also recognised its intuitive appeal as a practical test of the rightness of actions. He suggested several modifications which greatly strengthen the theory.

First, he recognised that we need qualitative moral criteria to distinguish between higher and lower pleasures, according to whether they serve the ultimate well-being of the individual. Second, he stressed the complexity of moral decisions, where the choice may not be between pleasure and pain but between different kinds of pain, or different kinds of pleasure:

The principle of utility does not mean that any given pleasure, as music, for instance, or any given exemption from pain, as for example health, are to be looked upon as means to a collective something called

happiness and to be derived on that account. They are desired and desirable in and for themselves; besides being a means, they are part of an end (Lindsay 1957).

Third, Mill stressed that the things which count as contributing to the greatest happiness for the greatest number are to be measured by the criterion of greatest benefit to all. The shift from what Bentham called a 'felicific calculus' to cost–benefit analysis of the likely or actual consequences of actions in promoting the common good is what is definitive of his 'utilitarianism'.

The first modification introduces the principle of totality – the good of the whole rather than the part – to supplement the pleasure principle. The second suggests the need for some kind of hierarchy of pleasures, or qualitative criteria for prioritising pleasures, or for discriminating between desirable and undesirable pleasures. The third introduces covertly the concept of good, or benefit, combining both ultimate value to the individual and justice in terms of promoting the common good of society.

Frankena (1973) and other modern philosophers have introduced a useful distinction between *act utilitarianism* and *rule utilitarianism*.

Bentham's simple formula, in so far as it is applied as a criterion to determine the *rightness or wrongness of particular acts* by considering their effects or consequence, and whether these obtain the maximum amount of happiness for the greatest number, could be taken as an example of act utilitarianism. On the basis of past experience, it attempts to predict the likely outcomes of alternative courses of action, or it attempts to assess or evaluate the actual psychological consequences of actions already performed. *Rule utilitarianism* would not judge an action right or wrong according to its consequences in a particular case, but rather would judge an action right if it is based on a general rule, the following of which would be likely to lead to the best consequence for all. Mill's modified version of Bentham's General Happiness Theory lends itself to interpretation as rule utilitarianism, since actions which serve the principle of totality observe hierarchical distinctions between pleasures and serve the common good, and are not simply determined by attempts to measure degrees of pain or happiness. Rather, what is to count as 'happiness' or 'pain' is determined by one or other or all three of these additional rules.

Utilitarianism has a continuing popular appeal in business, with its focus on costs and benefits, and in health care, because health professionals consider that they are in business to prevent or reduce pain, where possible, and to promote the health and well-being of patients. Because health professionals are expert at estimating what the likely consequences or side-effects of treatment may be, judging by consequences (act utilitarianism) appears scientific and reinforces their sense of authority in direct one-to-one clinical relationships. They feel less comfortable if asked to define 'health', 'quality of life' or 'happiness' – which would be necessary to apply a form of rule utilitarianism. However, when the nurse or doctor has to consider wider responsibilities to other patients, to the hospital, to the cause of nursing or medical research, to public health, then rule utilitarianism is the more appealing, for health professionals often believe they know how the greatest benefit for the greatest number is to be achieved. The problem is that defining 'justice' or 'the common good' is another matter, as well as having to justify the connection between their clinical and moral authority. Campbell (1984b) developed a strong argument for an historical link between the utilitarian tradition in Britain and its influence on the development of the welfare state, including the National Health Service. Here, the justification for the socialisation of medical services is to achieve justice by maximising benefits for the majority. Attempts to sustain the welfare state on utilitarian grounds alone, however (whether measured in terms of the costs and benefits of alternative forms of welfare provision, or the cost-effectiveness of different systems or practical services), raise fundamental questions about how utilitarian administrative policies for rationalising the distribution of health services are reconciled with patients' needs and rights and the demands of beneficence and justice in providing urgently needed treatment.

Despite their limitations, teleological and utilitarian theories appear to be common-sensical because they do emphasise certain important things about moral experience. First, goals are important in human life, whether they are conceived as built into our very natures as human beings, chosen by us individually, or determined by contract or social agreement. Secondly, these theories emphasise that consideration of the demands of the specific situation and the consequences of actions have to be taken into account in determining whether they are right and good. Thirdly, they emphasise that actions must have clear objectives and will only succeed if we choose the most appropriate and efficient means to achieve our objectives.

John Rawls on justice

If we leave aside the growing worldwide influence of socialism and Marxism from the time of the 1917 Russian Revolution onwards, the predominant influence in politics and moral philosophy in the English-speaking world has been that of the great English utilitarians. Against this trend, the work of John Rawls is significant.

While there was a brief revival of natural law thinking after World War II, Rawls turns to social contract theory rather than arguments based on 'human nature' to ground his theory of justice. What he shares in common with the classical tradition, however, is a belief in justice as the most fundamental principle of both ethics and law. In his now famous paper, 'Justice as fairness',[12] he argues that classical and modern forms of utilitarianism (including 'economic rationalism') are unable to account adequately for the concept of justice:

The fundamental idea in the concept of justice is that of fairness. It is this aspect of justice for which utilitarianism, in its classical form, is unable to account, but which is represented, even if misleadingly so, in the idea of the social contract.

He suggests that there are two principles, which he implies are intuitively self-evident, that must serve as the basis for the foundational concept of justice as fairness:

The **first principle** is that each person participating in a practice, or affected by it, has an equal right to the most extensive liberty compatible with a like liberty for all; and the **second** is that inequalities are arbitrary unless it is reasonable to expect that they will work out for every-one's advantage and unless the offices to which they attach, or from which they may be gained, are open to all.

While utilitarianism would appear, on the surface, to be the ideal moral theory to match the expectations of free market capitalist societies, Rawls argues that utilitarianism is unable to provide a satisfactory basis for a modern theory of rights, or the associated theory of justice as it applies to our life and work within either public sector or private institutions. Throughout, he discusses justice as a *virtue of institutions* rather than as relating to particular actions or persons.

Against the trend towards 'privatisation' of ethics, Rawls' emphasis on the importance of justice as a virtue of institutions has particular relevance to business ethics. As he points out, justice is not the sole virtue of institutions, for these may have a tradition of inefficiency, or be degrading, but not be unjust. Justice, in his terms, is concerned with how institutions 'define offices and powers, and assign rights and duties'. In this sense, he emphasises, as we have done, the importance of the concept of power-sharing as the basis for ethics. He suggests that 'essentially justice is the elimination of arbitrary distinctions and the establishment, within the structure of practice, of a proper balance between competing claims'.

His central concern is how to develop an adequate theory of justice that would be relevant to developing a theory of rights in a modern democratic and capitalist society. His approach shares in common with Kant the idea that certain fundamental ethical principles are intuitively self-evident. Unlike Kant, who suggests one should act on one's duty *because one perceives it to be the rational thing to do*, Rawls suggests that one should do one's duty because one consents to the terms on which rights are cashed out in one's society or place of work. In this sense, one must be a party to the process of developing ethical policy and rules for the moral community within which one works. He argues against the utilitarian principle of simply maximising happiness for the greatest number, in that this may well lead to further disadvantaging the disadvantaged. Minority group rights cannot be adequately protected within the

utilitarian theory, except on the basis of an assumed altruism. He contends that people intuitively understand when things are unfair, and even when they do not fully understand the structures of power in institutions, or the way authority is exercised in relation to their interests, people will, as a matter of common sense, choose the principles of justice, viz.:

- equal liberty, i.e. the maximum liberty compatible with the liberty of others
- equality of access, or fair and impartial access to social benefits and resources
- equality of opportunity for employment, status and position in society
- and further, that changes in public policy should benefit those most disadvantaged.

Rawls develops a kind of intuitionist social contract theory, but this differs in significant ways from the traditional social contract theorists. Hobbes and Rousseau[13] each postulates an original 'state of nature' without law and government, without ethics. They then proceed to develop their theories of law and morality on the basis of what is required to meet the deficiencies of human nature. Rawls, on the other hand, invites us to engage in a 'thought experiment' in which we have to imagine we are ignorant of our actual circumstances, advantages or disadvantages. Without making assumptions about the depravity of human nature (like Hobbes) or the innocence of man in a state of nature (like Rousseau's 'noble savage'), Rawls asks us to imagine how basically self-interested but reasonable people would set ground rules for their moral community. On the basis of his intuitive notions of fundamental common sense concepts of fairness, he argues that people will seek equality and the maximum degree of liberty that does not conflict with the liberty of others, or serve to increase inequalities and disadvantage to others. These notions of fairness he believes are basic to any rational moral community.

Thus, he argues, there has to be a deontological aspect to every functioning system of ethics. As moral communities address the demand to review their core values, apply principles or existing rules to ethical decision-making and seek to reach agreement about new policies or rules, they have to address the commonalities that underlie human experience or human nature. Given the common features of the human condition, variations of culture, time and place are perhaps much less important than the common needs and requirements for human flourishing.

While utilitarian theories focus on desirable goals and assessment of ethical value by determining our success or failure in attaining our goals, deontological theories emphasise those universal principles and requirements that are basic to determining ground rules in any moral community. They focus attention on the antecedent conditions, the prevailing circumstances, the underlying causes and principles relating to the situation, the pre-existing rules that apply, and the motives and intentions of the moral agent. No adequate moral theory can afford to ignore these factors and to concentrate exclusively on either means and methods or ends and consequences. However, by the same token, a deontological theory cannot, by itself, do justice to the other aspects of moral acts.

MORAL THEORY AND THE STRUCTURE OF MORAL ACTION

If it makes sense to analyse the process of moral and ordinary practical decision-making in terms of the stages of assessment, planning, implementation and evaluation (as in the Nursing Process and many other problem-solving methods), then it is perhaps not surprising to suggest that moral actions have a recognisable form or rational structure. In classical and mediaeval thought, philosophers spoke of human acts having an intentional character, i.e. that they have a purpose and direction. This purposeful direction of acts is dictated partly by our own purposes and goals, and partly by the nature of the world in which we act, and in which laws of cause and effect operate. Human acts, whether mental acts of judgement or performative acts of doing and making, have a structure which reflects this functional interdependence of agent and world.

This structure was analysed by Aristotle in terms of four kinds of conditions – material and formal conditions, goals or ends, and the efficient cause of something happening. Aquinas analysed the intentional structure of acts in terms of the complex relations between causes, means and ends (Gilson 1994):

- *Causes* in this analysis stood for both the objective conditions (or physical causes) prevailing or operative in a given situation and the subjective conditions (including moral principles and personal aims or motives) introduced by the agent.
- *Means* represented possible options or alternative practical courses of action, the personal skills and physical resources available, and the particular means chosen to execute an action plan.
- *Ends,* here, covered both the practical objectives or goals of the agent as subject, and the actual consequences or effects of an action.

What this kind of analysis suggests is that in considering the nature of human action, we have to take account of all three – causes, means and ends – and in reaching a responsible moral decision we would have to take proper account of the relevant causes, means and ends applying to a particular act in a particular situation. If called upon to justify a particular action, we should be able to do so after having made a proper assessment of the prevailing subjective and objective conditions, having made an informed and realistic plan based on available means and resources, and having anticipated correctly the likely consequences of the action taken to attain a goal. Bearing in mind the causes–means–ends structure of intentional and moral acts may enable us to make more sense of different moral theories, by recognising that they each tend to draw attention to particular features of moral judgement and action. It may be too simplistic to suggest that some of the perennial disputes in moral philosophy could be resolved if only the different protagonists would recognise that they each focus on real but partial aspects of the process, and that from a wider perspective we can recognise that their respective approaches are not irreconcilable but complementary. However, there is some truth and plausibility in this view, and we intend to explore it here.

For example, protagonists of natural law theory (namely that moral laws are somehow grounded in nature) focus attention on the dimension of causes – the prevailing objective conditions in the circumstances of human action generally. Situation ethics (or the theory that we should act spontaneously in the light of the demands of the given situation) also interprets principles for action in terms of given circumstances. Intuitionism (or the theory which seeks to ground moral duty in pre-reflexive apprehension of moral principles) appeals to subjective reasons as motives or causes for action.

By contrast, pragmatism (the theory that something is right because it works) confines attention to means – to rational planning based on the calculation of available means and resources – to achieve aims. Existentialist ethics (Sartre: 'people make themselves by their decisions') also stresses that in seeking to act morally people should not allow their actions to be predetermined by external causes or principles, or be influenced unduly by unpredictable consequences, but 'should act authentically in the given situation'.

Teleological theories of morals focus on ends. If we make assumptions, as Plato and Aristotle did, that there are inherent tendencies in nature and in human beings to seek their fulfilment or some ultimate goal, then the concept of 'end' is being interpreted at both a physical and a metaphysical level. At a more mundane level, utilitarianism grounds judgements of what is good or bad in terms of an assessment of the consequences or effects of an action. Actions are to be judged by their results, i.e. by their utility in promoting certain ends or general human happiness.

In a sense, what each of these types of theory does is to isolate and draw attention to one aspect of the intentional structure of human acts and then attempts to make this partial perspective normative and definitive for the interpretation of all human action. The seemingly interminable debates among philosophers about the ultimate basis of moral judgements suggests that each of these theories may be true, in the sense that they emphasise some genuine (if partial) aspect of our moral experience; but also that they are false and distort the reality of moral experience, by failing to take account of other complementary perspectives. We may need to balance emphasis on one aspect of our moral experience with emphasis on other aspects of the whole causes–means–ends structure of moral acts, in order to get a dynamic and three-dimensional picture of the reality (Downie & Calman 1987, Chs 1–4).

Figure 11.1 and Table 11.1 illustrate some of the relationships we have summarised here.

Table 11.1 How ethical theories relate to aspects of the structure of moral acts

Aspect of action	Type of moral theory	Relates to:
Prior conditions Objective conditions	**Deontological and natural law** e.g. natural law theory (Aristotle/Aquinas)	**Principles, rules and duties** Rights derived from reflection on human nature and needs
Subjective conditions	e.g. rational intuitionism (Kant, Rawls)	Principles deduced from the requirements for a rational ethic
Means and methods Objective conditions	**Pragmatic and virtue-based** e.g. pragmatism (Dewey, James, Marx)	**Instruments, action, agent** Trial and error serve to define what is right/wrong, good/bad
Subjective conditions	e.g. virtue ethics (Macintyre, Plato, Aristotle)	The moral character of the agent seen as crucial in ethics
Ends/outcomes Objective conditions	**Teleological and utilitarian** e.g. teleological eudaemonism (Aristotle, Aquinas)	**Costs/benefits, outcomes** The ultimate end of human life is happiness/human fulfilment
Subjective conditions	e.g. utilitarianism and hedonism (Bentham, Mill)	All human action is driven by self-interest or pleasure

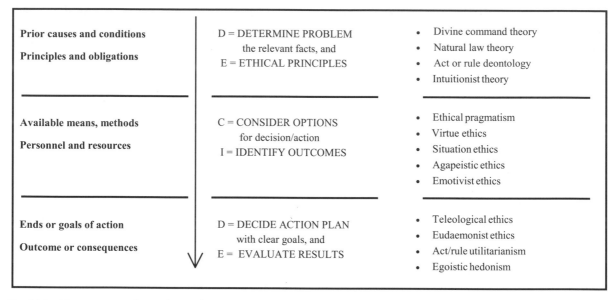

Fig. 11.1 The structure of moral acts, the DECIDE model, and its relation to ethical theories.

MORAL THEORY AND THE GOAL OF SOCIAL CONSENSUS

The range and variety of theories developed to justify moral principles, the most important and abiding of which have been outlined above, may leave the impression that there can be no real moral agreement or that it is a matter of indifference which theory one chooses. This would be to misunderstand the kind of impulse which has led to the formulation of these theories.

What all these theories have in common is a belief that rational grounds for our moral principles can and must be found, that public agreement and objective decision-making in law and the moral life are important and cannot be based on whim and arbitrary judgement. Each of the theories produces powerful arguments for the rationality of moral principles, whether we see the principles of respect for persons, justice and beneficence as being based on natural law, the demands of love, intuition, the requirements for the pursuit and achievement of happiness or the concept of duty. Each of these theories marshals certain kinds of evidence taken from moral experience and attempts to generalise its significance for an understanding of the nature of principles. It is tempting to say that each of these theories repre-

sents a complementary aspect of moral experience and that, while each has some value, it is limited to the extent that it is generalised as a basis for the interpretation of all or every aspect of human moral life. However, there are some irreconcilable aspects of these theories and we cannot rest in such an embracing 'ecumenical' view.

We cannot do without rules or principles to organise our lives and moral experience. Society cannot function without some kind of moral consensus on which to base its social institutions. Law and order ultimately rest on government by consent, even under tyranny. No tyrant can succeed in isolation: he has to be able to persuade others to support his cause. Choice between might and right, between government by force and government by consent, if there is to be a choice, has to be based on reasoned argument. If we surrender our faith in reasoned argument, public debate and the possibility of social agreement, then we are lost to the forces of irrationalism, prejudice and anarchy.

The only way to arrive at social consensus is by reasoning together – whether as a whole society or as a medical care team at ward level (Veatch 1981, Boyd et al 1986). While we may be born into already structured moral communities, or take up employment in organisations with a defined ethical culture and their own rules and regulations for professional conduct, nevertheless no such communities are static or unable to be changed. A living, healthy and responsible moral community has to be constantly recreated, by the review, reform or reaffirmation of its values by its members. If the values and rules of a moral community are imposed on people, they do not 'own' them and will almost certainly either disregard them or rebel against them. Negotiating and renegotiating the scope and nature of the boundaries of the moral community is the heart of its life, as it is the life-blood of real democracy. There is nothing to be afraid of in this process, or in the need for change. On the contrary, there is more to fear from moral communities that are not real communities, which are 'stuck in a time warp', dead, unable to either grow or adapt to changing circumstances, roles and responsibilities.

In practice, day-to-day decision-making does not often involve discussion of this level of moral theory. We operate, for the most part, within the existing social consensus and do not question the basis of fundamental moral principles – unless challenged to do so. Perhaps the first time we begin to think critically about our moral beliefs is when we leave home and go to school and encounter people with different cultural or religious backgrounds. When we enter training for adult and professional life, we are introduced to a complex set of professional and institutional values which may challenge personal and moral beliefs based on family upbringing, education and conviction. When we encounter painful conflicts of duty in professional life (e.g. between the duty to keep secrets and the duty to share information for the benefit of patients, or to choose between the rights of the mother and the father, or to preserve life or to alleviate pain), we are forced to examine the rational basis for our moral beliefs, and other people may demand that we justify them. When we move from junior to administrative responsibilities in large institutions, we have to find criteria in terms of which to choose between the rules we use for dealing with individuals and the rules applicable to large groups of people. When we move out into public life – representing our colleagues in a union or taking part in local government or national politics – we have to begin to think through the connections between morality and law, ethics and politics.

In all these situations, if we think critically and systematically about things, aspects of moral theory become relevant. We do not have to be philosophers to be concerned about these questions. We are drawn to think philosophically if we take seriously the quest for objectivity in ethical and legal debate, and this means adducing the best possible reasons and evidence we can for believing in moral principles at all. The moral theories we have outlined are only a guide to the way in which some great philosophers have thought about these questions in the past. We may learn a great deal from their wisdom, but we should not be seduced into thinking that they can do our thinking for us, or give us packaged 'answers' to the ultimate questions in life.

Reaching ultimate moral agreement may be an unobtainable goal but it is one of the grandest ambitions and most noble ideals of human beings. If it means agreement in the three senses we discussed earlier, agreement between what we profess and what we do, rational consensus or agreement among people about the ultimate goals and principles of social life, and agreement between our principles and the ultimate demands implicit in the structures and dynamics of being, then moral agreement is a noble goal indeed. It is a symbol of a fully mature, fully human and genuinely humane society.

further reading

Freewill and determinism
Augustine (354–430 AD) (Pontifex M, tr) 1955 The problem of free choice (de libero arbitrio). Newman Press, Westminster, MD

Downie R S, Calman K C 1987 Healthy respect: ethics in health care. Faber, London, chs 1–4

Hare R M 1963 Freedom and reason. Oxford University Press, Oxford, ch 4

Montefiore A 1958 A modern introduction to moral philosophy. Routledge & Kegan Paul, London, ch 12

Justification of our moral principles
Dancy J 1993 Moral reasons. Blackwells, Oxford

Hare R M 1952 The language of morals (reprinted 1964). Oxford University Press, Oxford

Hare R M 1963 Freedom and reason. Oxford University Press, Oxford

Korsgaard C M, Cohen G A 1996 The sources of normativity. Cambridge University Press, Cambridge

Toulmin S 1958 The place of reason in ethics. Cambridge University Press, Cambridge, chs 11–14

General references on moral philosophy or ethical theory
Foot P 1967 Theories of ethics. Oxford University Press, Oxford

Hare R M 1981 Moral thinking: its levels, methods and point. Oxford University Press, Oxford

Johnson O A (ed) 1994 Ethics: selections from classical and contemporary writers, 7th edn. Harcourt Brace, New York

Macintyre A 1967 A short history of ethics. Routledge & Kegan Paul, London

Maritain J 1963 Moral philosophy. Bles, London

Rachels J 1993 The elements of moral philosophy, 2nd edn. McGraw-Hill, New York

Raphael D D 1980 Moral philosophy. Oxford University Press, Oxford

Deontological theories (and divine command theories)
Frankena W K 1973 Ethics, 2nd edn. Prentice Hall, Englewood Cliffs, NJ

Maritain J 1963 Moral philosophy. Bles, London

Paton H J (tr) 1969 The moral law: Kant's groundwork to the metaphysic of morals. Hutchinson, London

Ross W D 1930 The right and the good. Oxford University Press, Oxford

Ross W D 1969 Kant's ethical theory. Oxford University Press, Oxford

Natural law theories
d'Entreves A P 1951 Natural law: an introduction to legal philosophy. Hutchinson, London

Finnis J M 1999 Natural law and natural rights. Clarendon Press, Oxford

Gilson E (Shook L K, tr) 1994 The Christian philosophy of St Thomas Aquinas. University of Notre Dame Press, Notre Dame, IN

Maritain J 1943 The rights of man and natural law. C Scribner's Sons, New York

Wild J 1953 Plato's modern enemies and the theory of natural law. University of Chicago Press, Chicago

Intuitionist ethics
Broad C D 1930 Five types of ethical theory. Routledge & Kegan Paul, London

Carritt E F 1928 Theory of morals. Oxford University Press, Oxford

Moore G E 1962 Principia ethica, revised edn. Cambridge University Press, Cambridge, chs 1, 3

Moore G E 1966 Ethics, 2nd edn. Oxford University Press, Oxford

Virtue ethics and ethics of prudence
Crisp R, Slote M 1997 Virtue ethics. Oxford University Press, Oxford

Macintyre A 1981 After virtue, 2nd edn. Notre Dame University Press, Notre Dame, IN

Nelson D M 1992 The priority of prudence: virtue and natural law. Pennsylvania State University, University Park, PA

Pieper J 1959 Prudence: the first cardinal virtue. Faber, London

Agapeistic or caring ethics theories
Baier A C 1995 Moral prejudices. Harvard University Press, Cambridge, MA

Bowden P 1997 Caring: gender-sensitive ethics. Routledge, London

Brown J, Kitson A, McKnight T J 1992 Challenges in caring: explorations in nursing and ethics. Chapman & Hall, London

Fletcher J 1979 Situation ethics. SCM Press, London

Frankena W K 1964 Love and principle in Christian ethics. In: Plantinga A (ed) Faith and philosophy. Eerdmans, Grand Rapids, MI

Ramsey P 1983 Deeds and rules in Christian ethics. University of America Press, New York

Teleological or utilitarian theories
Campbell A V, Charlesworth M, Gillett G, Jones D G 1997 Medical ethics. Oxford University Press, Oxford

Foot P 1967 Theories of ethics. Oxford University Press, Oxford

Gillon R 1986 Philosophical medical ethics. Wiley, Chichester, ch 4

Smart J J C, Williams B 1973 Utilitarianism for and against. Cambridge University Press, Cambridge

 end
notes

1   Wittgenstein L 1971 *Tractatus Logico-Philosophicus* (new edition in English & German). Routledge & Kegan Paul, London, 4.112.
2   See Hume D (Selby-Bigge L A, ed) 1978 *A Treatise of Human Nature* (1738). Oxford University Press, Oxford; and his later work, Hume D (Beauchamp T L, ed) 1998 *An Enquiry Concerning the Principles of Morals* (1770). Oxford University Press, Oxford.
3   See Kant I (Abbot T K, tr) 1909 *Critique of Pure Practical Reason*. Everyman, Dent, London, para 58, p 122.
4   These *cardinal virtues* were taken over by the Christian West from the Greeks. Although there are some minor differences of emphasis in Plato and Aristotle, they both recognise these virtues as fundamental to moral competence. See: Aristotle (Thomson J A K, tr) 1976 *Nicomachean Ethics*. In: *The Ethics of Aristotle* (revised edn) Penguin Books, Harmondsworth; Plato (Rouse W D, tr) 1984 *Plato's Republic*. In: *The Great Dialogues of Plato*. Mentor Books, Gateway Press, New York.
5   See discussion of the virtues in Pieper J 1959 *Prudence: the First Cardinal Virtue*. Faber & Faber, London.
6   See *Aristotle's Nicomachean Ethics*, Bk VI.
7   Jonsen A R, Toulmin S 1988 *The Abuse of Casuistry: a History of Moral Reasoning*. University of California Press, Berkeley; Hobbes T (Tuck R, ed) 1996 *Leviathan*. Cambridge University Press, Cambridge; Rousseau, J.J (tr. Cole G D H, revised by Brumfitt J H & Hall J C) 1973 *Social Contract and Discourses*. Dent, London.
8   Nygren A (Watson P S, tr) 1953 *Agape and Eros*. Westminster Press, Philadelphia; D'Arcy M 1962 *The Heart and Mind of Love* Collins, London; Levinas E. 1982 *Responsibility for Others* Duquesne University Press, USA; Levinas E 1985 *Ethics and Infinity*. Duquesne University Press, USA.
9   Cf. Hume D 1738 *A Treatise of Human Nature*, Part 2; and Ayer A J 1958 *Language, Truth and Logic*. Gollancz, London.
10   See *Aristotle's Nicomachean Ethics*, Bk I.
11   See Everyman Classics: Jeremy Bentham, *An Introduction to the Principles of Morals and Legislation*, first published in 1789, revised in 1822; John Stuart Mill, *Essay on Liberty* and *Essay on Utilitarianism*, first published in 1861.
12   Rawls J 1957 Justice as fairness. *Journal of Philosophy* 54: 653–662.
13   See works cited above in end note 7.

some suggestions on method

What is the nature of policy?
The issue of why a sound process of ethical policy development is necessary can be made intelligible and relevant to students by getting the class to address the question of how they might develop a class policy on plagiarism, or on smoking in the college. If the class is divided into two groups to work on the same issue and then charged with the responsibility of 'selling' their policy to the other group, then out of the ensuing discussion it is usually possible to illustrate the needs for all the steps in the POLICY model.

Why the variety of moral theories?
Students could be asked to write down some issue on which they hold a strong moral position. They could then be asked to work in pairs and each question the other in turn, recording the answers given for later analysis and discussion. The form the questioning should take is as follows:

- Why do you feel so strongly about this issue?
- Why do you believe your position on this is right?
- How do you justify the claim you make for your moral beliefs on this issue?
- Is this a matter of principle? Based on experience? Or related to what you believe should be our goals?

What is the appeal of deontological ethics?
Students could be divided into three groups to discuss what they consider the strengths and weaknesses of each of the following types of theory: religious ethics (divine command theory); natural law and natural rights; and the obligation to do one's duty come what may.

In giving feedback, the groups should be encouraged to tabulate their views on the strengths and weaknesses of each theory and then to summarise what they all have in common.

Why should we be virtuous?
Students should be encouraged first to identify what they consider the desirable virtues or competencies of nurses and/or nurse managers. This could be done either by group brainstorm or in small groups. Secondly, in either case, the students should be divided into small groups with the task of clarifying the kinds of reason which can be advanced to justify the claim that we must strive to be virtuous rather than morally incompetent or wicked. (Alternatively, students could be presented with a case involving a practical nursing problem in which a nurse has to make a difficult ethical decision. The task would be to identify the skills and resources that may be necessary to act effectively and responsibly in the given situation.)

Considering the outcomes, costs and benefits
Here the group could be presented with a case of a patient requesting termination of life support, because he has lost the will to live. The task students could be asked to address is how far one could go in attempting to decide whether to comply with the patient's wishes, by considering only the consequences – for the patient, for the relatives, for oneself as the responsible nurse, for the other patients on the ward, for the hospital, etc. Alternatively, they could be asked to discuss the potential benefits for the various stakeholders in the drama.

Nursing ethics – retrospect and prospect

SECTION CONTENTS

12

Nursing and nursing ethics into the 21st century

RETROSPECT AND PROSPECT

Since the publication of the first edition of this work, one of the first books on nursing ethics in the field, there have been many dramatic changes and developments in health care, nationally in the UK and internationally in both the high-income and developing countries. The past 20 years have witnessed new discoveries and developments in medicine, rapid professionalisation of nursing, shifts in health policy nationally and internationally, including 'organisational and management reforms' in many countries, and associated restructuring of the delivery of health care – all changes which have impacted on nursing itself. Worldwide, these developments have been driven by a variety of factors: scientific advances in health care, shifts in economic theory affecting the political economy of health service provision, and movement towards international agreement on health priorities to achieve 'health for all by the year 2000'. (Project 2000, which aimed specifically to enhance the knowledge, skills and expertise of nurses so that they could contribute more effectively to this ambitious global project, is a case in point.) All these changes and developments have impacted on the debate in nursing about the nature and scope of nursing ethics.

It is almost 150 years since 'the lady with the lamp' first set about organising nursing care for British soldiers in the field hospitals of the Crimean War, and later reflected on the need for a permanent cohort of trained and dedicated

327

nurses to continue the work of caring for the sick and dying in peace-time hospitals and clinics. As we mentioned in the preface to the first edition, an American nurse, Isabel Hampton Robb, published in 1900 a book with the same title as ours. In her *Nursing Ethics*, she said of ethics that 'it teaches men the practice of duties of human life and the reasons for what they do and of what they should leave undone'. As far as nurses were concerned, this was summed up for her in 'implicit and unquestioning obedience' and conformity to the requirements of conventional respectability.

During the past 100 years, nursing ethics has undergone a revolution, both in perception of its form and scope, and in the sophistication of the debate among nurses themselves. Nursing ethics has left behind the view that ethics is simply a matter of observing the right social etiquette, or the view that ethics is simply a matter of adherence to a disciplinary code, or that nursing ethics is just an echo of biomedical ethics. We believe that nurses have come to recognise that ethics is central to their profession as a caring profession; that the moral virtues are fundamental competencies required by nurses to perform their duties effectively and well; and, furthermore, that ethics encompasses the whole gamut of nursing – the values and standards of nursing practice, nursing management, and the collaboration of nurses in the organisation and delivery of health care services generally.

Where nursing is and where it is going, as it stands on the threshold of the third millennium, is the subject on which we seek to reflect in this postscript to the fourth edition of our book on nursing ethics. What is most significant for our purposes is the remarkable development of nursing ethics itself – reflected in the much greater emphasis given to teaching ethics in basic and post-basic training of nurses, in the growing body of academic and practical literature in the field contributed by a variety of experts in law, ethics, behavioural and social sciences and by nurses themselves (many of whom have acquired qualifications in ethics). There has been a profound shift in both the form and content of the debate about ethics in nursing. This has

been driven by the factors mentioned above, but also by the needs of nurses themselves. As they have taken on greater responsibility in decision-making, and new clinical roles, they have demanded assistance to meet the challenges with which they find themselves confronted. This book was written originally in response to such demands, and in its various editions we have attempted to keep pace with the changes mentioned above and dealt with in the body of the book.

In this book we have sought to highlight how these changes have exerted a direct influence on the nature of ethical debates within nursing. An understanding of where nursing has come from and some view of the direction in which it is moving are important if we are to follow and take an informed and responsible part in contemporary ethical debate, not only about new and challenging problems presented for nursing by scientific innovation, but also, more fundamentally, about clarification of the values which should be driving health care, and nursing in particular, as we move into the 21st century. The ethical issues which are of concern to the nursing profession cannot be divorced from the deeper value and policy questions in the ethics of health care generally.

DEMOGRAPHIC, ECONOMIC AND SOCIAL CHANGE

Changes over the past few decades affecting health care provision include significant demographic trends – an increasingly ageing population, with fewer employed to support the elderly and sick. Technological advances have taken place in many fields, perhaps the most far reaching being those which carry massive social and ethical implications, such as the new reproductive technologies and the mapping of the human genome, genetic screening and the developments in the field of immunology. The way in which the world was taken by surprise in the early 1980s by the arrival of HIV/AIDS is perhaps the most pervasive of the challenges, both clinical and moral, faced by health care workers. Political, economic and societal changes, therefore, all impact on health care and this gives us some clue as to the nature of health care provision required for the 21st century and nursing's place within it. As Strong & Robinson (1990) put it:

Life is a precondition of all human action. Perhaps because of this, health care provision is among the most intricate of all human phenomena. Here is the quintessential interface of the biological and the social realms, both of them extraordinarily complex and in their interaction doubly so.

Porter (1997, p. 595) summed up the state of health care at the end of the 20th century:

... Basic research, clinical science and technology working with one another have characterised the cutting edge of modern medicine. Progress has been made. For almost all diseases something can be done; some can be prevented or fully cured. Nevertheless, a century which has brought the most intense concentration of attention and resources on medical research ends with many of the major killers of western society – particularly heart and vascular disease, cancer, and chronic degenerative illnesses – largely incurable and in many cases increasing in incidence.

As the demands on the health care system have grown, so have the importance of cost-effectiveness and efficiency. Accountability for clinical practice comes in the shape of a demand for professional openness, increasing litigation and, on the part of the health care professionals, a move towards evidence-based practice. A more educated public and a society in which watchdog organisations, lobbying and whistleblowing are commonplace, mean that health care is delivered under much more public and media scrutiny than once was the case.

RESPECTING LAY VIEWS ON HEALTH AND ILLNESS

In the past 30 years, particularly since the World Health Assembly at Alma Ata in Russia in 1978, discussion about health care has moved from being a disease and medically dominated debate to one which takes more account of behavioural and social dimensions of health, and the lay view of health and illness in particular. The World Health Assembly's Alma Ata Declaration reaffirmed the wider definition of health included in the original 1947 WHO definition, recognising the need to shift priorities from a 'medical model' to a 'community health model', and from an emphasis on hospital medicine to primary care health and nursing services (WHO 1978).

The emergence of a plethora of self-help groups and popular interest in 'alternative medicine' worldwide present a challenge to nurses and nursing as a profession. WHO, in noting these trends, has emphasised the key role which nurses can play in sound health education and in teaching and transferring skills to lay people to enable them to do more at home and in the community to address the problems of delivering health services to the growing world population, especially where resources are constrained and limited, as in developing countries (see Fig. 8.1, p. 203).

Developments within the field of medical sociology and sociological research demonstrate this shift away from naïve dependence on medical science (Mackay et al 1998, p. 5):

Stacey widened the agenda for the field of medical sociology. She noted how the origins of medical sociology rested in the rather practical concerns of medical practitioners and health administrators. Stacey proposed a sociology of health and illness rather than of medicine as a way of breaking free of medical dominance in the research enterprise. More specifically, Stacey wanted to see a sociology surrounding the problems of health, illness and of suffering. Hence, she was beginning to articulate the task of medical sociology to be patient-oriented rather than doctor-oriented.

Stacey's call in 1978 for a move from medical sociology to the sociology of health and illness was motivated by the belief that an understanding of health and illness would be better served by a move away from a medically oriented study of disease and illness behaviour, and by more attention being paid to the social factors which influence health and illness (Stacey & Homans 1978). It is likely that the debates about medical ethics would benefit from a similar shift of emphasis – in this case away from medical and nursing ethics towards a more patient-centred health care ethics.

Throughout the 20th century, the concerns of the nursing profession have been very much focused upon nurse education and the occupational organisation of nursing. The professional development of medicine had an important influence on the occupational organisation of nursing and upon nursing's own professionalising ambitions. In many parts of the world in recent years, great progress has been made in moving towards training more graduate nurses, and there is a move to locate nursing within a higher education context. Nursing also has made a determined effort to identify and produce a body of knowledge which it can call its own. Developments in the sociology of health and illness have been significant for the development of nursing as an academic discipline. In this, the focus upon the individual patient has become paramount. These developments fit well with the growing interest in nursing ethics and would serve equally well if we move towards a generic ethics of health care.

Nursing outnumbers the other health care professions, and the salaries budget for nurses constitutes a good proportion of the health service bill. Nevertheless, such is the nature of health care that the activities and preoccupations of one professional group have an impact on others. In the case of nursing, what happens in the practice of medicine clearly will have implications for nursing and may also give rise to ethical questions. Aside from the effect other occupational groups exert, however, the nursing profession's own thinking and development of practice also dictate to a large extent the ethical agenda of nursing.

In addition, more general issues of political policy have an effect upon the ways in which health care professions develop. In the UK, for instance, the nursing profession has been shaped by the growing demand for health care services and the attempted political solutions of the governments of the day. In reality, the distinctions between nurse aids or auxiliaries, and the various routes to accreditation have been shaped as much by these issues of political economy as by the professional aspirations of nurse reformers. So, for example, when the registration of nurses came about early in the 20th century, this was largely as a part of wider plans for social reconstruction after World War I (Rafferty 1996).

NURSING ETHICS OR HEALTH CARE ETHICS?

In the Preface to this edition, we reaffirm our belief that 'nursing ethics' represents a valid area for investigation and study in its own right, and that it represents a distinctive locus and perspective for thinking about the ethical responsibilities of caring. However, it is increasingly being argued that the divisions between medical ethics, nursing ethics and the ethics of the various paramedical professions are unhelpful in collaborative activity in health care delivery, and that we should be moving towards an inclusive and generic ethics of health care.

For example, it has been argued (Melia 1994) that while nursing has a specific contribution to make to the ethics of health care, this contribution need not necessarily entail the development of a specifically occupationally based nursing ethics, set up either in opposition to medical ethics or simply confined to the 'domestic' concerns of nursing. The challenge, Melia argues, is for nursing to build on the fact that the actual day-to-day work of nurses involves close and prolonged contact with patients, and this sustained and direct experience means that nurses' insights here can help to ensure that greater consideration is given to the patient's perspective in modern health care generally. A similar point is made by Benner & Wrubel (1989). They argue that nurses bring a distinctive professional perspective to bear on the ethics of health care delivery. From both points of view it is possible to maintain that a wider concept of health care ethics would help to place the emphasis on the patient or client, rather than the doctor or nurse, and draws attention away from the professions and their narrower concerns.

The fact is that there are pros and cons to each position. Clearly, each group of health care professionals contributes its own particular insights, values and ethical stances to health care. Consequently, the codes of conduct for each profession not only must embody general ethical principles applicable to all the caring professions, but they must also relate to the specific responsibilities of each occupational group. If they are too global and aspirational (heavenly minded), they may be of no earthly good. If they do not relate meaningfully to the occupationally specific tasks and responsibilities of each group then they will be of little practical value – regardless of whether they have a 'customer focus' or are directed more at the needs of the patient recipient of health care than its providers.

The literature on caring and the ethics of care, particularly that sparked by the controversies around the work of Kohlberg and Gilligan (see Ch. 10), has gained a prominent place in the nursing curriculum. Carol Gilligan's (1982) work set off a train of publications concerned with gender differences and moral reasoning. This work is important for nursing and parallels can be drawn with debates about medical dominance, the caring role of nursing versus the curing activity of medicine and the gendered stereo-typing of the two occupational groups. Kohlberg's controversial claims about the differences in the pattern of moral development in men and women provoked a great deal of critical research on the teaching of ethics and the role of gender and gender stereotyping in ethical discourse. However, as we pointed out earlier, the ethics of care and the philosophical exploration of the nature of caring as distinct from a more rational justice ethic is not new. Nor is the debate entirely new to health care, where the relation of care and cure, of medicine as an art to medicine as a science, and the contribution of caring to therapy and the healing process is almost as old as medicine itself.

There are several ways in which the focus on 'caring ethics' has influenced ethical debate in nursing. First, the cure/care dichotomy has been used here, as in the past, to distinguish the 'object-ive and scientific medical model' of health from 'a more personal nursing perspective'. In this way, it has often become the focus or a central theme in claims made for a specialised body of nursing knowledge or arguments for the application of distinctive methods of research to nursing. Secondly, it has generated a whole literature by feminist writers, analysing the pattern of ethics and relationships in hospitals and other health care institutions, as constructed on a pattern of 'master discourse' that is patriarchal, impersonal

and determined by a 'justice perspective', to which the 'caring perspective' of the nurse must be opposed. Thirdly, it has raised some interesting questions about the nature of ethics itself and whether the pursuit of a universal framework of principles, rights and duties is to be preferred to a more phenomenological and exist-entially grounded approach which attends to the specific situation, particular relationships and the demands inherent in the exercise of personal moral responsibility.

Growing importance of research in nursing and nursing ethics

Nursing is concerned to establish a research base and so has also become very much preoccupied with evidence-based practice. While this makes good sense in terms of ensuring sound practice and good quality patient care, there are difficulties with achieving a balance between the demands of research and those of patient needs. Nursing, like other professions in health care, is concerned with quality of care but is also under pressure to pro-duce value for money. The nursing profession exists in order to provide public service and so there is a tension between the cost–benefit of the service and the autonomy of the individual patients. The same tension exists even within the private care sector where there are profit margins to be met and value for money is sought.

There are parallels to be drawn between the ways in which nursing research is developing and debates about the nature of nursing, the philo-sophy of nursing and the art of nursing. Much of this new thinking has been accepted by the profes-sion and has found a place within the curriculum. This raises important questions for the profession and for nursing ethics, in so far as these debates shape the curriculum and so ultimately have their influence on the nature of practice, and indeed the kind of practitioner that the system produces. Since moving into the universities, nursing has developed a more academic programme of train-ing for those seeking registration as a qualified nurse. This is reflected in the literature, in the form of empirically based research and in the produc-tion of 'models' and 'theories' of nursing – in other words, nursing has followed other disciplines in laying down its own body of knowledge.

A great deal of practical research has been done on the applicability of Kohlberg's model of cognitive development to the teaching of ethics in nursing, to establish whether his theory holds for the experience of nurses. At best this research has brought home the fact that like all human learning the processes are complex and multifactorial in their causation. Like Socrates' famous question 'Can virtue be taught?', the real question is not can we teach ethics as a body of information, or even as a set of decision-making skills, but can we engage nurses in the process of personal growth and development in which they can be assisted to internalise ethical values, make them their own, and demonstrate them in the way they relate to people and do their job (see Fry 1989a,b, McAlpine 1998).

An area of nursing ethics which begs for more rigorous research is not so much in the cognitive/psychological field as in the area of management practice and the administration of nursing and health services. Here the challenge is not only to evaluate how effectively quality management programmes are developed and implemented, but whether the processes by which they are evaluated are honest, fair and respect the rights of practitioners as well as patients and other 'stakeholders'.

Nursing knowledge is being developed in two main ways – through enquiry and debate on what can be described as 'the nature of nursing' and through empirical research. For a long time there has been discussion about the nature of nursing, focusing on the question of whether it is an art or a science, and these debates are rehearsed again in discussions of nursing research. The phenomenological approach to a study of the lived experience of the patient has clearly produced some interesting insights into their experience of health and illness and shed some light on some of the difficult aspects of nursing practice, as experienced by the nurse. Critics of this phenomenological approach to the study of nursing, along with publications on nursing as art and the philosophy of nursing, maintain that it has tended to be more speculative than practically useful and does not

sit well with a greater emphasis on evidence-based practice.

However, we believe this is a false dichotomy. Throughout this book we have taken an approach which draws upon the arguments of ethics and philosophy, on the one hand, and evidence taken from nursing research and experience on the other. We have based our arguments on real cases and situations drawn from the everyday practice of nursing, but we have also sought to interpret these in the light of normative theories. This is not surprising, for there is no human science that is value-free, except in the minds of naïve positivists. The normative questions asked by the philosophy of nursing, which are also the focus of attention of those concerned with nursing as an art, concern both what nursing is and what it ought to be. In a sense, every answer we give to the question 'What is nursing?' is implicitly normative. Here the task of philosophy is, as has often been said, to make the implicit explicit; that is, its task is to make the values presupposed in a particular operational definition of nursing clear, to critically examine these and to determine whether they are adequate or not. Conversely the question 'What is nursing?' cannot be asked without regard to the facts, without taking account of the history of nursing, and the evidence of where it stands today, and where it might be going – given many other facts and trends: epidemiological, demographic, economic, sociological, etc. There must be a relationship between the theoretical discussion of nursing – the 'What is nursing?' debate – and the evidence base that we need to develop for practice and nursing ethics.

Research work itself is never value-neutral. We may begin with the apparently neutral question: 'Can this project be undertaken?' (i.e. methodologically speaking). However, we soon have to proceed to the question 'Should it be undertaken?' (i.e. ethically speaking). Once we undertake the research itself, then we confront a whole series of further ethical questions: issues of informed consent, confidentiality, risks and benefits, the value of the research to society at large.

Epistemological questions about the scientific validity of the research and the methods used are also ethical to the extent that they affect the truth value of the research and its practical outcomes. The application of phenomenological methods to nursing research has been partly provoked by the need for an alternative to a naïve positivist philosophy of science, with its pretended value-neutrality and objectivity. What phenomenology has done has been to encourage the use of more qualitative methods for studying and analysing the structure of lived experience on the part of those involved in the situation of nursing care. Phenomenology is concerned with understanding the subjective experiences of everyday life from the perspective of those experiencing them, and there is a risk that such methods may be subjective and not impartial in the way they are applied. Further, there is a tendency for exaggerated claims to be made for this kind of qualitative research, that it has uncovered meanings and revealed truths inaccessible to other forms of scientific research. Unless the results of phenomenological research are subject to the same tests of public verification or falsification applicable to other research then their validity must be open to question.

While 'evidence-based' practice and research must be criticised for its tendency to avoid making its epistemological and normative presuppositions explicit, phenomenological method can be disingenuous about its objectivity as a method so long as it does not submit to the tests of inter-subjective validity and scientific agreement. Ultimately, research ethics itself is about fidelity to the truth and the canons of logical validity of arguments and the correspondence of truth-claims with the facts. If evidence-based practice is the goal, then the evidence – or nursing knowledge – has itself to be scientifically sound, but also phenomenologically true to the nature of nursing experience, not attempting to force it onto the Procrustean bed of a preconceived method.

This methodological as well as philosophical debate will continue as long as nurses continue to ask the question 'What is nursing?'. That is a question which nurses, like any other profession, must continue to ask if they are not to become rigid and ossified. The postmodern debates and critique of scientism within the social sciences have not passed nursing by. A postmodern view of nursing would have it that there are no grand theories or explanations to be had about the nature of nursing, and that everything is a matter of different types of discourse and different constructions of reality. Nursing has been through an era of near-grand theory building! This was not uniformly popular, especially among practitioners, but it has had an effect upon nursing's history, which even the postmoderns would have to accept. Whether it took the development of nursing education any further forward is a matter for debate. For a variety of reasons, nursing and nursing education have always had to be flexible, and this is still as true today as it ever was. It is essential for nurses to be able to plan and deliver care in a changing social environment, in a way that is responsive to demographic changes, and in the light of fast developing medical science and technology. The education process will only be successful if it produces nurses with analytic skills and a capacity to adapt.

THE FUTURE OF NURSING AND NURSING ETHICS

With the publication of *Health for All in the 21st Century* (WHO 1999b) we are faced with the challenge of where nursing should be going. The role of nursing in the health care systems of the 21st century is likely, however, to preserve many features of its past, in so far as seeing patients through experiences of altered health state to some resolution or accommodation will still be a major feature of the work of the main carer, whether or not this person is still called a nurse.

Nursing in many countries is now a well established occupation, having a place among the respected professions, with a university-based education, and seeking to lay a strong research base for its practice. There are ongoing debates in nursing research circles about the basic premises upon which nursing knowledge is founded. As in any other discipline, there is a relationship between the epistemological foundations of research methodology, research work and the nature of the knowledge produced. This may require some choices to be made about the kind of research and nursing knowledge which is to be developed, and perhaps more explicitly, there are choices to be made concerning the kind of professional practice to be developed for the future service of humanity.

What should be the ambitions of nursing in the 21st century? Has the professional goal that nursing has been moving towards become less appropriate, and is the activity of caring now more important than professional status? The long-term project to professionalise nursing as a single profession is probably impossible due to the sheer size of the occupational group. One way out would be to develop an academic elite, whose role is to supervise the work done by a more numerous group of assistants. Here the emphasis would be on graduate nurse managers who would administer services according to the best scientific management principles. An alternative model would be to reconstruct nursing as an occupation with the status of a skilled craft. In this way, rather than emphasising the 'elitist model' of nursing as a profession, nursing could adopt the model of the autonomy of the self-employed craft worker, performing a trade with considerable judgement, self-direction and skill with the support of assistants and apprentices, and in partnership with others.

The tack which nursing in the UK would appear to be adopting is following the American experience where routine management of patients is taken over by nurse specialists and where the specialisms mirror those to be found in medicine. The specialist practitioner is very likely to be taking on a range of tasks which are on the borderline between medical and nursing practice. For nursing to be taking over work which was at one time the province of medicine is not new (the measurement of blood pressure being a mundane case in point). It is the motives and the overall benefit to the health care enterprise that we need to consider when suggestions of role expansion and extension come up. Nursing should be very careful of venturing into the territory that medicine is all too willing to give up, because it is very likely that it will be the elderly and the chronic sick who will pay the price for this cheap doctoring solution to the problem.

In the closing paragraph of their work on the social history of nursing, Dingwall et al (1988) say that 'if we ask who will be standing beside the patient's bed in the year 2000, it is difficult to resist the conclusion that it will still be the handywoman class in the new guise of support workers'. In the 21st century, any shift of emphasis to the community should allow nursing to exploit what knowledge and experience it already has. For, while some of the challenges of the closing decades of the 20th century were new, many had been seen before, albeit in different guises. The global HIV/AIDS pandemic has resulted, in many countries, in moral panic and in denial by the politicians and the public which parallel responses to pandemics in the past. While some features of the HIV/AIDS pandemic are arguably new, nurses have discovered that the responses required of them are similar to those made when infectious diseases were rife, such as TB, syphilis and, further back, plagues. Public health measures and many community responses that have been mounted in past times are again relevant and appropriate. The lessons nursing has learnt, for instance, from oncology, palliative care, pain relief and the hospice movement have their place in caring for the end stages of AIDS. Health care professionals, however, may become less inclined to make distinctions between acute and chronic conditions in the future, because this distinction will be less helpful if the boundary between hospital and community becomes more flexible.

Nursing is at present at a crossroads in its development. It is a relatively young, fast-growing academic discipline and comprises an occupational group numerically larger than any other in health care. It has a legacy of being in a subordinate relationship to a dominant medical profession. However, nurses are developing a sense of identity and confidence of their own. This is based not only on 150 years or more of accumulated experience of nursing – in wartime and in times of peace and stability – but also on more secure knowledge arising from the application of the methods of the behavioural and social sciences (as well as medicine) to nursing research. All this adds further impetus to the desire of nurses to articulate what unique insights they bring to health care, and to develop a body of knowledge and area of practice for nursing which nurses can claim as their own. In other words, nursing is engaged in the activity described much earlier by Hughes (1958) as the typical approach taken by a young and new occupational group striving to attain professional status. Among the hallmarks of a profession, and required in many countries for its formal registration, is the possession of a code of professional ethics and evidence that this is applied and monitored in practice. It is clear, then, that the current debates in nursing, concerned with clarifying its nature, scope, practical functions and relevance for the future, will not only be critical for the direction of health care, but also central to defining the content and form of nursing ethics, and the significance of the contribution of nurses to the wider debates about biomedical ethics.

further reading

Benner P, Wrubel J 1989 The primacy of caring: stress and copying in health and illness. Addison Wesley, Menlo Park, CA

Dingwall R, Rafferty A M, Webster C 1988 An introduction to the social history of nursing. Routledge, London

Fry S 1989a Teaching ethics in nursing curricula: traditional and contemporary models. Nursing Clinics of North America 24(2): 485–497

Fry S 1989b The role of caring in a theory of nursing ethics. Hypatia 4(2): 88–103

Gilligan C 1982 In a different voice – psychological theory and women's development. Harvard University Press, Cambridge, MA

Hughes E C 1958 Men and their work. Free Press, New York

Kohlberg L 1984 Essays on moral development: the psychology of moral development. Nature and validity of moral stages, Vol 2. Harper & Row, New York

Mackay L, Soothill K, Melia K 1988 Classic texts in health care. Butterworth Heinemann, Oxford

McAlpine H 1988 Ethical reasoning of practising nurses: does ethics education make a difference? [Unpublished PhD thesis], Murdoch University, Western Australia

Melia K M 1994 The task of nursing ethics. Journal of Medical Ethics 20(4): 7–11

Porter R 1997 The greatest benefit to mankind – a medical history of humanity from antiquity to the present. Harper Collins, London

Rafferty A M 1996 The politics of nursing knowledge. Routledge, London

Robb I H 1990 Nursing ethics. Cleveland, Ohio

Stacey M, Homans H 1978 The sociology of health and illness: its present state, future prospects and potential for health research. Sociology 12(2): 281–307

Strong P, Robinson J 1990 The NHS under new management. Open University Press, Milton Keynes

WHO 1978 Primary health care. Report of international conference held at Alma Ata, USSR. World Health Organisation, Geneva

WHO 1999 Health for all in the 21st Century. World Health Organization, Geneva

Appendices

SECTION CONTENTS

APPENDIX 1

Traditional codes of medical ethics

HIPPOCRATIC OATH (c. 420 BC)

I swear by Apollo the physician, by Aesculapius, Hygeia and Panacea, and I take to witness all the gods, all the goddesses, to keep according to my ability and my judgements the following Oath:

To consider dear to me as my parents him who taught me this art; to live in common with him and if necessary to share my goods with him; to look upon his children as my own brothers, to teach them this art if they so desire without fee or written promise; to impart to my sons and the sons of the master who taught me and the disciples who have enrolled themselves and have agreed to the rules of the profession, but to these alone, the precepts and the instruction. I will prescribe regimen for the good of my patients according to my ability and my judgement and never do harm to anyone. To please no one will I prescribe a deadly drug, nor give advice which may cause his death. Nor will I give a woman a pessary to procure abortion. But I will preserve the purity of my life and my art. I will not cut for stone, even for patients in whom the disease is manifest; I will leave this operation to be performed by practitioners (specialists in this art). In every house where I come I will enter only for the good of my patients, keeping myself far from all intentional ill doing and all seduction, and especially from the pleasure of love with women or with men, be they free or slaves. All that may come to my knowledge in the exercise of my profession or outside of my profession or in daily commerce with men, which ought not to be spread abroad, I will keep secret and will never reveal. If I keep this oath faithfully, may I enjoy my life and practise my art, respected by all men and in all times; but if I swerve from it or violate it, may the reverse be my lot.

(Reprinted by permission: *Dorland's American Illustrated Medical Dictionary*, 28th edn. Saunders, Philadelphia, 1994.)

DECLARATION OF GENEVA

(World Medical Association 1948, 1968, 1983)

AT THE TIME OF BEING ADMITTED AS MEMBER OF THE MEDICAL PROFESSION:

I SOLEMNLY PLEDGE myself to consecrate my life to the service of humanity;

I WILL GIVE to my teachers the respect and gratitude which is their due;

I WILL PRACTISE my profession with conscience and dignity;

THE HEALTH OF MY PATIENTS will be my first consideration;

I WILL RESPECT the secrets which are confided in me;

I WILL MAINTAIN by all the means in my power, the honour and the noble traditions of the medical profession;

MY COLLEAGUES will be my brothers;

I WILL NOT PERMIT considerations of religion, nationality, race, party politics or social standing to intervene between my duty and my patient;

I WILL MAINTAIN the utmost respect for human life, from the time of conception; even under threat, I will not use my medical knowledge contrary to the laws of humanity.

I MAKE THESE PROMISES solemnly, freely and upon my honour.

(Adopted by the General Assembly of the World Medical Association, Geneva, 1948, 1968, 1983.)

(Reprinted by permission: World Medical Association.)

INTERNATIONAL CODE OF MEDICAL ETHICS

(World Medical Association 1949, 1968, 1983)

Duties of Physicians in General

A physician should always maintain the highest standards of professional conduct.

A physician shall not permit motives of profit to influence the free and independent exercise of professional judgement on behalf of all patients.

A physician shall, in all types of medical practice, be dedicated to providing competent medical services in full technical and moral independence, with compassion and respect for human dignity.

A physician shall deal honestly with patients and colleagues, and strive to expose those physicians deficient in character or competence, or who engage in fraud or deception.

THE FOLLOWING PRACTICES are deemed to be unethical conduct:

a) Self advertisement by physicians, unless permitted by the laws of the country and the Code of Ethics of the National Medical Association.
b) Paying or receiving any fee or any other consideration solely to procure the referral of a patient or for prescribing or referring a patient to any source.

A physician shall respect the rights of patients, of colleagues, and of other health professionals, and shall safeguard patient confidences.

A physician shall act only in the patient's interest when providing medical care which might have the effect of weakening the physical and medical condition of the patient.

A physician shall use great caution in divulging discoveries or new techniques or treatment through non-professional channels.

A physician shall certify only that which he has personally verified.

Duties of Physicians to the Sick

A physician shall always bear in mind the obligation of preserving human life.

A physician shall owe his patients complete loyalty and all the resources of his science. Whenever an examination or treatment is beyond the physician's capacity he should summon another physician who has the necessary ability.

A physician shall preserve absolute confidentiality on all he knows about his patient even after the patient has died.

A physician shall give emergency care as a humanitarian duty unless he is assured that others are willing and able to give such care.

Duties of Physicians to Each Other

A physician shall behave towards his colleagues as he would have them behave toward him.

A physician shall not entice patients from his colleagues.

A physician shall observe the principles of 'The Declaration of Geneva' approved by the World Medical Association.

(Adopted by the third General Assembly of the World Medical Association, London, 1949.)

(Reprinted by permission: World Medical Association.)

DECLARATION OF HELSINKI

(World Medical Association 1964, 1975, 1983, 1989, 1996)

Introduction

It is the mission of the physician to safeguard the health of the people. His or her knowledge and conscience are dedicated to the fulfillment of this mission.

The Declaration of Geneva of the World Medical Association binds the physician with the words, 'The Health of my patient will be my first consideration,' and the International Code of Medical Ethics declares that, 'A physician shall act only in the patient's interest when providing medical care which might have the effect of weakening the physical and mental condition of the patient.'

The purpose of biomedical research involving human subjects must be to improve diagnostic, therapeutic and prophylactic procedures and the understanding of the aetiology and pathogenesis of disease.

In current medical practice most diagnostic, therapeutic or prophylactic procedures involve hazards. This applies especially to biomedical research.

Medical progress is based on research which ultimately must rest in part on experimentation involving human subjects.

In the field of biomedical research a fundamental distinction must be recognized between medical research in which the aim is essentially diagnostic or therapeutic for a patient, and medical research, the essential object of which is purely scientific and without direct diagnostic or therapeutic value to the person subjected to the research.

Special caution must be exercised in the conduct of research which may affect the environment, and the welfare of animals used for research must be respected.

Because it is essential that the results of laboratory experiments be applied to human beings to further their scientific knowledge and to help suffering humanity, the World Medical Association has prepared the following recommendations as a guide to every physician in biomedical research involving human subjects. They should be kept under review in the future. It must be stressed that the standards as drafted are only a guide to physicians all over the world. Physicians are not relieved from criminal, civil and ethical responsibilities under the laws of their own countries.

I. Basic principles

1. Biomedical research involving human subjects must conform to generally accepted scientific principles and should be based on adequately performed laboratory and animal experimentation and on a thorough knowledge of the scientific literature.
2. The design and performance of each experimental procedure involving human subjects should be clearly formulated in an experimental protocol which should be transmitted for consideration, comment and guidance to a specially appointed committee independent of the investigator and the sponsor provided that this independent committee is in conformity with the laws and regulations of the country in which the research experiment is performed.
3. Biomedical research involving human subjects should be conducted only by scientifically qualified persons and under the supervision of a clinically competent medical person. The responsibility for the human subject must always rest with a medically qualified person and never rest on the subject of the research, even though the subject has given his or her consent.
4. Biomedical research involving human subjects cannot legitimately be carried out unless the importance of the objective is in proportion to the inherent risk to the subject.
5. Every biomedical research project involving human subjects should be preceded by careful assessment of predictable risks in comparison with foreseeable benefits to the subject or to others. Concern for the interests of the subject must always prevail over the interests of science and society.
6. The right of the research subject to safeguard his or her integrity must always be respected. Every precaution should be taken to respect the privacy of the subject and to minimize the impact of the study on the subject's physical and mental integrity and on the personality of the subject.
7. Physicians should abstain from engaging in research projects involving human subjects unless they are satisfied that the hazards involved are believed to be predictable. Physicians should cease any investigation if the hazards are found to outweigh the potential benefits.

8. In publication of the results of his or her research, the doctor is obliged to preserve the accuracy of the results. Reports of experimentation not in accordance with the principles laid down in this Declaration should not be accepted for publication.
9. In any research on human beings, each potential subject must be adequately informed of the aims, methods, anticipated benefits and potential hazards of the study and the discomfort it may entail. He or she should be informed that he or she is at liberty to abstain from participation in the study and that he or she is free to withdraw his or her consent to participation at any time. The doctor should then obtain the subject's freely given informed consent, preferably in writing.
10. When obtaining informed consent for the research project the doctor should be particularly cautious if the subject is in a dependent relationship to him or her or may consent under duress. In that case the informed consent should be obtained by a doctor who is not engaged in the investigation and who is completely independent of this official relationship.
11. In the case of legal incompetence, informed consent should be obtained from the legal guardian in accordance with national legislation. Where physical or mental incapacity makes it impossible to obtain informed consent, or when the subject is a minor, permission from the responsible relative replaces that of the subject in accordance with national legislation. Whenever the minor child is in fact able to give consent, the minor's consent must be obtained in addition to the consent of the minor's legal guardian.
12. The research protocol should always contain a statement of the ethical considerations involved and should indicate that the principles enunciated in the present Declaration are complied with.

II. Medical research combined with professional care (clinical research)

1. In the treatment of the sick person, the doctor must be free to use a new diagnostic and therapeutic measure, if in his or her judgement it offers hope of saving life, re-establishing health or alleviating suffering.
2. The potential benefits, hazards and discomfort of a new method should be weighed against the advantages of the best current diagnostic and therapeutic method.
3. In any medical study, every patient – including those of a control group, if any – should be assured of the best proven diagnostic and therapeutic method. This does not exclude the use of inert placebo in studies where no proven diagnostic or therapeutic method exists.
4. The refusal of the patient to participate in a study must never interfere with the doctor–patient relationship.
5. If the physician considers it essential not to obtain informed consent, the specific reasons for this proposal should be stated in the experimental protocol for transmission to the independent committee. (1. 2)
6. The physician can combine medical research with professional care, the objective being the acquisition of new medical knowledge, only to the extent that medical research is justified by its potential diagnostic or therapeutic value for the patient.

III. Non-therapeutic biomedical research involving human subjects (non-clinical biomedical research)

1. In the purely scientific application of medical research carried out on a human being, it is the duty of the physician to remain the protector of the life and health of that person on whom biomedical research is being carried out.
2. The subjects should be volunteers – either healthy persons or patients for whom the experimental design is not related to the patient's illness.
3. The investigator or the investigating team should discontinue the research if in his/her or their judgement it may, if continued, be harmful to the individual.
4. In research on man, the interest of science and society should never take precedence over considerations related to the well being of the subject.

(Adopted by the Third General Assembly of the World Medical Association, London, 1964; revised 1975, 1983, 1989, 1996.)

(Reprinted by permission: World Medical Association.)

APPENDIX 2

Traditional codes of ethics for nurses

CODE FOR NURSES: ETHICAL CONCEPTS APPLIED TO NURSING

(ICN 1973, revised 1992)

The fundamental responsibility of the nurse is fourfold: to promote health, to prevent illness, to restore health and to alleviate suffering. The need for nursing is universal. Inherent in nursing is respect for life, dignity and rights of man. It is unrestricted by considerations of nationality, race, creed, colour, age, sex, politics or social status. Nurses render health services to the individual, the family and the community and co-ordinate their services with those of related groups.

Nurses and people

The nurse's primary responsibility is to those people who require nursing care.

The nurse, in providing care, promotes an environment in which the values, customs and spiritual beliefs of the individual are respected.

The nurse holds in confidence personal information and uses judgement in sharing this information.

Nurses and practice

The nurse carries personal responsibility for nursing practice and for maintaining competence by continual learning.

The nurse maintains the highest standards of nursing care possible within the reality of a specific situation.

The nurse uses judgement in relation to individual competence when accepting and delegating responsibilities.

The nurse when acting in a professional capacity should at all times maintain standards of personal conduct which reflect credit upon the profession.

Nurses and society

The nurse shares with other citizens the responsibility for initiating and supporting action to meet the health and social needs of the public.

Nurses and co-workers

The nurse sustains a co-operative relationship with co-workers in nursing and other fields.

The nurse takes appropriate action to safeguard the individual when his care is endangered by a co-worker or any other person.

Nurses and the profession

The nurse plays the major role in determining and implementing desirable standards of nursing practice and nursing education.

The nurse is active in developing a core of professional knowledge.

The nurse, acting through the professional organisations, participates in establishing and maintaining equitable social and economic working conditions in nursing.

(Reprinted by permission: International Council of Nurses 1973, revised 1992.)

NURSES AND HUMAN RIGHTS

(International Council for Nurses 1983, revised 1993)

ICN position statement: nurses and human rights

Human rights in health care involve both recipients and providers. The International Council of Nurses (ICN) views health care as a right of all individuals, regardless of financial, political, geographic, racial or religious considerations. This right includes the right to choose or decline care, including the right to accept or refuse treatment or nourishment, informed consent, confidentiality, and dignity, including the right to die with dignity.

Human rights and the nurse's role

Nurses have an obligation to safeguard people's health rights at all times and in all places. This includes assuring that adequate care is provided within the resources available and in accordance with nursing ethics. As well, the nurse is obliged to ensure that patients receive appropriate information prior to consenting to treatment or procedures, including participation in research.

ICN advocates inclusion of human rights issues and the nurse's role in all levels of nursing education programmes.

As professionals, nurses are accountable for their own actions in safeguarding human rights. National nurses' associations have a responsibility to participate in the development of health and social legislation related to patient rights.

Nurses' rights

Nurses have the right to practise in accordance with the nursing legislation of the country in which they work and to adopt the ICN *Code for Nurses* or their own national ethical code. Nurses also have a right to practise in an environment that provides personal safety, freedom from abuse and violence, threats or intimidation.

National nurses' associations need to ensure an effective mechanism through which nurses can seek confidential advice, counsel, support and assistance in dealing with difficult human rights situations.

Background

Nurses deal with human rights issues daily, in all aspects of their professional role. Nurses may be pressured to apply their knowledge and skills in ways that are detrimental to patients and others. There is a need for increased vigilance, and a requirement to be well informed, about how new technology and experimentation can violate human rights. Furthermore, nurses are increasingly facing complex human rights issues, arising from conflict situations within jurisdictions, political upheaval and wars. The application of human rights protection should emphasise vulnerable groups such as women, children, elderly people, refugees and stigmatised groups.

ICN has developed a Health and Human Rights fact sheet, addressing the major areas where human rights impact on the health of populations, including public health, health care reform, access to care and gender perspectives. Other ICN publications are accessible on their website: <http://www.icn.org>.

(ICN endorses the Universal Declaration of Human Rights, adopted by the United Nations General Assembly in 1948.)

CODE OF PROFESSIONAL CONDUCT FOR THE NURSE, MIDWIFE AND HEALTH VISITOR

(UKCC 1992)

Each registered nurse, midwife and health visitor shall act, at all times, in such a manner as to:

- safeguard and promote the interests of individual patients and clients;
- serve the interests of society;
- justify public trust and confidence and
- uphold and enhance the good standing and reputation of the professions.

As a registered nurse, midwife or health visitor, you are personally accountable for your practice and, in the exercise of your professional accountability, must:

1. act always in such a manner as to promote and safeguard the interests and well being of patients and clients;
2. ensure that no action or omission on your part, or within your sphere of responsibility, is detrimental to the interests, condition or safety of patients and clients;
3. maintain and improve your professional knowledge and competence;
4. acknowledge any limitations in your knowledge and competence and decline any duties or responsibilities unless able to perform them in a safe and skilled manner;
5. work in an open and co-operative manner with patients, clients and their families, foster their independence and recognise and respect their involvement in the planning and delivery of care;

6. work in a collaborative and co-operative manner with health care professionals and others involved in providing care, and recognise and respect their particular contributions within the care team;

7. recognise and respect the uniqueness and dignity of each patient and client, and respond to their need for care, irrespective of their ethnic origin, religious beliefs, personal attributes, the nature of their health problems or any other factor;

8. report to an appropriate person or authority, at the earliest possible time, any conscientious objection which may be relevant to your professional practice;

9. avoid any abuse of your privileged relationships with patients and clients and of the privileged access allowed to their person, property, residence or workplace;

10. protect all confidential information concerning patients and clients obtained in the course of professional practice and make disclosures only with consent, where required by the order of a court or where you can justify disclosure in the wider public interest;

11. report to an appropriate person or authority, having regard to the physical, psychological and social effects on patients and clients, any circumstances in the environment of care which could jeopardise standards of practice;

12. report to an appropriate person or authority any circumstances in which safe and appropriate care for patients and clients cannot be provided;

13. report to an appropriate person or authority where it appears that the health or safety of colleagues is at risk, as such circumstances may compromise standards of practice and care;

14. assist professional colleagues, in the context of your own knowledge, experience and sphere of responsibility, to develop their professional competence, and assist others in the care team, including informal carers, to contribute safely and to a degree appropriate to their roles;

15. refuse any gift, favour or hospitality from patients or clients currently in your care which might be interpreted as seeking to exert influence to obtain preferential consideration and

16. ensure that your registration status is not used in the promotion of commercial products or services, declare any financial or other interests in relevant organisations providing such goods or services and ensure that your professional judgement is not influenced by any commercial considerations.

Notice to all Registered Nurses, Midwives and Health Visitors

The Code of Professional Conduct for the Nurse, Midwife and Health Visitor is issued to all registered nurses, midwives and health visitors by the United Kingdom Central Council for Nursing, Midwifery and Health Visiting. The Council is the regulatory body responsible for the standards of these professions and it requires members of the professions to practise and conduct themselves within the standards and framework provided by the Code.

(Reprinted by permission: United Kingdom Central Council for Nursing, Midwifery and Health Visiting. Original text document June 1992.)

CONFIDENTIALITY

(UKCC 1984b, 2nd edn)

Summary of the principles on which to base professional judgement in matters of confidentiality.

1. That a patient/client has a right to expect that information given in confidence will be used only for the purpose for which it was given and will not be released to others without their consent.

2. That practitioners recognise the fundamental right of their patients/clients to have information about them held in secure and private storage.

3. That, where it is deemed appropriate to share information obtained in the course of professional practice with other health or social work practitioners, the practitioner who obtained the information must ensure, as far as is reasonable, before its release that it is being imparted in strict professional confidence and for a specific purpose.

4. That the responsibility to either disclose or withhold confidential information in the public interest lies with the individual practitioner, that he/she cannot delegate the decision, and that he/she cannot be required by a superior to disclose or withhold information against his/her will.

5. That a practitioner who chooses to breach the basic principle of confidentiality in the belief that it is necessary in the public interest must have considered the matter sufficiently to justify that decision.

6. That deliberate breaches of confidentiality other than with the consent of the patient/client should be exceptional.

(Reprinted by permission: United Kingdom Central Council for Nursing, Midwifery and Health Visiting. UKCC 1984, 2nd edn (Clause 9))

INTERNATIONAL CODE OF ETHICS FOR MIDWIVES

(International Confederation of Midwives 1993)

Preamble

The aim of the International Confederation of Midwives (ICM) is to improve the standard of care provided to women, babies and families throughout the world through the development, education, and appropriate utilization of the professional midwife. In keeping with its aim of women's health and focus on the midwife, the ICM sets forth the following code to guide the education, practice and research of the midwife. This code acknowledges women as persons, seeks justice for all people and equity in access to health care, and is based on mutual relationships of respect, trust, and the dignity of all members of society.

The Code

I.   Midwifery relationships

A. Midwives respect a woman's informed right of choice and promote the woman's acceptance of responsibility for the outcomes of her choices.

B. Midwives work with women, supporting their right to participate actively in decisions about their care, and empowering women to speak for themselves on issues affecting the health of women and their families in their culture/society.

C. Midwives, together with women, work with policy and funding agencies to define women's needs for health services and to ensure that resources are fairly allocated considering priorities and availability.

D. Midwives support and sustain each other in their professional roles, and actively nurture their own and others' sense of self-worth.

E. Midwives work with other health professionals, consulting and referring as necessary when the woman's need for care exceeds the competencies of the midwife.

F. Midwives recognize the human interdependence within their field of practice and actively seek to resolve inherent conflicts.

II.   Practice of midwifery

A. Midwives provide care for women and childbearing families with respect for cultural diversity while also working to eliminate harmful practices within those same cultures.

B. Midwives encourage realistic expectations of childbirth by women within their own society, with the minimum expectation that no women should be harmed by conception or childbearing.

C. Midwives use their professional knowledge to ensure safe birthing practices in all environments and cultures.

D. Midwives respond to the psychological, physical, emotional and spiritual needs of women seeking health care, whatever their circumstances.

E. Midwives act as effective role models in health promotion for women throughout their life cycle, for families and for other health professionals.

F. Midwives actively seek personal, intellectual and professional growth throughout their midwifery career, integrating this growth into their practice.

III.   The professional responsibilities of Midwives

A. Midwives hold in confidence client information in order to protect the right to privacy, and use judgement in sharing this information.

B. Midwives are responsible for their decisions and actions, and are accountable for the related outcomes in their care of women.

C. Midwives may refuse to participate in activities for which they hold deep moral opposition; however, the emphasis on individual conscience should not deprive women of essential health services.

D. Midwives participate in the development and implementation of health policies that promote the health of all women and childbearing families.

IV.   Advancement of midwifery knowledge and practice

A. Midwives ensure that the advancement of midwifery knowledge is based on activities that protect the rights of women as persons.

B. Midwives develop and share midwifery knowledge through a variety of processes, such as peer review and research.

C. Midwives participate in the formal education of midwifery students and midwives.

(Reprinted by permission: International Confederation of Midwives 1993.)

APPENDIX 3

Patients' rights and Ottawa Charter for Health Promotion

A PATIENT'S BILL OF RIGHTS

(American Hospital Association 1973, revised 1992)

Introduction

Effective health care requires collaboration between patients and physicians and other health care professionals. Open and honest communication, respect for personal and professional values and sensitivity to differences are integral to optimal patient care. As the setting for the provision of health services, hospitals must provide a foundation for understanding and respecting the rights and responsibilities of patients, their families, physicians, and other caregivers. Hospitals must ensure a health care ethic that respects the role of patients in decision making about treatment choices and other aspects of their care. Hospitals must be sensitive to cultural, racial, linguistic, religious, age, gender, and other differences as well as the needs of persons with disabilities.

The American Hospital Association presents *A Patient's Bill of Rights* with the expectation that it will contribute to more effective patient care and can be supported by the hospital on behalf of the institution, its medical staff, employees, and patients. The American Hospital Association encourages health care institutions to tailor this bill of rights to their patient community by translating and/or simplifying the language of this bill of rights as may be necessary to ensure that patients and their families understand their rights and responsibilities.

Bill of Rights

These rights can be exercised on the patient's behalf by a designated surrogate or proxy decision-maker if the patient lacks decision-making capacity, is legally incompetent, or is a minor.

1. The patient has the right to considerate and respectful care.
2. The patient has the right to and is encouraged to obtain from physicians and other direct caregivers relevant, current, and understandable information concerning diagnosis, treatment, and prognosis.

Except in emergencies when the patient lacks decision-making capacity and the need for treatment is urgent, the patient is entitled to the opportunity to discuss and request information related to the specific procedures and/or treatments, the risks involved, the possible length of recuperation, and the medically reasonable alternatives and their accompanying risks and benefits.

Patients have the right to know the identity of physicians, nurses, and others involved in their care, as well as when those involved are students, residents, or other trainees. The patient also has the right to know the immediate and long-term financial implications of treatment choices, insofar as they are known.

3. The patient has the right to make decisions about the plan of care prior to and during the course of treatment and to refuse a recommended treatment or plan of care to the extent permitted by law and hospital policy and to be informed of the medical consequences of this action. In case of such refusal, the patient is entitled to other appropriate care and services that the hospital provides or transfer to another hospital. The hospital should notify patients of any policy that might affect patient choice within the institution.

4. The patient has the right to have an advance directive (such as a living will, health care proxy, or durable power of attorney for health care) concerning treatment or designating a surrogate or proxy decision-maker with the expectation that the hospital will honour the intent of that directive to the extent permitted by law and hospital policy.

Health care institutions must advise patients of their rights under state law and hospital policy to make informed medical choices, ask if the patient has an advance directive and include that information in patient records. The patient has the right to timely information about hospital policy that may limit its ability to implement fully a legally valid advance directive.

5. The patient has the right to every consideration of privacy. Case discussion, consultation, examination, and treatment should be conducted so as to protect each patient's privacy.

6. The patient has the right to expect that all communications and records pertaining to his/her care will be treated as confidential by the hospital, except in cases such as suspected abuse and public health hazards when reporting is permitted or required by law. The patient has the right to expect that the hospital will emphasize the confidentiality of this information when it releases it to any other parties entitled to review information in these records.

7. The patient has the right to review the records pertaining to his/her medical care and to have the information explained or interpreted as necessary, except when restricted by law.

8. The patient has the right to expect that, within its capacity and policies, a hospital will make reasonable response to the request of a patient for appropriate and medically indicated care and services. The hospital must provide evaluation, service, and/or referral as indicated by the urgency of the case. When medically appropriate and legally permissible, or when a patient has so requested, a patient may be transferred to another facility. The institution to which the patient is to be transferred must first have accepted the patient for transfer. The patient must also have the benefit of complete information and explanation concerning the need for, risks, benefits, and alternatives to such a transfer.

9. The patient has the right to ask and be informed of the existence of business relationships among the hospital, educational institutions, other health care providers, or payers that may influence the patient's treatment and care.

10. The patient has the right to consent to or decline to participate in proposed research studies or human experimentation affecting care and treatment or requiring direct patient involvement, and to have those studies fully explained prior to consent. A patient who declines to participate in research or experimentation is entitled to the most effective care that the hospital can otherwise provide.

11. The patient has the right to expect reasonable continuity of care when appropriate and to be informed by physicians and other caregivers of available and realistic patient care options when hospital care is no longer appropriate.

12. The patient has the right to be informed of hospital policies and practices that relate to patient care, treatment, and responsibilities. The patient has the right to be informed of available resources for resolving disputes, grievances, and conflicts, such as ethics committees, patient representatives, or other mechanisms available in the institution. The patient has the right to be informed of the hospital's charges for services and available payment methods.

The collaborative nature of health requires that patients, or their families/surrogates participate in their care. The effectiveness of care and patient satisfaction with the course of treatment depend, in part, on the patient fulfilling certain responsibilities. Patients are responsible for providing information about past illnesses, hospitalizations, medications, and other matters related to health status. To participate effectively in decision making, patients must be encouraged to take responsibility for requesting additional information or clarification about their health status or treatment when they do not fully understand information and instructions. Patients are also responsible for ensuring that the health care institution has a copy of their written advance directive if they have one. Patients are responsible for informing their physicians and other caregivers if they anticipate problems in following prescribed treatment.

Patients should also be aware of the hospital's obligation to be reasonably efficient and equitable in providing care to other patients and the community. The hospital's rules and regulations are designed to help the hospital meet this obligation. Patients and their families are responsible for making reasonable accommodations to the needs of the hospital, other patients, medical staff and hospital employees. Patients are responsible for providing necessary information for insurance claims and for working with the hospital to make payment arrangements, when necessary.

A person's health depends on much more than health care services. Patients are responsible for recognizing the impact of their life-style on their personal health.

Conclusion

Hospitals have many functions to perform, including the enhancement of health status, health promotion, and the prevention and treatment of injury and disease; the immediate and ongoing care and rehabilitation of patients; the education of health professionals, patients, and the community; and research. All these activities must be conducted with an overriding concern for the values and dignity of patients.

(A Patient's Bill of Rights was first adopted by the American Hospital Association in 1973.)

(This revision was approved by the AHA Board of Trustees on October 21, 1992. © 1992 by the American Hospital Association, One North Franklin Street, Chicago, IL 60606. Printed in USA all rights reserved. Catalog no. 157759.)

THE OTTAWA CHARTER FOR HEALTH PROMOTION

(World Health Organisation 1986)

The first International Conference on Health Promotion, meeting in Ottawa this 21st day of November 1986, hereby presents this CHARTER for action to achieve Health for All by the Year 2000 and beyond.

This conference was primarily a response to growing expectations for a new public health movement around the world. Discussions focused on the needs in industrialised countries, but took into account similar concerns in all other regions. It built on the progress made through the *Declaration on Primary Health Care at Alma- Ata*, the World Health Organization's Targets for Health for All document, and the recent debate at the World Health Assembly on inter-sectoral action for health.

Health promotion

Health promotion is the process of enabling people to increase control over, and to improve, their health. To reach a state of complete physical, mental and social well-being, an individual or group must be able to identify and to realise aspirations, to satisfy needs, and to change or cope with the environment. Health is, therefore, seen as a resource for everyday life, not the objective of living. Health is a positive concept, emphasising social and personal resources, as well as physical capacities. Therefore, health promotion is not just the responsibility of the health sector, but goes beyond healthy life-styles to well-being.

Pre-requisites for health

The fundamental conditions and resources for health are:

- Peace
- Shelter
- Education
- Food
- Income
- A stable eco-system
- Sustainable resources
- Social justice, and equity.

Improvement in health requires a secure foundation in these basic prerequisites.

Advocate

Good health is a major resource for social, economic and personal development and an important dimension of quality of life. Political, economic, social, cultural, environmental, behavioural and biological factors can all favour health or be harmful to it. Health promotion action aims at making these conditions favourable through advocacy for health.

Enable

Health promotion focuses on achieving equity in health. Health promotion action aims at reducing differences in current health status and ensuring equal opportunities and resources to enable all people to achieve their fullest health potential. This includes a secure foundation in a supportive environment, access to information, life skills and opportunities for making healthy choices. People cannot achieve their fullest health potential unless they be able to take control of those things which determine their health. This must apply equally to women and men.

Mediate

The pre-requisites and prospects for health cannot be ensured by the health sector alone. More importantly, health promotion demands co-ordinated action by all concerned: by governments, by health and other social and economic sectors, by non-governmental and voluntary organisations, by local authorities, by industry and by the media. People in all walks of life are involved as individuals, families and communities. Professional and social groups and health personnel have a major responsibility to mediate between differing interests in society for the pursuit of health.

Health promotion strategies and programmes should be adapted to the local needs and possibilities of individual countries and regions to take into account differing social, cultural and economic systems.

Health promotion action means:

Build healthy public policy

Health promotion goes beyond health care. It puts health on the agenda of policy makers in all sectors and at all levels, directing them to be aware of the health consequences of their decisions and to accept their responsibilities for health.

Health promotion policy combines diverse but complementary approaches including legislation, fiscal measures, taxation and organisational change. It is co-ordinated action that leads to health, income and social policies that foster greater equity. Joint action contributes to ensuring safer and healthier goods and services, healthier public services and cleaner, more enjoyable environments.

Health promotion policy requires the identification of obstacles to the adoption of healthy public policies in non-health sectors, and ways of removing them. The aim must be to make the healthier choice the easier choice for policy makers as well.

Create supportive environments

Our societies are complex and interrelated. Health cannot be separated from other goals. The inextricable links between people and their environment constitutes the basis for a socio-ecological approach to health. The overall guiding principle for the world, nations, regions and communities alike is the need to encourage reciprocal maintenance – to take care of each other, our communities and our natural environment. The conservation of natural resources throughout the world should be emphasised as a global responsibility.

Changing patterns of life, work and leisure have a significant impact on health. Work and leisure should be a source of health for people. The way society organises work should help create a healthy society. Health promotion generates living and working conditions that are safe, stimulating, satisfying and enjoyable.

Systematic assessment of the health impact of a rapidly changing environment – particularly in areas of technology, work, energy production and urbanisation – is essential and must be followed by action to ensure positive benefit to the health of the public. The protection of the natural and built environments and the conservation of natural resources must be addressed in any health promotion strategy.

Strengthen community action

Health promotion works through concrete and effective community action in setting priorities, making decisions, planning strategies and implementing them to achieve better health. At the heart of this process is the empowerment of communities – their ownership and control of their own endeavours and destinies.

Community development draws on existing human and material resources in the community to enhance self-help and social support, and to develop flexible systems for strengthening public participation in and direction of health matters. This requires full and continuous access to information, learning opportunities for health, as well as funding support.

Develop personal skills

Health promotion supports personal and social developments through providing information, education for health, and enhancing life skills. By so doing, it increases the options available to people to exercise more control over their own health and over their environments, and to make choices conducive to health.

Enabling people to learn, throughout life, to prepare themselves for all of its stages and to cope with chronic illness and injuries is essential. This has to be facilitated in school, home, work and community settings. Action is required through educational, professional, commercial and voluntary bodies, and within the institutions themselves.

Reorient health services

The responsibility for health promotion in health services is shared among individuals, community groups, health professionals, health service institutions and governments. They must work together towards a health care system which contributes to the pursuit of health.

The role of the health sector must move increasingly in a health promotion direction, beyond its responsibility for providing clinical and curative services. Health services need to embrace an expanded mandate which is sensitive and respects cultural needs. This mandate should support the needs of individuals and communities for a healthier life, and open channels between the health sector and broader social, political, economic and physical environmental components.

Reorienting health services also requires stronger attention to health research as well as changes in professional education and training. This must lead to a change of attitude and organisation of health services which refocuses on the total needs of the individual as a whole person.

Moving into the future

Health is created and lived by people within the settings of their everyday life; where they learn, work, play and love. Health is created by caring for oneself and others, by being able to take decisions and have control over one's life circumstances, and by ensuring that the society one lives in creates conditions that allow the attainment of health by all its members.

Caring, holism, and ecology are essential issues in developing strategies for health promotion. Therefore, those involved should take as a guiding principle that, in each phase of planning, implementation and evaluation of health promotion activities, women and men should become equal partners.

Commitment to health promotion

The participants in this Conference pledge:

- To move into the arena of healthy public policy, and to advocate a clear political commitment to health and equity in all sectors;
- To counteract the pressures towards harmful products, resource depletion, unhealthy living conditions and environments, and bad nutrition; and to focus attention on public health issues such as pollution, occupational hazards, housing and settlements;
- To respond to the health gap within and between societies, and to tackle the inequities in health produced by the rules and practices of these societies;
- To acknowledge people as their main health resource; to support and enable them to keep themselves, their families and friends healthy through financial and other means, and to accept the community as the essential voice in matters of its health, living conditions and well-being
- To re-orient health services and their resources towards the promotion of health; and to share power with other sectors, other disciplines, and, most importantly, with people themselves;
- To recognise health and its maintenance as a major social investment and challenge; and to address the overall ecological issue of our ways of living.

The Conference urges all concerned to join them in their commitment to a strong public health alliance.

Call for international action

The Conference calls on the World Health Organization and other international organisations to advocate the promotion of health in all appropriate forums and to support countries in setting up strategies and programmes for health promotion.

The Conference is firmly convinced that if people in all walks of life, non-governmental and voluntary organisations, governments, the World Health Organization and all other bodies concerned join forces in introducing strategies for health promotion, in line with the moral and social values that form the basis of this CHARTER, Health For All by the Year 2000 will become a reality.

(The CHARTER was adopted at an International Conference on Health Promotion, 'The Move Towards a New Public Health', 17–21 November 1986, Ottawa, Ontario, Canada.)

(Co-sponsored by the Canadian Public Health Association, Health and Welfare Canada, and the World Health Organization.)

References

Albert M 1993 Capitalism against capitalism. Whurr, London

Aldridge D 1998 Suicide: the tragedy of hopelessness. Jessica Kingsley, London

Allan P, Jolley M 1982 Nursing, midwifery and health visiting, since 1900. Faber & Faber, London

Allsopp J 1996 Health policy and the National Health Service: towards 2000. Longmans, London

Altschul A 1989 Let's have some real change for a change. Annual Mental Health Guest Lecture, Scottish Association for Mental Health, Edinburgh

American Hospital Association (AHA) 1973 A patients's bill of rights (revised 1992). American Hospital Association, Chicago

American Nurses Association 1977 Code for nurses (1950, revised 1976) [Reproduced and discussed in Tait 1977]

Appleby J, Little B, Ranade W, Robinson R, Smit H P 1992 Implementing the reforms: a second national survey of general managers, project paper 7. National Association of Health Authorities and Trusts, Birmingham

Aquinas, St Thomas (1225–1274) Summa theologiae, 2a–2ae.xxiii. 3 ad1; and 2a–2ae. lvii, 1 & 2 [cf. McDermott T 1989 Summa theologiae: a concise translation. Christian Classics, Westminster, MD, part II, ch 11, p 382–398]

Arendt H 1967 The origins of totalitarianism. 3E World Publishing, London

Aristotle (384–322 BC) (Thomson J A K, tr) 1976 Nicomachean ethics. In: The ethics of Aristotle, revised edn. Penguin Books, Harmondsworth

Armstrong D 1983 An outline of sociology as applied to medicine. Wright, Bristol

Ashford D E 1986 The emergence of the welfare states. Blackwells, Oxford

Ashley J 1976 Hospitals, paternalism and the role of the nurse. Teachers' College Press, New York

Audi R (ed) 1995 The Cambridge dictionary of philosophy. Cambridge University Press, Cambridge

Augustine (354–430 AD) (Healey J, tr) 1968 The city of God. Dent, London

Augustine (354–430 AD) Homily on the First Epistle of John, 7, viii [see Clark M (tr) 1984 Augustine of Hippo, selected writings. Paulist Press, New York]

Augustine (354–430 AD) (Pontifex M, tr) 1955 The problem of free choice (de libero arbitrio). Newman Press, Westminster, MD

Ayer A J 1958 Language, truth and logic. Gollancz, London

Bacon R, Eltis W 1976 Britain's economic problem: too few producers. Macmillan, London

Baggott R 1994 Health and health care in Britain. Macmillan, London

Baier A C 1995 Moral prejudices. Harvard University Press, Cambridge, MA

Baker N, Urquhart J 1987 The balance of care for adults with a mental handicap in Scotland. ISD Publications, Edinburgh

Balzer-Riley J, Smith S 1996 Communication in nursing. Mosby, St Louis, MO

Bandman E, Bandman B 1995 Nursing ethics through the life-span, Prentice Hall, Englewood Cliffs, NJ

Baric L 1974 Acquisition of the smoking habit and the model of smokers' careers. Journal of the Institute of Health Education 12(1): 9–18

Baric L 1982 Measuring family competence in the health maintenance and health education of children. World Health Organization, Copenhagen

Barnett L, Abbatt F 1994 District action research and education: resource book for problem-solving in health systems. Macmillan, London

Bayles M D 1989 Professional ethics, 2nd edn. Wadsworth, Belmont, CA

Beardshaw V 1981 Conscientious objectors at work. Social Audit, London, p 2

Beauchamp T L, Bowie N 1997 Ethical theory and business, 5th edn. Prentice Hall, Sydney

Beauchamp T L, Childress J F 1994 Principles of biomedical ethics, 4th edn. Oxford University Press, New York

Beauchamp T, Veatch R 1996 Ethical issues in death and dying. Prentice Hall, New York

Beck L W (tr) 1949 Kant I (1724–1804) Kant's critique of practical reason and other writings in moral philosophy. Chicago University Press, Chicago

Becker H S 1963 Outsiders: studies in the sociology of deviance. Free Press of Glencoe, New York

Benjamin M, Curtis J 1986 Ethics in nursing. Oxford University Press, New York

Benner P 1984 From novice to expert: excellence and power in clinical nursing practice. Addison-Wesley, Menlo Park, CA

Benner P, Wrubel J 1989 The primacy of caring: stress and coping in health and illness. Addison-Wesley, Menlo Park, CA

Bennett A E (ed) 1976 Communication between doctors and patients. Nuffield Provincial Hospitals Trust, London, ch 2

Benson S, Carr P 1994 The care assistant's guide to working with elderly mentally infirm people. Hawker, London

Bentham J (1748–1832) (Burns J A, Hart H L A, eds) 1970 An introduction to the principles of morals and legislation (first published in 1789, revised in 1822). Athlone Press, London.

Berlin I 1969 Four essays on liberty. Oxford University Press, Oxford

Berne E 1966 The games people play. Deutsch, London

Berne E 1973 What do you say after hello? The psychology of human destiny. Bantam Books, New York

Beveridge W 1942 Report on the Committee on Social Insurance and Allied Services. Command paper no. 6404. HMSO, London

Bevis E 1988 New directions for a new age. In: National League for Nursing (ed) Curriculum revolution: mandated for change. National League for Nursing, New York

Bishop A, Scudder J (eds) 1985 Caring, curing, coping: nurse, physician, patient relationships. University of Alabama Press, Alabama

Bok S 1995 Common values. University of Missouri Press, Columbia, MO

Bond J, Bond S 1994 Sociology and health care: an introduction for nurses and other health care professionals, 2nd edn. Churchill Livingstone, Edinburgh

Bonhoeffer D 1955 Ethics. SCM Press, London

Boudreau F, Lambert P 1993 Compulsory community treatment? The collision of views and complexities involved: is it the 'best possible alternative'? Canadian Journal of Mental Health 2(1): 79–96

Bowden P 1997 Caring: gender-sensitive ethics. Routledge, London

Bowlby J 1979 The making and breaking of affectional bonds. Tavistock, London

Boyd K M 1979 The ethics of resource allocation. Edinburgh University Press, Edinburgh

Boyd K M, Callaghan B, Shotter E 1986 Life before death. SPCK, London

Boyd K M, Higgs R, Pinchin A J 1997 The new dictionary of medical ethics. BMJ Publishing, London

Bradley J C, Edinberg M A 1990 Communication in a nursing context. Appleton & Lange, California

Brahams D, Brahams M 1983 The Arthur case – a proposal for legislation. Journal of Medical Ethics 9: 12–15

Branmer L M 1993 The helping relationship, processes and skills. Allyn & Bacon, Boston

Braun J V, Lipson S 1993 Toward a restraint-free environment. Health Professionals' Press, Baltimore, MD

British Association for Counselling 1999 Codes of ethics for counselling and practice. BAC, Rugby

British Association of Social Workers (BASW) 1971 Discussion paper no. 1: confidentiality in social work. BASW, London

British Association of Social Workers (BASW) 1977 The social work task. BASW, Birmingham

British Association of Social Workers 1996 The code of ethics for social workers. BASW, London

British Medical Association (BMA) 1984 Handbook of medical ethics. BMA, London

Broad C D 1930 Five types of ethical theory. Routledge & Kegan Paul, London

Brown J, Kitson A, McKnight T J 1992 Challenges in caring: explorations in nursing and ethics. Chapman & Hall, London

Buchanan A E, Brock D W 1989 Deciding for others: the ethics of surrogate decision-making. Cambridge University Press, Cambridge

Bullough V L, Bullough B 1984 History, trends and politics of nursing. Appleton-Century-Crofts, Norwalk, CT

Burdekin B, Guilfoyle M, Hall D (eds) 1993 Human rights and mental illness, 'Burdekin Report'. Report of the national enquiry into the human rights of people with mental illness. Australian Government Publishing Service, Canberra, ACT

Burnard P, Morrison P 1994 Nursing research in action: developing basic skills. Macmillan, Basingstoke

Burns N, Grove S K 1999 Understanding nursing research. WB Saunders, Philadelphia

Butler Bishop Joseph 1970 Sermons, 'On conscience', iii. In: Roberts T A (ed) Fifteen Sermons preached at the Rolls Chapel. SPCK, London

Campbell A V 1972 Moral dilemmas in medicine. Churchill Livingstone, Edinburgh

Campbell A V 1978 Medicine, health and justice: the problem of priorities. Churchill Livingstone, Edinburgh

Campbell A V 1984a Moderated love: a theology of professional care. SPCK, London

Campbell A V 1984b Moral dilemmas in medicine, 2nd edn. Churchill Livingstone, Edinburgh

Campbell A V 1985 Paid to care. SPCK, London

Campbell A V, Higgs R 1982 In that case. Darton, Longman & Todd, London

Campbell J, Bunting S 1991 Voices and paradigms: perspective on critical and feminist theory in nursing. Advances in Nursing Science 13(3): 1–15

Caplan A H, Callahan D 1981 Ethics in hard times. Hastings Centre Series on Ethics. Hastings on Hudson, USA

Carpenter M 1977 The new managerialism and professionalism in nursing. In: Stacey M, Reid M, Heath C, Dingwall R (eds) Health and the division of labour. Croom Helm, London

Carritt E F 1928 Theory of morals. Oxford University Press, Oxford

Carroll L 1954 Alice's adventures in wonderland, through the looking glass and other writings. Collins, London

Cartwright A, Anderson R 1981 General practice revisited: a second study of patients and their doctors. Tavistock, London

Cartwright A, Smith C 1988 Elderly people, their medicines and their doctors. Routledge, London

Charlesworth M 1993 Bioethics in a liberal society. Cambridge University Press, Cambridge

Chesterton G K 1927 Orthodoxy. John Lane, Bodley Head

Church M 1982 How do they read you? Scottish Health Education Group, Edinburgh

Clare A W, Corney R (eds) 1982 Social work and primary health care. Academic Press, London

Clark B 1978 Whose life is it anyway? Amber Lane Press, Oxford

Clark C C 1986 Wellness nursing: concepts, theory, research and practice. Springer, New York

Clark C L, Asquith S 1985 Social work and social philosophy: a guide for practice. Routledge & Kegan Paul, London, p 84

Clark M (tr) 1984 Augustine of Hippo, selected writings. Paulist Press, New York

Clement G 1996 Care, autonomy and justice: feminism and the ethic of care. Westview Press, Boulder, CO

Cohen J M (tr) 1961 Pascal, Blaise: the pensées. Penguin, Harmondsworth

COHSE 1977 The management of violent or potentially violent patients. Confederation of Health Service Employees, London

Cole A 1993 Whistling in the wind? Nursing Times 89(26): 2

Collison P 1995 The democratic solution. In: Murley Sir R (ed) Patients or customers: are the NHS reforms working? Institute of Economic Affairs, Health and Welfare Unit, London

Copp L A 1981 Care of the ageing. Churchill Livingstone, Edinburgh

Couglan P B 1993 Facing Alzheimer's: family care givers speak. Ballantine, New York

Council of Working Party on Euthanasia 1999 Report on the protection of the human rights and dignity of the terminally ill or dying. Biomedical Ethics 4(1): 4–11

Cousins N 1979 Anatomy of an illness – as perceived by the patient. WW Norton, New York

Coutts L C, Hardy L K 1985 Teaching for health: the nurse as a health educator. Churchill Livingstone, Edinburgh

Cowan M (tr) 1955 Nietzsche F (1844–1900) Beyond good and evil. Henry Regnery, Chicago

Cowen D V 1961 The foundations of freedom. Oxford University Press, Oxford

Creek J 1997 Occupational therapy and mental health. Churchill Livingstone, Edinburgh

Crisp R, Slote M 1997 Virtue ethics. Oxford University Press, Oxford

Crittenden P 1993 Learning to be moral: philosophical thoughts about moral development. Humanities Press, London

Cummings J 1994 Care services and priority setting: the New Zealand experience. Health Policy 29: 41–60

Curtin L, Flaherty M J 1982 Nursing ethics: theories and pragmatics. Prentice Hall, Englewood Cliffs, NJ

D'Arcy E 1961 Conscience and its right to freedom. Sheed & Ward, London

D'Arcy M 1962 The heart and mind of love. Collins, London

d'Entrevres A P 1951 Natural law: an introduction to legal philosophy. Hutchinson, London

Dancy J 1993 Moral reasons. Blackwells, Oxford

Davey B, Popay J 1992 Dilemmas in health care. Open University Press, London

Davies C 1979 Rewriting nursing history. Croom Helm, Beckenham

Davis A J, Aroskar M A 1983 Ethical dilemmas and nursing practice, 2nd edn. Appleton-Century-Crofts, Norwalk, CT

Davis C 1995 Gender and the professional predicament in nursing. Open University Press, Buckingham

de Beauvoir S 1988 The second sex. Picador, London

de Beauvoir S 1991 The ethics of ambiguity. Carol Publishing, New York

DeBono E 1990 I am right – you are wrong. Penguin Books, Harmondsworth

Department of Health (DoH) 1988 Care in the community. HMSO, London

Department of Health (DoH) 1989a Working for patients. HMSO, London

Department of Health (DoH) 1989b Caring for people. Command paper no 849. HMSO, London

Department of Health (DoH) 1991a The health of the nation. HMSO, London

Department of Health (DoH) 1991b The patient's charter. HMSO, London

DHEW 1978 Protection of human subjects of biomedical and behavioral research. Federal Register 43 (53). US Departments of Health, Education and Welfare, Washington, DC

DHH & CS 1993 Communicable diseases intelligence. Department of Health, Housing and Community Services, Australian Government Publication Services, Canberra

DHSS 1976 Prevention and health – everybody's business. HMSO, London

DHSS 1980 Inequalities in health: report of a commission of enquiry into the National Health Service (Chairman: Sir Douglas Black). DHSS, London

DHSS 1983 NHS management inquiry (Griffiths report). HMSO, London

Dingwall R, Rafferty A M, Webster C 1988 An introduction to the social history of nursing. Routledge, London

Dorn N, Nortoft B 1982 Health careers. Institute for the Study of Drug Dependence, London

Downie R S 1971 Roles and values: an introduction to social ethics. Methuen, London

Downie R S, Calman K C 1987 Healthy respect: ethics in health care. Faber, London

Downie R, Tannahill C, Tannahill A 1996 Health promotion: models and values. Oxford University Press, Oxford

Doyle D (ed) 1984 Palliative care: the management of far advanced illness. Croom Helm, London

Doyle D (ed) 1994, Domiciliary palliative care: a handbook for family doctors and community nurses. Oxford University Press, Oxford

Draper P, Popay J 1980 Medical charities, prevention and the media. British Medical Journal 280: 110

Dryden W, Charles-Edwards D, Woolfe R 1989 Handbook of counselling in Britain. Routledge & Kegan Paul, London

Duncan A S, Dunstan G R, Welbourn R B 1981 Dictionary of medical ethics. Darton, Longman & Todd, London (see Declarations of the World Medical Association)

Durham M 1997 Conjuring trick, no magic pill for the NHS. The Observer, 14 December 1997

Durkheim E 1952 Suicide: a study in sociology. Routledge & Kegan Paul, London

Dworkin G 1977 Strikes and the National Health Service. Journal of Medical Ethics 3(2): 75–85

Dworkin R 1977 Taking rights seriously. Harvard University Press, Cambridge, MA

Eadie H A 1975 The helping personality. Contact 49(Summer)

Egan G 1986 The skilled helper, 3rd edn. Brooks/Cole, Monterey, CA

Eggland E T, Heineman D S 1994 Nursing documentation: charting, recording and reporting. J B Lippincott, Philadelphia

Ehrenreich B, English D 1973 Witches, midwives and nurses: a history of women healers. Readers and Writers Cooperative, London

Eide A 1992 Universal declaration of human rights: a commentary. Oxford University Press, Oxford

Eliot T S 1944 Four quartets. Faber & Faber, London

Emmet D 1966 Rules, roles and relations. Macmillan, London

Enthoven A 1986 Reflections on the management of the National Health Service. Nuffield Provincial Hospitals Trust, London

Erwin E 1978 Behavior therapy: scientific, philosophical and moral foundations. Cambridge University Press, Cambridge

Ewles L, Simnett I 1985 Promoting health: a practical guide to health education. Wiley, Chichester

Faden R R, Beauchamp T L 1981 A history and theory of informed consent. Oxford University Press, New York

Fagles R, Knox B (trs) 1982 Sophocles' Antigone. In: Three Theban plays: Antigone, Oedipus the King and Oedipus at Colonus. Allen Lane, London

Faulder C 1985 Whose body is it? The troubled issue of informed consent. Virago, London

Faulkner A 1984 Communication. Churchill Livingstone, Edinburgh

Feifel H (ed) 1977 New meanings of death. McGraw Hill, New York

Feifel H et al 1967 Physicians consider death. Proceedings of the American Psychological Association

Fewell J, Woolfe R 1991 Groupwork skills. Health Education Board for Scotland, Edinburgh

Field D 1984 'We didn't want him to die on his own.' (Nurses' accounts of nursing dying patients.) Journal of Advanced Nursing 9: 59–70

Field D 1989 Nursing the dying. Tavistock, London

Field D, James N 1993 Where and how people die. In: Clarke D (ed) The future for palliative care. Open University Press, Buckingham

Finnis J M 1999 Natural law and natural rights. Clarendon Press, Oxford

Fletcher C 1967 Situation ethics: the new morality. SCM Press, London

Fletcher C M 1971 Communication in medicine. Nuffield Provincial Hospitals Trust, London

Fletcher J 1979a Situation ethics. SCM Press, London

Fletcher J 1979b Humanhood: essays in biomedical ethics. Prometheus Books, New York

Foot P 1967 Theories of ethics. Oxford University Press, Oxford

Frankena W K 1964 Love and principle in Christian ethics. In: Plantinga A (ed) Faith and philosophy. Eerdmans, Grand Rapids, MI

Frankena W K 1973 Ethics, 2nd edn. Prentice Hall, Englewood Cliffs, NJ

Freidson E 1970a Profession of medicine. Dodd Mead, New York

Freidson E 1970b Professional dominance. Dodd Mead, New York

Freidson E 1994 Professionalism reborn: theory, prophecy and policy. Polity Press, Cambridge

French P A 1995 Corporate ethics. Harcourt Brace College Publishers, London

Freund K 1977 The 'right' to strike. Journal of Medical Ethics 3(2): 1977

Fry S 1989a Teaching ethics in nursing curricula: traditional and contemporary models. Nursing Clinics of North America 24(2): 485– 497

Fry S 1989b The role of caring in a theory of nursing ethics. Hypatia 4(2): 88–103

George V, Taylor-Gooby P 1996 European welfare policy: squaring the circle. Macmillan, Basingstoke

Giddens A 1993 Sociology, 2nd edn. Polity Press, London

Gilby T 1964 St Thomas Aquinas – philosophical texts. Oxford University Press, London

Gill R 1985 A textbook of Christian ethics. T & T Clark, Edinburgh

Gilligan C 1977 In a different voice: women's conceptions of self and morality. Harvard Educational Review 47(4): 481–517

Gilligan C 1982 In a different voice: psychological theory and women's development. Harvard University Press, Cambridge, MA

Gillon R 1981 Medical ethics and medical education (editorial). Journal of Medical Education 7: 171–172

Gillon R 1986 Philosophical medical ethics. Wiley, Chichester

Gilmore M, Bruce N, Hunt M 1974 The work of the nursing team in general practice. Council for the Education and Training of Health Visitors, London

Gilson E (Shook L K, tr) 1994 The Christian philosophy of St Thomas Aquinas. Notre Dame University Press, Notre Dame, IN

Glaser B G, Strauss A L 1965 Awareness of dying. Aldine, Chicago

Glazer G 1995 The impact of NHS reforms on patient care: a view from a London teaching hospital. In: Murley Sir R (ed) Patients or customers: are the NHS reforms working? Institute of Economic Affairs, Health and Welfare Unit, London

Glennerster H, Matsaganis M 1992 The English and the Swedish health care reforms. Welfare state discussion paper WSP/79. London School of Economics, London

Glennerster H, Matsaganis M, Owens S 1994 Implementing GP fundholding: wildcard or willing hand? Open University Press, Buckingham

Glover J 1977 Causing death and saving lives. Penguin, Harmondsworth

GNC 1980 Guidelines on health education. General Nursing Council for Scotland, Edinburgh

Goffman E 1968 Asylums: essays on the social situation of mental patients and other inmates. Penguin, Harmondsworth

Goffman E 1969 The presentation of self in everyday life. Penguin, Harmondsworth

Golding P, Middleton S 1981 Images of welfare. Blackwell, Oxford

Goldman J 1982 Inconsistency and institutional review boards. Journal of the American Medical Association 248(2): 197–202

Goodare H, Smith R 1995 The rights of patients in medical research. British Medical Journal 310: 1277–1278

Gough I 1979 The political economy of the welfare state. Macmillan, London

Grace D, Cohen S 1997 Business ethics, 2nd edn. Australian problems and cases. Oxford University Press, Oxford

Grayson S 1993 The ideology of fertility. In: Hetherington P, Maddern P (eds) Sexuality and gender in history, selected essays. Optima Press, Western Australia, ch 16

Green J, Green M 1992 Dealing with death: practices and procedures. Chapman & Hall, London

Gregory T S (ed) 1955 Spinoza B (1632–1677) Ethics. Dent, London

Griffiths R 1983 NHS management inquiry (letter to Secretary of State). HMSO, London

Griffiths R 1988 Community care: agenda for action. HMSO, London

Gross P F 1985 Nursing care in the 1980's and beyond: the challenge to be relevant, ethical and accepted. Australian Nurses Journal 15(1): 46–48

Growe S 1991 Who cares? The crisis in Canadian nursing. McClelland & Stewart, Toronto

Hamberger L K, Burge S K, Graham A V, Costa A J 1997 Violence issues for health care educators and providers. Haworth Maltreatment and Trauma Press, New York

Hamilton W (tr) 1950 Plato (427–347 BC) The Gorgias. Penguin, Harmondsworth

Hare R M 1963 Freedom and reason. Oxford University Press, Oxford

Hare R M 1964 The language of morals. Oxford University Press, Oxford

Hare R M 1981 Moral thinking: its levels, methods and point. Oxford University Press, Oxford

Häring B 1975 Ethics of manipulation: issues in medicine, behaviour control and genetics. Seabury Press, New York

Harris J 1981 Ethical problems in the management of some severely handicapped children. Journal of Medical Ethics 7(3): 114–117

Harrison S, Hunter D J, Pollitt C 1990 The dynamics of British health policy. Unwin Hyman, London

Hawkins J M 1996 Oxford reference dictionary. Clarendon Press, Oxford

Healey J (tr) 1968 Augustine (354–430 AD) The city of God. Dent, London

Health Department of Western Australia 1997 A clinician's guide to the Mental Health Act 1996. HDWA, Perth, Western Australia

Hellman S 1995 The patient and the public good. Nature Medicine 1(5): 400–402

Henderson V 1966 The nature of nursing. Collier Macmillan, London

Hetherington P, Maddern P 1993 Sexuality and gender in history, selected essays. Optima Press, Western Australia

Hill E (tr) & Rotelli J E 1990 Works of St Augustine of Hippo. New City Press, Brooklyn, NY

Hill L, Smith N 1990 Self-care nursing: promotion of health. Appleton-Century-Crofts, Norwalk, CT

Hill T E 1991 Autonomy and self-respect. Cambridge University Press, Cambridge

Hinton J 1979 Comparison of places and policies for terminal care. Lancet 1: 29

HMSO 1976 Prevention and health – everybody's business. HMSO, London

HMSO 1978a Report of enquiry into Normansfield Hospital. Command paper no. 7357. HMSO, London

HMSO 1978b Report of Royal Commission on the National Health Service. HMSO, London

HMSO 1992a Social trends. HMSO, London

HMSO 1992b Annual abstract of statistics. Central Statistical Office, HMSO, London

HMSO 1997a The new NHS: modern, dependable. The Stationery Office, London

HMSO 1997b Designed to care (Scotland). The Stationery Office, Edinburgh

Hobbes T (Tuck R, ed) 1996 Leviathan. Cambridge University Press, Cambridge

Hornblum A H 1997 They were cheap and available: prisoners as research subjects in twentieth century America. British Medical Journal 315: 1437–1441

Horne E M, Cowan T 1992 Effective communication: some nursing perspectives. Wolfe, London

HPSS 1990/91/92 Health and personal social services statistics, for England (1992), Wales (1992) and Northern Ireland (1990/91). HMSO, London

Hudson B 1994 Making sense of markets in health and social care. Business Education Publishers, Sunderland

Hughes E C 1958 Men and their work. Free Press, New York

Hume D (1711–1776) (Selby-Bigge L A, ed) 1978 A treatise of human nature (1738). Oxford University Press, Oxford

Hume D (1711–1776) (Beauchamp T L, ed) 1998 An enquiry concerning the principles of morals (1770). Oxford University Press, Oxford

Illich I 1977 The limits of medicine. Medical nemesis: the expropriation of health. Penguin Books, Harmondsworth

Illsley R, Svensson P G 1984 The health burden of social inequalities. World Health Organization (European Office), Copenhagen

International Confederation of Midwives 1993 International code of ethics for midwives

International Council of Nurses (ICN) 1973 Code for nurses: ethical concepts applied to nursing. ICN, Geneva [This code was adopted in May 1973 in Mexico. It replaces the ICN Code of Ethics, adopted in São Paolo, Brazil, in 1953 and revised in 1965. See International Nursing Review 20(25), 1973]

International Council of Nurses 1983 Statement of nurse's role in safeguarding human rights. ICN, Geneva

ISD 1991 Scottish health statistics. Common Services Agency, Edinburgh

ISD 1997 Scottish health statistics. Common Services Agency, Edinburgh

Jackson M P 1987 Strikes. St Martin's Press, New York

James P 1996 Total quality management – introductory text. Prentice Hall, New York

Jaspers K 1962 The great philosophers: the foundations. Rupert HartDavis, London

Johnson N 1990 Reconstructing the welfare state: a decade of change. Harvester Wheatsheaf, London

Johnson O A (ed) 1994 Ethics: selections from classical and contemporary writers, 7th edn. Harcourt Brace, New York

Johnstone M-J 1991 Ethical issues in nursing research: a broad overview. Faculty of Nursing, RMIT, Bundoora, Victoria

Johnstone M-J 1994 Bioethics: a nursing perspective. WB Saunders/Baillière Tindall, London

Jonsen A R, Toulmin S 1988 The abuse of casuistry: a history of moral reasoning. University of California Press, Berkeley, CA

Jonsen A, Siegler M, Winslade W 1992 Clinical ethics: a practical approach to ethical decisions in clinical medicine. Macmillan, New York

Joss R, Kogan M 1995 Advancing quality: total quality management in the National Health Service. Open University Press, Buckingham

Jowell R, Brook L, Taylor B (eds) 1995 British social attitudes: the twelfth report. Dartmouth, Aldershot

Kagan K, Evans J 1995 Professional and inter-personal skills for nurses. Chapman & Hall, London

Kant I (1724–1804) (Abbot T K, tr) 1909 Critique of practical reason. Everyman, Dent, London

Kemp Smith N (tr) 1973 Kant I (1724–1804) Critique of pure reason. Macmillan, London

Kennedy R, Nicols J C 1995 The effects of the purchaser/provider split on patient care. In: Murley Sir R (ed) Patients or customers: are the NHS reforms working? Institute of Economic Affairs Health and Welfare Unit, London

Keown J 1995 Euthanasia examined: ethical, clinical and legal aspects. Cambridge University Press, Cambridge

Kerridge I, Lowe M, McPhee J 1998 Ethics and law for the health professions. Social Science Press, Katoomba, NSW

Kersbergen Kees van 1995 Social capitalism: a study of Christian democracy and the welfare state. Routledge, London

Ketefian S, Ormond L 1988 Moral reasoning and ethical practice in nursing: an integrative review. National League for Nursing, New York

Kiersky J H, Caste N J 1995 Thinking critically: techniques for logical reasoning. West, New York

Kirby M 1995 Patients' rights – why the Australian courts have rejected Bolam. Journal of Medical Ethics 21: 5–8

Kitson A 1987 An analysis of lay-caring and professional [nursing] caring relationships. International Journal of Nursing Studies 24: 160–161

Kitson A 1993 Nursing art and science. Chapman & Hall, London

Kitson A, Campbell R 1996 The ethical organisation: ethical theory and corporate behaviour. Macmillan Business, Basingstoke

Klein R 1989 The politics of the NHS, 2nd edn. Longman, London

Kohlberg L 1973 Continuities in childhood and adult moral development revisited. In: Boltes P B, Schaie K W (eds) Life span developmental psychology, 2nd edn. Academic Press, New York

Kohlberg L 1976 Moral stages and moralization. In: Lickona T (ed) Moral development and behaviour. Reinhart & Winston, NY

Kohlberg L 1984 Essays on moral development: the psychology of moral development: nature and validity of moral stages. Harper & Row, New York, vol 2

Kohnke M F 1982 Advocacy: risk and reality. CV Mosby, St Louis, MI

Korsgaard C M, Cohen G A 1996 The sources of normativity. Cambridge University Press, Cambridge

Kurtines W, Gewirtz J (eds) 1984 Morality, moral behaviour and moral development. John Wiley, New York

Laing R D, Esterson A 1970 Sanity, madness and the family. Penguin, Harmondsworth

Lamb M 1987 Nursing ethics and nursing education: past perspectives and recent developments. Perspectives in nursing, 1985–1987. National League for Nursing, New York, p 3–21

Laschinger H K, Goldenberg D 1993 Attitudes of practising nurses as predictors of intended care behaviour with persons who are HIV positive. John Wiley, New York

Lawler J 1991 Behind the screens. Churchill Livingstone, Edinburgh

Lebacqz K 1999 A time to die. Biomedical Ethics 4(1): 16

Lemert E M 1951 Social pathology. McGraw Hill, New York

Levinas E 1982 Responsibility for the other. Duquesne University Press, USA

Levinas E 1985 Ethics and infinity. Duquesne University Press, USA

Ley P 1976 Towards better doctor–patient communication. In: Bennett A E (ed) Communication between doctors and patients. Oxford University Press, Oxford

Lindley R 1986 Autonomy. Macmillan, Basingstoke

Lindsay A D (ed) 1951 Hume D (1711–1776) A treatise on human nature. Dent, London, vol 1, p 3

Lindsay A D (ed) 1957 Mill J S (1806–1873) Utilitarianism, liberty, and representative government. Dent, London

Lipson J G, Steiger N J 1996 Self-care nursing in a multi-cultural context, Sage, Thousand Oaks, CA

Lock S 1990 Monitoring research ethics committees. British Medical Journal 300: 61–62

MacAdam A I, Pyke J 1998 Judicial reasoning and doctrine of precedent in Australia. Butterworths, Sydney

McAlpine H 1996 Critical reflection about professional ethical stances: have we lost sight of the major objectives? Journal of Nursing Education 35(3): 119–126

McAlpine H 1998 Ethical reasoning of practising nurses: does ethics education make a difference? Unpublished PhD thesis, Murdoch University, Western Australia

McCall-Smith A 1991 Sexuality and the law. (Occasional Paper) Health Education Board for Scotland, Edinburgh

McCall-Smith S 1977 Royal College of Nursing code of professional conduct (discussion). Journal of Medical Ethics 3(3): 122

McClymont A, Thomas S E, Denham M J 1991 Health visiting and elderly people. Churchill Livingstone, Edinburgh

McCormick R 1974 Proxy consent in the experimental situation. Perspectives in Biology and Medicine 18: 2–20

McCormick R 1976 Experiments in children: sharing in sociality. Hastings Centre Report No. 6: 41–46

McHale J, Tingle J, Cribb A 1995 Law and nursing. Butterworth-Heinemann, Oxford

Macintyre A 1967 A short history of ethics (reprinted 1993). Routledge & Kegan Paul, London

Macintyre A 1981 After virtue, 2nd edn. Notre Dame University Press, Notre Dame, IN

Macintyre A 1988 Whose justice? Whose rationality? Notre Dame University Press, Notre Dame, IN

Macintyre A 1990 Three rival versions of moral enquiry. Notre Dame University Press, Notre Dame, IN

Mackay L 1989 Nursing a problem. Open University Press, Milton Keynes

Mackay L, Soothill K, Melia K 1998 Classic texts in health care. Butterworth-Heinemann, Oxford

McKeown T 1976 The role of medicine. Nuffield Provincial Hospitals Trust, London

McKeown T 1979 The role of medicine: dream, mirage or nemesis. Blackwell, Oxford

McNeill P M 1993 The ethics and politics of human experimentation. Cambridge University Press, Cambridge

McNeill P M, Berglund C A, Webster I W 1990 Reviewing the reviewers: a survey of institutional ethics committees in Australia. Medical Journal of Australia 152: 289–296

McNeill P M, Berglund C A, Webster I W 1994 How much influence do various members have within research ethics committees? Cambridge Quarterly of Health Care Ethics 3: 522–532

Maggs C 1987 Nursing history: the state of the art. Croom Helm, London

Maritain J 1943 The rights of man and natural law. C Scribner's Sons, New York

Maritain J 1963 (reprinted 1994) Moral philosophy. Bles, London

Matthies B K, Kreutzer J S, West D D 1997 The behaviour management handbook. Therapy Skill Builders, San Antonio, TX

May W 1975 Code, covenant, contract or philanthropy. Hastings Center Report No. 5

May W 1983 The physician's covenant. Westminster, Philadelphia

Mays N 1991 Origins and development of the National Health Service. In: Scambler G (ed) Sociology as applied to medicine. Baillière Tindall, London

Mayston 1969 Report of the working party on management structure of the local authority nursing services (Mayston Report). HMSO, London

Mead G H 1934 Mind, self and society. University of Chicago Press, Chicago

Mears P 1994 Health care teams: building continuous quality improvement. St Lucie Press, Delroy Beach, FL

Mele A R 1995 Autonomous agents: from self-control to autonomy. Oxford University Press, New York

Melia K M 1981 Student nurses' accounts of their work and training: a qualitative analysis. Unpublished PhD thesis, University of Edinburgh

Melia K M 1983 1. Students' views of nursing, 2. Just passing through. Nursing Times May 18: 26–27

Melia K M 1984 Student nurses' construction of occupational socialisation. Sociology of Health and Illness 6(2): 132–151

Melia K M 1987 Learning and working: the occupational socialisation of nurses. Tavistock, London

Melia K M 1989 Everyday nursing ethics. Macmillan Education, Basingstoke

Melia K M 1994 The task of nursing ethics. Journal of Medical Ethics 20(4): 7–11

Mill J S (1806–1873) (Acton H B, ed) 1972 Utilitarianism, liberty, and representative government (1861). Everyman, Dent, London

Mishra R 1984 The welfare state in crisis: social thought and social change. St Martin's Press, New York

Mishra R 1990 The welfare state in capitalist society. Harvester Wheatsheaf, London

Mitchell B 1970 Morality religious and secular. Oxford University Press, Oxford

Montefiore A 1958 A modern introduction to moral philosophy. Routledge & Kegan Paul, London

Mooney G 1992 Economics, medicine and health, 2nd edn. Harvester Wheatsheaf, Hampshire

Moore G E 1962 Principia ethica, revised edn. Cambridge University Press, Cambridge

Moore G E 1966 Ethics, 2nd edn. Oxford University Press, Oxford

Morris R et al (eds) 1971 Profession of social work: code of ethics. In: Encyclopaedia of social work, 16th issue. National Association of Social Workers, New York

Munro A 1996 Contracting, health care and the internal market. Paper given in the Department of Social Policy, University of Edinburgh, 28/10/1996

Murley R (ed) 1995 Patients or customers: are the NHS reforms working? Institute of Economic Affairs, Health and Welfare Unit, London

Murray R B, Zilner J P 1989 Nursing concepts for health promotion. Prentice Hall, London

National Health and Medical Research Council (Australia) 1995 Report on the functioning of research ethics committees. AusInfo, GPO Box 1920, Canberra, ACT 2601

National Health and Medical Research Council (Australia) 1999 National statement on ethical conduct in research involving humans. Cat. No. 9818566. AusInfo, GPO Box 1920, Canberra, ACT 2601

Nelson D M 1992 The priority of prudence: virtue and natural law. Pennsylvania State University, University Park, PA

Nietzsche F (1844–1900) (Cowan M, tr) 1955 Beyond good and evil. Henry Regnery, Chicago

Nolan Committee 1995 Reports on standards in public life, vols 1–3: no 1. On standards (1995 CM2850–I); no. 2. Local government (1996 CM3702–I0); and no 3. Local public spending bodies (1997 CM3270–I). HMSO, London

Norton D 1975 Research and the problem of pressure sores. Nursing Times 140: 65–67

Nowell Smith P 1957 Ethics. Blackwell, Oxford

Nygren A (Watson P S, tr) 1953 Agape and Eros. Westminster Press, Philadelphia

O'Keeffe T M 1984 Suicide and self-starvation. Philosophy 59: 349–363

OECD 1987 Financing and delivery of health care, a comparative study of OECD countries. Organization for Economic Cooperation and Development, Paris

Olsson S E 1990 Social policy and welfare state in Sweden. Arkiv förlag, Lund, Sweden

OPCS 1991 OPCS monitor. Office of Population Censuses and Surveys, HMSO, London

Pappworth M H 1967 Human guinea pigs: experimentation in man. Routledge & Kegan Paul, London

Parker J H 1977 Of professional conduct. (Reprinted from: Thomas Percival 1849 Medical ethics, 3rd edn. Oxford, p 27–68.) In: Reiser S J, Dyck A, Curran W J (eds) Ethics in medicine. MIT Press, Cambridge, MA, p 18–25

Parkes C M 1966 The patient's right to know the truth. Proceedings of the Royal Society of Medicine 66: 536

Parkes C M, Markus A 1998 Coping with loss: helping patients and their families. BMJ Books, London

Parsons T 1970 The social system. Routledge & Kegan Paul, London

Pascal B (Cohen J M, tr) 1961 The pensées. Penguin Books, Harmondsworth

Paton H J (tr) 1969 Kant I (1724–1804) The moral law: Kant's Groundwork to the metaphysic of morals. Hutchinson, London

Pender N 1996 Health promotion in nursing practice. Prentice Hall International, London

Peterson C, Maier S F, Seligman M E P 1993 Learned helplessness: a theory for the age of personal control. Oxford University Press, New York

Phillips C (ed) 1988 Logic in medicine. BMJ Publications, London

Phillips S S, Benner P 1996 The crisis of care: affirming and restoring caring practices in the helping professions. Georgetown University Press, Washington, DC

Pieper J 1959 Prudence: the first cardinal virtue. Faber, London

Plato (427–347 BC) (Hamilton W 1950, tr) The Gorgias. Penguin, Harmondsworth

Plato (427–347 BC) (Rouse W H D, tr; Warmington E H, Rouse P G, eds) 1984 Great dialogues of Plato. Mentor, New York

Pontifex M (tr) 1955 Augustine (354–430 AD) The problem of free choice (de libero arbitrio). Newman Press, Westminster, MD

Pope John XXIII 1963 Pacem in terris (Human rights and world peace). Holy See, Vatican City

Porritt L 1990 Interaction strategies: an introduction for health professionals. Churchill Livingstone, Edinburgh

Porter R 1997 The greatest benefit to mankind – a medical history of humanity from antiquity to the present. Harper Collins, London

Preston N (ed) 1994 Ethics for the public sector – education and training. The Federation Press, Sydney

Pritchard P, Pritchard J 1992 Developing teamwork in primary health care: a practical workbook. Oxford University Press, London

Pyne R 1998 Professional discipline in nursing, midwifery and health visiting – including a treatise on professional regulation. Blackwell, Oxford

Rachels J 1993 The elements of moral philosophy, 2nd edn. McGraw-Hill, New York

Rafferty A M 1996 The politics of nursing knowledge. Routledge, London

Ramsey P 1970 The patient as person. Yale University Press, New Haven, CT

Ramsey P 1976 The enforcement of morals: non-therapeutic research on children. Hastings Centre Report no. 6: 29–31

Ramsey P 1977 Children as research subjects: a reply. Hastings Centre Report No. 7: 40–42

Ramsey P 1978 Ethics at the edges of life. Yale University Press, New Haven

Ramsey P 1980 Basic Christian ethics. University of Chicago Press, Chicago

Ramsey P 1983 Deeds and rules in Christian ethics. University of America Press, New York

Ranade W 1994 A future for the NHS? Health care in the 1990s. Longman, London

Raphael D D 1980 Moral philosophy. Oxford University Press, Oxford

Rathbone-McCuan E, Fabian D R 1992 Self-neglecting elders: a clinical dilemma. Auburn House, New York

Rawls J 1971 A theory of justice. Harvard University Press, Cambridge, MA

RCN 1977 Code of professional conduct: a discussion document. Journal of Medical Ethics 3(3): 121

Reed J, Lomas G 1984 Psychiatric services in the community: developments and innovations. Croom Helm, London, ch 4

Reuter L 1999 Euthanasia and subjectivity: ethical reflections on the post-modern concept of personhood. Biomedical Ethics 4(1): 14–16

Reverby S 1987 Ordered to care: the dilemma of American nursing, 1850–1945. Cambridge University Press, Cambridge

Robb I H 1900 Nursing ethics. Cleveland, OH

Robertson A 1996 The internal market reform of the British NHS. The Italian National Research Council (CNR) conference, Rome, 16– 17 December 1996 (Proceedings to be published: Health service reforms in Europe: international comparisons.) Meanwhile an abridged version was published in 1998, as: Robertson A 1998 Markets, planning and the interests of the patient: an evaluation of the British health reform and its implications for Italy. Sociologica e Professione 31–32: 56–77

Robertson A 1997 Welfare: the European dimension'. In: Morton A R (ed) The future of welfare. University of Edinburgh Centre for Theology and Public Issues, Edinburgh

Robertson A, Thompson I E, Porter M 1992 Social policy and administration. Keele University, Keele, Staffordshire

Robertson A, Gilloran A, McGlew T, McKee K, McKinley A, Wright D 1995 Nurses' job satisfaction and the quality of care received by patients in psychogeriatric wards. International Journal of Geriatric Psychiatry 10: 575–584

Robinson R, LeGrande J 1995 Contracting and the purchaser/provider split. In: Saltman R B, Von Otter C (eds) Implementing planned markets in health care. Open University Press, Buckingham

Robinson V 1946 White caps. Lippincott, New York

Roe M 1995 Working together to improve health: a team handbook. Queensland Primary Health Care Reference Centre, Herston, Queensland

Rogers C 1961 On becoming a person. Constable, London

Rokeach M 1976 Beliefs, attitudes and values: a theory of organisation and change. Jossey-Bass, San Francisco

Roper N, Logan W, Tierney A 1981 Learning to use the nursing process. Churchill Livingstone, Edinburgh

Rosenberg W, Donald A 1995 Evidence based medicine: an approach to clinical problem solving. British Medical Journal 310: 1122– 1126

Ross T 1981 Thought control. Nursing Mirror, April 23(see also other articles on psychiatric ethics in the same series)

Ross W D 1930 The right and the good. Oxford University Press, Oxford

Ross W D 1969 Kant's ethical theory. Oxford University Press, Oxford

Rouse W D (ed, tr) 1984 Plato (429–347 BC) Great dialogues of Plato (revised edn). Mentor Books, New York

Rousseau J-J (Cole G D H, tr) 1973 Social contract and discourses (revised by Brumfitt J H, Hall J C). Dent, London

Royal College of Nursing (RCN) 1977a Code of ethics: a discussion document. RCN, London

Royal College of Nursing (RCN) 1977b Ethics related to research in nursing. RCN, London

Royal College of Nursing 1979 Code of professional conduct: discussion document. RCN, London

Royal College of Psychiatrists 1977 Guidelines on the care and treatment of mentally disturbed offenders. British Journal of Psychiatry Bulletin, April

Ruddick S 1989 Maternal thinking: towards a politics of peace. Beacon Press, Boston

Rumbold G 1993 Ethics in nursing practice, 2nd edn. Baillière Tindall, London

Salmon 1966 Report of the committee on senior nursing staff structure (Salmon report). HMSO, London

Saltman R B, von Otter C V 1995 Balancing social and economic responsibility. In: Saltman R B, von Otter C V (eds) Implementing planned markets in health care: balancing social and economic responsibility. Open University Press, Buckingham

Sartre J-P 1948 (Mairet P, tr) Existentialism and humanism. Methuen, London

Sartre J-P 1956 No exit and three other plays. Vintage Books, London

Sartre J-P 1957, 1969, 1973 Being and nothingness. Methuen, London

Scull A 1992 Museums of madness. St Martin's Press, New York

Seedhouse D 1986 Health – the foundations for achievement. Wiley, Chichester

Seligman M E P 1975 Helplessness: on depression, development and death. Scribners, New York

Shaw B 1994 The ragged edge: the disability experience from the first fifteen years of the disability rag. The Avocado Press, Louisville, KY

SHHD 1980 Scottish health authorities' priorities for the eighties (SHAPE report). HMSO, Edinburgh

SHHD 1990 Scottish health authorities revised priorities for the eighties and nineties (SHARPEN report). HMSO, Edinburgh

Sidell M 1997 Debates and dilemmas in promoting health: a reader. Macmillan (with The Open University), Basingstoke, England

Simon S B, Howe L W, Kirchenbaum H 1995 Values clarification. Warner Books, New York

Smart J J C, Williams B 1973 Utilitarianism for and against. Cambridge University Press, Cambridge

Smee C H 1995 Self-governing trusts and GP fundholders: the British Experience. In: Saltman R B, von Otter C V (eds) Implementing planned markets in health care: balancing social and economic responsibility. Open University Press, Buckingham

Smith R 1996 GPs – fundholders or commissioners? In: Bayley H, Jewell T (eds) Health crisis – what crisis? Fabian Society (in conjunction with the Socialist Health Association), London

Smithson M, Amato P R, Pearce P 1983 Dimensions of helping behaviour. Pergamon Press, New York

Solomon R C 1994 Above the bottom line, 2nd edn. Harcourt Brace, New York

Sommers T, Shields L 1987 Women take care: the consequences of care-giving in today's society. Triad, Gainsville, FL

Sophocles (496–406 BC) (Fagles R, Knox B, tr) 1982 Antigone. In: Three Theban plays: Antigone, Oedipus the King and Oedipus at Colonus. Allen Lane, London

Spinoza B de (1632–1677) (Gregory T S, ed) 1955 Ethics. Dent, London

Stacey M, Homans H 1978 The sociology of health and illness: its present state, future prospects and potential for health research. Sociology 12(2): 281–307

Stanley F 1992 New health boss says IVF a waste. The West Australian, 22 July 1992

Staunton P, Whyburn B 1997 Nursing and the law, 4th edn. Harcourt Brace, New York

Stebbing L S 1950 Modern introduction to logic. Methuen, London

Steele S M, Harmon V M 1983 Values clarification in nursing, 2nd edn. Appleton-Century-Crofts, Norwalk, CT.

Stevens E 1980 Making moral decisions. Paulist Press, New York

Stevenson J, Tripp-Reimer T (eds) 1990 Knowledge about care and caring: state of the art and future developments. American Academy of Nursing, Kansas City, MO

Stinson R, Stinson P 1981 On the death of a baby. Journal of Medical Ethics 7(1): 5–18

Strong P, Robinson J 1990 The NHS under new management. Open University Press, Milton Keynes

Stuart H F (tr) 1950 Pascal B (1623–1662) Pensées. Routledge, London, IV, p 227

Szasz T 1974 The myth of mental illness. Harper & Row, New York

Szasz T 1987 Insanity: the idea and its consequences. Wiley, New York

Tait B L 1977 The nurse's dilemma: ethical considerations in nursing practice. International Council of Nurses, Geneva

Talmon J L 1966 The origins of totalitarian democracy. Mercury Books, London

Taylor C 1992 Sources of the self – the making of modern identity. Cambridge University Press, Cambridge

Taylor-Gooby P 1985 Public opinion, ideology and state welfare. Routledge & Kegan Paul, London

Taylor-Gooby P 1986 Privatisation, power and the welfare state. Sociology 20: 228–246

Thomas M 1990 Final report: development and improvement of primary health care teams. Centre for Medical Education, Dundee University Medical School, Dundee

Thompson A 1993 Caring about carers. Research report for the West Australian Council of Social Service. Submitted to the WA Health Department in 1993

Thompson I E 1976 Suicide and philosophy. Contact 54(3): 9–23

Thompson I 1979a Dilemmas of dying – a study in the ethics of terminal care. Edinburgh University Press, Edinburgh

Thompson I E 1979b The nature of confidentiality. Journal of Medical Ethics 5(2): 57–64

Thompson I E 1980 Teaching medical ethics – a reply to Arbuthnot. Journal of Medical Ethics 4

Thompson I E 1984 Ethical issues in palliative care. In: Doyle D (ed) Palliative care: the management of far advanced illness. Croom Helm, London, ch 22

Thompson I E 1987a Personal rights and public policy: dilemmas in health education and prevention. In: Proceedings of the Twelfth World Conference on Health Education. International Union for Health Education, Health Education Bureau, Dublin

Thompson I E 1987b Fundamental ethical principles in health care. British Medical Journal 295: 1461–1465 [Reproduced in Phillips C (ed) Logic in medicine. BMJ Publications, London]

Thompson I E, Harries M 1997 Putting ethics to work. Public Sector Standards Commission, Perth, WA

Thompson J, Thompson H 1985 Bioethical decision-making for nurses. Appleton-Century-Crofts, Norwalk, CT

Thomson D 1991 Selfish generations? The ageing of New Zealand's welfare state. Bridget Williams Books, Wellington

Thomson D 1992 Welfare states and the problem of the common. CIS Occasional Papers 43, Social Research Programme, Centre for Independent Studies, Australia

Thomson J A K (tr) 1976 Aristotle (384–322 BC) Nicomachean ethics. In: The ethics of Aristotle, revised edn. Penguin Books, Harmondsworth, bks 2, 3, 4

Tice C J, Perkins K 1996 Mental health issues and ageing: building on the strengths of older persons. Brookes/Cole, Pacific Grove, CA

Tillich P 1952 The courage to be. Yale University Press, New Haven, CT

Tillich P 1954 Love, power and justice. Oxford University Press, Oxford

Tingle J, Cribb A 1995 Nursing law and ethics. Blackwell Scientific, Oxford

Tones K, Telford S, Keeley-Robinson Y 1994 Health education: efficiency, effectiveness and equity. Chapman & Hall, London

Toulmin S 1957 Metaphysical beliefs. Contemporary Scientific Mythology. SCM, London, Pt 1

Toulmin S 1958 The place of reason in ethics. Cambridge University Press, Cambridge

Toulmin S 1981 The tyranny of principles. Hastings Center Report 11(6): 31–39

Toulmin S 1986 The place of reason in ethics (reprint). University of Chicago Press, Chicago

Townsend P, Davidson N 1982 Inequalities in health: the Black report. Penguin, Harmondsworth

Tschudin V 1986 Ethics in nursing: the caring relationship. Heinemann Nursing, London

UK Hansard 1947 National Health Service Act 1947. Hansard, London

UKCC 1984a Guidelines on confidentiality. UKCC, London

UKCC 1984b Code of professional conduct for the nurse, midwife and health visitor. UKCC, London

UKCC 1987 Advisory papers: confidentiality – an elaboration of Clause 9 of the 2nd edition of the Code. UKCC London

UKCC 1989 Advisory papers: exercising accountability. UKCC, London.

UKCC 1992 Code of professional conduct for the nurse, midwife and health visitor, 3rd edn. UKCC, London

UKCC 1993 Post registration education and practice project. UKCC, London

UNISON 1997 Violence at work: a guide to risk prevention for Unison branches and safety representatives. UNISON, London

United Nations Organization (UNO) 1947 United Nations Declaration of Human Rights. United Nations Organization, New York (reprinted in: Campbell A V 1978 Medicine, health and justice. Churchill Livingstone, Edinburgh)

United Nations Organisation (UNO) 1993 United Nations development programme. Human development report 1993. Oxford University Press, Oxford

Veatch R M 1977 Case studies in medical ethics. Harvard University Press, London, p 351–356

Veatch R 1981 A theory of medical ethics. Basic Books, New York

Waldron J (ed) 1984 Theories of rights. Oxford University Press, Oxford

Walsh P 1982 Why I am opposing the doctors (interview by Cherrill Hicks). Nursing Times Sept 22: 1579–1580

Watson D 1985 A code of ethics for social work: the second step. Routledge & Kegan Paul, London

Webb P 1997 Health promotion and patient education: a professional's guide. Stanley Thornes, Cheltenham

Whincup M 1982 The duties of a health visitor. Nursing Times 77(13): 567–568 (Legal issues are often intrinsically bound up with ethical ones. Two useful references in this area are: Young A P 1961 Legal problems in nursing practice. Harper & Row, London; Pyne R H 1981 Professional discipline in nursing – theory and practice. Blackwell, Oxford)

White R 1970 Social change and the development of nursing. Kimpton, London

White R 1985 Political issues in nursing. Wiley, Chichester, vols 1 and 2

Whitehead M 1987 The health divide. Health Education Council, London

Whittaker E, Olesen V 1964 The faces of Florence Nightingale: functions of the heroic legend in an occupational subculture. Human Organisation 23: 123–130

WHO 1947 Constitution of the World Health Organization. United Nations Organisation, New York

WHO 1978 Primary health care. Report of international conference held at Alma Ata, USSR. World Health Organization, Geneva

WHO 1979 Primary health care in Europe. Euro reports on studies no. 14. World Health Organization, Copenhagen

WHO 1981 Regional programme in health education and life styles (31st Session of Regional Committee for Europe), EUR/RC31/10. World Health Organization, Copenhagen

WHO 1984 Discussion document on health promotion: concepts and principles. World Health Organization, Copenhagen

WHO 1985 Targets for health for all. World Health Organization, Geneva

WHO 1986 The Ottawa charter. World Health Organization, Geneva

WHO 1990/91 World health statistics annual. World Health Organization, Geneva

WHO 1992 International classification of diseases, 10th revision. World Health Organization, Geneva, section F

WHO 1999a World health report. World Health Organization, Geneva

WHO 1999b Health for all in the 21st century. World Health Organization, Geneva

WHO 1999c ASD report on the global HIV/AIDS epidemic. World Health Organization, Geneva

Wicks M 1987 A future for all. Penguin, Harmondsworth

Wild J 1953 Plato's modern enemies and the theory of natural law. University of Chicago Press, Chicago

Wilding P 1982 Professional power and social welfare. Routledge & Kegan Paul, London

Wilkinson R 1996 Unhealthy societies: the affliction of inequalities. Routledge, London

Wilson M 1976 Health is for people. Darton Longman & Todd, London

Windt P Y, Appleby P C, Battin M P, Francis L P, Landesman B M 1989 Ethical issues in the professions. Prentice Hall, Englewood Cliffs, NJ

Wittgenstein L (Anscombe G E M, tr) 1958 Philosophical investigations. Blackwells, Oxford

Wittgenstein L 1971 Tractatus logico-philosophicus (new edition in English and German). Routledge & Kegan Paul, London

Woozley A D 1981 Law and the legislation of morality. In: Caplan A H, Callahan D (eds) Ethics in hard times. Hastings Center Series on Ethics, Hastings on Hudson, USA

World Bank 1993 Investing in health – 1993 world development report. Oxford University Press, Oxford

World Medical Association 1964 Declaration of Helsinki (as amended at 48th General Assembly 1996). WMA Secretariat, 28 Avenue des Alpes – B.P. 63, F-01212, Ferney-Voltaire, Cedex

Yovich J, Grudzinskas G 1990 The management of infertility – a manual of gamete handling procedures. Heinemann Medical, London

Glossary of ethical terms

Accountability
Having to account for your actions to someone else in a position of authority over you, or public accountability before the courts.

Act utilitarianism
Moral theory that would justify individual acts by whether they increase your pleasure or reduce the risk of pain. [Cf: Rule utilitarianism.]

Act deontology
Moral theory that justifies individual acts by whether they are done in accordance with your duty [Greek *deon*], or based on fundamental principles. [Cf: Rule deontology.]

Action theory
A philosophical approach which analyses the common features of human acts, that is, conscious, voluntary and intentional acts, and distinguishes these from automatic or reflexive behaviour.

Algorithm
A process or rule for calculation, or rule to be followed in decision making.

Altruism
A principle for action based on unselfish regard for other people.

Attitudes
Attitudes are generally 'inherited' dispositions or ways of regarding or reacting to other people, groups, things or ideas. However they may become 'ingrained' as internalised prejudices or opinions about other people both inside and outside our own group, or towards the external world. Attitudes can include cognitive, affective and behavioural components learned from parents, one's peer group or culture, e.g. racism, sexism, ageism.

Autonomy
Literally, to be a law unto oneself [Cf: Greek *autos* = self, and *nomos* = law], but while 'being a law unto oneself' usually has derogatory connotations of lawlessness, it was introduced by Kant to emphasise that the responsible moral agent must internalise and make the moral law their own, and not merely act from some duty imposed on them by authority. [Cf: Heteronomy.]

Beliefs
A belief is a personal judgement for which one makes a truth-claim, and which one should be prepared to defend – by producing sound reasons or evidence. While attitudes are generally acquired from others, beliefs comprise the sub-set of attitudes for which we personally make truth claims. To say that we believe something to be true does not mean that we know for certain that it is true, so we do not give beliefs unconditional assent.

Bench-marking
An approach to management and strategic planning which involves setting base-line criteria against which to measure progress.

Beneficence
The principle that we should do good to others [Latin: *beneficio*] rather than harm [Latin *maleficio*], means responsible care or having a duty of care.

Bill of Rights
A statement of human rights claimed to be universally applicable to human beings in virtue of sharing the same 'human nature', however defined.

Binary system
A system of thought or logic that allows two and only two values, e.g: true/false, right/wrong, and does not admit of degrees of comparison.

Bourgeoisie
Term used to describe the new commercial class of upwardly mobile townspeople who, from the 16th century onwards, played an increasing part in the politics of Europe, a term also used by Karl Marx to describe the educated middle class from which the capitalist entrepreneurs emerged in opposition to the aristocracy and working class labourers.

Business ethic
An approach to trade and commercial practice based on a claimed right to seek one's own commercial advantage through free competition and the private

accumulation of wealth, based on faith in a self-regulating free market.

Capping liability
Limit imposed by statute on auditors' liability to third parties for negligent acts or mis-statements.

Caring ethic
An individualistic approach based on responsibility for others and the exercise of protective beneficence in a caring role towards vulnerable people.

Deontological theory
A general approach to the justification of ethical behaviour, in which priority is given to fundamental principles, rights and duties. [Greek *deon* = duty.]

Determinism
The theory that all our actions are determined by unexceptionable causal laws and that these laws of nature constrain our actions to such a degree that they prevent the possibility of free choice or action. [Cf: Freewill.]

Dilemma
In general a situation in which a difficult choice has to be made between two equally attractive or undesirable options. In ethics, a moral dilemma is an apparent or actually irresolvable clash of competing principles or duties. However, genuine or serious dilemmas are rare and most situations which present as dilemmas can be reframed as problems amenable to treatment by problem-solving methods. To describe all moral quandaries as dilemmas often represents an unwillingness to accept responsibility for making decisions.

Duties/obligations
What one is bound to do to fulfil one's contractual commitments to clients or one's employer, or what one is required to do by virtue of one's function, for example, to exercise due authority as a parent, leader, manager, etc. Duties usually correlate with the rights or entitlements of others and may be either moral or legal duties, and may or may not be enforceable.

Economic rationalism
Is the term used in Australia for the type of neo-conservative economic theory which claims to make value-neutral economic decisions, based on measurable criteria of effectiveness and efficiency, profitability and cost reduction.

Effectiveness
A measure of the impact of a policy in achieving long-term strategic goals.

Efficiency
A measure of productivity by examining operational systems and processes.

Emotivism
The theory that a moral judgement is nothing more than an expression of a person's feelings of approval or disapproval of a another's actions, sometimes called the "Boo- Hurrah theory of value".

Empiricism
The theory that all knowledge is derived from experience, or more specifically from sense-experience, scientific observation and experiment.

Enlightenment [The]
The period of the 18th and early 19th Centuries in European history in which emphasis on reason and scientific method had a great influence on culture.

Epicureanism
The philosophy of life based on the pursuit of pleasure, where the aim is to minimise pain and achieve a positive balance of pleasure over pain by self-control and avoiding excess of any kind. [Cf: Hedonism.]

Ethics
In general, ethics, from the Greek *ethos*, means the spirit of a community. It refers to the formal cooperative endeavour of a moral community to define its values, the necessary conditions, practical requirements, and protective rules which will ensure its well-being and the flourishing of its members. 'An ethic' refers to the 'belief-and-value system' of any moral community, or to the formal code of practice of a corporate body, or profession. [Cf: Ideology.]

'Ethics' [applied]
Skill in applied ethics means being able to act responsibly, appropriately and effectively in various situations, and it also means being able to provide a clear, coherent and reasoned justification for one's decisions and actions, with reference to commonly accepted standards. This requires the following skills:

● knowledge of the basic principles which express our fundamental values and from which we derive practical moral rules

● competence in the practical problem-solving and the decision- making skills required for dealing with moral problems

● discretion in formulating sound ethical policies and choosing relevant decision procedures for use in different types of situations.

- sound habits and stable dispositions [competencies] to ensure that one acts effectively as a responsible moral agent.

Etiquette/social mores

These terms refer to the traditions or social customs that define one's social comportment or acceptable ways of relating to others, e.g. rules of dress; manners; culture-specific practices in a society, sect, club or group; court ceremonial and procedure; business and professional courtesies. All social groups have such rules, whether written down or simply taken for granted, and modern professional groups and business corporations are no exception. [Cf: French *tiquette* = ticket of entry, and Latin *mores* = manners or fashion.]

Eudaimonism

Eudaimonism refers to a type of philosophy in which the pursuit of happiness, rather than mere pleasure, is the highest goal [Cf: Greek *eudaimonia* = happiness or well- being]. Aristotle's ethics is called teleological eudaimonism because he believed all things, and especially living things, have a built-in tendency, or drive, to fulfil their potentialities, which, in the case of human beings, is striving for happiness, well-being or fulfilment.

Felicific calculus

Literally, a calculus for measuring the degree of happiness produced by an action or policy. A concept introduced by Bentham in his version of utilitarianism – sometimes referred to as psychological hedonism because it is concerned with attainment of sustained feelings of pleasure. Attempts by modern economists to measure the 'quality of life' owe something to Bentham.

Fiduciary duties

A protective duty of care owed to a client by someone in a consulting role as a result of a person entrusting themselves, their affairs or their secrets to you. [From the Latin *fiducia* = trust.]

Force-field analysis

Method for clarifying the forces that are operating on a situation or giving rise to a problem, by systematically examining four related fields: the present reality, the hoped for ideal, forces resistant to change and forces promoting change. The object is to identify and prioritise those resistant forces that need to be addressed and the supportive forces that should be exploited to achieve desired change.

Freewill

The belief that despite the influences on us of heredity and environment, human beings have the capacity for free choice or self-determinism, because we have the ability to gain insight into the operation of causal laws, and therefore can direct the course of events by becoming causes ourselves.

Fundamentalism

Strict maintenance of the letter of the law of traditional religious beliefs, often associated with the belief in the infallibility of religious authority or the authority of sacred Scriptures. In ethics, fundamentalism is associated with unquestioning acceptance of traditional systems of moral rules.

Golden Rule

Variously expressed in different religious and cultural traditions around the world, but generally expressed as 'Do to others as you would wish that they should do to you' or in negative and stronger terms as 'Never do to others what you would not wish them to do to you in similar circumstances'.

Ground rules

The foundational rules [or constitution] of a group, sports club, society or moral community, which are agreed to and observed by members.

Hedonism

A philosophy in which the pursuit of pleasure [and avoidance of pain] are the primary objectives. [Cf: Greek *hedone* = pleasure.]

Heteronomy

Submission to the rule of an externally imposed authority, or to laws imposed by some outside power. [Cf: Greek *hetero* = alien or other, and *nomos* = law.]

Ideologue

Proponent of some ideology.

Ideology

A comprehensive world-view, framework of meaning, or belief-and-value system that enables people to organise, make sense of, and change their world, both social and physical.

in loco parentis

Responsibility to act on behalf of an [absent] parent.

Inalienable right

A right claimed to be intrinsic to one's nature as a human being and therefore not able to be removed [though it may be subject to restriction by others].

Individualism

Belief that individual rights should not be restricted in any way, and which correspondingly underplays the importance of society and societal duties.

Innate knowledge
Knowledge claimed to be in born in us and accessible by either introspection or direct intuition. Some advocates of deontology claim we can directly intuit our rational duty, because the notion is innate in rational beings.

Integrity
A virtue that implies sound character or the wholeness of the moral person, combining consistency, reliability, honesty and fairness. [Cf Latin *integer* = whole, undivided, uncontaminated.]

Intellectual virtues
Traditionally, according to Aristotle, these comprise theoretical and practical knowledge [of a discipline], acquired skill and practical expertise, judgement, intelligence, self-insight, resourcefulness, persistence and wisdom.

Intentional acts
Purposeful actions that have a clear goal or objective.

Intentionality
The characteristic of all conscious acts, namely that they refer to [intend] some object independent of consciousness – that 'object' may be some thing or person or an 'object' in the sense of a goal or objective.

Intuitionism
The theory that we can achieve knowledge [particularly of moral truths] by direct inspection of our own minds [or consciences].

Liberalism
Belief in achievement of the autonomy of the individual as the ultimate objective of moral and political action, alternatively in the economic sphere it refers to the *laissez faire* doctrine of unrestricted free trade and unregulated open competition.

Logic
The intellectual discipline that studies the forms of consistent and coherent thought and the rules that ensure that this is possible.

Meta-ethics
See 'Moral philosophy' below.

Mission
The given task or reason for the existence of a group or organisation. The term has been adopted to encourage business organisations to identify the primary nature of their business, who are its primary customers and what goals should direct its strategic and operational planning [Cf: Latin *missio* = to send.]

Morals/morality
The terms 'morals' and 'morality' generally refer in English to the goodness or badness of a person's character or dispositions, or to their personal conduct. 'Moral'/'immoral', have thus come to refer to a person's private standards, values and lifestyle as well. For this reason the paired terms 'morality'/'immorality' are commonly applied to people's sexual behaviour, or personal standards [or lack of standards] of behaviour. However the terms are not restricted to the private sphere, for in any family or community, morality tends to be grounded in more universal cultural, ethnic, religious or ideological beliefs. [Cf: Latin *moralis* = custom or convention.]

Moral autonomy
See Autonomy.

Moral philosophy/meta ethics
For many who have studied philosophy, their introduction to ethics has not been to ethics as a practical discipline, but to moral philosophy, or meta-ethics. Both refer to the critical and academic study of different moral theories or different 'belief and value systems' ('the science of morals'). Moral philosophy, is not so much concerned with practical moral decision-making or the justification of actual decisions and actions. It is concerned rather with equipping us to understand the general philosophical grounds on which we can justify our principles and belief-and-value systems, both on theoretical grounds, and when faced with practical challenges from sceptics. In this sense 'meta-ethics' is a higher level or 'second-order' study of the theoretical underpinnings of our moral systems [e.g. Deontology, Virtue Ethics or Utilitarianism].

Moral community
Term used to refer to any group of people who are united in their commitment to a set of common groundrules for action and dealing with other people.

Moral majority
Term used in the media to refer to those conservative religious or moral pressure groups that claim to represent the 'silent majority'.

Moral theory
See 'Moral philosophy' above.

Moral virtues
Traditionally, following Plato and Aristotle and the Christian tradition, the most important or 'cardinal' moral virtues have been regarded as Temperance [self-control or self-mastery], Courage, Justice [or Fairness] and Prudence [or practical wisdom].

Natural justice
Generally refers to the requirements of due process and fair and public trial in court, but can be applied more generally to the entitlement to be treated fairly and equitably, based on the assumption of universal human rights.

Norm, normative
A norm is a standard or scale by which we check, compare, or measure things, or assess people's performance and the consistency of their actions. A norm or standard allows degrees of comparison to be made, [e.g. 'bad', 'worse', 'worst', 'good', 'better', 'best'] on a continuum where terms like 'good' and 'bad' mark the limits of the scale at either end. Norms point to a scale of performance indicators by which we make qualitative or quantitative assessments based on the available evidence. [Cf: Latin *norma* = carpenter's square.]

Objectivity
The claim to achieve a detached and independent point of view. Whether this ideal is attainable can be debated, and the term is often used tendentiously to recommend one's opinions as superior-in debate with someone else.

Operational plan
In the strategic planning process broad objectives are clarified and goals set. Operational plans are then determined as the means by which we make sure our strategic objectives are met within a determined timeframe, budget, etc. Integrating ethics into the process of operationalising a strategic plan results in the formulation of operational ethical policy.

Option appraisal
Is the process of considering a variety of possible options, assessing their likely costs and benefits and determining which options are given priority.

Owner value
A term introduced by Elaine Sternberg to indicate that a sound business is not only concerned with maximising profits, but with promoting 'long-term owner value' – a term which is intended to include 'goodwill', investor confidence, reputation for sound business practice and equitable treatment of staff, being a good corporate citizen and having influence in the community.

Peer review
A form of performance appraisal where instead of the manager, members of a team, or of the profession, appraise one another's performance – giving both positive feedback and constructive criticism.

Performance appraisal
Assessment of your professional performance against previously negotiated targets and pre-determined criteria or 'performance indicators'. 'Bench-marking' is a process in which such performance indicators are set, so that you know what standard is expected of you in your work.

Personal autonomy
See Autonomy.

Personalist ethic
An approach to ethics in which a primary emphasis is given to personal considerations and maintaining caring relationships. [Cf: Individualism.]

Philosophy
Is not a body of theory but an activity in which we reflect on our ordinary life experience from a 'higher level'. For example, Philosophy is not just another science, but seeks to understand the fundamental pre-suppositions common to all sciences. It is reflective knowledge of knowledge, reflective consideration of the theoretical foundations of ethics as such and so on. It seeks to clarify the nature of the answers we give to ultimate questions about the nature of the Self, the Good Life and the Good Society. Philosophy demands the courage to subject all theories given in the past to critical scrutiny in the quest for ultimate truth.

Pragmatism
A theory of truth and value that maintains that all truth and valuations are necessarily provisional and should be subject to revision in the light of experience, trial and error. If they work and prove useful, then we may be more confident that they are true or valuable, but we can never be certain.

Principle [moral]
A statement of a basic and universal moral truth, or general moral requirement that serves as the starting point for moral reasoning. Alternatively it may be a fundamental belief that is the source of inspiration or direction for moral action, and basis for reasoning about moral priorities. [Cf: Latin *principium* = beginning or starting point from which to proceed.]

Privatisation [ethics]
The tendency to treat all ethical matters as personal and private to the individual, something that contradicts our moral tradition which has emphasised that ethics is about power and power-sharing among people and responsibility and public accountability within a moral community.

Probity
Uprightness and honesty in one's dealings with others.

Process improvement
A systematic approach to the review of management systems within an organisation in which opportunities for improvement are identified, support from colleagues obtained, data collected and needs investigated, the problems identified and analysed, planned intervention undertaken and its impact evaluated and then standardised if appropriate. The whole 'continuous improvement cycle' can be repeated as frequently as necessary.

Problem
A doubtful or difficult matter requiring solution, something hard to understand or to deal with, an exercise, test or challenge set for us, or 'thrown up' by life or experience. However, 'problems' in principle have 'solutions'. Problems may be difficult, but we make the assumption that they are soluble. [Cf: Greek *problema* from *pro-ballo* = throw towards.]

Protective beneficence
See Beneficence and Duty of care.

Quandary
A perplexed state, a state of practical uncertainty or puzzlement over alternative choices, a practical difficulty, which may be resolved with help or access to additional resources. [Origin unknown.]

Rationalism
A type of philosophy which emphasises the role of reason rather than sense experience as the ultimate arbiter of truth and value, and one which assumes that we can know certain self-evident [innate] truths by introspection.

Reductionism
The attempt to explain everything in terms of one simple hypothesis, or to reduce all theories to one basic theory.

Regulative criteria
Those rules which regulate an activity, in contrast to constitutive criteria which set up the framework for the activity in question. In tennis, for example, the constitutive criteria define the size and shape of the court, the nature of the ball, rackets used and height of the net. Regulative criteria determine how you score points and what actions result in penalties. In ethics the concepts of freedom, responsibility and the existence of a moral community would be constitutive, regulative criteria determine what actions are considered good/bad or right/wrong.

Relativism
The philosophical position that no objective truth or values can exist for these are relative to the unique experience of each individual [inter-personal relativism] or are distinctive to each society or culture [cultural relativism], or are bound up with the ideology that you adopt [philosophical relativism]

Revelation
The belief that there are certain truths or moral rules given by God and revealed to human beings by super-natural means, or disclosed in sacred writings.

Respect for persons
The fundamental moral principle that embodies the demand that we show due regard to the rights and dignity of other human beings and seek to empower them to achieve their full human potential-to our mutual benefit.

Retribution
Punishment given as punishment, not for some other perhaps well-intended reason, such as to reform the criminal, to protect others, or to deter crime.

Rights
Justified legal or moral entitlements which may be based on particular agreements [such as promises, bets, oaths, vows, covenants or contracts] or claimed universal entitlements of human beings as human beings [such as the rights embodied in the UNO Universal Declaration of Human Rights].

Rights [negative]
A right to demand that someone desist from doing something to you that harms your interests, causes you pain, damage or inconvenience. Negative rights do not make any positive demands on others, simply require that they stop doing something that is causing you harm.

Rights [positive]
A right that entitles you to demand that someone else [or more generally society] gives you some benefit [such as education, welfare, employment] but where the willingness and ability of the other person/s to give you your entitlements will depend on their generosity and available resources. Rights usually correlate with duties, my rights may impose duties on you and your rights impose duties on me as would be the case with contractual agreements. [Cf: Duties and obligations.]

Role
Socially determined function, or function defined by professional status, as in the role of an actor determined by the script of the playwright.

Rule
A rule is a statement of what can, should or ought to be done [or not done]. A rule is a prescription which seeks to regulate or govern what we do. Rules define our duties, and are based on some source of 'legislative' authority [e.g. parents, church, school, government]. Rules create a binary universe of discourse in which only two predicates can be applied to things, actions, or opinions, i.e. they must be either 'right' or 'wrong'.

Rule deontology
The moral theory that requires that any moral rule, in order to be morally binding must be universally applicable to all people. For example, Kant's Categorical Imperative; 'Always act so that the rule on which you act could become the basis for a universal law'.

Rule utilitarianism
The moral theory that requires that we should always act on the rule that our action should be designed to bring the greatest happiness to the greatest number, and minimise harm to the others.

Second order
A statement about a statement would be a 'second order' statement, and thus moral philosophy stands in a second order relation to ethics as an exploration of the theoretical basis of everyday ethics.

Situation ethics
The ethical theory that maintains that ethics should not have rules and that we should not be bound by rules, but respond to every situation on its own terms and apply our general principles and values as best we can to the unique circumstances. The Christian love ethic is sometimes expressed this way, namely: 'Just do what is the most loving thing in the situation'.

Social contract theory
The philosophical position which maintains that there are no natural human rights we have by virtue of being human beings, but rather that all rights and duties arise from contracts between people and between societies. Hobbes and Rousseau argued that some kind of priordial social contract was necessary to prevent anarchy and social conflict.

Species being
The common nature we possess by virtue of belonging to the same species, and which distinguishes us from, say, chimpanzees and crocodiles.

Stakeholders
All those who have an interest [stake] in any enterprise, community or business, and to be distinguished from 'stockholders', namely those with a direct financial investment in a company or business.

State of nature
An assumed condition of either innocence [Rousseau] or brute competition and violence [Hobbes] before people enter into a social contract to form civil or political society and accept both rights and duties to others.

Statutory duties
Duties prescribed by law or regulation.

Strategic planning
An approach to management in which corporate planning for the longer term is undertaken with a view to getting away from 'short-termism', 'ad-hockery' and 'crisis management', where setting long-term goals and objectives can help redirect operational planning and provide a framework for assessment of success in achieving the flourishing of the business as a whole.

Subjective
Usually used in a dismissive way to indicate that something is based on personal whim or fancy, without reference to public standards or without exposing your beliefs or actions to the criticism of others. However, all actions are obviously 'subjective' insofar as they are the actions of a subject.

Systems analysis
An approach to corporate management which starts with defining the core business of an organisation and then analyses what systems are required to operate the business effectively and efficiently, including a critique of existing systems within the overall objectives of the business.

Tautology
An expression which essentially repeats in the predicate part what is already contained in the subject part of a sentence, without adding anything new, e.g. all bachelors are unmarried men; they came in succession, one after another.

Teleological ethics
Theories which focus on the goal of an action, or its consequences, to define whether actions are morally justifiable, rather than focusing on the ethical principles or means adopted to achieve the end.

Teleological theories may focus either on the specific goal of an action, or maintain, like Aristotle, that all human action aims towards some end and that we are driven by a tendency to seek our own happiness or fulfilment. [Cf: Greek *telos* = end or goal.]

Teleological eudaimonism
See Eudaimonism.

Total quality management [TQM]
An approach to corporate management which combines strategic planning with an emphasis on values as integral to defining the goals of an organisation and therefore central to the well-being of a corporation.

Utilitarianism
The theory advocated in particular by Bentham and Mill that the guiding principle for all conduct should be to achieve the greatest happiness for the greatest number, and that the criterion of the rightness or wrongness of an action is whether it is useful in furthering this goal [utility principle].

Validity [logical]
A quality of arguments of the correct logical form, where it is not the truth of premises but the correct pattern or structure of an argument that validates it.

Value judgements
Judgements where an assessment has to be made of the relative importance or value of something or some action, often involving option appraisal.

Values
While beliefs do not necessarily commit us to action, values do, for we stake our lives on our choice of values. We make a commitment to values as our chosen means to attain our life goals. Values are based on beliefs, and may encourage us to change some inherited attitudes and to cultivate other attitudes, e.g. To be more tolerant of people with a different religious, or cultural background. Values serve as the basis from which we make personal assessments of the worth, importance, or efficacy of things as means to achieve our life-goals or the wellbeing of others.

Values clarification
A method of reviewing one's personal and professional values, assessing their relative importance for your life and work, and determining your future goals in the light of this exercise in prioritising your values. The process can be applied to organisations as well as individuals.

Virtue
A stable state of moral excellence achieved through habitual practice of appropriate dispositions and behaviours.

Virtue ethics
An ethical theory which focuses attention on the possession of sound moral qualities by the moral agent as necessary for consistent ethical behaviour. A theory which rejects the apparent dichotomy between deontological [duty based] and utilitarian [consequentialist] theories, in favour of emphasis on the agent as having primary responsibility for implementing principles in action.

Vision
A term used in management and strategic planning to describe the collective view of stakeholders in an organisation as to where it is going and what its goals should be.

Whistle-blowing
A term used to describe action taken by an employee to inform senior management [or some outside authority] of activity which they regard as fraudulent, dishonest, criminal or dangerous to others. There is a general requirement of the common law that one has a duty to inform the appropriate authorities if you have evidence of the commission of a crime, but protection of 'whistle-blowers' has become an issue because of the apparent inadequacy of statutory protections for public-minded individuals who disclose misconduct and who may suffer dismissal from employment as a result.

Author Index

Subject Index